A Contemporary Approach to Chinese Medicine

A Contemporary Approach to Chinese Medicine

Edited by Patrick Lampard

SYRAWOOD
PUBLISHING HOUSE
New York

Published by Syrawood Publishing House,
750 Third Avenue, 9th Floor,
New York, NY 10017, USA
www.syrawoodpublishinghouse.com

A Contemporary Approach to Chinese Medicine
Edited by Patrick Lampard

International Standard Book Number: 978-1-68286-567-5 (Hardback)

Cataloging-in-Publication Data

A contemporary approach to Chinese medicine / edited by Patrick Lampard.
p. cm.
Includes bibliographical references and index.
ISBN 978-1-68286-567-5
1. Medicine, Chinese. 2. Alternative medicine. I. Lampard, Patrick.
R602 .C66 2018
610.951--dc23

Printed in China.

TABLE OF CONTENTS

Preface .... **IX**

Chapter 1 **Selection and validation of reference genes for normalization of quantitative real-time reverse transcription PCR analysis in *Poria cocos* (Schw.) Wolf (*Fuling*)** **1**
Xin Zhang, Zhi-Chao Xu, Jiang Xu, Ai-Jia Ji, Hong-Mei Luo, Jing-Yuan Song, Chao Sun, Yuan-Lei Hu and Shi-Lin Chen

Chapter 2 **Attenuation of blood pressure in spontaneously hypertensive rats by acupuncture was associated with reduction oxidative stress and improvement from endothelial dysfunction** **18**
Sin Bond Leung, Hongwei Zhang, Chi Wai Lau and Zhi-Xiu Lin

Chapter 3 **Discriminating from species of *Curcumae* Radix (*Yujin*) by a UHPLC/Q-TOFMS-based metabolomics approach** **36**
Fang Liu, Xu Bai, Feng-Qing Yang, Xiao-Jing Zhang, Yuanjia Hu, Peng Li and Jian-Bo Wan

Chapter 4 **Influence of sulfur fumigation on glycoside profile in Platycodonis Radix (*Jiegeng*)** **47**
Xiao-Qing Ma, Su-Mei Li, Chi Leung Chan, Tao Su, Wei-Dong Li, Hui Cao, Wang-Fun Fong and Zhi-Ling Yu

Chapter 5 **Phytochemicals and potential health effects of *Sambucus williamsii* Hance (*Jiegumu*)** **60**
Hui-Hui Xiao, Yan Zhang, Raymond Cooper, Xin-Sheng Yao and Man-Sau Wong

Chapter 6 **Herb-partitioned moxibustion upregulated the expression of colonic epithelial tight junction-related proteins in Crohn's disease model rats** **76**
Rong Ji, Anqi Wang, Haixia Shang, Liu Chen, Chunhui Bao, Luyi Wu, Huangan Wu and Yin Shi

Chapter 7 **Inhibitory effect of *trans*-ferulic acid on proliferation and migration of human lung cancer cells accompanied with increased endogenous reactive oxygen species and β-catenin instability** **86**
Yao Fong, Chia-Chun Tang, Huei-Ting Hu, Hsin-Yu Fang, Bing-Hung Chen, Chang-Yi Wu, Shyng-Shiou Yuan, Hui-Min David Wang, Yen-Chun Chen, Yen-Ni Teng and Chien-Chih Chiu

Chapter 8 **Synergistic effects of melphalan and *Pinus kesiya* Royle ex Gordon (*Simaosong*) extracts on apoptosis induction in human cancer cells** **99**
Natthida Weerapreeyakul, Sasipawan Machana and Sahapat Barusrux

Chapter 9 **Combination of cisplatin and bromelain exerts synergistic cytotoxic effects against breast cancer cell line MDA-MB-231 in vitro** **109**
Ahmad Zaim Mat Pauzi, Swee Keong Yeap, Nadiah Abu, Kian Lam Lim, Abdul Rahman Omar, Suraini Abdul Aziz, Adam Leow Thean Chow, Tamilselvan Subramani, Soon Guan Tan and Noorjahan Banu Alitheen

Chapter 10 ***Gastrodia and Uncaria* (tianma gouteng) water extract exerts antioxidative and antiapoptotic effects against cerebral ischemia in vitro and in vivo** 120
Jia Wen Xian, Angus Yiu-Ting Choi, Clara Bik-San Lau, Wing Nang Leung, Chun Fai Ng and Chun Wai Chan

Chapter 11 **Effects of intra-articular SHINBARO treatment on monosodium iodoacetate-induced osteoarthritis in rats** 132
Won Kyung Kim, Hwa-Jin Chung, Yuna Pyee, Tae Jun Choi, Hyen Joo Park, Ji-Young Hong, Joon-Shik Shin, Jin Ho Lee, In-Hyuk Ha and Sang Kook Lee

Chapter 12 **Acupuncture as an intervention to reduce alcohol dependency** 142
Charlotte Southern, Charlie Lloyd, Jianping Liu, Congcong Wang, Tingting Zhang, Martin Bland and Hugh MacPherson

Chapter 13 **Chinese herbal medicine for constipation: *zheng*-based associations among herbs, formulae, proprietary medicines, and herb-drug interactions** 154
Linda L. D. Zhong, Guang Zheng, Li Da Ge, Cheng Yuan Lin, Tao Huang, Ling Zhao, Cheng Lu, Ai Ping Lu and Zhao Xiang Bian

Chapter 14 **Induction of apoptosis in human hepatocellular carcinoma cells by extracts of *Lannea coromandelica* (Houtt.) Merr. and *Diospyros castanea* (Craib) Fletcher** 165
Natthida Weerapreeyakul, Cholpajsorn Junhom, Sahapat Barusrux and Thaweesak Thitimetharoch

Chapter 15 **Conservation and sustainable use of medicinal plants: problems, progress, and prospects** 175
Shi-Lin Chen, Hua Yu, Hong-Mei Luo, Qiong Wu, Chun-Fang Li and André Steinmetz

Chapter 16 **Anti-inflammatory activities of *Ganoderma lucidum* (*Lingzhi*) and *San-Miao-San* supplements in MRL/lpr mice for the treatment of systemic lupus erythematosus** 185
Zhe Cai, Chun Kwok Wong, Jie Dong, Delong Jiao, Man Chu, Ping Chung Leung, Clara Bik San Lau, Ching Po Lau, Lai Shan Tam and Christopher Wai Kei Lam

Chapter 17 **Rapid differentiation of *Xihuangcao* from the three *Isodon* species by UPLC-ESI-QTOF-MS/MS and chemometrics analysis** 198
Lai Lai Wong, Zhitao Liang, Hubiao Chen and Zhongzhen Zhao

Chapter 18 **An investigation of fungal contamination on the surface of medicinal herbs in China** 214
Run-sheng Zheng, Wen-li Wang, Jing Tan, Hui Xu, Ruo-ting Zhan and Wei-wen Chen

Chapter 19 **Quality control of *Lycium chinense* and *Lycium barbarum cortex* (*Digupi*) by HPLC using kukoamines as markers** 222
Yuan-Yuan Li, Rui Di, Wing-Leung Hsu, Ye-Qing Huang and Hon-Yeung Cheung

Chapter 20 **The neuroprotective effects of *Tao-Ren-Cheng-Qi Tang* against embolic stroke in rats** 230
Ling-Wei Hsu, Wei-Cheng Shiao, Nen-Chung Chang, Meng-Che Yu, Ting-Lin Yen, Philip Aloysius Thomas, Thanasekaran Jayakumar and Joen-Rong Sheu

Chapter 21 **Electroacupuncture for the prevention of postoperative gastrointestinal dysfunction in participants undergoing vascular laparotomy under general anesthesia: a randomized controlled trial** **238**
Meng-yue Liu, Cheng-wei Wang, Zhou-peng Wu and Ning Li

Permissions

List of Contributors

Index

PREFACE

This book has been an outcome of determined endeavour from a group of educationists in the field. The primary objective was to involve a broad spectrum of professionals from diverse cultural background involved in the field for developing new researches. The book not only targets students but also scholars pursuing higher research for further enhancement of the theoretical and practical applications of the subject.

Chinese medicine or traditional Chinese medicine (TCM) refers to the form of traditional medicine that cures diseases with methods that are orthodox. These methods generally include acupuncture, massage, qigong, etc. Common diseases treated with Chinese medicine include menopause, indigestion, hormonal imbalance, high blood pressure, headaches, fatigue, arthritis, etc. This book provides significant information of this discipline to help develop a good understanding of Chinese medicine and its related fields. Some of the diverse topics covered in it address the varied branches that fall under this category. Researchers and students actively engaged in this field will find the text full of crucial and unexplored concepts.

It was an honour to edit such a profound book and also a challenging task to compile and examine all the relevant data for accuracy and originality. I wish to acknowledge the efforts of the contributors for submitting such brilliant and diverse chapters in the field and for endlessly working for the completion of the book. Last, but not the least; I thank my family for being a constant source of support in all my research endeavours.

Editor

1

Selection and validation of reference genes for normalization of quantitative real-time reverse transcription PCR analysis in *Poria cocos* (Schw.) Wolf (*Fuling*)

Xin Zhang[1], Zhi-Chao Xu[1], Jiang Xu[2], Ai-Jia Ji[1], Hong-Mei Luo[1*], Jing-Yuan Song[1,3], Chao Sun[1], Yuan-Lei Hu[4] and Shi-Lin Chen[1,2*]

Abstract

Background: Quantitative real-time reverse transcription PCR (qRT-PCR) requires a stable internal control to avoid misinterpretation of data or errors for gene expression normalization. However, there are still no validated reference genes for stable internal control in *Poria cocos* (Schw.) Wolf (*Fuling*). This study aims to validate the reference genes of *P. cocos*.

Methods: This study firstly collected the 14 candidate reference genes by BLASTP from the genome of *P. cocos* for qRT-PCR analysis to determine the expression levels of 14 housekeeping genes (*GAPDH, MAPK, β-Act, RPB2, RPB1-1, RPB1-2, his3-1, his3-2, APT, SAMDC, RP, β-Tub, EIF*, and *CYP*) under different temperatures and in response to different plant hormones (indole-3-acetic acid, abscisic acid, 6-benzylaminopurine, methyl jasmonate, and gibberellic acid), and the threshold cycle (C_t) values. The results were analyzed by four programs (i.e., geNorm, NormFinder, BestKeeper, and RefFinder) for evaluating the candidate reference genes.

Results: *SAMDC, his3-2, RP, RPB2*, and *his3-1* were recommended as reference genes for treating *P. cocos* with indole-3-acetic acid, abscisic acid, 6-benzylaminopurine, methyl jasmonate, and gibberellic acid, respectively. Under different temperatures *RPB2* was the most stable reference gene. *CYP* was the most stable gene for all 90 samples by RefFinder.

Conclusion: *SAMDC, his3-2, RP, RPB2*, and *his3-1* were evaluated to be suitable reference genes for *P. cocos* following different treatments. *RPB2* was the most stable reference gene under different temperatures and *CYP* was the most stable gene in the mycelia under all six evaluated conditions.

Background

Quantitative real-time reverse transcription PCR (qRT-PCR) is used for determining the abundance of mRNAs in molecular biology studies. Suitable reference genes are necessary to ensure accuracy and to avoid bias. Typically, reference genes are housekeeping genes necessary for cellular metabolism. The genes for cyclophilin (*CYP*), tubulin, ubiquitin, glyceraldehyde-3-phosphate dehydrogenase (*GAPDH*), actin, 18S ribosomal RNA, 28S ribosomal RNA, and albumin are among the most frequently used reference genes [1].

However, the expression levels of reference genes may not be stable in different species [2], different tissues [3], or even identical cells under different culture conditions [4]. For example, the biosynthesis of triterpenes was induced by methyl jasmonate (MeJA) in *Ganoderma lucidum* (Leyss. ex Fr.) P. Karst (*Lingzhi*) [5, 6]. However, the stability of fungal reference genes in the presence of plant hormones has not been properly evaluated by the gene expression levels of enzymes involved in the triterpene biosynthesis pathway.

*Correspondence: hmluo@implad.ac.cn; slchen@implad.ac.cn
[1] Institute of Medicinal Plant Development, Chinese Academy of Medical Sciences and Peking Union Medical College, Beijing 100193, China
Full list of author information is available at the end of the article

Little research has been conducted on reference genes in fungi. In *Hemileia vastatrix* Berk. and Br. (*Toubaoxiujun*), the cytochrome *b*, 40S ribosomal protein and *Hv00099* genes have been selected as reference genes in vitro; however, the 40S ribosomal protein, *GAPDH*, and *Hv00099* genes were the most stable genes *in planta* [7]. In *Hypocrea jecorina* Berk. and Br. (*Hongherouzuojun*), the gene encoding a GTPase was recommended as a reference gene [8]. Reference genes for qRT-PCR under different culture conditions and at different developmental stages in *G. lucidum* were reported [9].

Poria cocos (Schw.) Wolf (*Fuling*) is medicinal fungi and nutrition food widely distributes in East Asia, particularly in China, North America, Africa, and Australia [10, 11]. Pharmaceutically active constituents extracted from *P. cocos*, including polysaccharides, triterpene derivatives, lanostane derivatives, and poricoic acid, exhibited anti-oxidant [12, 13], anti-inflammatory [14], anti-tumor [15–17], anti-emetic [18], anti-nephritic [19], anti-rejection [20], diuretic [21], and anti-hyperglycemic activities [22]. The nematicidal activity of *P. cocos* was investigated and the active compounds were isolated [23]. Studies on the molecular biology of *P. cocos* were limited, including the basic molecular studies such as gene expression analysis and gene function identification [24]. qRT-PCR method was effective to detect the candidate genes involved in secondary metabolite biosynthesis. For example, the genes are most likely involved in the biosynthesis of pachymic acid in *P. cocos* was identified by qRT-PCR [25]; however, contigs and singletons were used instead of reference genes. The stability of potential internal control genes in *P. cocos* has not been evaluated.

This study aims to discover and obtain the stable reference genes of *P. cocos* for normalization of qRT-PCR analysis.

Methods

Sampling and culture conditions

The *P. cocos* strain CGMCC5.78 was purchased from the Institute of Microbiology, Chinese Academy of Sciences and was stored in the Institute of Medicinal Plant Development at −80 °C. We identified the strain using the DNA barcoding method with *ITS2* primers. Ninety mycelial samples under different culture conditions were used in this study. Vegetative mycelia were cultured in two different media: potato dextrose agar medium (AOBOX, Beijing, China) and sucrose medium. The components of the sucrose medium were as follows: vitamin B1, 0.05 g/L; $MgSO_4{\cdot}7H_2O$, 0.5 g/L; $KH_2PO_4{\cdot}H_2O$, 1 g/L; yeast extract, 2.5 g/L; peptone, 5 g/L; and sucrose, 35 g/L. The strain was maintained in potato dextrose agar medium. In the preculture stage, 40-mL sucrose medium was inoculated with mycelia and shaken (Thermo Fisher Scientific 491, Waltham, MA, USA) at 50 rpm in the dark in an incubator at 28 °C for 1 week. Subsequently, all of the mycelia were spread and were shaken at 120 rpm for an additional week in the dark at 28 °C. Finally, all cultures, including the culture broth, were incubated under various conditions (Table 1), including different concentration of hormones and different temperatures for 24 h.

The samples were arbitrarily allocated into six groups for analysis (Table 1). The samples in groups A, B, C, D, and E were cultured in the media supplemented with different concentrations of indole-3-acetic acid (IAA; Sangon, Shanghai, China), abscisic acid (ABA; Sangon), 6-benzylaminopurine (6-BA;Sigma, St Louis, MO, USA), methyl jasmonate (MeJA; Sigma), and gibberellic acid (GA; Sangon), respectively. Group F comprised samples collected from cultures incubated at five different temperatures. The mycelia were collected by double gauze filters (CWBio, Beijing, China). Each experiment was performed in triplicate. A total of 90 samples were collected, and all of the samples were frozen in liquid nitrogen and stored at −80 °C.

Total RNA extraction, DNase treatment, and cDNA synthesis

The liquid nitrogen frozen samples were ground into fine powder by a mortar and pestle. The total RNA of each sample was extracted by the Polysaccharide and Polyphenol Total RNA Isolation Kit (spin column; BioTeke, Beijing, China) according to the manufacturer's instructions. The total RNA integrity and quality were confirmed by 1 % agarose gel electrophoresis by ethidium bromide staining. The RNA concentration was determined by a NanoDrop2000 spectrophotometer (Thermo Fisher Scientific, Waltham, MA, USA). One microgram of total RNA of each sample was reverse transcribed by the FastQuant RT Kit (with gDNase; TIANGEN, Beijing, China) according to the manufacturer's protocol. All templates were diluted 30-fold for PCR and qRT-PCR.

Candidate gene selection, primer design, and validation

Based on previous studies [1, 3, 4] of reference genes determined in other species, 14 genes were evaluated

Table 1 Different treatment conditions applied to the mycelia of *P. cocos*

Treatment	Group	Treatment conditions				
IAA (mg/L)	A	10	20	30	40	50
ABA (mg/L)	B	10	20	30	40	50
6-BA (mg/L)	C	0.01	0.1	1	5	10
MeJA (μm/L)	D	5	10	50	100	200
GA (mg/L)	E	10	20	30	40	50
Temperature (°C)	F	4	15	20	28	40

in the present study, including multiple-copy genes. These genes include glyceraldehyde-3-phosphate dehydrogenase (*GAPDH*), mitogen-activated protein kinase (*MAPK*), beta actin (*β-Act*), RNA polymerase subunit2 (*RPB2*), RNA polymerase subunit1 (*RPB1*), histone 3 (*his3*), adenine phosphoribosyl transferase (*APT*), *S*-adenosyl methionine decarboxylase (*SAMDC*), ribosomal protein (*RP*), beta tubulin (*β-Tub*), eukaryotic translation initiation factor (*EIF*), and cyclophilin (*CYP*). The primer sequences, amplicon size and number of gene copies in the genome are summarized in Table 2. The candidate genes were selected from the *P. cocos* genome sequence database (SRA: PRJNA42921) by the BLASTP program (National Library of Medicine, USA) and a threshold *E*-value $<1 \times 10^{-50}$.

Primer Premier 6.0 (PREMIER Biosoft, USA) and DNAMAN (LynnonBiosoft, USA) were used for primer design with the following criteria: an amplicon size ranging from 130 to 180 bp, an optimal T_m of 53–55 °C, and a primer length from 18 to 22 bp. The primers were synthesized by Sangon Biotech (Shanghai, China). The specificity of each primer pair was measured by 2 % agarose gel electrophoresis following PCR (95 °C for 5 min; 35 cycles of 95 °C for 15 s and 60 °C for 1 min; 72 °C for 10 min) by the 90 cDNA sample mixture. Additionally, qRT-PCR was performed and the melting curve was determined for primers specific validation.

Real-time PCR performance and C_t data collection

The expression level of each gene was determined in 96-well plates by an Applied Biosystems 7500 Real-Time PCR system (Life Technologies, Grand Island, NY, USA). Each reaction mixture contained 200 nM of each primer, 2 μL of the prepared cDNA template, 4.9-μL ddH_2O, and 7.5-μL Ultra SYBR Mixture with ROX (CWBio, Beijing, China) in a final volume of 15 μL. The amplifications were performed by an initial denaturation step of 95 °C for 5 min, followed by 45 cycles of 95 °C for 15 s and 60 °C for 1 min. A temperature ramp step was added after 45 amplification cycles for specificity analysis (melting curve), with 95 °C for 15 s, 60 °C for 1 min, 95 °C for 15 s, and a final temperature of 60 °C for 15 s. There were three biological duplicate samples, and each biological duplicate sample was evaluated in triplicate.

Table 2 Descriptions of the 14 candidate reference genes and their primer sequences for qRT-PCR

Gene	Gene description	Primer sequences (forward/reverse)	Amplicon length (bp)	Access number	Total copy numbers
GAPDH	Glyceraldehyde 3-phosphate dehydrogenase	TGTTCGTCTGCGGTGTCA/AGTGGACG GTGGTCATCAG	150	KJ716556	1
MAPK	Mitogen-activated protein kinase	CACATCCAGCACGAGAACAT/GGAG GATCTGGTAGAGGAAGTA	163	KJ716546	10
β-Act	Beta actin	ATGCGAGGTTATGCGTTCA/CCGAC CATCTGGGAGTGTAT	156	KJ716554	2
RPB2	RNA polymerase subunit 2	ACCAACTTCCTCGTCAGAATG/TCCT GATTGTATCCGCTGTAAC	161	KJ716552	1
RPB1-1	RNA polymerase subunit 1	GGCTTACAACAGGTCGTCAA/CGTG GCGTCCTCAATAACTT	153	KJ716547	2
RPB1-2	RNA polymerase subunit 1	AGGATGACGAAGCAGAGGAA/ TGGCATTGGGCAGGTTCT	168	KJ716548	
his3-1	Histone 3	AGTCCACGGAACTCCTAATCA/AGCG GCTAAGTTGGTGTCT	167	KJ716557	3
his3-2	Histone 3	CGACGGAGTTGCTCATCAG/GTG GATCGCAGCCAGATTC	170	KJ716544	
APT	Adenine phosphoribosyltransferase	ACCTGAGGAGTCTGCTGAAG/TTGTG GAATAGTGTGCGATGT	149	KJ716549	1
SAMDC	*S*-adenosylmethionine decarboxylase	GCTTCTACTCTCGCAAGGC/GATATACA GCAGCCAGTGGTC	155	KJ716550	1
RP	Ribosomal protein	TGTCGCTCTCCTCAAGTCC/CGGAATGC CTTGACGATACC	165	KJ716551	1
β-Tub	Beta tubulin	GCCAACATACGGTGATCTGAA/GAAGAA GTGAAGACGAGGGAAT	142	KJ716555	1
EIF	Eukaryotic translation initiation factor	TGACGATGACAGCGATGAAG/CACCTG GACTGCCTTATGC	145	KJ716545	1
CYP	Cyclophilin	CATGGCTTCGGCTACAAGG/TTGGTGT GCTTGAGCTTGAA	152	KJ716553	3

Data analysis

The C_t values from each reaction were used for analysis of the expression levels of all detected reference genes. The geNorm [26], NormFinder [27], BestKeeper [28], the Delta CT method [29] and the Web-based tool RefFinder [30] were used to determine the stability of the candidate reference genes. The default parameters of these software were applied.

Results

Expression profile of candidate reference genes

The mean C_t value was computed by three biological duplicates and three technical replicates for each independent experiment (the template generated from each condition of *P. cocos* was used in different independent experiment), and the three technical replicates were performed independently. A higher C_t value indicates decreased transcription of the target gene. The average C_t value of each candidate gene under conditions ranged from 22.45 ± 0.97 to 32.86 ± 0.86 cycles (Table 3). The average C_t value of six of the 14 genes was higher than 30.00. *RPB1-2* and *CYP* demonstrated the lowest and highest relative expression levels, with average C_t values of 31.21–33.21 and 22.37–23.91, respectively. The variation in the C_t value was determined by the maximum and minimum C_t values. The variation in the C_t value of each candidate reference gene in all 90 samples ranged between 3.22 and 7.89. *RPB1-1* exhibited the lowest variation in C_t value followed by *CYP* (3.24). In contrast, *EIF* exhibited the highest variation in C_t value (7.89).

Stability ranking of candidate reference genes

geNorm ranks the potential reference genes on the basis of their average pairwise variation in expression of one gene compared with each other gene of the set [26]. geNorm recommends 1.5 as the M-value cutoff. An M-value of less than 1.5 indicates stable expression, with the lowest M-value corresponding to the highest stability, and *vice versa*. Two reference genes were recommended for an ideal relative quantitative analysis. The M-values of candidate genes under different conditions generated by geNorm are listed in Table 4. The stability of the genes under different treatment conditions analyzed by geNorm is shown in Figs. 1, 2, 3. In group A, *his3-1* and *CYP* were the most stable genes, and *his3-2* was the most unstable gene. In group B, *MAPK* and *EIF* exhibited the highest stability, and *β-Act* exhibited the lowest stability. Under different temperatures, the expression levels of *RPB1-2* and *RPB2* were the most stable in the cultured mycelia, and *SAMDC* exhibited a performance that was worse than those of the other 13 genes. When treated with different concentrations of 6-BA, *RP* and *CYP* were the most stable reference genes, and *RPB1-2* exhibited the highest M-value. Following treatment with MeJA, an inducer of secondary metabolism [5, 6], the best reference genes were *RPB1-2* and *his3-1*, whereas *GAPDH* was the most unstable. Following GA treatment, the expression level of *MAPK* exhibited the most variation, whereas *RPB2* and *SAMDC* were considered suitable reference genes. Following treatment with IAA, ABA, different temperatures, 6-BA, MeJA, and GA, the average M-values were 0.517–0.871, 0.768–1.36, 0.734–1.242, 0.857–1.333, 0.521–0.849, and 0.602–1.058, respectively. These values suggested that 6-BA contributed the most to the variation in expression levels of the reference genes. A geNorm analysis using all samples indicated that *his3-1* and *RP* were the most stable genes with the lowest M-values, and *APT* was the most variable gene.

NormFinder is an Excel-based program for evaluating the expression stability of candidate reference genes based on the expression values, which enables estimation not only of the overall variation of the candidate normalization genes but also of variation between sample subgroups of the sample set [27]. NormFinder shows less sensitivity toward coregulation of the candidate normalization genes. A lower stability value indicates a higher stability. In group A, *SAMDC* was the most stable gene, with a stability value of 0.135, whereas *his3-2* was the most unstable gene, with a stability value of 0.769. In group B, *his3-2* exhibited the lowest stability value of 0.088, and *β-Act* exhibited the highest stability value of 1.586. Under different temperatures, *his3-2* was the most stable, with a stability value of 0.069, and *SAMDC* was the least stable, with a stability value of 1.428. In group C, *RP* exhibited the best performance with a stability value of 0.183, and the expression level of *RPB1-2* varied the most under different concentrations of 6-BA, with a stability value of 1.228. Following MeJA treatment, *RPB2* exhibited the lowest variation, with a stability value of 0.106, and *GAPDH* exhibited the lowest stability value of 0.887. In group E, *his3-1* was recommended as the reference gene for GA treatment, with a stability value of 0.244, and *MAPK* was the most unstable gene among the 14 genes, with a stability value of 1.119. When all of the samples were analyzed, *CYP* exhibited the lowest stability value of 1.320, whereas *EIF* exhibited the highest stability value at 13.240.

Gene expression stability was evaluated by BestKeeper using the standard deviation (SD), percentage covariance (CV), and correlation coefficient (*r*) [28]. BestKeeper can determine the best suited standards, out of 10 candidates, and combine them into an index. The candidate reference genes with SD >1 are considered unstable, and a higher

Table 3 The average C_t value (mean ± SD) of each candidate gene under different conditions

	GAPDH	*MAPK*	*β-Act*	*RPB2*	*RPB1-1*	*RPB1-2*	*his3-1*	*his3-2*	*APT*	*SAMDC*	*RP*	*β-Tub*	*EIF*	*CYP*
IAA	22.88 ± 1.26	29.49 ± 0.94	30.13 ± 0.83	29.60 ± 1.30	31.31 ± 1.19	32.10 ± 0.97	26.49 ± 1.06	25.53 ± 1.43	29.11 ± 1.05	32.57 ± 0.97	28.21 ± 0.80	27.98 ± 0.89	28.57 ± 0.96	22.45 ± 0.97
ABA	23.69 ± 0.73	30.76 ± 0.74	30.66 ± 1.50	29.71 ± 2.03	31.58 ± 1.34	31.83 ± 1.54	27.04 ± 0.82	26.22 ± 0.62	29.43 ± 0.88	32.44 ± 0.87	28.39 ± 0.70	28.18 ± 1.05	28.92 ± 0.66	23.35 ± 0.48
6-BA	22.66 ± 1.23	27.48 ± 0.81	31.00 ± 0.87	29.81 ± 1.06	31.57 ± 1.01	32.51 ± 1.27	26.53 ± 0.68	22.37 ± 0.92	32.06 ± 1.01	28.40 ± 1.19	27.96 ± 0.69	24.12 ± 1.05	24.51 ± 1.09	23.26 ± 0.74
MeJA	23.91 ± 1.23	30.85 ± 1.18	29.97 ± 0.78	32.45 ± 1.00	30.69 ± 0.81	32.86 ± 0.86	26.91 ± 0.91	26.73 ± 0.86	31.65 ± 0.95	33.24 ± 1.18	28.20 ± 1.15	28.13 ± 1.23	29.95 ± 0.92	23.53 ± 0.67
GA	24.33 ± 1.32	31.47 ± 0.61	30.36 ± 1.28	31.82 ± 1.26	30.60 ± 1.20	32.06 ± 0.96	26.52 ± 1.23	25.66 ± 1.27	31.48 ± 1.34	32.58 ± 1.22	27.48 ± 1.61	27.72 ± 1.64	29.22 ± 1.53	23.48 ± 0.96
Temperature	23.16 ± 1.01	27.08 ± 1.18	30.37 ± 0.68	29.94 ± 0.88	31.50 ± 0.93	31.90 ± 0.94	25.87 ± 1.56	22.30 ± 0.77	32.12 ± 1.08	28.64 ± 1.17	27.37 ± 1.77	24.27 ± 1.11	25.08 ± 1.04	22.80 ± 0.93

Table 4 The M value of each candidate gene under different conditions generated by geNorm

	GAPDH	*MAPK*	*β-Act*	*RPB2*	*RPB1-1*	*RPB1-2*	*his3-1*	*his3-2*	*APT*	*SAMDC*	*RP*	*β-Tub*	*EIF*	*CYP*
IAA	0.745	0.845	0.637	0.732	0.730	0.698	0.556	0.879	0.668	0.508	0.824	0.644	0.704	0.546
ABA	0.984	0.809	1.644	1.324	1.274	1.583	0.932	0.784	0.842	1.045	0.853	1.189	0.789	0.848
6-BA	1.352	0.971	1.032	1.178	1.120	1.392	1.023	1.022	1.290	0.985	0.798	1.125	1.177	0.861
MeJA	0.981	0.766	0.537	0.506	0.715	0.520	0.554	0.592	0.937	0.793	0.686	0.842	0.551	0.617
GA	0.950	1.237	0.707	0.716	0.691	0.872	0.658	0.703	1.007	0.732	0.934	0.891	0.730	0.795
Temperature	0.857	0.887	0.852	0.730	0.964	0.753	1.286	0.750	0.808	1.057	1.414	1.132	1.135	0.758

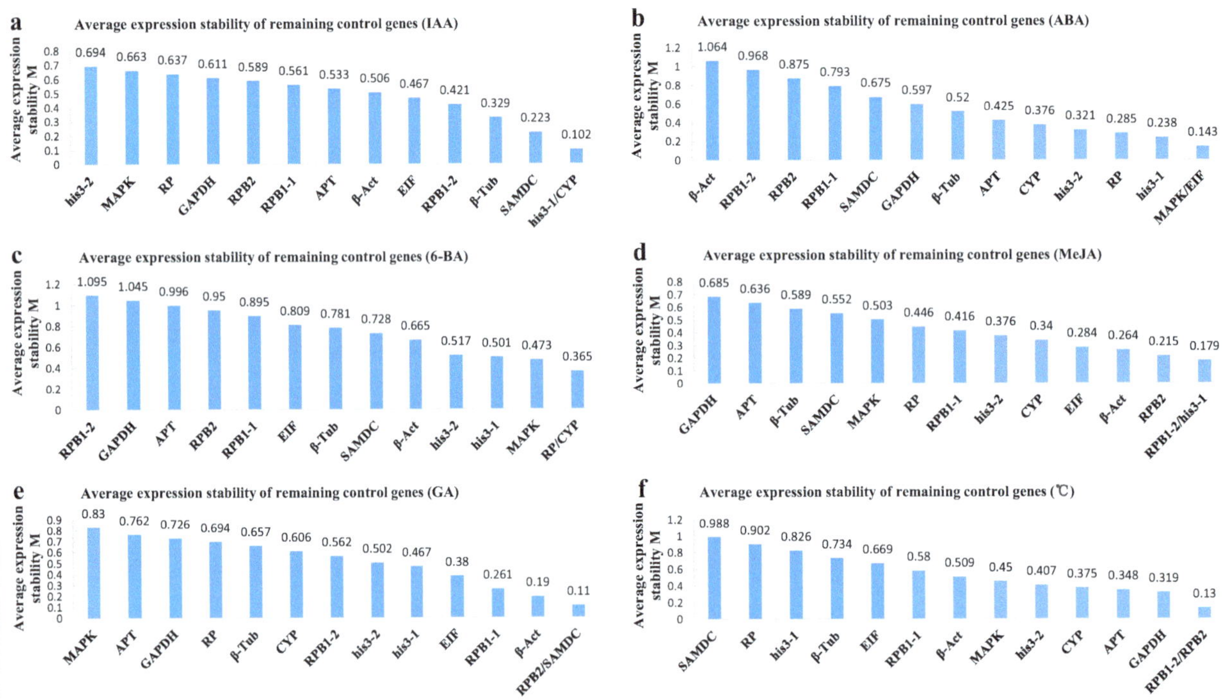

Fig. 1 Stability values of the candidate reference genes calculated using geNorm under different treatment conditions. **a**, **b**, **c**, **d**, and **e** Stability values of the 14 candidate genes treated with IAA, ABA, 6-BA, MeJA, and GA, respectively. **f** Stability values of the14 candidate genes under different temperatures

SD value indicates greater variation. From groups A to F, the recommended reference genes were *β-Tub*, *CYP*, *RP*, *his3-2*, *MAPK*, and *EIF*, with SD values of 0.397, 0.171, 0.234, 0.420, 0.345, and 0.297, respectively. In addition, the genes exhibiting the highest SD values in groups A, B, C, D, E, and F were *his3-2* (SD = 1.115), *RPB1-2* (SD = 1.137), *GAPDH* (SD = 0.842), *MAPK* (SD = 0.949), *RP* (SD = 1.468), and *RP* (SD = 1.491), respectively. When all 90 samples were considered, the expression level of *CYP* was the most stable, whereas *EIF* was the most unstable, with SD values of 0.608 and 1.980, respectively.

RefFinder analysis integrates four different methods (i.e., Delta CT, geNorm, NormFinder, and BestKeeper). The C_t values were input into RefFinder directly, and the ranking of the four methods was calculated. Based on the rankings from each method, RefFinder assigns an appropriate weight to an individual gene and calculates the geometric mean of their weights for the overall final ranking [30]. The rankings of the candidate reference genes used in Delta CT were according to the repeatability of the gene expression differences among the samples. The results analyzed by RefFinder are summarized in Tables 5, 6, 7, 8, 9, 10. In group A, *SAMDC* was recommended as the most stable reference gene. In group B, *his3-2* exhibited the best performance, whereas *his3-1* exhibited the best performance in group E. Under different treatment temperatures and different concentrations of MeJA, *RPB2* maintained a stable expression level.

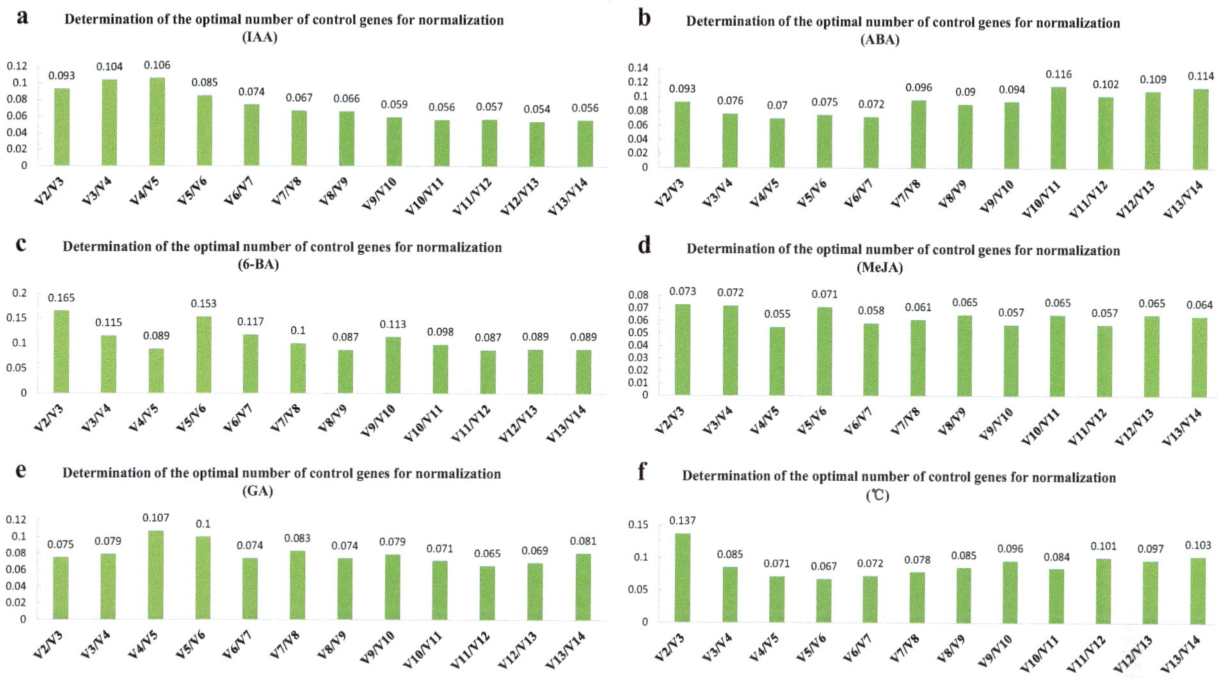

Fig. 2 Determination of the optimal number of control genes for normalization under different treatment conditions. If the V_2/V_3 value is less than 0.15, two genes are suitable for normalization as recommended by geNorm. Otherwise, more genes are needed until the V_n/V_{n+1} value is less than 0.15, and the suitable gene number for normalization is *n*. **a**, **b**, **c**, **d**, and **e** Optimal number of control genes for normalization after IAA, ABA, 6-BA, MeJA, and GA treatment, respectively. **f** Optimal number of control genes for normalization under different temperatures

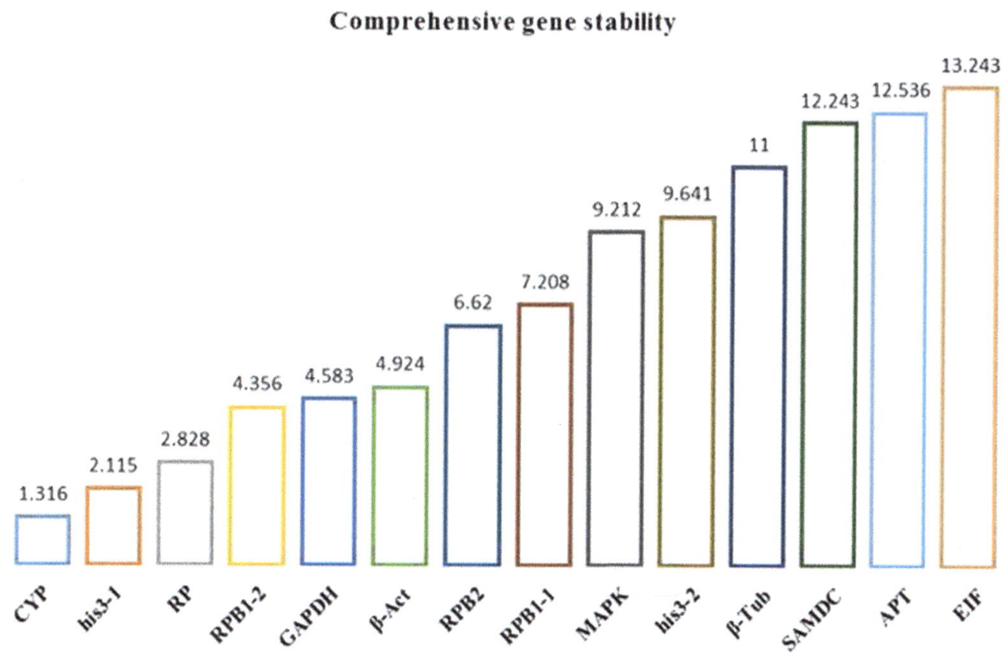

Fig. 3 Comprehensive gene stability. Ranking order of gene stability in all samples under the various conditions using Delta CT, geNorm, NormFinder, and BestKeeper

Table 5 Ranking order of the reference genes with IAA treatment (Better-Good-Average)

Method	1	2	3	4	5	6	7	8	9	10	11	12	13	14
DeltaCT	*SAMDC*	*CYP*	*his3-1*	*β-Act*	*β-Tub*	*APT*	*RPB1-2*	*EIF*	*RPB1-1*	*RPB2*	*GAPDH*	*RP*	*MAPK*	*his3-2*
BestKeeper	*β-Tub*	*RP*	*RPB1-2*	*EIF*	*SAMDC*	*β-Act*	*CYP*	*MAPK*	*his3-1*	*RPB2*	*APT*	*RPB1-1*	*GAPDH*	*his3-2*
NormFinder	*SAMDC*	*CYP*	*his3-1*	*β-Act*	*β-Tub*	*APT*	*EIF*	*RPB1-2*	*RPB2-3*	*RPB1-1*	*GAPDH*	*RP*	*MAPK*	*his3-2*
geNorm	*his3-1/CYP*		*SAMDC*	*β-Tub*	*RPB1-2*	*EIF*	*β-Act*	*APT*	*RPB1-1*	*RPB2*	*GAPDH*	*RP*	*MAPK*	*his3-2*
Recommended comprehensive ranking	*SAMDC*	*CYP*	*his3-1*	*β-Tub*	*β-Act*	*RPB1-2*	*EIF*	*APT*	*RP*	*RPB2*	*RPB1-1*	*GAPDH*	*MAPK*	*his3-2*

Table 6 Ranking order of the reference genes with ABA treatment (Better-Good-Average)

Method	1	2	3	4	5	6	7	8	9	10	11	12	13	14
DeltaCT	*his3-2*	*EIF*	*MAPK*	*APT*	*CYP*	*RP*	*his3-1*	*GAPDH*	*SAMDC*	*β-Tub*	*RPB1-1*	*RPB2*	*RPB1-2*	*β-Act*
BestKeeper	*CYP*	*his3-2*	*RP*	*MAPK*	*EIF*	*his3-1*	*GAPDH*	*APT*	*β-Tub*	*SAMDC*	*RPB1-1*	*β-Act*	*RPB2*	*RPB1-2*
NormFinder	*his3-2*	*APT*	*EIF*	*CYP*	*MAPK*	*RP*	*GAPDH*	*his3-1*	*SAMDC*	*β-Tub*	*RPB1-1*	*RPB2*	*RPB1-2*	*β-Act*
geNorm	*MAPK/EIF*		*his3-1*	*RP*	*his3-2*	*CYP*	*APT*	*β-Tub*	*GAPDH*	*SAMDC*	*RPB1-1*	*RPB2*	*RPB1-2*	*β-Act*
Recommended comprehensive ranking	*his3-2*	*EIF*	*MAPK*	*CYP*	*RP*	*APT*	*his3-1*	*GAPDH*	*β-Tub*	*SAMDC*	*RPB1-1*	*RPB2*	*RPB1-2*	*β-Act*

Table 7 Ranking order of the reference genes with 6-BA treatment (Better-Good-Average)

Method	1	2	3	4	5	6	7	8	9	10	11	12	13	14
DeltaCT	*RP*	*CYP*	*MAPK*	*SAMDC*	*his3-2*	*his3-1*	*β-Act*	*RPB1-1*	*β-Tub*	*EIF*	*RPB2*	*APT*	*GAPDH*	*RPB1-2*
BestKeeper	*RP*	*CYP*	*SAMDC*	*his3-2*	*his3-1*	*β-Act*	*MAPK*	*RPB1-1*	*EIF*	*RPB2*	*β-Tub*	*APT*	*RPB1-2*	*GAPDH*
NormFinder	*RP*	*CYP*	*SAMDC*	*MAPK*	*β-Act*	*his3-2*	*his3-1*	*RPB1-1*	*β-Tub*	*RPB2*	*EIF*	*APT*	*GAPDH*	*RPB1-2*
geNorm	*RP/CYP*		*MAPK*	*his3-1*	*his3-2*	*β-Act*	*SAMDC*	*β-Tub*	*EIF*	*RPB1-1*	*RPB2*	*APT*	*GAPDH*	*RPB1-2*
Recommended comprehensive ranking	*RP*	*CYP*	*SAMDC*	*MAPK*	*his3-2*	*his3-1*	*β-Act*	*RPB1-1*	*β-Tub*	*EIF*	*RPB2*	*APT*	*GAPDH*	*RPB1-2*

Table 8 Ranking order of the reference genes with MeJA treatment (Better-Good-Average)

Method	1	2	3	4	5	6	7	8	9	10	11	12	13	14
DeltaCT	*RPB2*	*RPB1-2*	*β-Act*	*EIF*	*his3-1*	*his3-2*	*CYP*	*RP*	*RPB1-1*	*MAPK*	*SAMDC*	*β-Tub*	*APT*	*GAPDH*
BestKeeper	*his3-2*	*CYP*	*EIF*	*RPB1-1*	*RPB1-2*	*APT*	*RPB2*	*SAMDC*	*β-Act*	*his3-1*	*GAPDH*	*RP*	*β-Tub*	*MAPK*
NormFinder	*RPB2*	*β-Act*	*RPB1-2*	*EIF*	*his3-1*	*his3-2*	*CYP*	*RP*	*RPB1-1*	*MAPK*	*SAMDC*	*β-Tub*	*APT*	*GAPDH*
geNorm	*RPB1-2/his3-1*		*RPB2*	*β-Act*	*EIF*	*CYP*	*his3-2*	*RPB1-1*	*RP*	*MAPK*	*SAMDC*	*β-Tub*	*APT*	*GAPDH*
Recommended comprehensive ranking	*RPB2*	*RPB1-2*	*β-Act*	*EIF*	*his3-1*	*his3-2*	*CYP*	*RPB1-1*	*RP*	*SAMDC*	*APT*	*MAPK*	*β-Tub*	*GAPDH*

Table 9 Ranking order of the reference genes with GA treatment (Better-Good-Average)

Method	1	2	3	4	5	6	7	8	9	10	11	12	13	14
DeltaCT	*his3-1*	*RPB1-1*	*his3-2*	*β-Act*	*RPB2*	*EIF*	*SAMDC*	*CYP*	*RPB1-2*	*β-Tub*	*RP*	*GAPDH*	*APT*	*MAPK*
BestKeeper	*MAPK*	*RPB1-2*	*CYP*	*RPB1-1*	*RPB2*	*SAMDC*	*GAPDH*	*APT*	*his3-2*	*his3-1*	*β-Act*	*EIF*	*β-Tub*	*RP*
NormFinder	*his3-1*	*his3-2*	*RPB1-1*	*EIF*	*β-Act*	*RPB2*	*CYP*	*SAMDC*	*RPB1-2*	*β-Tub*	*GAPDH*	*RP*	*APT*	*MAPK*
geNorm	*RPB2/SAMDC*		*β-Act*	*RPB1-1*	*EIF*	*his3-1*	*his3-2*	*RPB1-2*	*CYP*	*β-Tub*	*RP*	*GAPDH*	*APT*	*MAPK*
Recommended comprehensive ranking	*his3-1*	*RPB1-1*	*RPB2*	*SAMDC*	*his3-2*	*β-Act*	*RPB1-2*	*EIF*	*CYP*	*MAPK*	*GAPDH*	*β-Tub*	*APT*	*RP*

Table 10 Ranking order of the reference genes under different temperatures (Better-Good-Average)

Method	1	2	3	4	5	6	7	8	9	10	11	12	13	14
DeltaCT	*RPB2*	*his3-2*	*RPB1-2*	*CYP*	*APT*	*β-Act*	*GAPDH*	*MAPK*	*RPB1-1*	*β-Tub*	*EIF*	*his3-1*	*RP*	*SAMDC*
BestKeeper	*EIF*	*β-Act*	*RPB2*	*RPB1-1*	*RPB1-2*	*β-Tub*	*his3-2*	*SAMDC*	*GAPDH*	*CYP*	*APT*	*MAPK*	*his3-1*	*RP*
NormFinder	*his3-2*	*RPB2*	*CYP*	*RPB1-2*	*APT*	*β-Act*	*GAPDH*	*MAPK*	*RPB1-1*	*β-Tub*	*EIF*	*his3-1*	*RP*	*SAMDC*
geNorm	*RPB1-2/RPB2*		*GAPDH*	*APT*	*CYP*	*his3-2*	*MAPK*	*β-Act*	*RPB1-1*	*EIF*	*β-Tub*	*his3-1*	*RP*	*SAMDC*
Recommended comprehensive ranking	*RPB2*	*RPB1-2*	*his3-2*	*β-Act*	*CYP*	*APT*	*EIF*	*GAPDH*	*RPB1-1*	*MAPK*	*β-Tub*	*SAMDC*	*his3-1*	*RP*

Following 6-BA treatment, *RP* ranked as a suitable reference gene (Table 7). Following comprehensive analysis of all of the samples under the various conditions by Delta CT, geNorm, NormFinder, and BestKeeper, *CYP* was recommended as the reference gene.

The results obtained using these different methods were not identical. In group C, *RP* was recommended as the most stable gene by all of these methods, whereas in group F, *RPB2* was recommended as the reference gene by Delta CT, geNorm and RefFinder. However, in the remaining groups, Delta CT, NormFinder and RefFinder recommended the same gene as the reference gene; *SAMDC, his3-2, RPB2* and *his3-1* in groups A, B, D, and E, respectively. Following comprehensive analysis of all of the samples under the various conditions, *CYP* was recommended as the reference gene by Delta CT, BestKeeper, NormFinder, and RefFinder, although not with geNorm. According to the above-mentioned results, RefFinder was likely the most comprehensive and scientific of these methods.

Evaluation of the combination of reference genes

Pairwise variation (V) determines the optimal number of control genes for normalization and proposes 0.15 as a cutoff value [26]. If the V_n/V_{n+1} value is less than 0.15, the suitable gene number for normalization is n. Additional control genes were not necessary in the six groups except for group C (i.e., the 6-BA treatment group),as indicated by V_2/V_3 values below 0.15 [26]. Three reference genes were recommended for group C, as indicated by a V_3/V_4 value of 0.115, which is consistent with the M-value ranking for this group.

Discussion

Validation of the stability of candidate reference genes under different experimental conditions [31], with different tissues [32, 33], at different stages, and in different species [34] is necessary. In the present study, *EIF* was the most unstable gene in *P. cocos*; however, *EIF1* and *EIF3* were recommended as reference genes in *Ammopiptanthus mongolicus* (Maxim. ex Kom.) S.H. Cheng [35]. In contrast, *CYP* was the most stable gene in leaves of *Deschampsia antarctica* É. Desv. [36] under three abiotic stresses (salt, cold, and PEG treatment), whereas the *EF-1α* gene was recommended for roots. In banana fruit, the expression levels of two widely used reference genes, actin and *GAPDH*, were not stable [34].

The candidate reference gene rankings for the individual groups evaluated in this study may differ slightly from the ranking for all samples because, under specific circumstances, more accurate rankings would be established. Moreover, most of the M-values of the 14 genes were less than 1.5 except for *SAMDC, EIF,* and *APT*, indicating that most of the candidate reference genes were stable. As one of the least stable genes, the instability of *APT* has been reported in papaya under six experimental conditions [37]. It was contradictory that *CYP* was the best overall reference gene but did not exhibit the best performance in any single group. *CYP* was the most stable reference gene using Delta CT, NormFinder, and BestKeeper but not geNorm (Table 11). In addition, *CYP* was the third-most stable reference gene by geNorm. Moreover, *CYP* frequently ranked among the top five reference genes (Tables 5, 6, 7, 8, 9, 10), particularly under 6-BA treatment, in which *CYP* exhibited the highest average M-value when using geNorm for analysis. In group C, *CYP* ranked firmly as the second-most stable reference gene. In contrast, the ranking of other candidate genes in the six groups varied greatly. A similar phenomenon has been observed in *Ammopiptanthus mongolicus* [35]. *EIF1* and *EIF3* were selected as reference genes across all of the samples, whereas these two genes were the most stable only under drought stress among the four evaluated abiotic stresses. Following acibenzolar-*S*-methyl treatment, the combination of *CYP* and *eIF4B* was most suitable as an internal control in *Eucalyptus* L'Hér. In addition to *P. cocos* and *Eucalyptus* [38], *CYP* has been selected as an internal control for several animal cells. In human peripheral blood, *CYP* was a more suitable housekeeping gene than *β-Act* and *GAPDH* [39]. *CYP* was also recommended as one of the reference genes for neurons of the central nervous system [40] and in atopic human bronchial epithelial cells [41]. Moreover, *CYP* was considered to be an RNA normalization control in rats [42].

NormFinder, BestKeeper and geNorm are widely used for selection of reference genes, although the results generated by the different methods may be slightly different [43, 44]. Our results displayed the same tendency as those of previous studies [26–30]. Moreover, the validity of the results might be related to the materials used or even to potential experimental errors. The importance of systematic evaluation before candidate genes are used as reference genes, especially under different conditions were observed in the study.

Conclusion

SAMDC, his3-2, RP, RPB2, and *his3-1* were evaluated to be suitable reference genes for *P. Cocos* following different treatments. *RPB2* was the most stable reference gene under different temperatures and *CYP* was the most stable gene in the mycelia under all six evaluated conditions.

Table 11 Ranking order of the reference genes for all treatment conditions (Better-Good-Average)

Method	1	2	3	4	5	6	7	8	9	10	11	12	13	14
DeltaCT	*CYP*	*his3-1*	*GAPDH*	*RP*	*RPB1-2*	*RPB2*	*β-Act*	*his3-2*	*RPB1-1*	*MAPK*	*β-Tub*	*SAMDC*	*EIF*	*APT*
BestKeeper	*CYP*	*RPB1-2*	*β-Act*	*RP*	*his3-1*	*RPB1-1*	*GAPDH*	*RPB2*	*APT*	*MAPK*	*β-Tub*	*his3-2*	*SAMDC*	*EIF*
NormFinder	*CYP*	*his3-1*	*GAPDH*	*RP*	*RPB2*	*RPB1-2*	*β-Act*	*MAPK*	*his3-2*	*RPB1-1*	*β-Tub*	*SAMDC*	*EIF*	*APT*
geNorm	*his3-1/RP*		*CYP*	*β-Act*	*RPB1-1*	*RPB1-2*	*GAPDH*	*RPB2*	*MAPK*	*his3-2*	*β-Tub*	*SAMDC*	*EIF*	*APT*
Recommended comprehensive ranking	*CYP*	*his3-1*	*RP*	*RPB1-2*	*GAPDH*	*β-Act*	*RPB2*	*RPB1-1*	*MAPK*	*his3-2*	*β-Tub*	*SAMDC*	*APT*	*EIF*

Abbreviations

GAPDH: glyceraldehyde-3-phosphate dehydrogenase; MAPK: mitogen-activated protein kinase; β-Act: beta actin; RPB2: RNA polymerase subunit 2; RPB1-1: RNA polymerase subunit 1; RPB1-2: RNA polymerase subunit 1; his3-1: histone 3; his3-2: histone 3; APT: adenine phosphoribosyl transferase; SAMDC: S-adenosyl methionine decarboxylase; RP: ribosomal protein; β-Tub: beta tubulin; EIF: eukaryotic translation initiation factor; CYP: cyclophilin; IAA: indole-3-acetic acid; ABA: abscisic acid; 6-BA: 6-benzylaminopurine; MeJA: methyl jasmonate; GA: gibberellin acid; qRT-PCR: quantitative real-time PCR; PCR: polymerase chain reaction.

Authors' contributions

JX designed the study. XZ and ZCX performed RNA extraction. XZ performed qRT-PCR. XZ, ZCX, AJJ, CS and YLH analyzed the data. XZ, JYS, HML and SLC wrote the manuscript. All authors read and approved the final manuscript.

Author details

[1] Institute of Medicinal Plant Development, Chinese Academy of Medical Sciences and Peking Union Medical College, Beijing 100193, China. [2] Institute of Chinese Materia Medica, China Academy of Chinese Medical Sciences, Beijing 100700, China. [3] Chongqing Institute of Medicinal Plant Cultivation, Chongqing 408435, China. [4] State Key Laboratory of Protein and Plant Gene Research, College of Life Sciences, Peking University, Beijing 100871, China.

Acknowledgements

Dr. Xu Guo (Shandong Academy of Agricultural Sciences) is acknowledged for providing the *P. cocos* strain CGMCC5.78 used in this work. This work was supported by the National Key Technology R&D Program (Grant no. 2012BAI29B01) and the Program for Innovative Research Team at the Institute of Medicinal Plant Development (IMPLAD).

Competing interests

The authors declare that they have no competing interests.

References

1. Czechowski T, Stitt M, Altmann T, Udvardi MK, Scheible WR. Genome-wide identification and testing of superior reference genes for transcript normalization in *Arabidopsis*. Plant Physiol. 2005;139:5–17.
2. Sun Y, Li Y, Luo D, Liao DJ. Pseudogenes as weaknesses of ACTB (Actb) and GAPDH (Gapdh) used as reference genes in reverse transcription and polymerase chain reactions. PLoS ONE. 2012;7:e41659.
3. Marum L, Miguel A, Ricardo CP, Miguel C. Reference gene selection for quantitative real-time PCR normalization in *Quercus suber*. PLoS ONE. 2012;7:e35113.
4. Chooi WH, Zhou R, Yeo SS, Zhang F, Wang DA. Determination and validation of reference gene stability for qPCR analysis in polysaccharide hydrogel-based 3D chondrocytes and mesenchymal stem cell cultural models. Mol Biotechnol. 2013;54:623–33.
5. Ren A, Qin L, Shi L, Dong X, da Mu S, Li YX, Zhao MW. Methyl jasmonate induces ganoderic acid biosynthesis in the basidiomycetous fungus *Ganoderma lucidum*. Bioresour Technol. 2010;101:6785–90.
6. Shang CH, Shi L, Ren A, Qin L, Zhao MW. Molecular cloning, characterization, and differential expression of a lanosterol synthase gene from *Ganoderma lucidum*. Biosci Biotech Bioch. 2010;74:974–8.
7. Vieira A, Talhinhas P, Loureiro A, Duplessis S, Fernandez D, Silva Mdo C, Paulo OS, Azinheira HG. Validation of RT-qPCR reference genes for in planta expression studies in *Hemileia vastatrix*, the causal agent of coffee leaf rust. Fungal Biol. 2011;115:891–901.
8. Steiger MG, Mach RL, Mach-Aigner AR. An accurate normalization strategy for RT-qPCR in *Hypocrea jecorina* (Trichoderma reesei). J Biotechnol. 2010;145:30–7.
9. Xu J, Xu Z, Zhu Y, Luo H, Qian J, Ji A, Hu Y, Sun W, Wang B, Song J, et al. Identification and Evaluation of Reference Genes for qRT-PCR Normalization in *Ganoderma lucidum*. Curr Microbiol. 2014;68:120–6.
10. Zhao YY, Feng YL, Bai X, Tan XJ, Lin RC, Mei Q. Ultra performance liquid chromatography-based metabonomic study of therapeutic effect of the surface layer of *Poria cocos* on adenine-induced chronic kidney disease provides new insight into anti-fibrosis mechanism. PLoS ONE. 2013;8:e59617.
11. Mantovani MS, Bellini MF, Angeli JP, Oliveira RJ, Silva AF, Ribeiro LR. beta-Glucans in promoting health: prevention against mutation and cancer. Mutat Res. 2008;658:154–61.
12. Wu SJ, Ng LT, Lin CC. Antioxidant activities of some common ingredients of traditional chinese medicine, *Angelica sinensis*, *Lycium barbarum* and *Poria cocos*. Phytother Res. 2004;18:1008–12.
13. Zhou L, Zhang Y, Gapter LA, Ling H, Agarwal R, Ng KY. Cytotoxic and anti-oxidant activities of lanostane-type triterpenes isolated from *Poria cocos*. Chem Pharm Bull. 2008;56:1459–62.
14. Yasukawa K, Kaminaga T, Kitanaka S, Tai T, Nunoura Y, Natori S, Takido M. 3 beta-p-hydroxybenzoyldehydrotumulosic acid from *Poria cocos*, and its anti-inflammatory effect. Phytochemistry. 1998;48:1357–60.
15. Lin Y, Zhang L, Chen L, Jin Y, Zeng F, Jin J, Wan B, Cheung PC. Molecular mass and antitumor activities of sulfated derivatives of alpha-glucan from *Poria cocos* mycelia. Int J Biol Macromol. 2004;34:289–94.
16. Ukiya M, Akihisa T, Tokuda H, Hirano M, Oshikubo M, Nobukuni Y, Kimura Y, Tai T, Kondo S, Nishino H. Inhibition of tumor-promoting effects by poricoic acids G and H and other lanostane-type triterpenes and cytotoxic activity of poricoic acids A and G from *Poria cocos*. J Nat Prod. 2002;65:462–5.
17. Gapter L, Wang Z, Glinski J, Ng KY. Induction of apoptosis in prostate cancer cells by pachymic acid from *Poria cocos*. Biochem Biophys Res Commun. 2005;332:1153–61.
18. Tai T, Akita Y, Kinoshita K, Koyama K, Takahashi K, Watanabe K. Anti-emetic principles of *Poria cocos*. Planta Med. 1995;61:527–30.
19. Hattori T, Hayashi K, Nagao T, Furuta K, Ito M, Suzuki Y. Studies on antinephritic effects of plant components (3): effect of pachyman, a main component of *Poria cocos* Wolf on original-type anti-GBM nephritis in rats and its mechanisms. Jpn J Pharmacol. 1992;59:89–96.
20. Zhang GW, Liu HY, Xia QM, Li JQ, Lu H, Zhang QH, Yao ZF. Anti-rejection effect of ethanol extract of *Poria cocos* wolf in rats after cardiac allograft implantation. Chin Med J. 2004;117:932–5.
21. Zhao YY, Feng YL, Du X, Xi ZH, Cheng XL, Wei F. Diuretic activity of the ethanol and aqueous extracts of the surface layer of *Poria cocos* in rat. J Ethnopharmacol. 2012;144:775–8.
22. Li TH, Hou CC, Chang CL, Yang WC. Anti-hyperglycemic properties of crude extract and triterpenes from *Poria cocos*. Evid-based Complement Alternat Med. 2011;2011.
23. Li GH, Shen YM, Zhang KQ. Nematicidal activity and chemical component of *Poria cocos*. J Microbiol. 2005;43:17–20.
24. Wang JR, Lin JF, Guo LQ, You LF, Zeng XL, Wen JM. Cloning and characterization of squalene synthase gene from *Poria cocos* and its up-regulation by methyl jasmonate. World J Microb Biot. 2013.
25. Shu S, Chen B, Zhou M, Zhao X, Xia H, Wang M. De novo sequencing and transcriptome analysis of *Wolfiporia cocos* to reveal genes related to biosynthesis of triterpenoids. PLoS ONE. 2013;8:e71350.
26. Vandesompele J, De Preter K, Pattyn F, Poppe B, Van Roy N, De Paepe A, Speleman F. Accurate normalization of real-time quantitative RT-PCR data by geometric averaging of multiple internal control genes. Genome Biol. 2002;3: RESEARCH0034.
27. Andersen CL, Jensen JL, Orntoft TF. Normalization of real-time quantitative reverse transcription-PCR data: a model-based variance estimation approach to identify genes suited for normalization, applied to bladder and colon cancer data sets. Cancer Res. 2004;64:5245–50.
28. Pfaffl MW, Tichopad A, Prgomet C, Neuvians TP. Determination of stable housekeeping genes, differentially regulated target genes and sample integrity: BestKeeper-Excel-based tool using pair-wise correlations. Biotechnol Lett. 2004;26:509–15.
29. Silver N, Best S, Jiang J, Thein SL. Selection of housekeeping genes for gene expression studies in human reticulocytes using real-time PCR. BMC Mol Biol. 2006;7:33.
30. Xie F, Sun G, Stiller JW, Zhang B. Genome-wide functional analysis of the cotton transcriptome by creating an integrated EST database. PLoS ONE. 2011;6:e26980.

31. Toegel S, Huang W, Piana C, Unger FM, Wirth M, Goldring MB, Gabor F, Viernstein H. Selection of reliable reference genes for qPCR studies on chondroprotective action. BMC Mol Biol. 2007;8:13.
32. Soes S, Sorensen BS, Alsner J, Overgaard J, Hager H, Hansen LL, Kristensen LS. Identification of accurate reference genes for RT-qPCR analysis of formalin-fixed paraffin-embedded tissue from primary non-small cell lung cancers and brain and lymph node metastases. Lung Cancer. 2013;81:180–6.
33. Nygard AB, Jorgensen CB, Cirera S, Fredholm M. Selection of reference genes for gene expression studies in pig tissues using SYBR green qPCR. BMC Mol Biol. 2007;8:67.
34. Chen L, Zhong HY, Kuang JF, Li JG, Lu WJ, Chen JY. Validation of reference genes for RT-qPCR studies of gene expression in banana fruit under different experimental conditions. Planta. 2011;234:377–90.
35. Shi J, Liu M, Shi J, Zheng G, Wang Y, Wang J, Chen Y, Lu C, Yin W. Reference gene selection for qPCR in *Ammopiptanthus mongolicus* under abiotic stresses and expression analysis of seven ROS-scavenging enzyme genes. Plant Cell Rep. 2012;31:1245–54.
36. Lee H, Kim JH, Park M, Kim I-C, Yim JH, Lee HK. Reference genes validation for qPCR normalization in *Deschampsia antarctica* during abiotic stresses. Antarct Sci. 2010;22:477–84.
37. Zhu X, Li X, Chen W, Chen J, Lu W, Chen L, Fu D. Evaluation of new reference genes in papaya for accurate transcript normalization under different experimental conditions. PLoS ONE. 2012;7:e44405.
38. Boava LP, Laia ML, Jacob TR, Dabbas KM, Goncalves JF, Ferro JA, Ferro MI, Furtado EL. Selection of endogenous genes for gene expression studies in *Eucalyptus* under biotic (Puccinia psidii) and abiotic (acibenzolar-S-methyl) stresses using RT-qPCR. BMC Res Notes. 2010;3:43.
39. Pachot A, Blond JL, Mougin B, Miossec P. Peptidylpropyl isomerase B (PPIB): a suitable reference gene for mRNA quantification in peripheral whole blood. J Biotechnol. 2004;114:121–4.
40. Chen J, Sochivko D, Beck H, Marechal D, Wiestler OD, Becker AJ. Activity-induced expression of common reference genes in individual cns neurons. Lab Invest. 2001;81:913–6.
41. He JQ, Sandford AJ, Wang IM, Stepaniants S, Knight DA, Kicic A, Stick SM, Pare PD. Selection of housekeeping genes for real-time PCR in atopic human bronchial epithelial cells. Eur Respir J. 2008;32:755–62.
42. Weisinger G, Gavish M, Mazurika C, Zinder O. Transcription of actin, cyclophilin and glyceraldehyde phosphate dehydrogenase genes: tissue- and treatment-specificity. Biochim Biophys Acta. 1999;1446:225–32.
43. Ceelen L, De Spiegelaere W, David M, De Craene J, Vinken M, Vanhaecke T, Rogiers V. Critical selection of reliable reference genes for gene expression study in the HepaRG cell line. Biochem Pharmacol. 2011;81:1255–61.
44. Wei L, Miao H, Zhao R, Han X, Zhang T, Zhang H. Identification and testing of reference genes for Sesame gene expression analysis by quantitative real-time PCR. Planta. 2013;237:873–89.

2

Attenuation of blood pressure in spontaneously hypertensive rats by acupuncture was associated with reduction oxidative stress and improvement from endothelial dysfunction

Sin Bond Leung[1], Hongwei Zhang[1], Chi Wai Lau[2] and Zhi-Xiu Lin[1*]

Abstract

Background: Hypertension can be treated effectively by acupuncture; however, the association between acupuncture and endothelial function remains unknown. This study aimed to investigate the effects of acupuncture on endothelial dysfunction and oxidative stress-related parameters in spontaneously hypertensive animals.

Methods: Eighteen-week-old Wistar–Kyoto rats (WKYs) and spontaneously hypertensive rats (SHRs) were arbitrarily divided into four groups: WKY control ($n = 8$), SHR control ($n = 8$), SHR sham-acupuncture ($n = 8$) and SHR acupuncture ($n = 8$). The SHR acupuncture group had electroacupuncture for 6 consecutive weeks on acupoints ST36 and LR3. Blood pressure was monitored during the treatment period, and animals were euthanized at the 6th week. Aortas were harvested for determination of angiotensin II levels, NADPH oxidase activity and nitrate/nitrite levels. The level of reactive oxygen species (ROS) was determined by dihydroethidium (DHE) imaging, and functional studies were performed to assess vascular reactivity. Endothelial nitric oxide synthase was measured by Western blot assay.

Results: Blood pressure at the end of treatment was significantly lower in the SHR acupuncture group (185.0 ± 5.6 mmHg) compared with the SHR sham-acupuncture and the SHR control groups (201.0 ± 5.4 and 197.4 ± 5.9 mmHg, respectively; $P < 0.001$). Serum angiotensin II level in the SHR control group was significantly higher than in the WKY control group ($P < 0.001$), while it was significantly attenuated by acupuncture treatment ($P = 0.023$). DHE staining showed that ROS level was reduced in the aortas ($P = 0.0017$) and carotid arteries ($P = 0.039$) of acupuncture-treated SHRs. Biochemical assays showed that acupuncture inhibited the NADPH oxidase activity ($P = 0.022$) and enhanced antioxidant capacity ($P = 0.0039$). In functional studies, endothelium-dependent relaxation of aortic rings ($P = 0.018$) and carotid arteries ($P = 0.022$) in response to acetylcholine was improved in the SHR acupuncture group. Aortas of SHRs receiving acupuncture also expressed an elevated level of eNOS ($P > 0.001$) and p-eNOS ($P = 0.012$) and a reduced nitrotyrosine level ($P = 0.0012$). The nitrate/nitrite level in aortic tissue was also attenuated after acupuncture ($P = 0.0018$).

Conclusion: The effects of acupuncture in treating hypertension were associated with reduced oxidative stress, increased nitric oxide bioavailability and endothelial function in SHRs.

Keywords: Acupuncture, Hypertension, Endothelial dysfunction, Spontaneously hypertensive rats

*Correspondence: linzx@cuhk.edu.hk
[1] School of Chinese Medicine, Faculty of Medicine, The Chinese University of Hong Kong, Shatin, N.T., Hong Kong, People's Republic of China
Full list of author information is available at the end of the article

Background

Acupuncture is recognized by the World Health Organization (WHO) for the management of many diseases, including hypertension [1]. Previous studies have showed that acupuncture reduces hypertension through diverse mechanisms [2, 3]. Acupuncture intervention re-modulated the activity of the renin-angiotensin-aldosterone system, endothelium-derived vasoactive substances, and vascular function [4–6]. The effects of acupuncture on hypertension might be associated with regulation of NO [1]. It was reported that NO levels increased after acupuncture treatment [7–9]. Moreover, acupuncture exhibited strong antioxidative effects in the treatment of cerebral ischemia, myocardial injury, and Parkinson's disease [10–14]. However, the effects of acupuncture on hypertension in relation to oxidative stress are not yet fully understood.

Endothelial dysfunction was found in cardiovascular diseases, including hypertension [15–17]. Normal endothelium secretes vasoactive substances to regulate vascular tone, and endothelium-derived nitric oxide (NO) to maintain healthy vasculature. However, under oxidative stress, the bioavailability of NO is decreased; this is one of the hallmarks of endothelial dysfunction [18–22]. Increased reactive oxygen species (ROS) level during hypertension has been observed clinically and in vivo [20–22]. Certain anti-hypertensive medications, such as nebivolol and carvedilol, possess antioxidative activity to improve NO bioavailability [23–25].

This study aimed to investigate the effects of acupuncture on endothelial dysfunction in spontaneously hypertensive rats, and to determine the association of the observed changes in blood pressure, and biochemistry of endothelial function, NO bioavailability, and oxidative stress.

Methods

Animals and artery preparation

Eighteen week-old spontaneously hypertensive rats (SHRs) and Wistar-Kyoto rats (WKYs) were supplied by the Laboratory Animal Service Centre, The Chinese University of Hong Kong. Rats were kept in a holding room with temperature control of 22–24 °C and 12-h light/dark cycle. Standard diet and water were provided ad libitum. The animals were divided into four groups, including the WKY control group (n = 8), SHR control group (n = 8), SHR sham-acupuncture group (n = 8) and SHR real acupuncture group (n = 8). After 6 weeks of treatment, the animals were sacrificed by carbon dioxide inhalation. Aortas and carotid arteries were dissected out and the surrounding connective tissues were removed. This study was approved by the Animal Experimentation Ethic Committee (Additional file 1), The Chinese University of Hong Kong and conformed to the guidelines of the *Principles of Laboratory Animal Care* (NIH publications No. 80-23, revised 1996). The project proposals and proposal revised history were provided (Additional files 2, 3, 4). The members of clinical research ethics committee was provided (Additional file 5). The animal studies were performed following the ARRIVE guideline (Additional file 6).

Acupuncture intervention

Electro-acupuncture was applied to SHRs in the SHR acupuncture group for 6 consecutive weeks. Acupuncture needles (13 mm in length and 0.14 mm in diameter) were inserted into the bilateral ST36 and LR3 acupoints. A regular manual manipulation of the needle was performed to elicit a gentle voluntary movement of the lower limbs of the rats, which was considered to be equivalent to the *deqi* (obtaining *qi*) sensation, typically felt by patients with the feelings of soreness, tingling, distension and heaviness. Needles were then connected to an electrical stimulator (Model E600 HAN Multi-Purpose Digital Electronic Acupunctoscope, Hong Kong), and the output of which was set to a continuous wave at 2 Hz, 400 μs band width with an intensity of 2 mA. The duration of each treatment was 20 min and acupuncture treatment was conducted once daily, 5 days every week for 6 consecutive weeks. In the SHR sham-acupuncture control group, intervention was adopted by pricking of a non-acupoint/non-meridian area using a blunted end needle without penetrating through the skin. The locations selected for the sham-acupuncture were over the posterolateral side of the calf muscle and lateral side of the feet approximately over the fifth metatarsal bone. The blunted end needle was removed immediately and no electric stimulation was applied; however, rats were restrained for 20 min as did in the acupuncture group. Both the SHR control and WKY control groups received no real or sham-acupuncture treatment during the 6-week period.

Blood pressure monitoring

Blood pressure was non-invasively measured by determining tail blood volume with a volume pressure recording sensor and an occlusion tail-cuff (CODA System, Kent Scientific, Torrington, CT, USA). The trend of blood pressure was recorded at several time points, i.e., prior to treatment, at the 2nd, 4th week and the end of interventions [26].

Measurement of isometric force

Aortic rings were suspended in organ bath filled with Krebs solution (pH7.4) containing 119 mM NaCl, 4.7 mM KCl, 2.5 mM $CaCl_2$, 1 mM $MgCl_2$, 25 mM

$NaHCO_3$, 1.2 mM KH_2PO_4, and 11 mM D-glucose, oxygenated with 95 % O_2–5 % CO_2, and kept at 37 °C. Aortic rings were fixed in one end to a metal hook and the other end connected to a force transducer under a basal tension of 25 mN as described previously [27]. Carotid arteries were suspended in wire myograph (Danish Myo Technology, Denmark) under a basal tension of 5mN. They were allowed to equilibrate for 30 min and then challenged by 60 mM KCl solution to ensure the viability of the aortas. Phenylephrine (0.3 μM) was used to induce a contraction followed by relaxation by acetylcholine (10 μM) for assessing the integrity of functional endothelium. After washout, phenylephrine (0.3 μM) was added again to produce a stable contraction, then acetylcholine (ACh) was applied cumulatively (3 nM–3 μM) to induce endothelium-dependent relaxations. In some rings treated with L-NAME (100 μM) for 30 min, endothelium-independent relaxations were examined in response to NO donor sodium nitroprusside (SNP).

Western blot analysis

Aortic rings were frozen in liquid nitrogen and homogenized in ice-cold RIPA lysis buffer (1 mg/mL leupeptin, 5 mg/mL aprotonin, 100 mg/mL PMSF, 1 mM sodium orthovanadate, 1 mM EGTA, 1 mM EDTA, 1 mM NaF, and 2 mg/mL b-glycerolphosphate). The lysates were centrifuged (Centrifuge 5430R, EppendorfAG, Hamburg, Germany) at 20,000×*g* for 20 min at 4 °C. The supernatants were collected and the protein concentration was determined by the Lowry method (BioRad, CA, USA). Samples containing 20 μg of protein was boiled for 10 min with 5 % β-mercaptoethanol and then separated on a 10 % SDS–polyacrylamide gel by electrophoresis. The resolved protein was transferred to an immobilion-P polyvinylidenedifluoride membrane (Millipore Corp., Bedford, MA, USA) and blocked with 1 % BSA for 20 min. Primary antibodies against eNOS (BD, Lexington, KY, USA), nitrotyrosine (Upstate, Lake Placid, NY, USA) and GAPDH (Ambion, Austin, TX, USA) were used for incubation at 4 °C overnight, followed by horseradish peroxidase-conjugated secondary antibodies (DakoCytomation, Glostrup, Denmark). An enhanced chemiluminescence detection system (ECL reagents, Amersham Pharmacia Biotech, Buckinghamshire, UK) was applied to develop the membranes and a documentation program (Fluochem, Alpha innotect Corp., San Leandro, CA, USA) was used for densitometry measurement [28].

Measurement of antioxidant capacity

After rat euthanasia, blood was collected and stored in tubes containing heparin. The samples were centrifuged at 1000×*g* for 10 min at 4 °C; plasma was then collected and stored on ice. The assay was performed using an antioxidant assay kit (Cayman Chemicals, Ann Arbor, MI, USA) according to the manufacturer's instructions. The principle of the assay is based on the antioxidant activity in the sample to inhibit the oxidation of 2,2′-azino-di-[3-ethylbenzthiazoline sulfonate] by metmyoglobin. The antioxidant capacity was compared with that of Trolox, a water-soluble tocopherol analogue, as the standard, and the absorbance at 750 nm was measured colorimetrically (ELX800; BioTek Instruments, Winooski, VT, USA) [29].

Measurement of serum angiotensin II level

After rat euthanasia, blood was collected and stored in tubes containing EDTA on ice. Blood samples were centrifuged at 3000×*g* for 20 min at 4 °C, and serum was extracted immediately. Angiotensin II level was assessed using an enzyme immunoassay kit (SPI-Bio, Massy, France) according to the manufacturer's instructions [30].

Measurement of NADPH oxidase activity

Aortic tissue was prepared and homogenized in lysis buffer as described above. The supernatant was used to measure the NADPH oxidase activity by a lucigenin chemiluminescence assay. We mixed 60 μg of sample with lucigenin (10 μM, final concentration) and NADPH (100 μM, final concentration) in a dark environment. The chemiluminescence signal was then measured every 1 min for 10 min using a luminometer (GloMax 20/20; Promega, Madison, WI, USA). An extra set of controls was designed by adding diphenyleneiodonium (DPI, 5 μM), a NADPH oxidase inhibitor, in the homogenate of the SHR control group [31].

Measurement of aortic nitrite/nitrate level

Aortic rings were prepared and homogenized in lysis buffer as described above. The supernatant was used to measure the serum nitrite/nitrate level by colorimetric assay kit (Cayman Chemicals, Ann Arbor, MI, USA). We used 30 μg of sample for the measurement according to the manufacturer's instructions [32].

Measurement of reactive oxygen species by dihydroethidium imaging

Dihydroethidium (DHE; Molecular Probes, Eugene, OR, USA) was used to evaluate the amount of oxidant formation [33]. Frozen sections of aortic rings and carotid arteries were sectioned at 10 μm thickness by cryostat microtome (Leica CM1100; Leica Instruments, Germany) and incubated in Krebs solution containing 5 μM DHE for 10 min at 37 °C. Samples were examined with a confocal microscope (FV1000; Olympus, Tokyo, Japan) at an excitation/emission of 488/605 nm. Fluorescence intensity was quantified by Fluoview version 1.5 (FV10-ASW1.5; Olympus, Tokyo, Japan).

Immunohistochemistry

Aortic rings were immunohistochemically stained. Aortas were fixed in 4 % paraformaldehyde overnight at 4 °C, and then processed and embedded in paraffin. Rings were cut into 5 μM cross-sections by microtome (Leica CM1100; Leica Instruments, Germany) and placed on glass slides. Slides were de-waxed, dehydrated, immersed in 5 % H_2O_2 in methanol, and boiled in 0.01 mol/L citrate buffer (pH 6.0) for 3 min in a microwave for antigen retrieval. Donkey serum (5 %; Jackson Immunoresearch, West Grove, PA, USA) was used to incubate the sections for 30 min for blocking. Primary antibody nitrotyrosine (1:500; Upstate, Lake Placid, NY, USA) diluted in donkey serum was used for overnight incubation at 4 °C. The slides were washed in phosphate-buffered solution (PBS) three times (5 min each time) and incubated with secondary biotin-SP conjugated goat anti-rabbit antibody (1:200; Jackson Immunoresearch, West Grove, PA, USA) for 1 h at room temperature. The slides were again washed three times in PBS, followed by incubation with streptavidin-HRP conjugate (ZymedLaboratories Inc., South San Francisco, CA, USA) at 1:200 dilution for 1 h at room temperature. Visualization was done by 3,3′-diaminibenzide tetrachloride (DAB) staining (Vector Laboratories Inc., Burlingame, CA, USA). DAB chromogen substrate was added and incubated for 2 min on the sections. Slides were rinsed in running water for 10 min and counterstained with hematoxylin. Dehydration and mounting were done and microscopic pictures were taken using Spot Advanced software (Diagnostic Instruments, Detroit, MI, USA). Images and intensity of signals were analyzed using ImageJ software (National Institutes of Health, Bethesda, MD, USA) [34].

Histological study and connective tissue assessment

Glass slides with sections of aortic rings were prepared by fixation in paraffin, cutting in sections, de-waxing and dehydration as for immunohistochemistry stain. Sections were directly stained for collagen and elastin contents, and histological study. After de-waxing, the sections were stained using the Weigert–Van Gieson method [35] for collagen content assessment. Slides were immersed in 2.5 % lithium carmine, or named solution A (25 g carmine in 100 mL saturated solution of lithium carbonate), for 5 min and washed in water for 2 min. The slides were then placed in Weigert's stain, or named solution B (basic fuchsin 2 g, resorcinol 4 g, distilled water 300 mL, 20 % ferric perchloride solution 40 mL, 95 % ethanol 280 mL, hydrochloric acid 2.8 mL), for another 5 min followed by washing in tap water for 2 min. Differentiation was carried out in 1 % acid alcohol, and sections were finally stained in Van Gieson's stain (saturated aqueous picric acid 80 mL, 1 % acid fuchsin 20 mL) for 10 min. Slides were counterstained with hematoxylin and then washed, dehydrated and mounted for microscopic assessment of collagen content and histological studies. Elastin content was assessed by the orcein technique [36]; synthetic orcein (1 g) was dissolved in 100 mL of 70 % alcohol with the aid of heat, followed by cooling and filtering. Hydrochloric acid (1 mL) was added in the last step of stain preparation. Slides were placed in the stain for 1 h at room temperature. They were then rinsed in 70 % alcohol and differentiated in acid alcohol, followed by washing in tap water for 2 min. Counterstaining was carried out using hematoxylin before the slides were washed, dehydrated and mounted for further analysis. Collagen and elastin contents were quantified using ImageJ software.

Under the same section area and using identical magnification, the areas of collagen and elastin stain were measured and expressed as fold change relative to WKY control sections. For collagen and elastin fractions, the same length of segments were selected in sections and the areas of collagen or elastin stain were measured over the total selected area [37].

Data analysis

Results were expressed as mean ± SD. The relaxation of aortic rings and carotid arteries was presented as percentage of the evoked tone. Data were analyzed using GraphPad Prism software (GraphPad Software Inc., San Diego, CA, USA). The cumulative concentration–response curve was analyzed with a non-linear curve fitting. The maximal relaxation response (E_{max}) and negative logarithm of the dilator concentrations to cause 50 % relaxation (pD_2) were calculated. The relaxation at different concentration of drugs was compared. Statistical analysis was performed by one-way ANOVA followed by the Newman–Keuls test for comparisons among all groups. $P < 0.05$ was considered statistically significant. Exact P values were shown, unless $P < 0.001$.

Results

Acupuncture attenuated blood pressure in spontaneously hypertensive rats

The blood pressure trends during 6 weeks of acupuncture treatment are shown in Fig. 1. At the beginning of the treatment, blood pressure was similar among the SHR control, SHR sham-acupuncture and SHR acupuncture groups (193.5 ± 5.8, 198.9 ± 4.5 and 197.4 ± 5.2 mmHg, respectively). Blood pressure in the WKY group was significantly lower than that in the SHR groups (133.1 ± 4.1 vs. 193.5 ± 5.8 mmHg, $P < 0.001$). At the end of treatment, blood pressure was significantly lower in the SHR

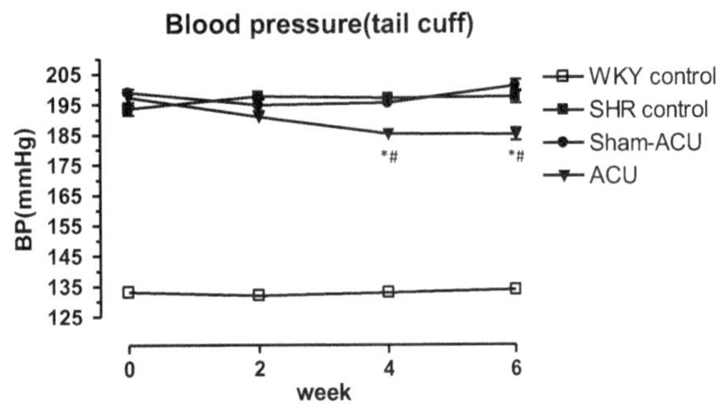

Fig. 1 Effect of acupuncture treatment on blood pressure in experimental rats. Data were expressed as means ± SD. (*,#$P < 0.001$ for ACU vs. SHR control and sham-acupuncture, respectively)

acupuncture group (185.0 ± 5.6 mmHg) compared with the SHR sham-acupuncture group (201.0 ± 5.4 mmHg) and SHR control group (197.4 ± 5.9 mmHg; $P < 0.001$). There was a significant reduction in blood pressure in the SHR acupuncture group compared with the three control groups (Table 1).

Acupuncture improved endothelium-dependent relaxations in aortas and carotid arteries

Acetylcholine-induced endothelium-dependent relaxation (EDR) in the aortas was significantly lower in the SHR control group (E_{max}% 38.5 ± 9.5) compared with the WKY control group (E_{max}% 81.3 ± 7.9; $P < 0.001$). Sham-acupuncture did not affect EDR in the SHRs (E_{max}% 42.5 ± 9.1). However, acupuncture treatment significantly improved EDR in the SHRs; E_{max}% in the SHR sham-acupuncture control group (54.3 ± 10.1) was significantly lower than that in the SHR control group (E_{max}% 42.5 ± 9.1; $P = 0.0191$) and the WKY control group (E_{max}% 38.5 ± 9.5; $P = 0.0238$) (Fig. 2; Table 2).

There were similar findings in the carotid arteries. The EDR of the SHR control group was significantly lower than that of the WKY control group ($P < 0.001$). Acupuncture treatment partially restored EDR, while sham-acupuncture exerted no effect. Endothelium-independent relaxation was similar in all four groups (Fig. 3; Table 3).

Acupuncture increased the eNOS expression and attenuated nitrotyrosine level

The eNOS expression in aortas of the SHR control group was significantly decreased, compared with the WKY control group ($P < 0.001$). Acupuncture significantly increased the eNOS expression ($P < 0.001$), but sham-acupuncture showed no effect. Nitrotyrosine was overexpressed in the SHR control group compared with the WKY control group; acupuncture, but not sham treatment, attenuated its expression (Figs. 4, 5).

Acupuncture enhanced the antioxidant capacity in the aortas

The serum of the WKY control group showed a significantly higher antioxidant capacity than that of the SHR control group ($P < 0.001$); neither sham-acupuncture nor acupuncture affected the antioxidant capacity. In aortic homogenate, the antioxidant capacity was significantly higher in the WKY control compared with the SHR control group ($P < 0.001$). Acupuncture promoted antioxidant capacity, while sham-acupuncture elicited no effect (Fig. 6).

Acupuncture reduced serum angiotensin II level

As shown in Fig. 2, the serum angiotensin II levels were significantly higher in both the SHR control group (324.4 ± 57.9 pg/mL) and the SHR sham-acupuncture group (327.1 ± 71.1 pg/mL) compared with the WKY control group (132.0 ± 27.2 pg/mL; $P < 0.001$). For the SHRs receiving 6 weeks of acupuncture, the angiotensin II level was significantly reduced (256 ± 49.1 pg/mL) compared with the sham-acupuncture control ($P = 0.036$) and the SHR control group ($P = 0.023$; Fig. 7).

Acupuncture attenuated NADPH oxidase activity in the aortas

The enzymatic activity was significantly lower in the WKY control group compared with the SHR control group ($P < 0.001$). Acupuncture on the SHRs significantly reduced NADPH oxidase activity in the aorta ($P = 0.022$), while sham-acupuncture exerted no effect. An extra control group created by incubating the aortas

Table 1 The blood pressures at the beginning, 4th and 6th week of treatment

	BP, mmHg (0 week)	BP, mmHg (4th week)	BP, mmHg (6th week)	Change in BP, mmHg
WKY control	133.1 ± 4.1	132.9 ± 4.0	133.8 ± 5.0	+0.6 ± 3.8
SHR control	193.5 ± 5.8	197.0 ± 4.6	197.4 ± 5.9	+3.9 ± 3.8
Sham-acupuncture	198.9 ± 4.5	195.4 ± 4.2	201.0 ± 5.5	+2.1 ± 4.0
Acupuncture	197.4 ± 7.5	185.3 ± 5.0*,#	185.0 ± 5.7*,#	−12.4 ± 6.3*,#

Data were expressed as means ± SD

*,# $P < 0.001$ for ACU vs. SHR control and sham-acupuncture respectively

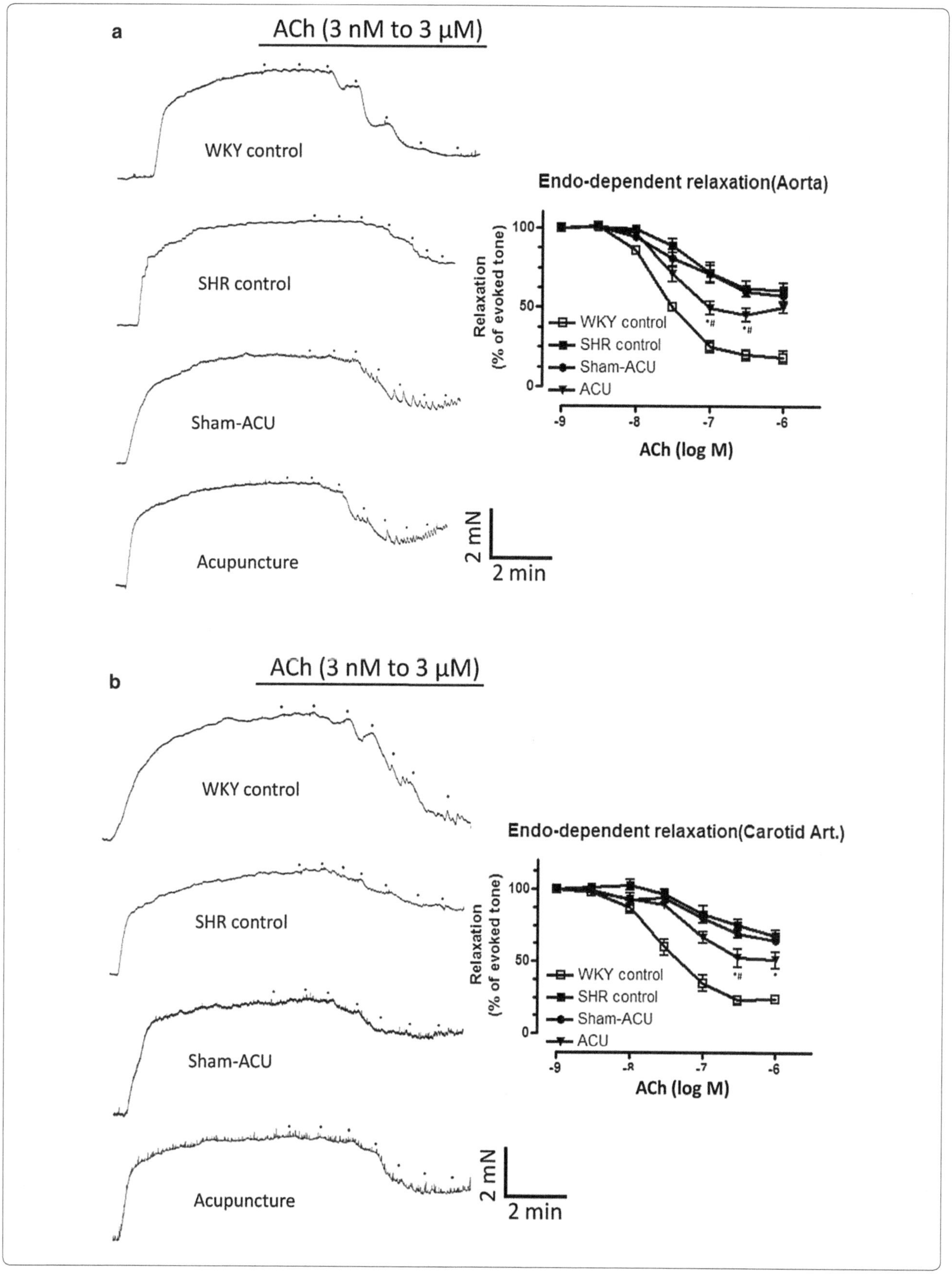
a
ACh (3 nM to 3 μM)
WKY control
SHR control
Sham-ACU
Acupuncture
2 mN
2 min
Endo-dependent relaxation(Aorta)
Relaxation (% of evoked tone)
100
50
0
WKY control
SHR control
Sham-ACU
ACU
-9
-8
-7
-6
ACh (log M)
b
ACh (3 nM to 3 μM)
WKY control
SHR control
Sham-ACU
Acupuncture
2 mN
2 min
Endo-dependent relaxation(Carotid Art.)
Relaxation (% of evoked tone)
100
50
0
WKY control
SHR control
Sham-ACU
ACU
-9
-8
-7
-6
ACh (log M)

(See figure on previous page.)

Fig. 2 The cumulative concentration–response curves for Ach-induced relaxations of different groups in aorta (**a**) and carotid (**b**) arteries. Data were expressed as means ± SD. (For aorta at ACh[log M] concentration of −6.5,*$P = 0.024$ for ACU vs. SHR control and #$P = 0.019$ for ACU vs. sham-acupuncture. At ACh[log M] concentration of −7, *$P = 0.018$ for ACU vs. SHR control and #$P = 0.0095$ vs. sham-acupuncture. For carotid artery at ACh[log M] concentration of −6,*$P = 0.045$ for ACU vs. SHR control. At ACh[log M] concentration of −6.5, *$P = 0.022$ for ACU vs. SHR control and #$P = 0.05$ for ACU vs. sham-acupuncture)

Table 2 ACh-induced relaxations in the aorta and carotid arteries of the rats in the acupuncture and control groups

	pD_2	E_{max} (%)
ACh relaxation of aortas		
WKY control	7.63 ± 0.22	81.3 ± 7.9
SHR control	7.27 ± 0.61	38.5 ± 9.5
Sham-acupuncture	7.36 ± 0.37	42.5 ± 9.1
Acupuncture	7.55 ± 0.83	54.3 ± 10.1*,#
ACh relaxation of carotid arteries		
WKY control	7.54 ± 0.29	76.7 ± 5.2
SHR control	7.04 ± 0.68	31.8 ± 7.3
Sham-acupuncture	7.00 ± 0.44	35.2 ± 4.3
Acupuncture	7.16 ± 0.54	48.9 ± 9.6*

Data were expressed as means ± SD. (*,# refer to Fig. 2)

with DPI showed a markedly reduced NADPH oxidase level in tissue homogenate ($P < 0.001$) (Fig. 8).

Acupuncture increased aortic nitrite/nitrate level

Nitrite/nitrate level was significantly higher in the WKY control group compared with the SHR control group ($P < 0.001$). Acupuncture on the SHRs attenuated the nitrite/nitrate level, while sham-acupuncture produced no effect (Fig. 9).

Acupuncture reduced reactive oxygen species in the aortas and carotid arteries

DHE fluorescence in the aortas was significantly elevated in the SHR control and the SHR sham-acupuncture group compared with the WKY control group ($P < 0.001$) (Fig. 10). Acupuncture treatment was able to mitigate aortic ROS production. Similar results were observed in carotid arteries.

Acupuncture reduced nitrotyrosine expression in the endothelial layer

The nitrotyrosine immunostaining was weak in the aortas of the WKY control group, while a prominent stain was observed in the intima of the SHR control and the SHR sham-acupuncture group. The intensity of staining was attenuated in the SHR acupuncture group (Fig. 11).

Acupuncture exerted no effect on vascular structure and connective tissues

The WKY control group had a thinner intima-media compared with that of the SHR groups; both sham-acupuncture and acupuncture had no effect on this. There was no statistical difference in the thickness of the lamella layer between the SHR acupuncture group, the SHR sham-acupuncture group, and the SHR control group ($P = 0.56$) (Fig. 12).

There was significantly more total collagen in the aortic ring sections of the SHRs than in the WKYs ($P < 0.001$). Both the SHR sham-acupuncture and SHR acupuncture groups had a similar amount of total collagen to the SHR control group ($P = 0.59$). The SHRs also had a significantly higher fraction of collagen compared with the WKYs ($P < 0.001$). Neither sham-acupuncture nor acupuncture affected the collagen fraction compared with the SHR control group ($P = 0.22$) (Fig. 13).

The elastin amount in the WKYs was significantly lower compared with that in the SHRs ($P < 0.001$). No difference was observed in the SHR sham-acupuncture and the SHR acupuncture group compared with the SHR control group ($P = 0.23$). The elastin fraction was significantly higher in the WKY control group than in the SHR control group ($P < 0.001$). The elastin fraction in the SHR sham-acupuncture and SHR acupuncture groups was similar to that in the SHR control group ($P = 0.44$) (Fig. 14).

Acupuncture exerted no effects on vascular inflammation

The effects of acupuncture on vascular inflammation were studied by measuring the intercellular adhesion molecule (ICAM) and vascular cell adhesion molecule (VCAM) expression by Western blot analysis. The WKY control group showed a significantly lower expression of both ICAM and VCAM compared with the SHR groups ($P < 0.001$); both sham-acupuncture and real acupuncture had no effect (Fig. 15).

Adverse effects and complications

No morbidity or mortality was observed in the rats during the course of acupuncture and sham-acupuncture treatment. In addition, there was no abnormality of lower limb movement in any animal while receiving acupuncture treatment; only occasional minimal bleeding from

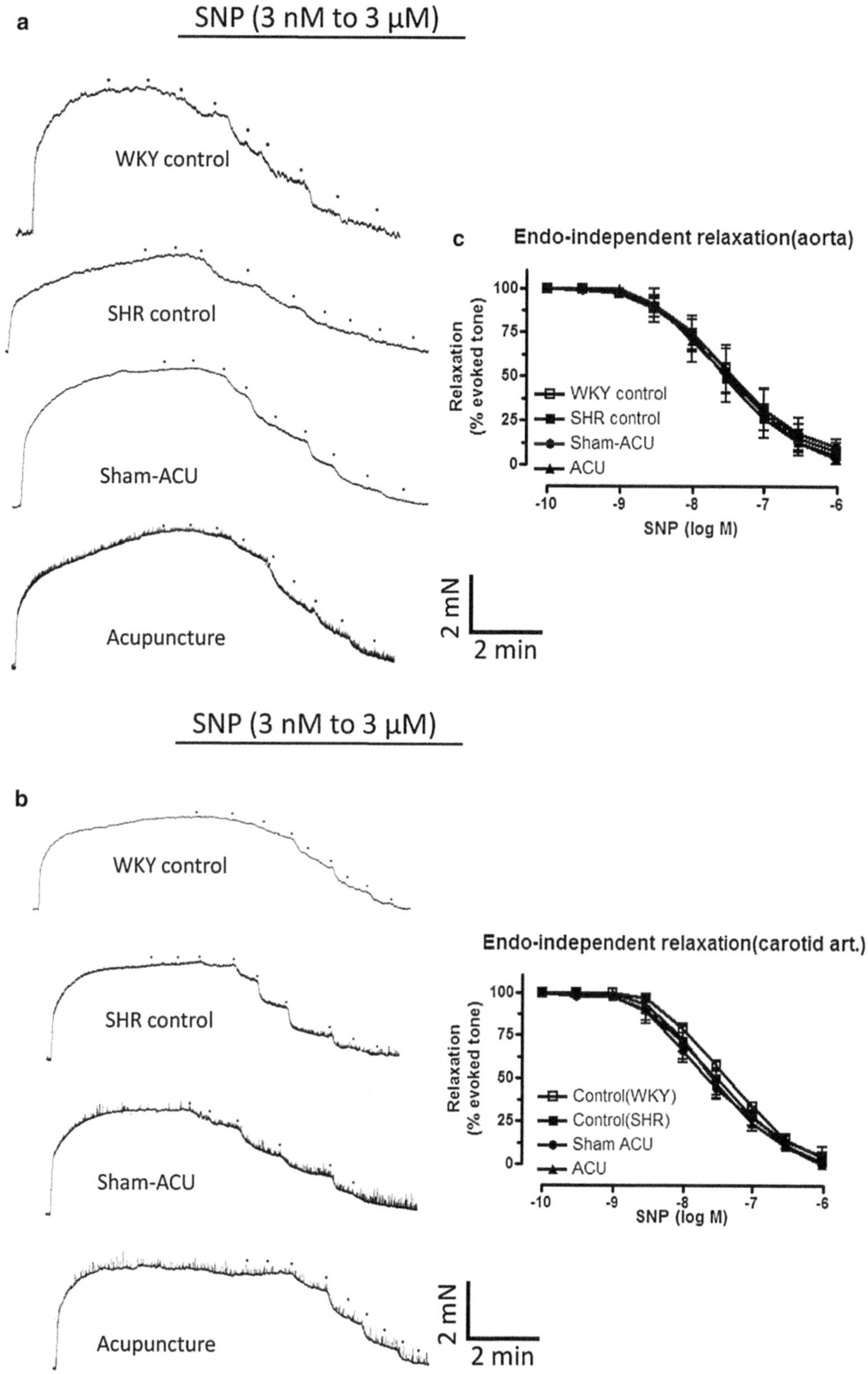

Fig. 3 The cumulative concentration–response curves for the SNP-induced relaxations of different groups in aorta (**a**) and carotid (**b**) arteries. Acupuncture did not restore endothelium-independent relaxation (**c**). Data were expressed as means ± SD

Table 3 The SNP-induced relaxations in the aorta and carotid arteries of the rats in the acupuncture and control groups

Treatment	pD_2	E_{max} (%)
SNP relaxation of aortas		
WKY control	7.47 ± 0.26	98.0 ± 19.8
SHR control	7.56 ± 0.18	97.7 ± 11.4
Sham-acupuncture	7.52 ± 0.26	93.3 ± 17.8
Acupuncture	7.51 ± 0.27	101.6 ± 23.1
SNP relaxation of carotid arteries		
WKY control	7.38 ± 0.07	100.3 ± 5.3
SHR control	7.48 ± 0.18	100.4 ± 16.1
Sham-acupuncture	7.63 ± 0.15	97.6 ± 8.8
Acupuncture	7.55 ± 0.15	101.8 ± 9.8

Data were expressed as means ± SD

the acupuncture site was seen, which was stopped by gentle manual pressure.

Discussion

Effective treatment to lower high blood pressure can reduce the risk of stroke and myocardial infarction by 40 and 15 % respectively [38]. Anti-hypertensive medications remain the mainstay of treatment, in addition to lifestyle modifications such as weight reduction, physical exercise, cessation of smoking, and adoption of healthy diet. A meta-analysis [39] on the effect of acupuncture on essential hypertension in humans reported that acupuncture without antihypertensive medications did not significantly improve blood pressure in hypertensive patients; however, the number of studies included was small, and each study had a relatively small sample size. Another review [40] showed that acupuncture could lower systolic and diastolic blood pressure in humans, but the results were limited by the unsatisfactory methodological quality of the identified trials.

Although the search is still ongoing for solid evidence regarding the essence of the meridian system, increasing clinical data has been accumulated to support the efficacy of acupuncture [41–43]. In 2003, a document published by the WHO stated that acupuncture is suitable for treating primary hypotension and early essential hypertension [1]. The influence of acupuncture on hypertension might be related to its regulatory effect on the level of serum NO [1]; for mild and moderate essential hypertension, the hypotensive effect of acupuncture was more potent than placebo, and was comparable to certain conventional hypotensive agents [1]. At present, the evidence-based support for acupuncture as a treatment for hypertension in humans is still inconclusive. There has

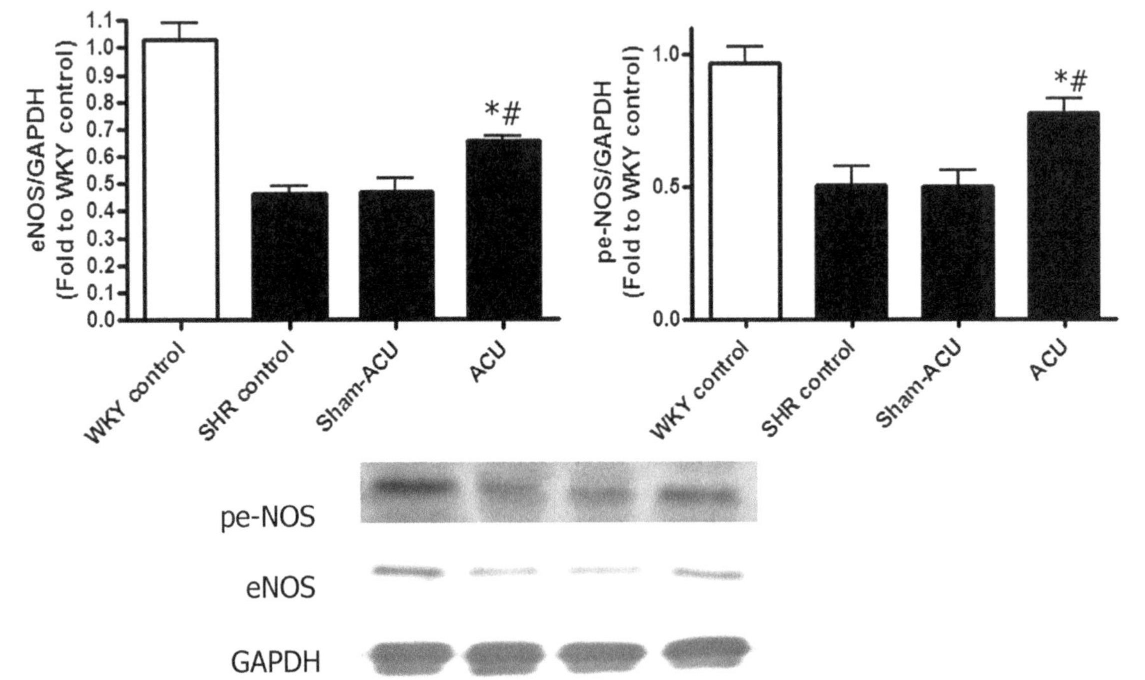

Fig. 4 Effects of acupuncture on eNOS and peNOS expressions in the aorta tissues. Acupuncture significantly enhanced the eNOS and peNOS expressions when compared with the SHR control and sham-acupuncture group. Data were expressed as means ± SD. (For eNOS expression, $^*P < 0.001$ for ACU vs. SHR control and $^\#P = 0.0053$ for ACU vs. sham-acupuncture. For peNOS expression, $P = 0.012$ for ACU vs. SHR control and $^\#P = 0.0073$ for ACU vs. sham-acupuncture)

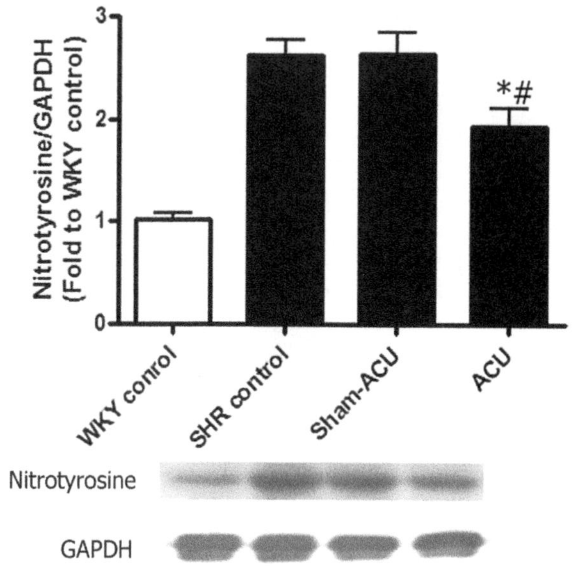

Fig. 5 Effects of acupuncture on nitrotyrosine expression in the aorta tissues. Both the SHR control and sham-acupuncture group showed an increased nitrotyrosine expression when compared with the WKY control. Acupuncture treatment markedly inhibited nitrotyrosine expression. Data were expressed as means ± SD (*$P = 0.0012$ for the SHR vs. the WKY control and #$P = 0.0073$ for ACU vs. sham-acupuncture)

been no review on the effect of acupuncture on hypertension in animals, but many studies have reported significant attenuation of blood pressure [8, 44–48].

NO regulates blood vessel remodeling and angiogenesis [49, 50], and is also a major endothelium-derived relaxing factor for maintenance of normal vascular tone. In endothelial dysfunction, the bioavailability of NO is compromised, resulting in increased vascular tone and resistance [51]. Oxidative stress is closely associated with the bioavailability of NO, as free radicals may directly scavenge NO and uncouple its production enzyme, NOS [52]. Angiotensin II is a potent vasoconstrictor, and also acts as an important hormone to promote fluid retention; it may also increase oxidative stress by upregulating the activity of NADPH oxidase to produce more ROS [53, 54].

Endothelial dysfunction of the vessels is well known in 18-week-old SHRs [55] According to acupuncture theory, there are many acupoints that can be used to treat hypertension; among them, ST36 and LR3 are two of the most commonly used acupoints that have demonstrated effectiveness in lowering blood pressure in animal studies [8, 44–46]. In electroacupuncture, different frequency and wave types have previously been shown to have positive results in managing hypertension [8, 47, 48].

The regimen in our study of using a continuous wave at 2 Hz is a commonly used setting in acupuncture treatment of both humans and animals. In humans, blinding of treatment allocation can be achieved by using different devices such as Streitberger's needle or Park's sham device [56, 57]. However, in animal studies, the blinding of the animals from knowing whether they are receiving real acupuncture is less critical. The pricking of non meridian non-acupoint locations by a blunt-ended needle can avoid the non-specific effect of needle penetration as well as the possible acupressure effect. In our study, there

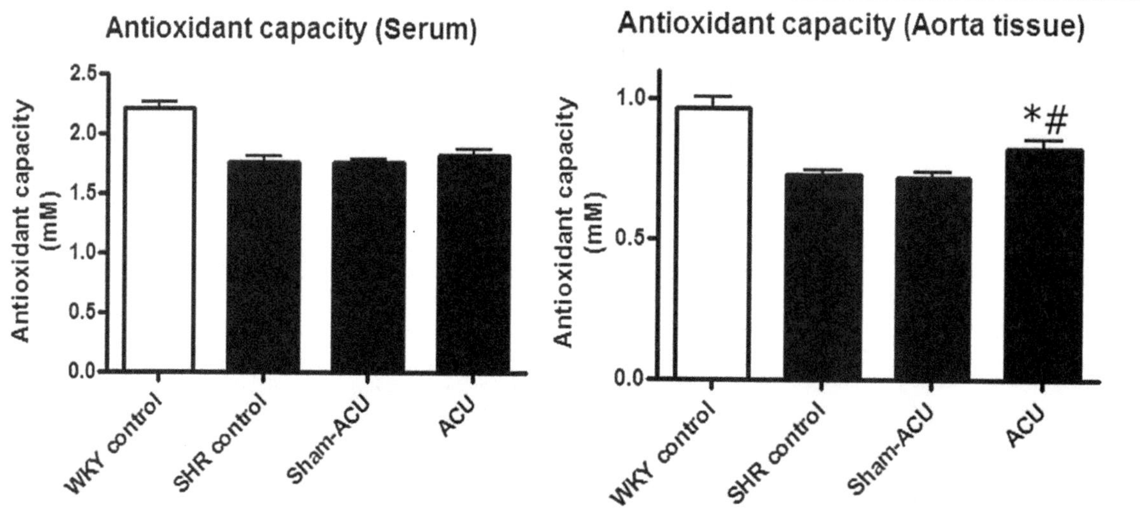

Fig. 6 Antioxidant capacity of different groups. Antioxidant capacity was lower in both serum and aorta tissues of the SHR control when compared with SHR. The aorta tissue in the acupuncture group showed an improved antioxidant capacity. Data were expressed as means ± SD (In aorta tissue, *$P = 0.0039$ for ACU vs. SHR control and #$P = 0.0032$ for ACU vs. sham-acupuncture)

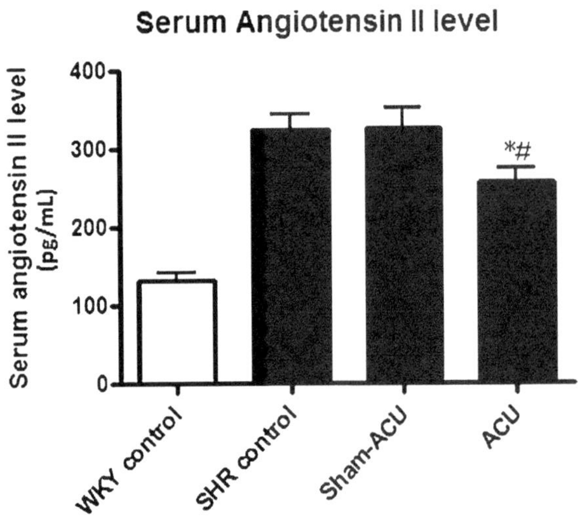

Fig. 7 Effects of acupuncture treatment on serum angiotensin II level as measured by EIA kit. The level was significantly attenuated after acupuncture treatment when compared with the SHR control and sham-acupuncture group. Data were expressed as means ± SD ($^*P = 0.023$ for ACU vs. SHR control and $^\#P = 0.035$ for ACU vs. sham-acupuncture)

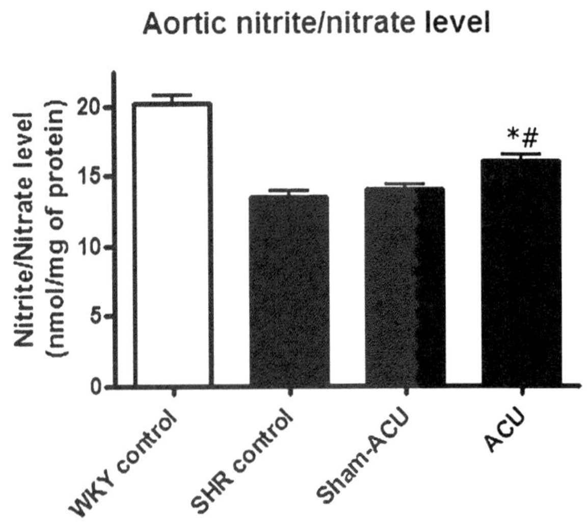

Fig. 9 Effects of acupuncture treatment on aortic nitrite/nitrate level. The level was significantly accentuated after acupuncture treatment when compared with the SHR control and sham-acupuncture group. Data were expressed as means ± SD ($^*P = 0.0018$ for ACU vs. SHR control and $^\#P = 0.0061$ for ACU vs. sham-acupuncture)

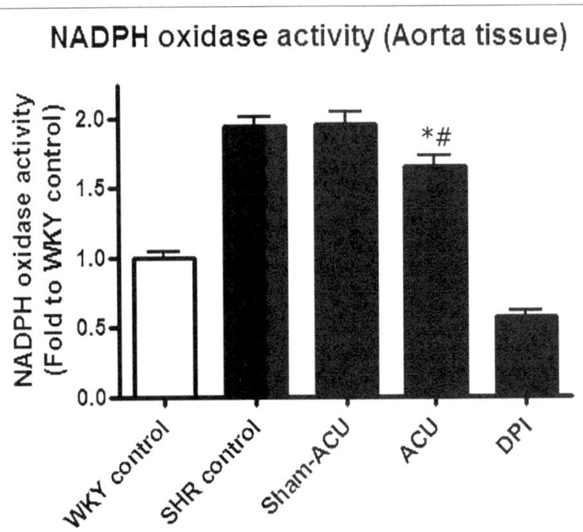

Fig. 8 Effects of acupuncture on NADPH oxidase activity. NADPH oxidase activity in the WKY control was lower than that in the SHR control. Sham-acupuncture did not affect the enzyme activity but real acupuncture significantly reduced it. DPI, a NADPH oxidase inhibitor that can markedly inhibit the enzyme's activity. Data were expressed as means ± SD ($^*P = 0.022$ for ACU vs. SHR control and $^\#P = 0.028$ for ACU vs. sham-acupuncture)

was no significant difference between the SHR control group that received no treatment and the SHR sham-acupuncture group.

In functional studies of aortas and carotid arteries, acupuncture improved the EDR but not the endothelial-independent relaxation in SHRs. eNOS is the NO-producing enzyme, and phosphorylated eNOS is the activated form of eNOS. The levels of both eNOS and phosphorylated eNOS were decreased in the SHRs compared with the WKYs. These assays could indirectly reflect the amount of NO in the vessel, and both expressions were promoted by real acupuncture treatment but not by sham-acupuncture. NO has a short half-life of only 4 s, and it undergoes a series of reactions in vivo to yield nitrite (NO_2_) and nitrate (NO_3_) [58]. As the proportion of these compounds varies in different physiological environments, we measured the total nitrite/nitrate level to assess the NO bioavailability. Aortic nitrite/nitrate levels of the SHRs were lower than that in the WKYs, and acupuncture treatment was able to further promote this reduction. Combined with the findings from the functional studies and protein blotting, it seemed that the beneficial effect of acupuncture on vascular reactivity was elicited via the enhancement of NO bioavailability.

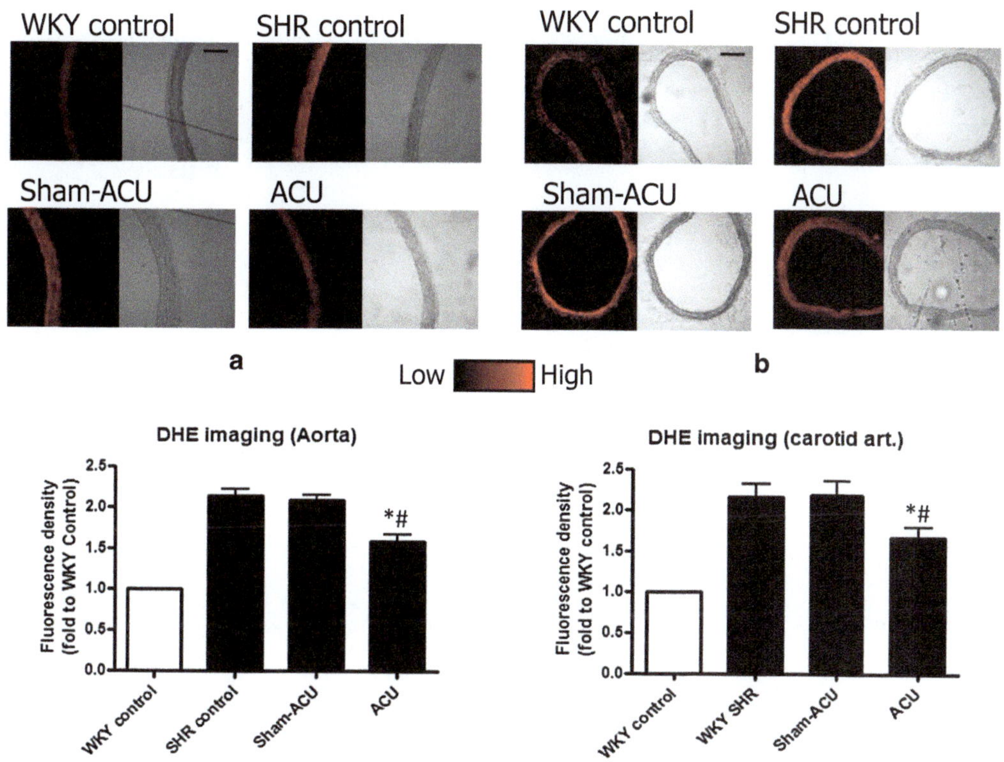

Fig. 10 ROS accumulation in aorta (**a**) and carotid arteries (**b**) as detected by DHE staining. Acupuncture treatment significantly lowered the ROS level in aorta. (*$P = 0.0017$ for ACU vs. SHR control and $^{\#}P = 0.0016$ for ACU vs. sham-acupuncture.) and carotid arteries (*$P = 0.039$ for ACU vs. SHR control and $^{\#}P = 0.0449$ for ACU vs. sham-acupuncture.). Data were expressed as means ± SD

The antioxidant capacity in aortic tissue homogenate was lower in the SHRs than in the WKYs, and acupuncture was able to promote this antioxidant capacity. The DHE signal from the aorta and carotid artery was stronger in the SHRs than the WKYs, suggesting that a higher level of superoxide anion was present in the vessels of the SHRs. The samples from the SHR acupuncture group revealed that the superoxide level was attenuated by acupuncture treatment. As it is difficult to measure peroxynitrite (i.e., oxidize lipoproteins or nitrate tyrosine residue of proteins), nitrotyrosine was used to indirectly indicate the peroxynitrite level and oxidative stress level. Western blotting revealed a significantly higher expression of the nitrotyrosine level in the SHRs than in the WKYs. Real acupuncture, not sham-acupuncture, attenuated nitrotyrosine expression.

Immunohistochemistry assays were performed to localize the nitrotyrosine. An increased intensity was clearly shown along the endothelial lining in the SHRs compared with the WKYs; a lighter staining was observed in the aortic ring from the SHR acupuncture group. Our results indicate that acupuncture was able to increase NO bioavailability in the rat vessels, and relieve oxidative stress.

The NADPH oxidase activity was higher in the SHRs than the WKYs, and acupuncture could attenuate this. As angiotensin II is one of the factors that stimulates NADPH oxidase, we also measured the serum angiotensin II and found that acupuncture treatment was able to reduce its level. It may be concluded that acupuncture treatment reduces blood pressure through altering a number of pathophysiological actions including fluid retention, vascular tone, NADPH oxidase activity, and oxidative stress.

Apart from the endothelium, acupuncture did not exert a significant effect on vascular structure in terms of wall thickness, number of lamellar layers, and the collagen and elastin content. Previous studies reported a reduced vessel wall thickness after acupuncture [59, 60], but we failed to reproduce similar results. This discrepancy could be owing to the difference in the experimental settings, including animal model, acupuncture technique, and treatment duration. Lastly, we investigated the anti-inflammatory effect of acupuncture, and observed a higher level of both ICAM-1 and VCAM-1 expression in the aortic tissues of the SHRs compared with that of the WKYs; however, both sham-acupuncture and acupuncture exerted no effect on ICAM-1 and

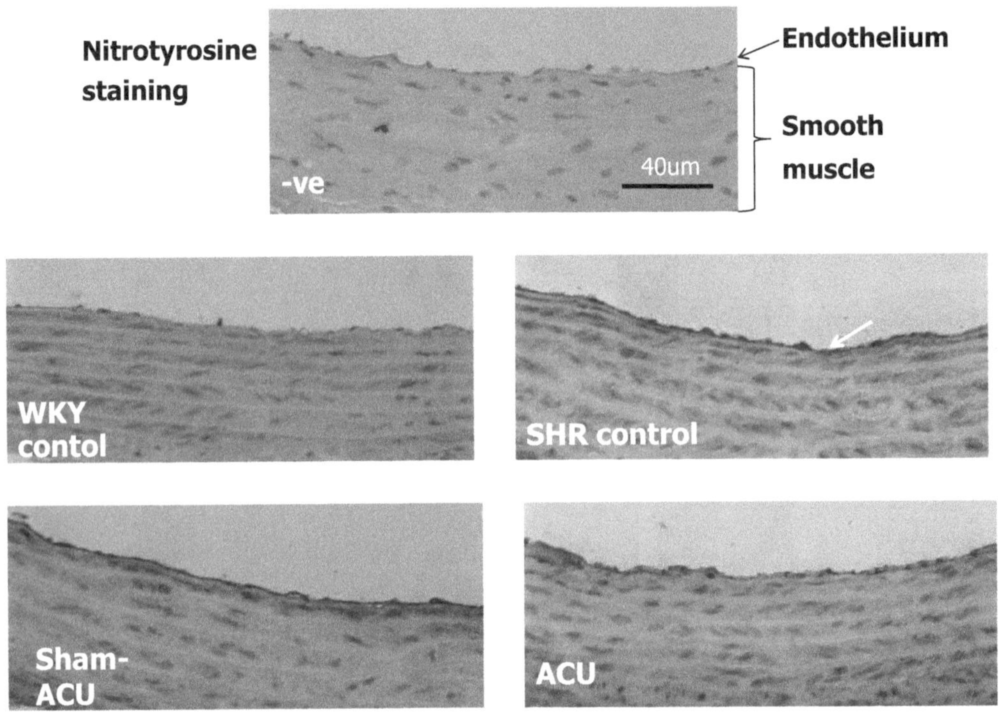

Fig. 11 Immunohistochemistry localization of nitrotyrosine expression in aorta tissues. The negative (−ve) control used no nitrotyrosine antibodies and yielded no staining of tissues. In the SHR control and sham-acupuncture group, a clear staining of the intima was observed. In the acupuncture group, the intensity of the staining was attenuated, while the WKY control group only showed a weak signal

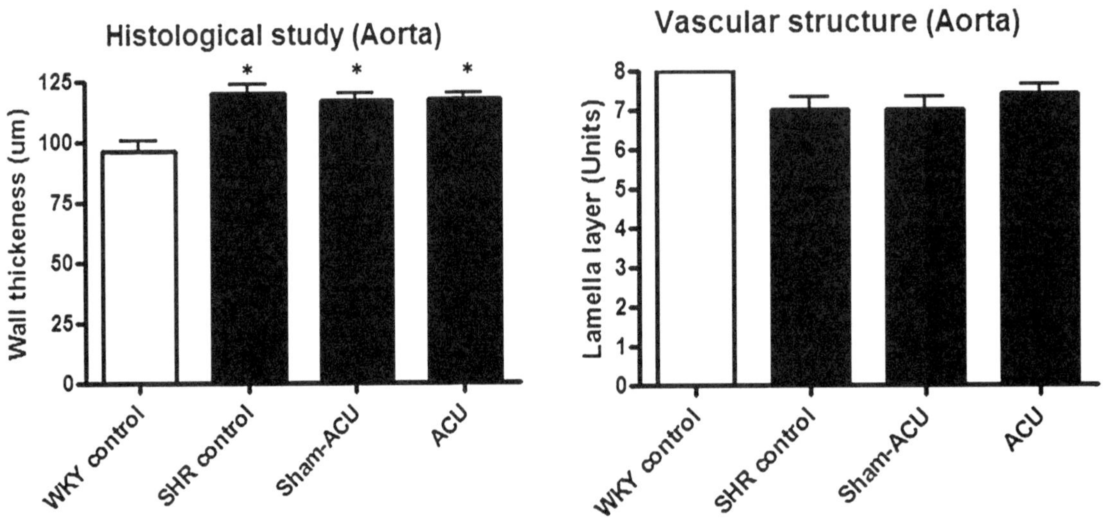

Fig. 12 Effects of acupuncture on vascular structure. The WKY rats had a thinner aorta wall than the SHRs and acupuncture exerted no effect on wall thickness. The number of lamella layer showed no difference among all four groups (*$P < 0.001$ for the WKY control vs. all other groups)

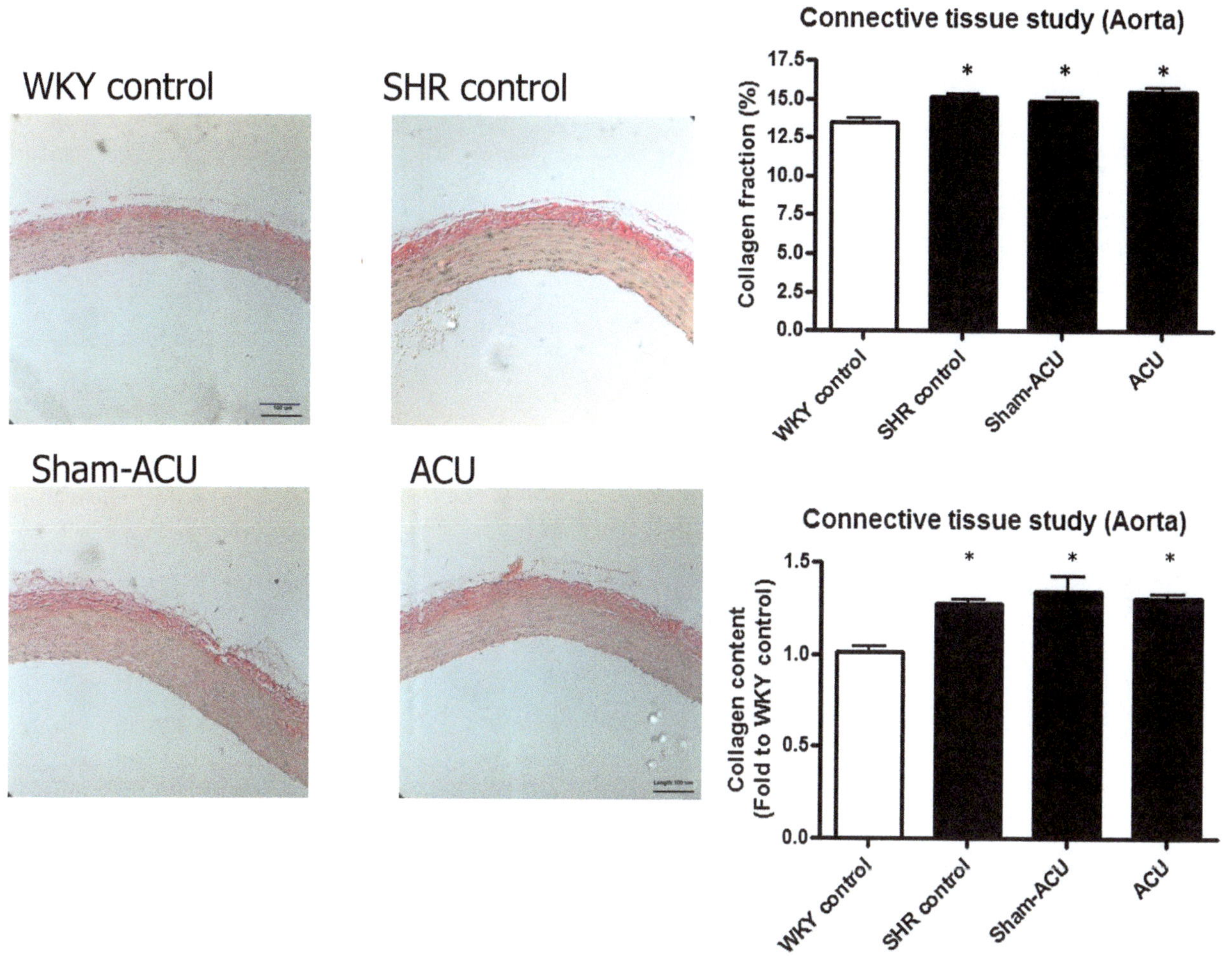

Fig. 13 Effects of acupuncture on collagen content. Collagen was stained in red by the Van Gieson's stain. The total collagen and fraction of collagen were lower in the WKY control. Acupuncture did not affect the collagen content. Data were expressed as means ± SD (*$P < 0.001$ for the WKY control vs. all other groups)

VCAM-1 expression. This is the first animal study to demonstrate the close relationship between the reduction in oxidative stress and improvement in bioavailability of nitric oxide by acupuncture. However, the effects of acupuncture on other pathways related to the reactive oxygen species production clearly warrants further investigation. Moreover, the remodulation of other endothelial derived vasoactive substances and their

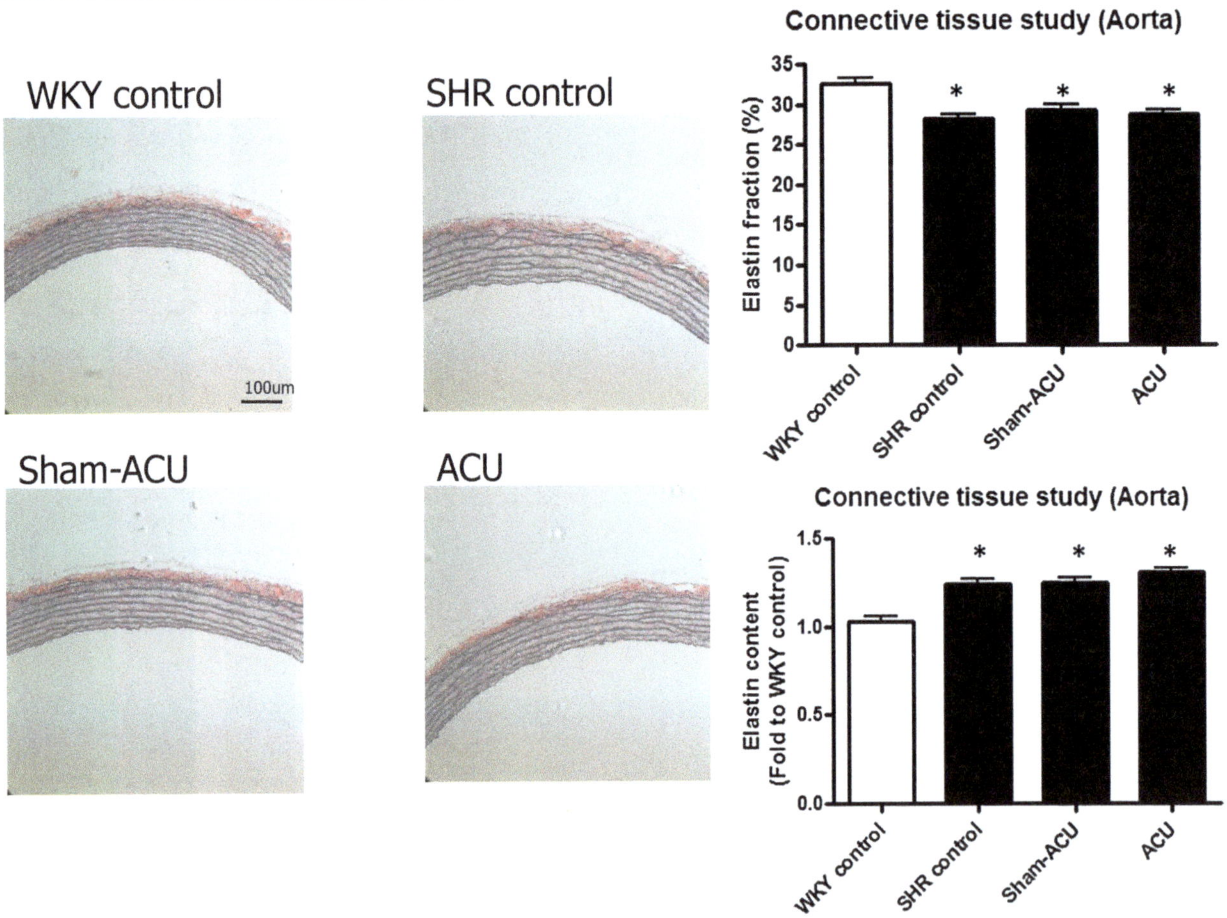

Fig. 14 Effects of acupuncture on elastin content. Elastin was stained blue by Orcein stain. The WKY control had a higher proportion of elastin but the total content of it in their aorta tissues was lower. Acupuncture and sham-acupuncture showed no effect on both elastin fraction and elastin content. Data were expressed as means ± SD (*$P < 0.001$ for the WKY control vs. all other groups)

mechanisms remained largely obscure. Our experimental findings provides a backbone for the investigation of the therapeutic action of acupuncture on hypertensive animals and the findings can help put the clinical use of acupuncture for hypertension on a solid scientific footing.

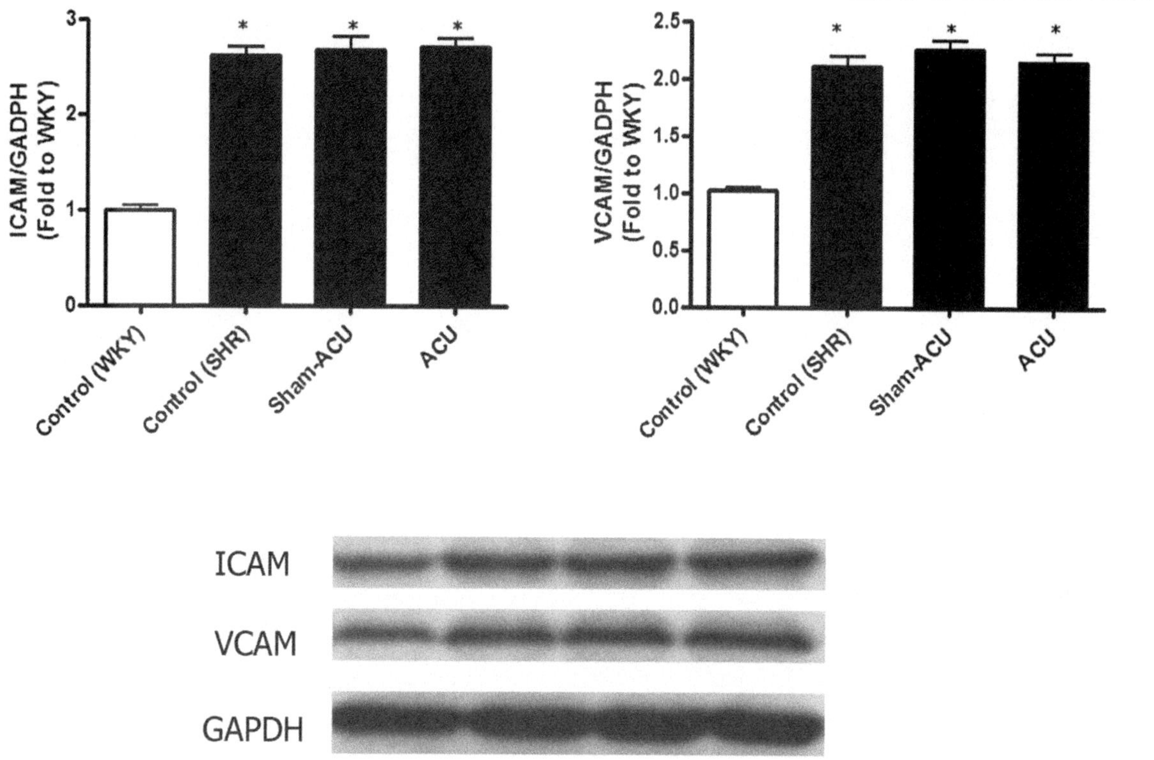

Fig. 15 Effects of acupuncture on the ICAM and VCAM expressions in the aorta tissues. The expressions of these inflammatory markers were lower in the WKY control. Sham-acupuncture and real acupuncture did not affect the level of ICAM and VCAM expression. Data were expressed as means ± SD (*$P < 0.001$ for the WKY control vs. all other groups)

Conclusion

Acupuncture treatment attenuated blood pressure in the SHRs. The effects of acupuncture in treating hypertension in the SHRs was associated with improvements in oxidative stress, NO bioavailability, and endothelial function.

Abbreviations

Ach: acetylcholine; DHE: dihydroethidium; DPI: diphenyliodonium; EDCF: endothelial-derived constricting factor; EDHF: endothelial-derived hyperpolarizing factor; EDR: endothelial-dependent relaxation; EDRF: endothelial-derived relaxing factor; Emax: maximal relaxation response; eNOS: endothelial nitric oxide synthase; ICAM: intracellular adhesion molecule; L-NAME: NG-nitro-L-arginine methyl ester; NADPH: nicotinamide adenine dinucleotide phosphate; NO: nitricoxide; NOS: nitric oxide synthase; PBS: phosphate buffered saline; pD2: dilator concentrations to cause 50 % relaxation; peNOS: phosphorylated endothelial nitric oxide synthase; Phe: phenylephrine; ROS: reactive oxygen species; SDS-PAGE: sodium dodecyl sulfate polyacrylamide gel by electrophoresis; SHR: spontaneously hypertensive rat; SNP: sodium nitroprusside; SOD: superoxide dismutase; VCAM: vascular adhesion molecule; WKY: Wistar Kyoto rat.

Authors' contributions

ZXL conceived the study and designed the experiments. SBL conducted all parts of the experiments. SBL and CWL performed the blood pressure measurement. SBL and HZ conducted the statistical analysis. SBL wrote the manuscript and ZXL revised the manuscript. All authors read and approved the final manuscript.

Author details

[1] School of Chinese Medicine, Faculty of Medicine, The Chinese University of Hong Kong, Shatin, N.T., Hong Kong, People's Republic of China. [2] School of Biomedical Sciences, Faculty of Medicine, The Chinese University of Hong Kong, Shatin, N.T., Hong Kong, People's Republic of China.

Acknowledgements

This study was supported by a Direct Grant of The Chinese University of Hong Kong (Project No. 2030434). We are grateful to Professor Huang Yu of the School of Biomedical Sciences, Faculty of Medicine, The Chinese University of Hong Kong for his guidance in the experimental design and execution, and his critical comments on the manuscript.

Competing interests

The authors declare that they have no competing interests.

References

1. World Health Organization. Acupuncture: review and analysis of reports on controlled clinical trials. 2002. http://whqlibdoc.who.int/publications/2002/9241545437.pdf.
2. Jin C, Zhang T, Ji L, Tian Y. Survey of studies on mechanisms of acupuncture and moxibustion in decreasing blood pressure. Zhongguo Zhen Jiu. 2007;6:467–70.
3. Chui S, Tang C. Progress in the research of neuroendocrine immunological mechanism of acupuncture in regulating blood pressure and protecting target organs in hypertension. Zhen Ci Yan Jiu. 2008;3:208–12.
4. Zhang Y, Liu Y, Pan K. Comparison of effects of different acupuncture-moxibustion methods on renin-angiotensin-aldosterone system (RAAS) and atrial natriuretic polypeptide (ANF). Hu BeiZhong Yi Xue Yuen XueBao. 2001;2:20–1.
5. Wu X, Li M, Lu Y. Influence of acupuncture treatment on nitrogen monoxide, endothelin, angiotensin and rennin levels of acute hypertension rats. Zhongguozhong Yi Yao Xin Xi ZaZhi. 2008;7:41–2.
6. Lee H, Kim J. Effect of acupuncture on blood pressure and plasma renin activity in two-kidney one-clip Goldblatt hypertensive rats. Am J Chin Med. 1994;4:215–9.
7. Chen YL, Mo SL. Effects of electroacupuncture 'Zusanli' on serum nitric oxide (NO) and plasma endothelin (ET) of spontaneously hypertensive rats. Chin J Nat Med. 2002;4:14–6.
8. Kim DD, Pica AM, Duran RG, Duran WN. Acupuncture reduces experimental renovascular hypertension through mechanisms involving nitric oxide synthases. Microcirculation. 2006;13:577–85.
9. Hwang HS, Kim YS, Ryu YH, Lee JE, Lee YS, Yang EJ, Lee MS, Choi SM. Electroacupuncture delays hypertension development through enhancing NO/NOS activity in spontaneously hypertensive rats. Evid Based Complement Altern Med. 2011;2011:130529. doi:10.1093/ecam/nen064.
10. Wang H, Pan Y, Xue B, Wang X, Zhao F, Jia J, Liang X, Wang X. The antioxidative effect of electro-acupuncture in a mouse model of Parkinson's disease. PLoS One. 2011;5:e19790.
11. Li ZR, Shen MH, Peng YJ. Progress in researches on the effect of acupuncture in antagonizing oxygen stress. Chin J Integr Med. 2005;2:156–60.
12. Yu YP, Ju WP, Li ZG, Wang DZ, Wang YC, Xie AM. Acupuncture inhibits oxidative stress and rotational behavior in 6-hydroxydopamine lesioned rat. Brain Res. 2010;1336:58–65.
13. Siua FK, Lob SC, Leung MC. Electro-acupuncture potentiates the disulphide-reducing activities of thioredoxin system by increasing thioredoxin expression in ischemia-reperfused rat brains. Life Sci. 2005;77:386–99.
14. Liu C, Yu J, Zhang X, Fub W, Wang T, Hana J. Acupuncture prevents cognitive deficits and oxidative stress in cerebral multi-infarction rats. Neurosci Lett. 2006;393:45–50.
15. Vanhoutte PM, Shimokawa H, Tang EH, Feletou M. Endothelial dysfunction and vascular disease. Acta Physiol. 2009;196(2):193–222.
16. Feletou M, Vanhoutte PM. Endothelial dysfunction: a multifaceted disorder (The Wiggers Award Lecture). Am J Physiol Heart Circ Physiol. 2006;3:985–1002.
17. Lockette W, Otsuka Y, Carretero O. The loss of endothelium-dependent vascular relaxation in hypertension. Hypertension. 1986;8:6166.
18. Higashi Y, Sasaki S, Nakagawa K, Matsuura H, Oshima T, Chayama K. Endothelial function and oxidative stress in renovascular hypertension. N Engl J Med. 2002;346:1954–62.
19. Redon J, Oliva MR, Tormos C, Giner V, Chaves J, Iradi A, Saez GT. Antioxidant activities and oxidative stress byproducts in human hypertension. Hypertension. 2003;41:1096–101.
20. Tanito M, Nakamura H, Kwon YW, Teratani A, Masutani H, Shioji K, Kishimoto C, Ohira A, Horie R, Yodoi J. Enhanced oxidative stress and impaired thioredoxin expression in spontaneously hypertensive rats. Antioxid Redox Signal. 2004;6:89–97.
21. de Champlain J, Wu R, Girouard H, Karas M, El Midaoui A, Laplante MA, Wu L. Oxidative stress in hypertension. Clin Exp Hypertens. 2004;7–8:593–601.
22. Wong WT, Wong SL, Tian XY, Huang Y. Endothelial dysfunction: the common consequence in diabetes and hypertension. J Cardiovasc Pharmacol. 2010;4:300–7.
23. Oettl K, Greilberger J, Zangger K, Haslinger E, Reibnegger G, Jürgens G. Radical-scavenging and iron-chelating properties of carvedilol, an antihypertensive drug with antioxidative activity. Biochem Pharmacol. 2011;2:241–8.
24. Van de Water A, Janssens W, van Neuten J, Xhonneux R, de Cree J. Pharmacological and haemodynamic profile of nebivolol, a chemically novel, potent and selective β1-adrenergic antagonist. J Cardiovasc Pharmacol. 1988;11:552–63.
25. Cockcroft JR, Chowienczyk PJ, Brett SE, Chen CP, Dupont AG, Van Nueten L, Wooding SJ, Ritter JM. Nebivololvasodilates human forearm vasculature: evidence for an L-arginine/NO-dependent mechanism. J Pharmacol Exp Ther. 1995;274:1067–71.
26. Feng M, Whitesall S, Zhang Y, Beibel M, D'Alecy L, DiPetrillo K. Validation of volume-pressure recording tail-cuff blood pressure measurements. Am J Hypertens. 2008;12:1288–91.
27. Chen ZY, Zhang ZS, Ho WK, Zhu M, Kwan KY, Huang Y. Endothelium-dependent relaxation induced by hawthorn extract in the rat isolated mesenteric artery. Life Sci. 1998;22:1983–91.
28. Yang Q, Xue H, Wong WT, Tian X, Huang Y, Tsui SK, Ng PK, Wohlfart P, Li H, Xia N, Tobias S, Underwood MJ, He G. AVE3085, an enhancer of endothelial nitric oxide synthase, restores endothelial function and reduces blood pressure in spontaneously hypertensive rats. Br J Pharmacol. 2011;163:1078–85.
29. Miller NJ, Rice-Evans C, Davies MJ. A new method for measuring antioxidant activity. Biochem Soc Trans. 1993;21:95.
30. Li JJ, Lu J, Kaur C, Sivakumar V, Wu CY, Ling EA. Expression of angiotensin II and its receptors in the normal and hypoxic amoeboid microglial cells and murine BV-2 cells. Neuroscience. 2009;4:1488–99.
31. Wind S, Beuerlein K, Eucker T, Müller H, Scheurer P, Armitage ME, Ho H, Schmidt HH, Wingler K. Comparative pharmacology of chemically distinct NADPH oxidase inhibitors. Br J Pharmacol. 2010;4:885–98.
32. Schiessl B, Strasburger C, Bidlingmaier M, Mylonas I, Jeschke U, Kainer F, Friese K. Plasma- and urine concentrations of nitrite/nitrate and cyclic Guanosinemonophosphate in intrauterine growth restricted and preeclamptic pregnancies. Arch Gynecol Obstet. 2006;3:150–4.
33. Cheang WS, Wong WT, Tian XY, Yang Q, Lee HK, He GW, Yao X, Huang Y. Endothelial nitric oxide synthase enhancer reduces oxidative stress and restores endothelial function in db/db mice. Cardiovasc Res. 2011;2:267–75.
34. Suzuki A, Fujii A, Jokura H, Tokimitsu I, Hase T, Saito I. Hydroxyhydroquinone interferes with the chlorogenic acid-induced restoration of endothelial function in spontaneously hypertensive rats. Am J Hypertens. 2008;1:23–7.
35. Luna LG (ed). Manual of histologic staining methods of the AFIP. 3rd ed. New York: McGraw-Hill; 1968. p. 76.
36. Sheehan D, Hrapchk B. Theory and practice of histotechnology. 2nd ed. Columbus: Battelle Press; 1987. p. 247–8.
37. Xu Q, Chakravorty A, Bathgate RA, Dart AM, Du XJ. Relaxin therapy reverses large artery remodeling and improves arterial compliance in senescent spontaneously hypertensive rats. Hypertension. 2010;5:1260–6.
38. Collins R, Peto R, MacMahon S, Hebert P, Fiebach NH, Eberlein KA, Godwin J, Qizilbash N, Taylor JO, Hennekens CH. Blood pressure, stroke, and coronary heart disease. Part 2, short-term reductions in blood pressure: overview of randomised drug trials in their epidemiological context. Lancet. 1990;8693:827–38.
39. Li DZ, Zhou Y, Yang YN, Ma YT, Li XM, Yu J, Zhao Y, Zhai H, Lao L. Acupuncture for essential hypertension: a meta-analysis of randomized sham-controlled clinical trials. Evid Based Complement Altern Med. 2014;2014:279478.
40. Wang J, Xiong X, Liu W. Acupuncture for hypertension. Int J Cardiol. 2013;169(5):317–26.
41. Liu AJ, Li JH, Li HQ, Fu DL, Lu L, Bian ZX, Zheng GQ. Electroacupuncture for acute ischemic stroke. Am J Chin Med. 2015;30:1550088.
42. Wu X, Chung VCh, Hui EP, Ziea ET, Ng BF, Ho RS, Tsoi KK, Wong SY, Wu JC. Effectiveness of acupuncture and related therapies for palliative care of cancer: overview of systematic reviews. Sci Rep. 2015;26(5):16776.
43. Lee A, Chan SK, Fan LT. Stimulation of the wrist acupuncture point PC6 for preventing postoperative nausea and vomiting. Cochrane Database Syst Rev. 2015;2(11):CD003281. doi:10.1002/14651858.CD003281.pub4.
44. Yang H, Zhong X, Liu T, Kuai L, Gao M. Impact of different emulated acupuncture-needle manipulations on blood pressure and myocardial angiotensin II content in spontaneous hypertension rats. Zhen Ci Yan Jiu. 2008;33(3):186–91.

45. Liu X, Han T, Lu Y, Wang X, Guo W, Jing H. Effects on serum ACE plasma Ang II content in hypertension model rats through the compatibility of chinese medicine and acupuncture. Liao Ningzhong Yi Yao Da Xue Xue Bao. 2011;13(8):106–7.
46. Zhi J, Wang Z, Wang L. Effect of different quantity of acupuncture stimulation on cervical sympathetic discharge in rats with stress-induced hypertension. Zhong Yi Zazhi. 2009;50(9):811–3.
47. Liu W, Jin L, Han D, Ren X, Zhu J, Zhang L. Effect of electroacupuncture of different acupoints on blood pressure, plasma angiotensin II, aldosterone and atrial natriuretic peptide in spontaneous hypertension rats. Zhen Ci Yan Jiu. 2009;34(6):393–7.
48. Huang D, Zhang L. Effect of needling quchi and zusanli on blood pressure and insulin resistance in spontaneously hypertensive rats. Liao Ningzhong Yi Yao Da Xue Xue Bao. 2009;12(4):224–5.
49. Rudic RD, Shesely EG, Maeda N, Smithies O, Segal SS, Sessa WC. Direct evidence for the importance of endothelium-derived nitric oxide in vascular remodeling. J Clin Invest. 1998;101:731–6.
50. Ziche M, Morbidelli L, Masini E, Amerini S, Granger HJ, Maggi CA, Geppetti P, Ledda F. Nitric oxide mediates angiogenesis in vivo and endothelial cell growth and migration in vitro promoted by substance P. J Clin Invest. 1994;94:2036–44.
51. Aicher A, Heeschen C, Mildner-Rihm C, Urbich C, Ihling C, Willerson JT, Kereiakes DJ. Endothelial dysfunction. Circulation. 2003;108:2060–1.
52. Cai H, Harrison DG. Endothelial dysfunction in cardiovascular diseases—the role of oxidant stress. Circ Res. 2000;87:840–4.
53. Jung O, Schreiber JG, Geiger H, Pedrazzini T, Busse R, Brandes RP. gp91phox-containing NADPH oxidase mediates endothelial dysfunction in renovascular hypertension. Circulation. 2004;109:1795–801.
54. Griendling KK, Sorescu D, Ushio-Fukai M. NAD(P)H oxidase: role in cardiovascular biology and disease. Circ Res. 2000;86:494–501.
55. Sunano S, Osugi S, Shimamura K. Blood pressure and impairment of endothelium-dependent relaxation in spontaneously hypertensive rats. Experientia. 1989;45(8):705–8.
56. Streitberger K, Kleinhenz J. Introducing a placebo needle into acupuncture research. Lancet. 1998;352(9125):364–5.
57. Park J, White A, Stevinson C, Ernst E, James M. Validating a new non-penetrating sham acupuncture device: two randomised controlled trials. Acupunct Med. 2002;20(4):168–74.
58. Vallance P, Chan N. Endothelial function and nitric oxide: clinical relevance. Heart. 2001;85(3):342–50.
59. Su Z, Xiao D, Ju J, Yu A, Yin Z. The effect of electro-acupuncture on blood pressure and aortic vascular remodeling in spontaneously hypertensive rats. Shang Hai Zhen Jiu Za Zhi. 2003;5:20–2.
60. Qian C. The effect of acupuncture on blood pressure and vascular remodeling in 2 kidney 1 clip hypertensive rat. PhD thesis. HuBeiDaXue (Zhen Jiu Tui Na). 2008.

3

Discriminating from species of *Curcumae* Radix (*Yujin*) by a UHPLC/Q-TOFMS-based metabolomics approach

Fang Liu[1], Xu Bai[2], Feng-Qing Yang[3], Xiao-Jing Zhang[1], Yuanjia Hu[1], Peng Li[1] and Jian-Bo Wan[1*]

Abstract

Background: Chinese medicinal herbs may use more than one species of *Curcumae* Radix (*Yujin*) is the tuberous roots of *Curcumae wenyujin*, *C. kwangsiensis*, *C. phaeocaulis* and *C. longa*. This study aimed to characterize the chemical profiles of these different species of *Curcumae* Radix, and develop a method for rapid discrimination of these species by ultra-high performance liquid chromatography–quadrupole time-of-flight mass spectrometry (UHPLC/Q-TOFMS) combined with multivariate statistical analysis.

Methods: The metabolomes of 33 different batches of *Curcumae* Radix derived from four *Curcumae* species were profiled by UHPLC/Q-TOFMS. The resulting sample codes, t_R–m/z pairs and ion intensities were processed by unsupervised principal component analysis (PCA) and supervised orthogonal partial least squared discriminant analysis (OPLS-DA) to characterize the chemical composition of *Curcumae* Radix across the four different species.

Results: Obvious differences were observed in the chemical compositions of the *Curcumae* Radix samples derived from the four different species according to PCA and OPLS-DA. These results suggested that curcumin, curcumenone, curcumenol and zederone could be used as unique chemical markers for *C. longa*, *C. wenyujin*, *C. phaeocaulis* and *C. kwangsiensis*, respectively.

Conclusions: This study developed a UHPLC/Q-TOFMS method coupled with multivariate statistical analysis to discriminate between *Curcumae* Radix samples from four different *Curcumae* species, i.e., *C. longa*, *C. wenyujin*, *C. phaeocaulis* and *C. kwangsiensis*. Notably, this new approach resulted in the identification of curcumin (**a**), curcumenone (**b**), curcumenol (**c**) and zederone (**d**) as unique chemical markers for the identification.

Background

Herbal medicines may be derived from specific single or multiple plant species, and a herb may have more than one species. The increasing popularity of multi-species herbs in medical use was documented in the 2010 edition of the Chinese Pharmacopoeia [1]. For instance, snow lotus herb (*Xuelian*), which has several health benefits, is mainly derived from *Saussurea involucrata*, *S. laniceps* and *S. medusa* [2], whereas dragon's blood (*Xuejie*), which is used as a medicine, is mainly derived from *Daemonorops draco* and *Dracaena cochinchinensis* [3]. Previous studies have demonstrated that the chemical characteristics of multi-species herbal medicines can vary considerably depending on the originating species [3–5]. However, despite these findings, multi-species herbs are still treated as though they are identical. Each species of herb has its own genetic traits and geographical origins, which manifest themselves as unique primary and secondary metabolite patterns (i.e., metabolome) [3–5].

Curcumae Radix (*Yujin*) is used to treat a variety of different diseases, including hepatitis, cholecystitis, hyperlipidaemia and cancer [6–8]. Essential oils and curcuminoids are considered to be the major bioactive ingredients of *Curcumae* Radix [9], which is obtained

*Correspondence: jbwan@umac.mo
[1] State Key Laboratory of Quality Research in Chinese Medicine, Institute of Chinese Medical Sciences, University of Macau, Macao, People's Republic of China
Full list of author information is available at the end of the article

from the dried tuberous roots of four *Curcuma* species, including *Curcuma wenyujin*, *C. kwangsiensis*, *C. phaeocaulis* and *C. longa*, as officially described in the Chinese Pharmacopoeia [10]. Given that *Curcumae* Radix can be derived from four different *Curcuma* species, there could be considerable differences in the chemical composition among these four species, which differences could affect their therapeutic effects. It is difficult to distinguish between the origins of raw materials in the clinic because of their similar morphological features. To date, several analytical methods, including liquid chromatography-mass spectrometry (LC-MS) [11, 12], high-performance liquid chromatography (HPLC) [13, 14], gas chromatography-mass spectrometry (GC-MS) [15, 16], thin layer chromatography (TLC) [17] and capillary electrophoresis (CE) [18], have been developed to discriminate among the different species of *Curcuma* based on the chemical diversity of several main ingredients, particularly sesquiterpenoids. Metabolomics could be readily used to qualitatively and quantitatively monitor variations in the chemical component profiles of herbal medicines derived from different species [19, 20], as well as those subjected to different processing methods [21, 22], cultivation times [23] and geographical locations [24]. Recently, a GC-MS-based metabolomics method was successfully established to discriminate three *Curcuma* species according to the global chemical difference in *Curcuma* rhizomes (*Ezhu*) [19]. However, several sesquiterpene compounds from *Curcuma* plants are heat-sensitive. For example, furanodiene degrades to curzerene via a [3,3]-sigmatropic reaction (Cope rearrangement) upon heat treatment [25], whereas (4*S*, 5*S*)-germacrone-4,5-epoxide cyclizes through a transannular reaction on exposure to heat [26].

The aim of this study was to characterize the chemical profiles of *Curcumae* Radix and develop a rapid method to discriminate between the species by ultra-high-performance liquid chromatography–quadrupole time-of-flight mass spectrometry (UHPLC/Q-TOFMS) combined with multivariate statistical analysis.

Methods

Plant materials and chemical reagents

Thirty-three batches of authentic *Curcumae* Radix were collected from Good Agricultural Practice (GAP)-certified farms located in Rui'an and Leqing, Zhejiang province (C. *wenyujin*, n = 12), Yulin and Linshan, Guangxi province (*C. kwangsiensis*, n = 6), and Leshan and Chengdu, Sichuan province (*C. phaeocaulis*, n = 6; and *C. longa*, n = 9) provinces of China during December, 2012. The botanical origins of the different *Curcumae* Radix samples were morphologically recorded [27] based on the whole plants when they were collected from the GAP-certified farms, and were subsequently identified by Dr. Fengqing Yang at the School of Chemistry and Chemical Engineering, Chongqing University, China. Voucher specimens of the *Curcumae* Radix samples from four different *Curcuma* species (No. YJ01-YJ33) were deposited at the Institute of Chinese Medical Sciences, University of Macau, Macao, China. HPLC-grade methanol and acetonitrile were purchased from Baker Company (Sanford, ME, USA). LC-MS grade formic acid was purchased from Sigma-Aldrich (St. Louis, MO, USA). All of the other chemicals and solvents used in the current study were purchased as the analytical grades and used as received. Ultra-high-purity water was prepared using a Millipore SAS-67120 (Molsheim, Cedex, France).

Pressurized liquid extractions (PLE)

Samples for analysis were prepared using a Dionex ASE 200 system (Dionex, Sunnyvale, CA, USA) according to a previously described procedure [28]. Briefly, *Curcumae* Radix was dried at 60 °C for 2 h, and then pulverized in a mill to give a homogeneous powder (60 mesh). A portion of the dried powder (approximately 0.5 g) was mixed with diatomaceous earth (0.5 g), and the resulting mixture was transferred to an 11-mL stainless steel extraction cell. The sample was subsequently extracted under the following conditions: solvent, methanol; pressure, 6.89×10^3 kPa (1000 psi); temperature, 100 °C; static extraction time, 5 min; number of extractions, 1; and flush volume, 40 %. After the extraction, the PLE extract was transferred to a 25-mL volumetric flask, which was made up to its volume with methanol. An aliquot of the extract was centrifuged (Heraeus Multifuge; Thermo Fisher Scientific, USA) at 11,200×*g* for 5 min, and the supernatant was filtered through a 0.22-μm polytetrafluoroethylene filter (Whatman, NJ, USA) prior to being injected into the UHPLC/Q-TOFMS system.

LC-MS analysis

UHPLC analysis was performed by an ACQUITY UHPLC system (Waters, Milford, MA, USA) equipped with a binary solvent delivery manager, auto-sampler and high temperature (HT) column oven. The UHPLC system was also equipped with an ACQUITY HSS T3 C_{18} column (100 × 2.1 mm i.d., 1.8 μm; waters) for the chromatographic separation of the sample mixture. The column was eluted with a binary gradient elution system consisting of (solvent A) acetonitrile and (solvent B) 0.1 % aqueous formic acid solution (containing 1 % acetonitrile). Chromatographic separation was achieved under the following elution conditions: isocratic 1 % solvent A (0–0.5 min); linear gradient from 1 % to 99 % solvent A (0.5–5 min); isocratic 99 % solvent A (5.0–6.0 min); and linear gradient from 99 % to 1 % solvent A (6.0–8.0 min). The flow rate and column temperature were set at

0.45 mL/min and 45 °C, respectively. An aliquot (5 μL) of each sample was injected into the column.

The UHPLC system was connected to a Xevo G2 quadrupole time-of-flight (Q-TOF) mass spectrometer (waters) with an electrospray ionization (ESI) source. Samples of the eluent from the UHPLC system were analyzed on this system under the following conditions: ionization mode, positive; source temperature, 120 °C; capillary voltage, 3000 V; sampling cone voltage, 30 V; extraction cone voltage, 4 V; cone gas flow, 20 L/h; desolvation gas flow, 800 L/h; and desolvation temperature, 450 °C. Mass data were collected in the range of *m/z* 50–1200 Da in the centroided mode. A lock-mass calibrant of leucine-enkephalin was continuously introduced to the mass spectrometer at a concentration of 200 ng/mL via a lock-spray interface at a flow-rate of 50 μL/min. This process generated a reference ion in the positive ionization mode (i.e., $[M+H]^+ = 556.2771$), which ensures a high level of accuracy during the MS analysis.

Method validation

A pooled sample of *Curcumae* Radix extracts was prepared by mixing 200 μL of each batch of *Curcumae* Radix extract in a single sample vial. The resulting mixture was used to provide a representative quality control (QC) sample containing all of the analytes at an average concentration. The QC sample was analyzed six times at the beginning of each run to ensure that the system was properly equilibrated. The QC sample was also analyzed after every three tested samples to further monitor the stability of the analytical process based on three representative ions in the chromatogram (i.e., t_R 2.50 min, *m/z* 312.1601; t_R 4.16 min, *m/z* 219.1744; and t_R 4.80 min, *m/z* 231.1385), which were selected for the validation of the method in the positive ionization mode. The relative standard deviations (RSDs) of peak intensity, retention time and molecular weight for the selected ions in the pooled QC samples were calculated (RSD = SD/mean)] to evaluate the reproducibility and stability of the method.

Data processing and pattern recognition

The raw UHPLC/Q-TOFMS data were imported to the Progenesis QI software (Waters) for peak detection and alignment using the following parameters: mass tolerance within 5 ppm; retention time tolerance within 0.3 min; and relative mass error of theoretical fragmentation within 5 ppm. All data were normalized to the summed total ion intensity per chromatogram and three-dimensional data matrices were generated consisting of variable ID numbers (retention time-*m/z* value), sample codes and normalized peak areas. These matrices were then entered into the SIMCA-P 13.0 software (Umetrics AB, Sweden) for multivariate statistical analysis, including unsupervised principal component analysis (PCA). The resulting PCA model was evaluated and interpreted in terms of the R^2X (cum) and Q^2 (cum) values in its score plot. The R^2X value represents the explanatory capacity of the variables, whereas Q^2 provides an indication of the predictive capability of the model. The R^2X and Q^2 values were both found to be close to 1.0, indicating the good fitness of this method. Various chemical components were extracted from the loading plot of the PCA and a scatter plot (*S*-plot) of OPLS-DA as being responsible for the difference between the *Curcuma* species. Furthermore, ions with high variable importance on projection (VIP) values from the *S*-plots were considered to be potential chemical biomarkers, and subsequently subjected to further structural identification. A one-way ANOVA was also employed to test the significance of any differences observed between these markers among the four different species of *Curcuma* Radix. Differences with $P \leq 0.05$ were considered statistically significant.

Results and discussion

Method development and validation

It can be difficult to distinguish between the different types of compound found in the different species of *Curcumae* Radix (e.g., the essential oils and curcuminoids) using the short analytic times associated with UHPLC. With this in mind, we conducted a small pilot study to optimize the chromatographic conditions used for the UHPLC analysis, including the column type and mobile phase, to achieve the highest possible resolution with the fastest separation time. Three ACQUITY UHPLC columns were evaluated in the current study, including BEH C18 (100 × 2.1 mm i.d., 1.7 μm), BEH HILIC (50 × 2.1 mm i.d., 1.7 μm) and HSS T3 C18 (100 × 2.1 mm i.d., 1.8 μm) columns. Among these columns, the ACQUITY HSS T3 C18 column was found to be the most suitable for the analysis of *Curcumae* Radix because it afforded good peak capacity and the best resolution of the major components. A variety of different mobile phases were evaluated for the elution of the column, including acetonitrile–water and methanol–water systems. These mobile phase systems were also evaluated in the presence of various modifiers, and the results were compared to determine which system gave the best resolution. The results of this screening process revealed that a combination of acetonitrile (organic mobile phase) and 0.1 % aqueous formic acid (containing 1 % acetonitrile; aqueous mobile phase) was optimal for the simultaneous separation of the major components in *Curcumae* Radix, as well as being compatible with the MS analysis (i.e., no ionization suppression from the formic acid). The addition of 1 % acetonitrile to the aqueous phase was found to be beneficial for stabilizing the baseline drift of instrument analysis. Ionization was conducted in the positive and negative ionizations modes to achieve maximum signal strength. It is noteworthy that higher levels of sensitivity and more structural information were obtained in the positive ionization mode. Having established the optimized chromatographic and MS conditions, we were able to successfully separate and identify the major chemical components in *Curcumae* Radix within 8 min (Fig. 1). To validate this method, we measured the RSD of the peak areas and *m/z* values (i.e., $[M+H]^+$) of selected peaks (i.e., t_R 2.50 min, *m/z* 312.1601; t_R 4.16 min, *m/z* 219.1744; and t_R 4.80 min, *m/z* 231.1385), which were less than 5.46 and 0.01 %, respectively. Furthermore, the retention times of these peaks remained exactly the same over 16 runs, which indicated that the established method was robust with good reproducibility and stability for the analysis of experimental *Curcumae* Radix samples.

Multivariate statistical analysis

Visual inspection of the results revealed that there were obvious differences among the four different *Curcumae* species. However, it was not possible to differentiate between these four groups based on visual inspection alone. We therefore applied multivariate statistical analysis to intuitively refine intergroup differences in the chemical components and identify potential chemical biomarkers that could be used to distinguish between the different groups.

The resulting dataset contained sample code, t_R–*m/z* pair and ion intensity data, which were processed by PCA to clearly discriminate between the four species based on the differences in their chemical compositions. It is noteworthy that a total of 2599 t_R–*m/z* pairs were extracted in the positive ion mode for all of the samples analyzed in this study. After Pareto scaling and mean-centering, these data were displayed as scores and loadings in a coordinate system of principal components resulting from data dimensionality reduction. The three-component PCA score plots (Fig. 2A) showed that the 33 *Curcumae* Radix samples could be clearly classified into four different clusters depending on their species, according to the differences in their global chemical profiles. Although the clusters corresponding to *C. wenyujin* and *C. phaeocaulis* were close to each other, they could be clearly distinguished by PC2. Sevenfold cross validation was used to assess the validity of the model. Notably, all of the observations in the current study fell within the Hotelling T2 (0.95) ellipse. Furthermore, the R^2X (cum) and Q^2 (cum) values were determined to be 0.788 and 0.724, respectively, thereby highlighting the quality of our PCA model.

Characterization of chemical markers

A loading plot of the PCA was constructed to identify the characteristic chemical components responsible for the differences observed across the four species of *Curcumae* Radix. Each point in the loading plot represents a chemical component (variable), and the further each variable moves away from the main cluster of the analyzed chemicals, the more likely it is that this component makes a significant contribution to the intergroup differences. As shown in Fig. 2B, the loading plot of the PCA revealed that seven ions, including **a** (t_R 4.11 min, *m/z* 369.1331), **b** (t_R 4.24 min, *m/z* 235.1696), **c** (t_R 4.31 min, *m/z* 235.1697), **d** (t_R 4.35 min, *m/z* 247.1333), **e** (t_R 4.48 min, *m/z* 237.1851), **f** (t_R 4.58 min, *m/z* 237.1853) and **g** (t_R 4.80 min, *m/z* 231.1383), were making significant contributions to the clusters. These ions were therefore considered to be potential chemical markers for discriminating between the four species of *Curcumae* Radix.

An *S*-plot of the OPLS-DA was constructed based on a comparison of the results for one species with those of the remaining three species to confirm the identities of the chemical markers obtained from the loading plots, as well as identifying the characteristic chemicals of each species (Fig. 3). In this particular case, we used *C. wenyujin* as an example. The 12 *Curcumae* Radix samples derived from *C. wenyujin* were defined as groups, whilst the remaining 21 samples were marked as the second group, which formed the basis of our OPLS-DA model. The resulting *S*-plot is shown in Fig. 3A, where each point indicates an ion t_R-*m/z* pair. The X and Y axes represent the contribution and confidence of the variables, respectively. In this plot, the further a specific data point is from zero on the X or the Y axis, the greater its contribution or confidence level for the two-group separation, respectively. The points at either ends of the S-shaped curve therefore represent potential chemical markers with the highest confidence [29]. In terms of the results, three ions (**b**, **e** and **f**) were found at the end of the S-shaped curve in the bottom-left corner of the graph, which were considered to be characteristic components that made the greatest contribution to distinguish *C. wenyujin* from the other three species. These components were responsible for the variance observed in the *Curcumae* Radix derived from *C. wenyujin* versus the other three species. Two ions (**d**, **g**) were found to be characteristic markers capable of discriminating *C. kwangsiensis* from the other species of *Curcumae* Radix (Fig. 3B). In contrast, ions **a** and **c** were found to be specific markers for the *Curcumae* Radix derived from *C. longa* and *C. kwangsiensis*, respectively.

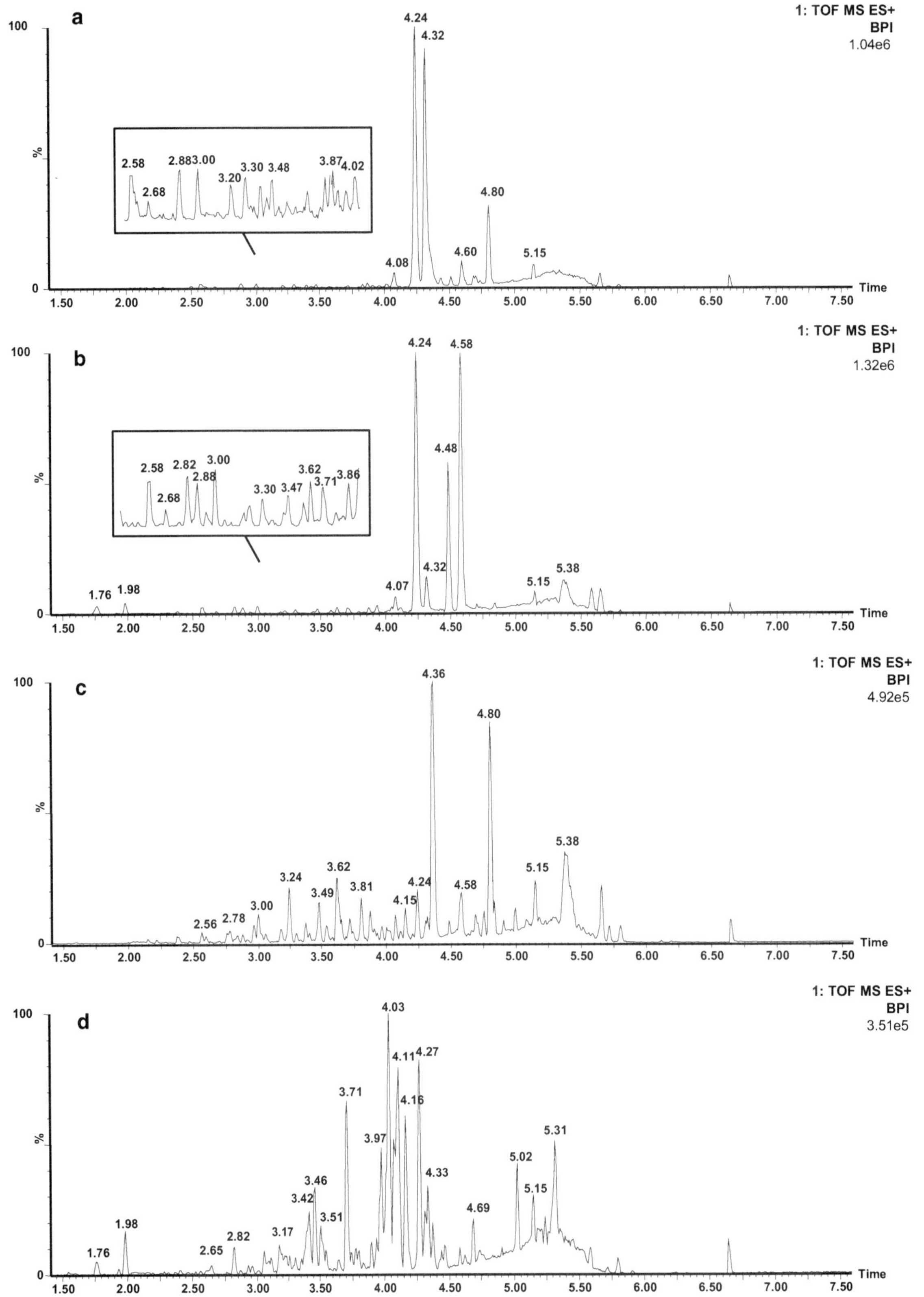

Fig. 1 Base peak intensity (BPI) chromatograms of representative *Curcuma* Radix derived from (**a**) *C. phaeocaulis*, (**b**) *C. wenyujin*, (**c**) *C. kwangsiensis* and (**d**) *C. longa*, analyzed by UPLC/Q-TOFMS in positive ion mode

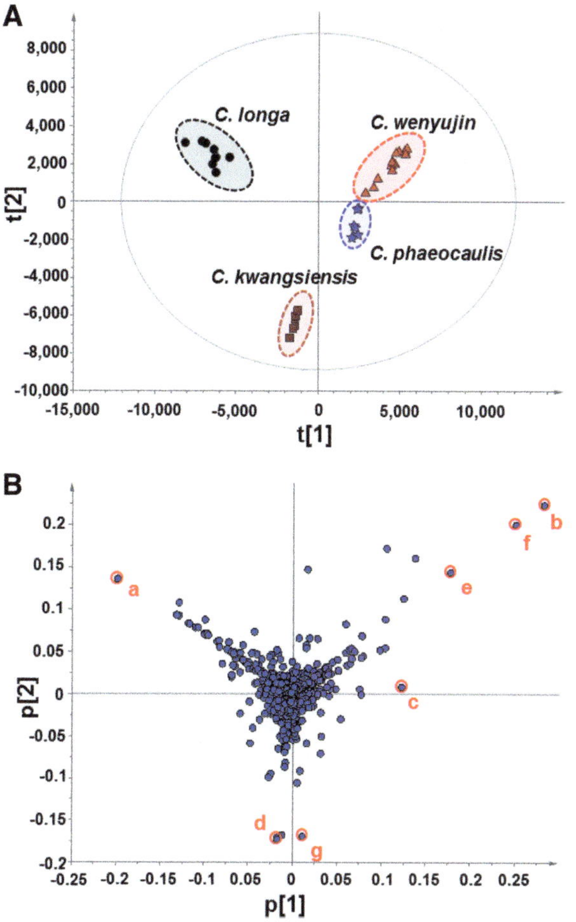

Fig. 2 PCA/Scores plot (**A**) and loading plot (**B**) based on the global chemical profiling of *Curcuma* Radix derived from four species. The components contributing most to the differences were marked as a *red circle*, including (*a*) t_R 4.11 min, *m/z* 369.1331; (*b*) t_R 4.24 min, *m/z* 235.1696; (*c*) t_R 4.31 min, *m/z* 235.1697; (*d*) t_R 4.35 min, *m/z* 247.1333; (*e*) t_R 4.48 min, *m/z* 237.1851; (*f*) t_R 4.58 min, *m/z* 237.1853; and (*g*) t_R 4.80 min, *m/z* 231.1383

Identification of chemical markers and their changes in relative intensities

The Mass Fragment™ software package from waters was used to elucidate the structures of the different chemical components based on their fragmentation patterns. In this study, we were only able to identify seven chemical markers using the loading plots and the *S*-plots (Fig. 4). Furthermore, these structures were only tentatively assigned based on a comparison of their molecular weights, molecular formulas and MS/MS fragment ions with those published in the literature for compounds [11–16] isolated from *Curcuma* species, as well a comparison with known biochemical databases, such as MassBank (http://www.massbank.jp/), PubChem (http://pubchem.ncbi.nlm.nih.gov/), and Respect for Phytochemicals (http://spectra.psc.riken.jp/). The error in the measured molecular mass values was determined to be less than 2 mDa based on a comparison with the theoretical exact mass values provided by the authoritative websites mentioned above. Representative MS/MS spectra, chemical structures and proposed fragmentation pathway details for chemical marker **a** are shown in Fig. 4a. MS analysis of chemical marker **a** revealed an *m/z* value of 369.1340 for $[M+H]^+$ in the positive ionization mode, which suggested that its empirical molecular formula was $C_{21}H_{20}O_6$. The differences in the mass of this parent ion and its two main fragment ions (*m/z* 285.1137 and 177.0555) were 80 and 192 Da, which corresponded to loss of the $C_4H_4O_2$ and $C_{11}H_{12}O_3$, respectively. These data suggested that this compound was curcumin, based on a comparison with data from the literature [12, 30]. The most plausible interpretation of this fragmentation pathway is shown in Fig. 4c, which is primarily based on the information from the MS/MS data. Similarly, MS analysis of ion **b** (Fig. 4b) revealed an *m/z* value of 235.1699 for $[M+H]^+$ in the positive ionization mode, which suggested that this compound had an empirical molecular formula of $C_{15}H_{23}O_2$. Ion **b** gave a fragment ion with an *m/z* value of 177.1273, representing a 58 Da mass difference compared with the parent ion, indicating the loss of C_3H_6O. This daughter ion (*m/z* 177.1273) afforded four main fragment ions with *m/z* values of 161.0966, 133.1015, 105.0861 and 91.0548, representing mass differences of 16, 44, 58 and 62 Da, respectively, which corresponded to the successive loss of the CH_4, CO, CH_2 and CH_2. These data therefore suggested that this compound was curcumenone and its fragmentation pathway is shown in Fig. 4d [31]. Based on the method described above, markers **c**–**g** were tentatively identified as curcumenol, zederone, neocurdione, curdione and curzerenone, respectively, by comparing their data with those from the literature [31, 32], as well as searching the biochemical databases listed above (Additional file 1).

The signal intensities of the chemical markers identified in the different *Curcumae* Radix samples were analyzed by one-way ANOVA to provide a further comparison of the differences among the four species of *Curcumae* Radix. The marker levels varied considerably among the different *Curcumae* Radix samples (Fig. 5). The intensity of curcumin was found to be significantly ($P < 0.0001$) higher in *C. longa* than it was in any of the other three species (Fig. 5a), suggesting that curcumin could be used as a specific marker for distinguishing *C. longa* from the other three species. *C. wenyujin* showed significantly higher levels ($P < 0.001$) of curcumenone (**b**), neocurdione (**e**) and curdione (**f**) than the other three species of *Curcumae* Radix (Fig. 5b, e and f). Furthermore, *C. wenyujin* contained higher levels of neocurdione and

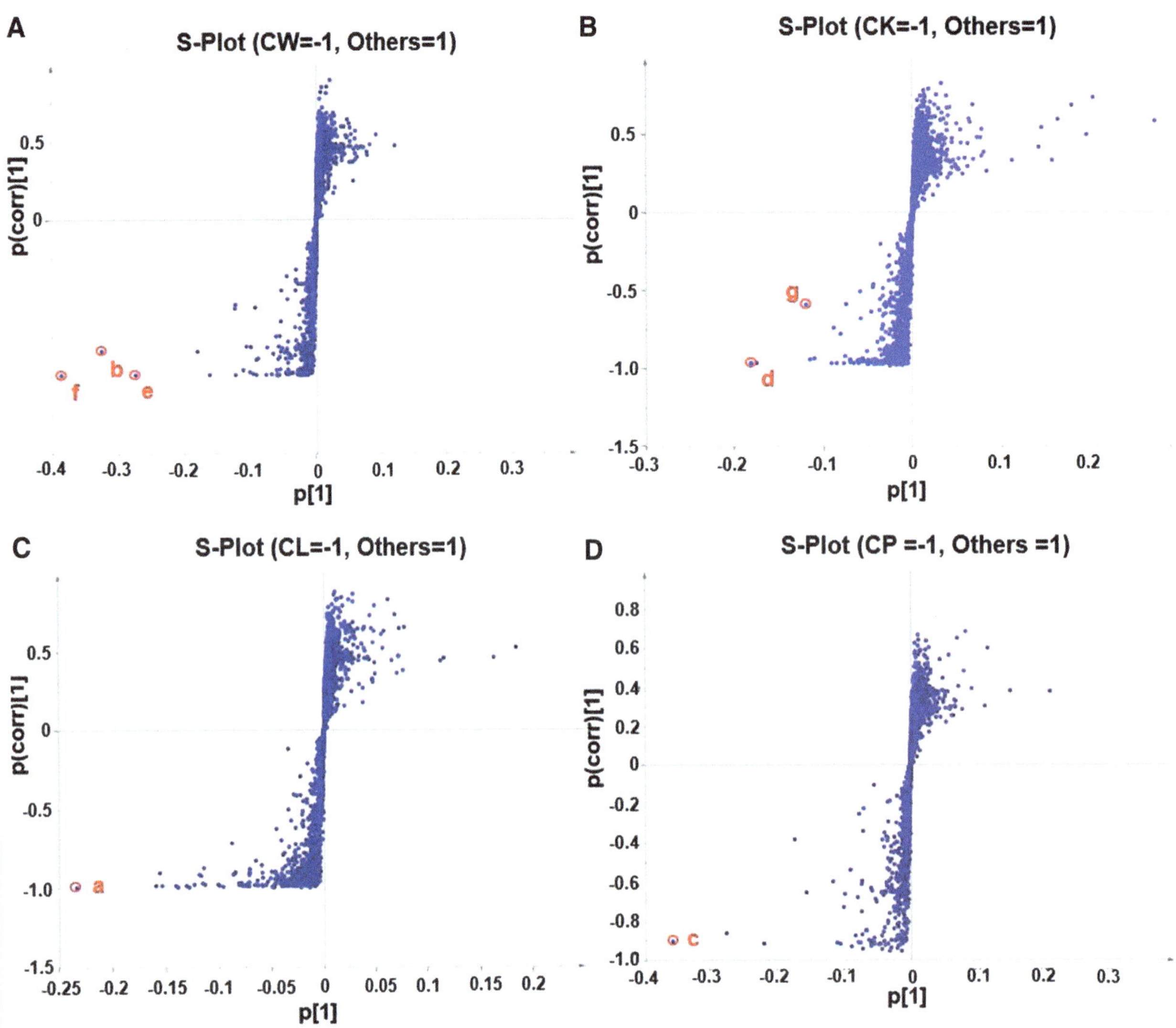

Fig. 3 S-plots of OPLS-DA constructed based on a comparison of *C. phaeocaulis* (CP, **A**), *C. wenyujin* (CW, **B**), *C. kwangsiensis* (CK, **C**) and *C. longa* (CL, **D**) with the remaining three species. (**a**) t_R 4.11 min, *m/z* 369.1331; (**b**) t_R 4.24 min, *m/z* 235.1696; (**c**) t_R 4.31 min, *m/z* 235.1697; (**d**) t_R 4.35 min, *m/z* 247.1333; (**e**) t_R 4.48 min, *m/z* 237.1851; (**f**) t_R 4.58 min, *m/z* 237.1853; and (**g**) t_R 4.80 min, *m/z* 231.1383

curdione (35- to 140-times higher) than any of the other three species of *Curcumae* Radix, suggesting that these compounds could be considered as markers for distinguishing *C. wenyujin* from the other three species. Curcuminoids and sesquiterpenoids are considered to be the main bioactive ingredients of *Curcumae* Radix [13, 14]. Curcuminoids, such as curcumin, have been reported to exhibit a wide range of interesting pharmacological activities, including antioxidative, anti-inflammatory, hypocholesterolemic, antihepatotoxic and anticancer effects [4]. Sesquiterpenoids, such as curcumenone, curdione and curzerenone, are the main components of the essential oils derived from *Curcumae* Radix, which have been reported to exhibit antioxidative, anti-tumor and antiviral activities [32].

PCA analysis based on the identified chemical markers

PCA was performed based on the seven chemical markers identified above to assess their ability to actively discriminate between the different species of *Curcumae* Radix. After normalizing the fused data, a 33 (objects) × 7 (variables) dataset was constructed and subjected to PCA. The resulting PCA bi-plot is shown in Fig. 6a, where the observations and variables of the multivariate data are represented in the same plot. These data showed that variables with similar loadings

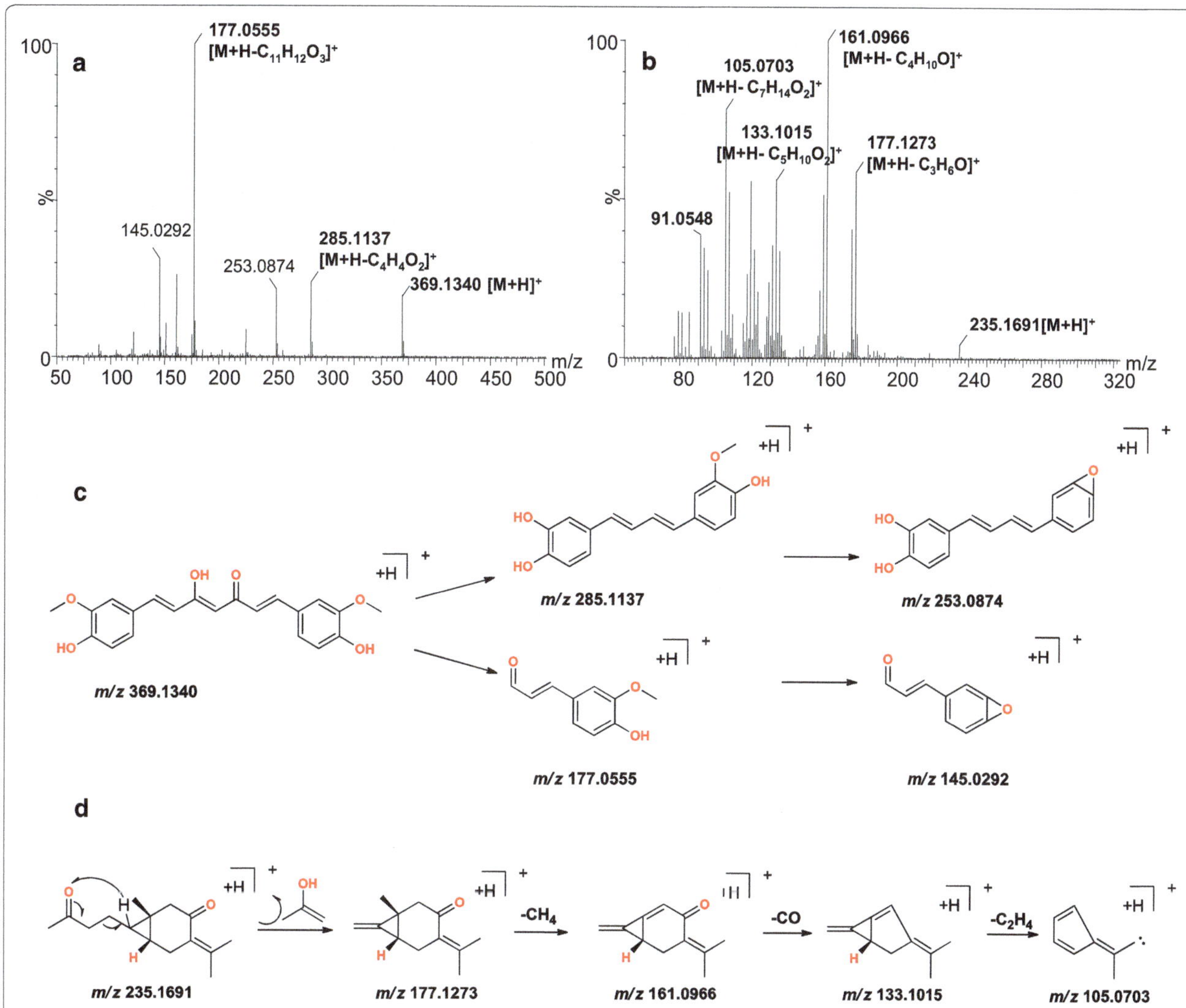

Fig. 4 Mass spectra for the proposed fragmentation pathways of curcumin (**a**, **c**) and curcumenone (**b**, **d**) in the positive ionization mode

appeared to be strongly correlated with the objects. In a similar manner to Fig. 2A, all of the *Curcumae* Radix samples were successfully separated into their correct species based on the differences in these seven chemical markers.

Based on the VIP values obtained from the *S*-plots of the OPLS-DA models (Fig. 3), curcumin (**a**), curcumenone (**b**), curcumenol (**c**) and zederone (**d**) were selected as unique markers for *C. longa*, *C. wenyujin*, *C. phaeocaulis* and *C. kwangsiensis*, respectively. PCA was also conducted based on these four unique markers using a 33 (objects) × 4 (variables) data matrix, and the resulting PCA bi-plot revealed that all of the *Curcumae* Radix samples evaluated in the current study were successfully separated into the correct species based on these four markers. It is noteworthy that the separation observed between *C. kwangsiensis* and *C. longa* (Fig. 6B) was much clearer for the four chemical markers than it was for the PCA bi-plot constructed using the seven chemical markers described above (Fig. 6A). Our data therefore suggest that curcumin (**a**), curcumenone (**b**), curcumenol (**c**) and zederone (**d**) are unique chemical markers for *C. longa*, *C. wenyujin*, *C. phaeocaulis* and *C. kwangsiensis*, respectively, which could be used to discriminate between different *Curcumae* Radix samples in terms of their species of origin.

Conclusions

This study developed a UHPLC/Q-TOFMS method coupled with multivariate statistical analysis to discriminate between *Curcumae* Radix samples from four different *Curcumae* species, i.e., *C. longa*, *C. wenyujin*, *C.*

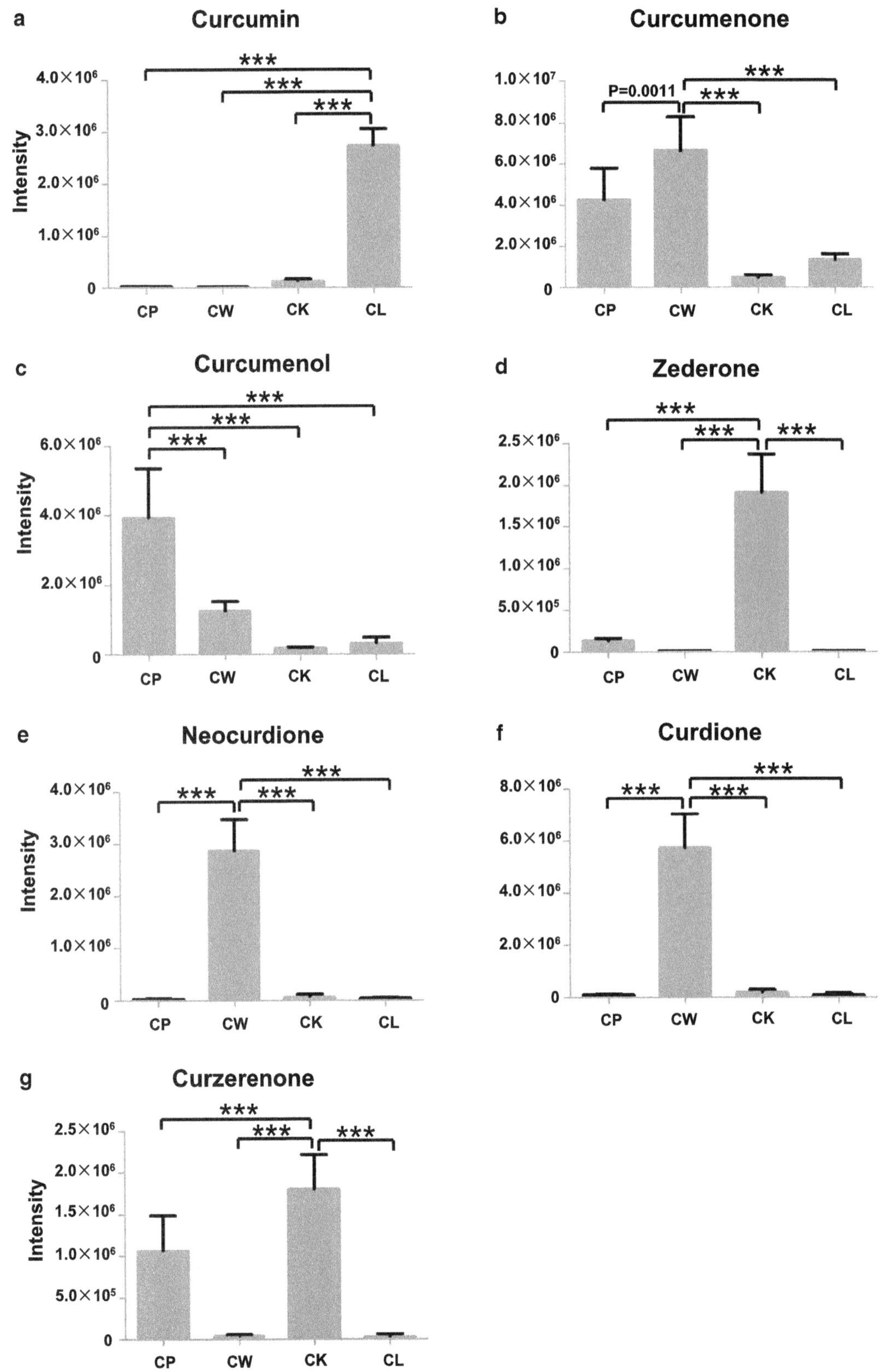

Fig. 5 Relative intensities of the chemical markers in *Curcuma* Radix derived from four species. (**a**) curcumin, (**b**) curcumenone, (**c**) curcumenol, (**d**) zederone, (**e**) neocurdione, (**f**) curdione and (**g**) curzerenone. Data represent the mean values ± SD (n = 3). ** and **** indicate $P < 0.01$ and $P < 0.0001$, respectively

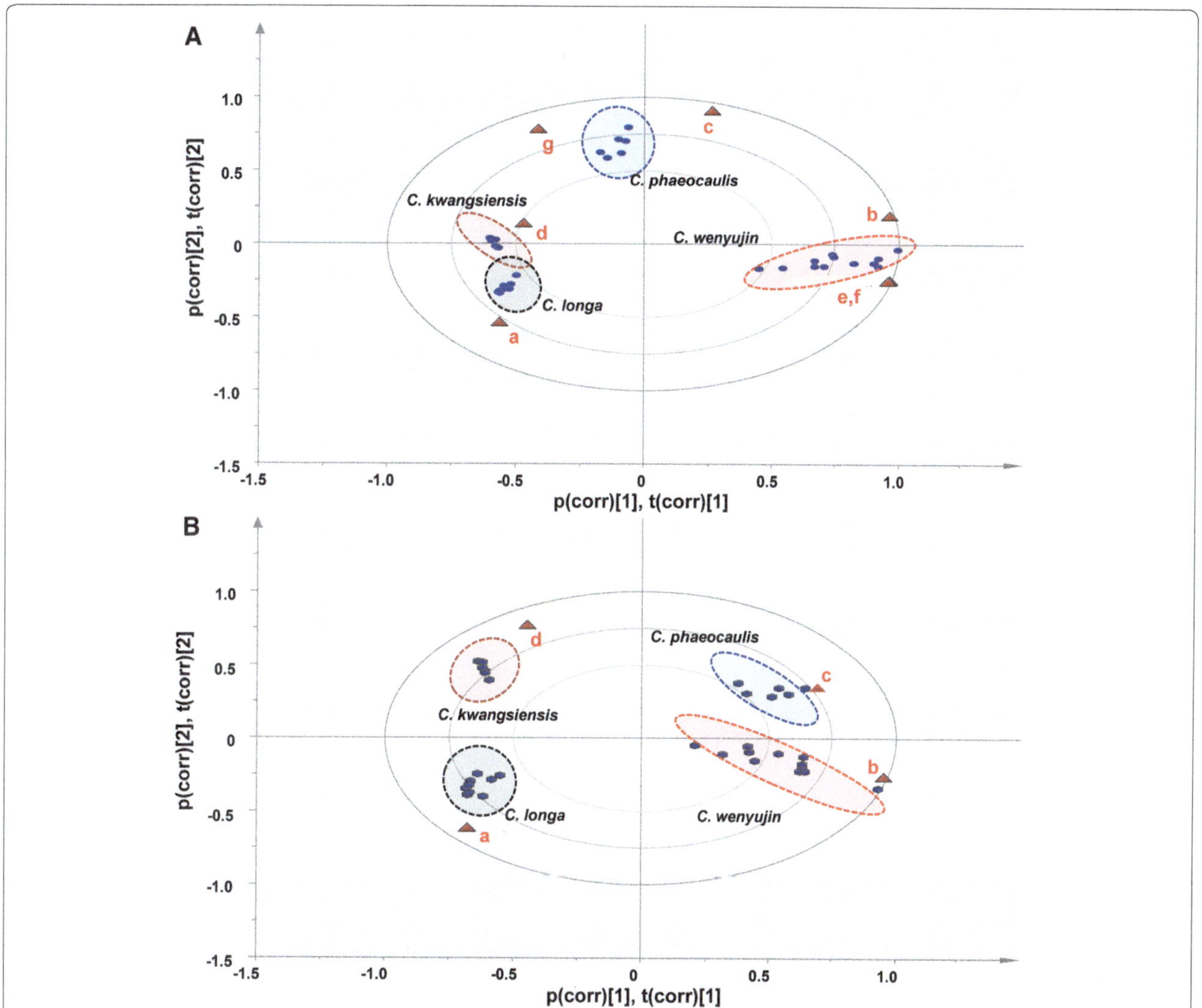

Fig. 6 PCA/bi-plots of the 33 *Curcuma* Radix samples constructed using (**A**) seven chemical markers (**a**–**g**) and (**B**) four unique chemical markers (**a**–**d**). (**a**) curcumin, (**b**) curcumenone, (**c**) curcumenol, (**d**) zederone, (**e**) neocurdione, (**f**) curdione and (**g**) curzerenone

phaeocaulis and *C. kwangsiensis*. This method was used to identify curcumin (**a**), curcumenone (**b**), curcumenol (**c**) and zederone (**d**) as unique chemical markers of four *Yujin*.

Abbreviations
BPI: based peak intensity; CE: capillary electrophoresis; GAP: good agricultural practice; GC-MS: gas chromatography-mass spectrometry; HPLC: high-performance liquid chromatography; TLC: thin layer chromatography; *m/z*: mass-to-charge ratio; OPLS-DA: orthogonal partial least squared discriminant analysis; PCA: principal component analysis; PLE: pressurized liquid extractions; QC: quality control; RSDs: relative standard deviations; RT or t_R: retention time; CMs: chinese medicines; UPLC/Q-TOFMS: ultra-performance liquid chromatography–quadrupole time-of-flight mass spectrometry; VIP: variable importance on projection.

Authors' contributions
JBW conceived and designed the study. XB performed the LC–MS analysis experiment and FL collected the data. FL and JBW wrote the manuscript. FQY, YJH and PL revised the manuscript. All authors read and approved the final manuscript.

Author details
[1] State Key Laboratory of Quality Research in Chinese Medicine, Institute of Chinese Medical Sciences, University of Macau, Macao, People's Republic of China. [2] Waters Technologies (Shanghai) Ltd., Shanghai, People's Republic of China. [3] School of Chemistry and Chemical Engineering, Chongqing University, Chongqing 400030, People's Republic of China.

Acknowledgements
This study was supported by the grants from the Research Committee of the University of Macau (MYRG123-ICMS12 and MYRG111-ICMS13 to JB Wan) and from the Macao Science and Technology Development Fund (010/2013/A1 to JB Wan).

Competing interests

Xu Bai is an employee of the Waters Technologies who is the manufacturer of the UHPLC-Q-TOFMS used in this study. Other authors have no competing interests.

References

1. Chinese Pharmacopoeia commission. Pharmacopoeia of the People's Republic of China. Beijing: China Medical Science Press; 2010.
2. Yi T, Chen HB, Zhao ZZ, Jiang ZH, Cai SQ. Comparative analysis of the major constituents in the traditional Tibetan medicinal plants Saussurea laniceps and S. medusa by LC-DAD-MS. Chromatographia. 2009;70:957–62.
3. Yi T, Chen HB, Zhao ZZ, Yu ZL, Jiang ZH. Comparison of the chemical profiles and anti-platelet aggregation effects of two "Dragon's Blood" drugs used in traditional Chinese medicine. J Ethnopharmacol. 2011;133:796–802.
4. Zhang XJ, Qiu JF, Guo LP, Wang Y, Li P, Yang FQ, Su H, Wan JB. Discrimination of multi-origin chinese herbal medicines using gas chromatography-mass spectrometry-based fatty acid profiling. Molecules. 2013;18:15329–43.
5. Chai XY, Li SL, Li P. Quality evaluation of Flos lonicerae through a simultaneous determination of seven saponins by HPLC with ELSD. J Chromatogr A. 2005;1070:43–8.
6. Lu B, Xu L, Yu L, Zhang L. Extract of radix curcumae prevents gastric cancer in rats. Digestion. 2008;77:87–91.
7. Lan FY. Pharmacological activity and clinical application of Yujing. Changchun Zhongyiyao Daxue Xuebao. 2009;25:27–8.
8. Tao W, Xu X, Wang X, Li B, Wang Y, Li Y, Yang L. Network pharmacology-based prediction of the active ingredients and potential targets of Chinese herbal Radix Curcumae formula for application to cardiovascular disease. J Ethnopharmacol. 2013;145:1–10.
9. Nishiyama T. Curcuminoids and Sesquiterpenoids in turmeric(*Curcuma longa* L.) suppress an increase in blood glucose level in type 2 diabetic KK-Ay Mice. J Agric Food Chem. 2005;53:959–63.
10. Commission CP. Pharmacopoeia of the People's Republic of China edition, In: Yujin. Beijing: China Medical Science Press; 2010. pp. 193–194.
11. Jiang H, Timmermann BN, Gang DR. Use of liquid chromatography-electrospray ionization tandem mass spectrometry to identify diarylheptanoids in turmeric (*Curcuma longa* L.) rhizome. J Chromatogr A. 2006;1111:21–31.
12. Shen Y, Han C, Chen X, Hou X, Long Z. Simultaneous determination of three Curcuminoids in *Curcuma wenyujin* Y.H.chen et C.Ling. by liquid chromatography-tandem mass spectrometry combined with pressurized liquid extraction. J Pharm Biomed Anal. 2013;81–82:146–50.
13. Ni Y, Mei M, Kokot S. One- and two-dimensional gas chromatography-mass spectrometry and high performance liquid chromatography-diode-array detector fingerprints of complex substances: a comparison of classification performance of similar, complex Rhizoma Curcumae samples with the aid of chemometrics. Anal Chim Acta. 2012;712:37–44.
14. Zhu JJ, An YW, Hu G, Yin GP, Zhang QW, Wang ZM. Simultaneous determination of multiple sesquiterpenes in *Curcuma wenyujin* herbal medicines and related products with one single reference standard. Molecules. 2013;18:2110–21.
15. An YW, Hu G, Yin GP, Zhu JJ, Zhang QW, Wang ZM, Peng J, Fan B. Quantitative analysis and discrimination of steamed and non-steamed rhizomes of *Curcuma wenyujin* by GC-MS and HPLC. J Chromatogr Sci. 2013;52:961.
16. Yang FQ, Li SP, Zhao J, Lao SC, Wang YT. Optimization of GC-MS conditions based on resolution and stability of analytes for simultaneous determination of nine sesquiterpenoids in three species of *Curcuma* rhizomes. J Pharm Biomed Anal. 2007;43:73–82.
17. Zhang JS, Guan J, Yang FQ, Liu HG, Cheng XJ, Li SP. Qualitative and quantitative analysis of four species of *Curcuma* rhizomes using twice development thin layer chromatography. J Pharm Biomed Anal. 2008;48:1024–8.
18. Lechtenberg M, Quandt B, Nahrstedt A. Quantitative determination of curcuminoids in *Curcuma* rhizomes and rapid differentiation of *Curcuma* domestica Val. and *Curcuma* xanthorrhiza Roxb. by capillary electrophoresis. Phytochem Anal. 2004;15:152–8.
19. Xiang Z, Wang XQ, Cai XJ, Zeng S. Metabolomics study on quality control and discrimination of three curcuma species based on gas chromatograph-mass spectrometry. Phytochem Anal. 2011;22:411–8.
20. Lee EJ, Shaykhutdinov R, Weljie AM, Vogel HJ, Facchini PJ, Park SU, Kim YK, Yang TJ. Quality assessment of ginseng by (1)H NMR metabolite fingerprinting and profiling analysis. J Agric Food Chem. 2009;57:7513–22.
21. Chan EC, Yap SL, Lau AJ, Leow PC, Toh DF, Koh HL. Ultra-performance liquid chromatography/time-of-flight mass spectrometry based metabolomics of raw and steamed Panax notoginseng. Rapid Commun Mass Spectrom. 2007;21:519–28.
22. Toh DF, New LS, Koh HL, Chan EC. Ultra-high performance liquid chromatography/time-of-flight mass spectrometry (UHPLC/TOFMS) for time-dependent profiling of raw and steamed Panax notoginseng. J Pharm Biomed Anal. 2010;52:43–50.
23. Yang SO, Shin YS, Hyun SH, Cho S, Bang KH, Lee D, Choi SP, Choi HK. NMR-based metabolic profiling and differentiation of ginseng roots according to cultivation ages. J Pharm Biomed Anal. 2012;58:19–26.
24. Sun J, Chen P. Differentiation of Panax quinquefolius grown in the USA and China using LC/MS-based chromatographic fingerprinting and chemometric approaches. Anal Bioanal Chem. 2011;399:1877–89.
25. Baldovini N, Tomi F, Casanova J. Identification and quantitative determination of furanodiene, a heat-sensitive compound, in essential oil by 13C-NMR. Phytochem Anal. 2001;12:58–63.
26. Ishii H, Tozyo T, Nakamura M, Takeda K. Components of the root of lindera strychnifolia Vill—XIII: structure of isogemafurene and lineroxide. Tetrahedron. 1968;24:625–31.
27. Zhonghua Bencao Editorial Committee Chinese State Administration of TCM, Zhonghua Bencao. Shanghai: Shanghai Scientific and Technical Press; 1999.
28. Yang FQ, Wang YT, Li SP. Simultaneous determination of 11 characteristic components in three species of *Curcuma* rhizomes using pressurized liquid extraction and high-performance liquid chromatography. J Chromatogr A. 2006;1134:226–31.
29. Wan JB, Bai X, Cai XJ, Rao Y, Wang YS, Wang YT. Chemical differentiation of Da-Cheng-Qi-Tang, a Chinese medicine formula, prepared by traditional and modern decoction methods using UPLC/Q-TOFMS-based metabolomics approach. J Pharm Biomed Anal. 2013;83:34–42.
30. He XGLLZ, Lian LZ, Lindenmaier M. Liquid chromatography–electrospray mass spectrometric analysis of curcuminoids and sesquiterpenoids in turmeric (*Curcuma longa*). J Chromatogr A. 1998;818:127–32.
31. Yang FQ, Wang HK, Chen H, Chen JD, Xia ZN. Fractionation of volatile constituents from *Curcuma* rhizome by preparative gas chromatography. J Autom Methods Manag Chem. 2011;2011:942467.
32. Qin NY, Yang FQ, Wang YT, Li SP. Quantitative determination of eight components in rhizome (Jianghuang) and tuberous root (*Yujin*) of *Curcuma longa* using pressurized liquid extraction and gas chromatography-mass spectrometry. J Pharm Biomed Anal. 2007;43:486–92.

4

Influence of sulfur fumigation on glycoside profile in Platycodonis Radix (*Jiegeng*)

Xiao-Qing Ma[1†], Su-Mei Li[1†], Chi Leung Chan[1], Tao Su[1], Wei-Dong Li[1], Hui Cao[2], Wang-Fun Fong[1] and Zhi-Ling Yu[1*]

Abstract

Background: Over recent decades, sulfur fumigation is becoming abused in processing some freshly harvested herbs used as both medicine and food, although it has been questioned whether sulfur fumigation will change the efficacy and safety of the herbs. One of the herbs commonly processed by sulfur fumigation is Platycodonis Radix (*Jiegeng* in Chinese). Glycosides are the main bioactive components of *Jiegeng*. Up to the present, no study has been carried out to evaluate the impact of sulfur fumigation on glycoside profile of *Jiegeng*.

Methods: A rapid and versatile ultra-high performance liquid chromatography coupled with ultra-high resolution quadrupole time-of-flight mass spectrometry (UHPLC UHD Q-TOF MS/MS) method was developed for comprehensive analysis of the glycoside profiles of sulfur-fumigated and air-dried *Jiegeng* samples.

Results: Twenty-three glycosides were detected in air-dried and sulfur-fumigated *Jiegeng* samples. After sulfur fumigation, the peak heights of eight glycosides, namely platycogenin A, platycodin D, platycodin D_2, platycodin D_3, polygalacin D, polygalacin D_2, deapio-platycodin D and 3″-*O*-acetylplatycodin D_2, remarkably decreased; while peak heights of five glycosides, namely syringin, lobetyolin, platycoside E, deapio-platycodin D_2 and deapio-platycoside E, slightly increased; in addition, peaks of ten glycosides, platycodin A, platycodin C, platycodin V, platycoside C, 16-oxo-platycodin D, 2″-*O*-acetylpolygalacin D, 2″-*O*-acetylpolygalacin D_2, 3″-*O*-acetylpolygalacin D, 3″-*O*-acetylpolygalacin D_2, and platycogenic acid B, disappeared.

Conclusion: Sulfur fumigation caused significant changes of glycoside components of *Jiegeng*. Further investigations are warranted to explore how these chemical changes occurred and whether these changes would affect the efficacy and safety of *Jiegeng*.

Keywords: Sulfur fumigation, *Jiegeng*, Glycosides, Processing

Background

Herbs used as medicines and/or foods need to be processed after harvest. One of the processing methods is sulfur fumigation, which was first applied in preparing a processed form of Dioscoreae Rhizoma (*Guangshanyao* in Chinese), in Henan province, China, in 1900. The sulfur dioxide (SO_2) generated during sulfur fumigation can bleach the herbs, and kill contaminated/parasitical microbes and insects on the herbs thus prolonging shelf life of the herbs. However, sulfur-fumigation would inevitably change the chemical components in the herbs. Recently, the disadvantages of sulfur fumigation have drawn much attention in Chinese medicine and food sectors. Since 1995, the number of sulfur-fumigated herbs has been gradually reduced in individual editions of Chinese Pharmacopeia (CP), and the sulfur-fumigation method for processing Chinese materia medicas (CMMs) was abolished in the 2005 edition of CP. Due to the benefit of sulfur fumigation on prolonging shelf life of CMMs,

*Correspondence: zlyu@hkbu.edu.hk
†Xiao-Qing Ma and Su-Mei Li contributed equally to this work
[1] School of Chinese Medicine, Hong Kong Baptist University, Kowloon Tong, Hong Kong, China
Full list of author information is available at the end of the article

some CMMs were still processed by sulfur fumigation after CP2005 was issued. In CP2010, the limits of SO_2 residue on sulfur fumigated herbs were settled. Nevertheless, some reports have shown that sulfur fumigation could cause dramatic changes in chemical profiles of various herbs [1–8].

Platycodonis Radix (the dried root of *Platycodon grandiflorum*, *Jiegeng* in Chinese), a Chinese medicinal herb traditionally used for dissipating phlegm, is commonly processed by sulfur fumigation. To the best of our knowledge, no study has been conducted to evaluate the influence of sulfur fumigation on the chemical constituents of *Jiegeng*. Glycosides are the main bioactive constituents of *Jiegeng*, responsible for a diversity of bioactivities such as anti-inflammation, anti-allergy, antitumor, augmentation of immune responses, anti-obesity, and anti-hyperlipidemia [9–13]. In this study, we compared the compositions of glycosides in sulfur-fumigated and air-dried *Jiegeng* samples using a newly developed ultra-high performance liquid chromatography coupled with ultra-high resolution quadrupole time-of-flight mass spectrometry (UHPLC UHD Q-TOF MS/MS) method. The UHPLC with sub-2-μ liquid chromatography provided strategies to improve resolution while maintained or even shortened the overall run time. Q-TOF MS enabled automated exact mass measurement of precursor and production spectra for structural elucidation with high confidence. The UHPLC UHD Q-TOF MS/MS offered superior chromatographic resolution with exact mass measurements for both MS and MS/MS modes.

Methods

Chemicals

Acetonitrile is of LC/MS grade (Fisher Scientific, Pittsburgh, PA, USA) and formic acid is of HPLC grade (Sigma-Aldrich, St. Louis, MO, USA). Ultra-pure water was prepared using a Milli-Q Plus water purification system (Millipore, Billerica, MA, USA). All other reagents used for extraction are of analytical grade.

Reference compounds

The reference compounds syringin, lobetyolin, platycodin D, platycodin D_2, deapio-platycodin D were from Sichuan Wei Keqi Biological Technology Co., Ltd. (Sichuan, China). Sulfur, complied with the Chinese Pharmacopoeia (2010 edition), was obtained from the Chinese Medicine Clinic of Hong Kong Baptist University.

Stock standard solutions of syringin, lobetyolin, platycodin D, platycodin D_2, deapio–platycodin D (each about 1 mg/mL) were separately prepared in methanol and were stored at 4 °C before use. A mixed reference standard solution was prepared by mixing and diluting the five stock standard solutions with methanol to get a concentration of 0.1 mg/mL for each standard. The solution was filtered through a 0.45 μm PTFE filter prior to UHPLC UHD Q-TOF MS/MS analysis.

Herbal samples

Fresh *Jiegeng* samples were collected from Inner Mongolia Autonomous Region, China. The identities of *Jiegeng* samples were authenticated to be the root of *Platycodon grandiflorum* by morphological methods according to the monograph in CP2010 by Dr. Zhi-Ling Yu. The voucher specimens were deposited in the Technology Development Division, School of Chinese Medicine, Hong Kong Baptist University.

Sulfur-fumigated *Jiegeng* samples were prepared separately from two batches of fresh *Jiegeng* samples according to the following procedures: 10 g of sulfur powder was heated until it was burned. The burning sulfur and 100 g of fresh *Jiegeng* slices (2–4 mm in thickness) were put into the lower and upper layers of a desiccator, respectively. The desiccator was then kept closed for 12 h. The sulfur fumigation was repeated twice with each 10 g of sulfur powder. After fumigation, the sulfur-fumigated *Jiegeng* slices and its corresponding fresh *Jiegeng* slices were air dried in a fume cupboard for 6 days. The SO_2 residues in sulfur fumigated *Jiegeng* samples were determined to be around 0.43 g/kg following the method described in CP2010.

All samples were first homogenized, pulverized in a mill, and passed through a 20-mesh sieve before analysis. The powdered sample (4.0 g) was accurately weighed in a 150 mL conical flask and extracted once with 40 mL of water by sonication (240 W) for 30 min. The extract was filtered and the supernatant was transferred to a 200 mL round-bottomed flask. The extraction procedure was repeated twice. All the extracts were combined and evaporated to dryness at reduced pressure in a rotary evaporator. The residue was dissolved in 16 mL of methanol. Diethyl ether (35 mL) was added to the methanolic solution and the precipitate was collected. The collected precipitate was extracted with methanol for three times (16, 8, 3 mL). The combined methanol extracts were evaporated to about 10 mL. The methanolic concentrate was washed twice with 35 mL of diethyl ether each time. The methanolic fraction was then transferred to a volumetric flask (10 mL) and was made up to the mark with methanol. All samples were filtered through a 0.45 μm PTFE membrane filter prior to UHPLC UHD Q-TOF MS/MS analysis.

Liquid chromatography

The UHPLC conditions for LC–MS analysis were as follows: chromatography was performed on an Acquity UPLC HSS T3 C_{18} column, 2.1 × 100 mm i.d., 1.8 μm

(Waters Corp., Milford, MA, USA); and the column temperature was maintained at 40 °C. A gradient elution of solvent A (Milli-Q water with 0.1 % formic acid) and solvent B (acetonitrile with 0.1 % formic acid) was applied as follows: 0–5 min, 10–20 % B; 5–10 min, 20–23 % B; 10–15 min, 23 % B; 15–18 min, 23–27 % B; 18–26 min, 27–32 % B; 26–26.1 min, 32–100 % B; 26.1–30 min, 100 % B. An equilibration period of 4.0 min was used between individual runs. The flow rate was 0.35 mL/min, and the injection volume was 0.5 μL.

Mass spectrometry

An Agilent 6450 UHD Accurate-Mass Q-TOF mass spectrometer (Agilent Technologies, Santa Clara, CA, USA) was connected to the Agilent 1290 Infinity UHPLC system via electrospray ionization (ESI) ion source with Jet-Stream technology for the LC/MS/MS analysis of *Jiegeng* samples. The ESI–MS spectra were acquired in both positive and negative modes. Ultra-pure nitrogen (N_2) was used as the nebulizing and sheath gas. Product ion scanning experiments were conducted using ultra-high-purity N_2 as collision gas. The ESI parameters were set as follows: the capillary voltage is 4.5 kV. The flow rate and temperature of sheath gas were 8 L/min and 350 °C, respectively. The flow rate and temperature of drying gas were 8 L/min and 300 °C, respectively. The pressure of nebulizer gas was 40 psi. The fragmentor voltage was 175 V. The mass analyzer scanned from 100 to 1700 (*m/z*). The Q-TOF acquisition rates were 2 and 3 Hz for full scanning and product ion scanning, respectively. The energies for collision-induced dissociation (CID) experiments were set at 10, 20, 30 and 40 eV, respectively.

The Q-TOF mass spectrometer was tuned in the low mass range (from 100 to 1700 Da) and in the extended dynamic range mode (2 GHz). To ensure the mass accuracy and reproducibility, all MS data were acquired with reference masses at *m/z* 112.9855 and 966.0007 in the negative ESI mode, and at *m/z* 121.0508 and 922.0097 in the positive ESI mode.

Results

Comparison of the chemical profiles of sulfur-fumigated and air-dried *Jiegeng* samples

To compare the chemical compositions of sulfur-fumigated and air-dried *Jiegeng* samples, chemical profiling was conducted by UHPLC UHD Q-TOF MS in both positive and negative ion modes. Two batches of air-dried *Jiegeng* samples (FX-JG-01, FX-JG-03) and their corresponding sulfur-fumigated ones (ZX-JG-02, ZX-JG-04) were analyzed using the established UHPLC UHD Q-TOF MS/MS method in this study. Within each sample group (air-dried and sulfur-fumigated), similar results were obtained from the two batches of samples. The results for samples FX-JG-01 and ZX-JG-02, which were from the same batch of fresh *Jiegeng* sample, were described and discussed in detail. The representative base peak ion (BPI) chromatograms of sample FX-JG-01 and ZX-JG-02 were shown in Fig. 1. It was found that the intensity of the major peaks (peaks 5, 7–23) detected in the air-dried *Jiegeng* sample (Fig. 1a, c) were obviously decreased or even disappeared in the corresponding sulfur-fumigated sample (Fig. 1b, d), whereas the peak heights of some components (peaks 1, 2, 3, 4, 6) were slightly higher in the sulfur-fumigated sample than in the air-dried sample. These results suggest that sulfur fumigation caused significant changes in the chemical profile of *Jiegeng*.

Structural elucidation and identification of chemical components in sulfur-fumigated and air-dried *Jiegeng* samples

For structural elucidation, the quasi-molecular ion peak of each compound was selected to obtain the product ion spectra with optimal collision energies (Table 1). Peak 2 showed a $[M+Na]^+$ ion at *m/z* 419.1664 ($C_{20}H_{28}O_8$) in positive ion mode and the ion could be further fragmented into ion *m/z* 257.1250 $[M+Na-C_6H_{10}O_5]^+$, the fragmented ions corresponded to the loss of one $C_6H_{10}O_5$. Moreover, a $[M+HCOO]^-$ ion at *m/z* 441.1756 in negative ion mode generated fragments at *m/z* 305.1301 $[M-H-C_7H_6]^-$ and 215.1107 $[M-H-C_6H_{12}O_6]^-$, resulting from the losses of C_7H_6 and one glycosyl moiety, successively. Therefore, peak 2 was tentatively assigned as lobetyolin (**2** in Fig. 2) and its identity was further confirmed by comparing the retention time and mass spectrum of reference standard. For peak 4, precursor ion $[M-H]^-$ was observed at *m/z* 1547.6719 ($C_{69}H_{112}O_{38}$) with product ions at *m/z* 1415.6044, 1283.5692 and 1005.4878 representing the loss of apiosyl, xylosyl and rhamnosyl+arabinosyl moieties attached at C-28 of triterpenoid core, respectively. Therefore, peak 4 was tentatively assigned as platycoside E (**4** in Fig. 2). Peak 6 (Fig. 3) displayed a precursor ion *m/z* 1255.5890 $[M+H]^+$ and product ions at *m/z* 1123.5478 $[M+H-C_5H_8O_4]^+$, *m/z* 961.5037 $[M+H-C_{11}H_{18}O_9]^+$ and *m/z* 799.4424 $[M+H-C_{11}H_{18}O_9-C_6H_{10}O_5]^+$, and was deduced as deapio-platycodin D_2 (**6** in Fig. 2). Peak 8 was tentatively assigned as deapio-platycodin D (**8** in Fig. 2) according to the following facts. In positive mode, molecular ion *m/z* 1093.5400 $[M+H]^+$ and the fragment ions at *m/z* 961.4949, 799.4453, 683.3975 and 521.3406 were due to glycosidic bond cleavage with sequential loss of xylosyl, rhamnosyl, arabinosyl and glucosyl moieties linked at C-28 and C-3 of the triterpenoid core, respectively. In negative mode, molecular ion *m/z* 1091.5265 $[M-H]^-$ and the fragment ions at

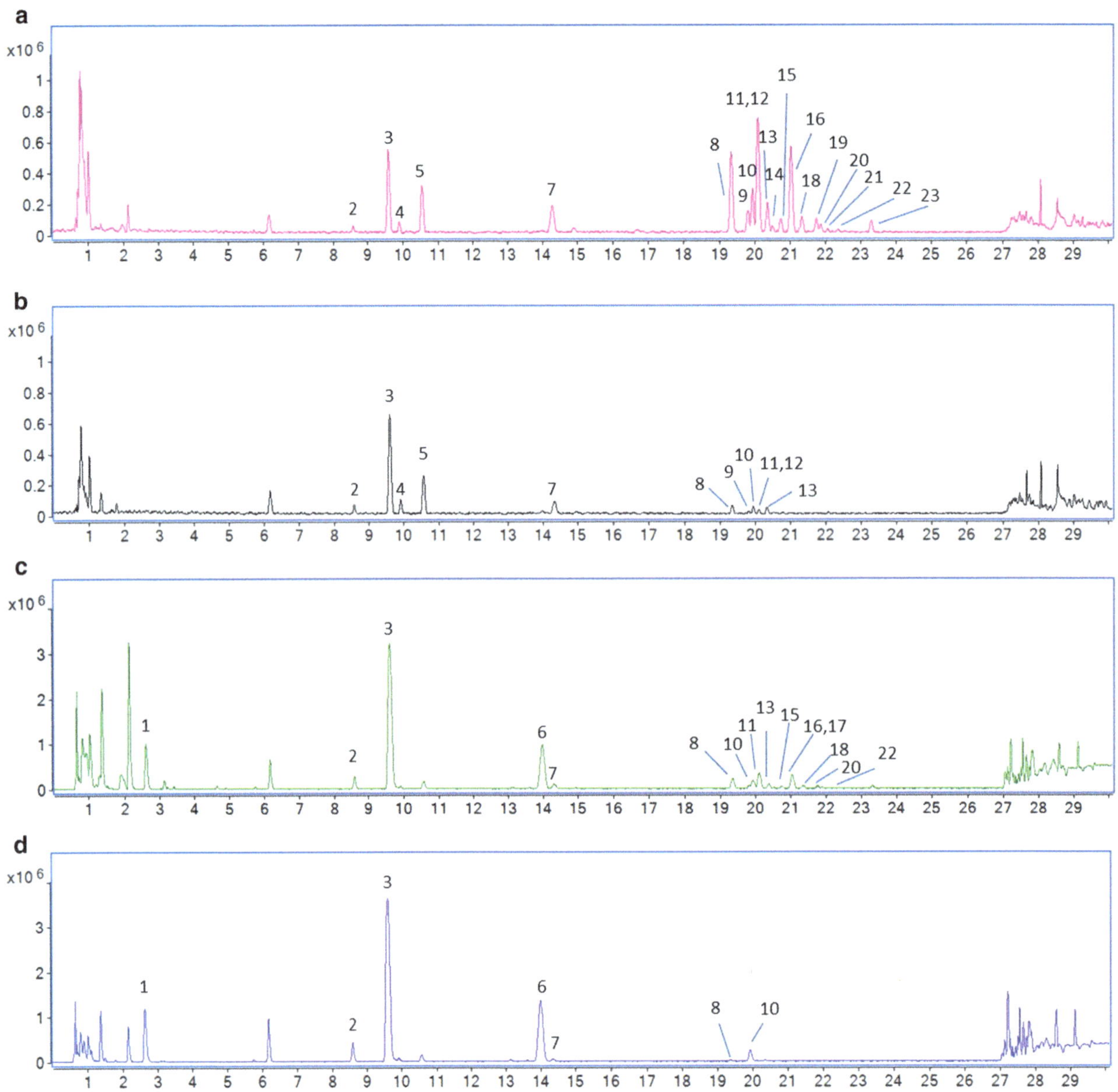

Fig. 1 Representative base peak chromatograms of *Jiegeng* samples. **a** Air-dried *Jiegeng* in negative ion mode; **b** Sulfur-fumigated *Jiegeng* in negative ion mode; **c** Air-dried *Jiegeng* in positive ion mode; **d** Sulfur-fumigated *Jiegeng* in positive ion mode

m/z 959.4430, 681.3620 could be sequential loss of xylosyl and rhamnosyl+arabinosyl respectively [11]. Peak 10 showed an $[M+Na]^+$ ion at *m/z* 1247.5620 and $[M-H]^-$ ion at *m/z* 1223.5669 ($C_{57}H_{92}O_{28}$). In TOF–MS/MS spectra, fragment ion at *m/z* 705.3831 $[M+Na-C_{21}H_{34}O_{16}]^+$ (positive ion mode), and fragment ion at *m/z* 681.3806 $[M-H-C_{21}H_{34}O_{16}]^-$ (negative ion mode) were both resulted from the loss of apiosyl+xylosyl+rhamnosyl+arabinosyl moiety. Moreover, by comparing with authentic reference standard, peak 10 was identified as platycodin D (**10** in Fig. 2). For peak 18 (Figs. 4, 5), molecular ion *m/z* 1135.5480 $[M+H]^+$ and its product ions *m/z* 1003.5055 $[M+H-C_5H_8O_4]^+$, *m/z* 841.4540 $[M+H-C_5H_8O_4-C_6H_{10}O_5]^+$, *m/z* 683.3916 $[M+H-C_{18}H_{28}O_{13}]^+$ and *m/z* 521.3454 $[M+H-C_{18}H_{28}O_{13}-C_6H_{10}O_5]^+$ were observed in positive ion mode. Meanwhile, molecular ion *m/z* 1133.5336 $[M-H]^-$ and fragment ions *m/z* 1091.5205 $[M-H-C_2H_2O]^-$ and *m/z* 681.3849 $[M-H-C_{18}H_{28}O_{13}]^-$ were observed in negative ion mode. Based on the literature information [14], peak 18 was tentatively assigned as platycoside C (**18** in Fig. 2). For peak 21, precursor ion $[M-H]^-$ was observed at *m/z* 1265.5750 ($C_{59}H_{94}O_{29}$)

Table 1 Components identified in sulfur-fumigated and air-dried *Jiegeng* samples

No.	Compound name	Formula	RT (min)	$[M+H]^+$ mass accuracy (ppm)	$[M-H]^-$ mass accuracy (ppm)	Positive ions $[M+H]^+$ and proposed CID fragment ions	Negative ions $[M-H]^-$ and proposed CID fragment ions	Ref.
1a	Syringin	$C_{17}H_{24}O_9$	2.725	3.33	–	395.1300 $[M+Na]^+$ 233.0841 $[M+Na-C_6H_{10}O_5]^+$	–	
2a	Lobetyolin	$C_{20}H_{28}O_8$	8.872	−0.55	1.88	419.1664 $[M+Na]^+$ 257.1205 $[M+Na-C_6H_{10}O_5]^+$ 203.0575 $[C_6H_{12}O_6Na]^+$	441.1756 $[M+HCOO]^-$ 305.1301 $[M-H-C_7H_6]^-$ 215.1107 $[M-H-C_6H_{12}O_6]^-$ 179.0565 $[C_6H_{11}O_6]^-$	
3	Platycoside G_1 (Deapio–platycoside E)	$C_{64}H_{104}O_{34}$	9.745	5.20	1.20	1417.6425 $[M+H]^+$ 503.3338 $[C_{30}H_{47}O_6]^+$ 485.3247 $[C_{30}H_{45}O_5]^+$	1415.6327 $[M-H]^-$ 1283.5692 $[M-H-C_5H_8O_4]^-$ 1005.4907 $[M-H-C_{16}H_{26}O_{12}]^-$ 519.3385 $[C_{30}H_{47}O_7]^-$	[11]
4	Platycoside E	$C_{69}H_{112}O_{38}$	9.922	–	1.63	–	1547.6719 $[M-H]^-$ 1415.6044 $[M-H-C_5H_8O_4]^-$ 1283.5692 $[M-H-(C_5H_8O_4)_2]^-$ 1005.4878 $[M-H-C_{21}H_{34}O_{16}]^-$	[11]
5	Platycogenin A	$C_{42}H_{68}O_{16}$	10.661	–	0.60	–	827.4433 $[M-H]^-$ 665.3907 $[M-H-C_6H_{10}O_5]^-$	[27]
6	Platycoside A (Deapio–platycodin D_2)	$C_{58}H_{94}O_{29}$	13.902	4.70	–	1255.5890 $[M+H]^+$ 1123.5478 $[M+H-C_5H_8O_4]^+$ 961.5037 $[M+H-C_{11}H_{18}O_9]^+$ 799.4424 $[M+H-C_{17}H_{28}O_{14}]^+$	–	[28]
7	Platycodin D_3	$C_{63}H_{102}O_{33}$	14.291	6.00	−0.18	1409.6130 $[M+Na]^+$ 867.4480 $[M+Na-C_{21}H_{34}O_{16}]^+$	1385.6239 $[M-H]^-$ 1253.5975 $[M-H-C_5H_8O_4]^-$ 843.4433 $[M-H-C_{21}H_{34}O_{16}]^-$	[11, 29]
8a	Deapio–platycodin D	$C_{52}H_{84}O_{24}$	19.323	3.70	1.31	1093.5400 $[M+H]^+$ 961.4949 $[M+H-C_5H_8O_4]^+$ 799.4453 $[M+H-C_{11}H_{18}O_9]^+$ 683.3975 $[M+H-C_{16}H_{26}O_{12}]^+$ 521.3406 $[M+H-C_{16}H_{26}O_{12}-C_6H_{10}O_5]^+$	1091.5268 $[M-H]^-$ 959.4430 $[M-H-C_5H_8O_4]^-$ 681.3620 $[M-H-C_{16}H_{26}O_{12}]^-$	[11]
9a	Platycodin D_2	$C_{63}H_{102}O_{33}$	19.829	–	−0.74	–	1385.6247 $[M-H]^-$ 843.4439 $[M-H-C_{21}H_{34}O_{16}]^-$	[30]
10a	Platycodin D	$C_{57}H_{92}O_{28}$	19.946	4.90	1.16	1247.5620 $[M+Na]^+$ 705.3831 $[M+Na-C_{21}H_{34}O_{16}]^+$	1223.5669 $[M-H]^-$ 681.3806 $[M-H-C_{21}H_{34}O_{16}]^-$	[11]

Table 1 continued

No.	Compound name	Formula	RT (min)	$[M+H]^+$ mass accuracy (ppm)	$[M-H]^-$ mass accuracy (ppm)	Positive ions $[M+H]^+$ and proposed CID fragment ions	Negative ions $[M-H]^-$ and proposed CID fragment ions	Ref.
11	3″-*O*-Acetylplatycodin D_2	$C_{65}H_{104}O_{34}$	20.088	4.70	2.22	1451.6250 $[M+Na]^+$ 867.4011 $[M+Na-C_{23}H_{36}O_{17}]^+$	1427.6282 $[M-H]^-$ 1295.5884 $[M-H-C_5H_8O_4]^-$ 843.4379 $[M-H-C_{23}H_{36}O_{17}]^-$ 663.3800 $[M-H-C_{23}H_{36}O_{17}-C_6H_{12}O_6]^-$	[29]
12	Polygalacin D_2	$C_{63}H_{102}O_{32}$	20.123	–	0.43	–	1369.6281 $[M-H]^-$ 1237.5581 $[M-H-C_5H_8O_4]^-$ 827.4438 $[M-H-C_{21}H_{34}O_{16}]^-$ 647.3782 $[M-H-C_{21}H_{34}O_{16}-C_6H_{12}O_6]^-$ 541.1819 $[C_{21}H_{33}O_{16}]^-$	[29]
13	Polygalacin D	$C_{57}H_{92}O_{27}$	20.510	–	1.36	–	1207.5738 $[M-H]^-$ 665.3726 $[M-H-C_{21}H_{34}O_{16}]^-$ 541.1728 $[C_{21}H_{33}O_{16}]^-$	[11]
14	Platycodin C (3″-*O*-Acetylplatycodin D)	$C_{59}H_{94}O_{29}$	20.344	4.30	4.64	1289.5730 $[M+Na]^+$ 705.3770 $[M+Na-C_{23}H_{36}O_{17}]^+$	1265.5720 $[M-H]^-$ 1133.5398 $[M-H-C_5H_8O_4]^-$ 681.3842 $[M-H-C_{23}H_{36}O_{17}]^-$	[29]
15	3″-*O*-Acetylpolygalacin D_2	$C_{65}H_{104}O_{33}$	20.723	4.30	1.25	1435.6290 $[M+H]^+$ 851.4342 $[M+Na-C_{23}H_{36}O_{17}]^+$	1411.6328 $[M-H]^-$ 1279.6025 $[M-H-C_5H_8O_4]^-$ 827.4424 $[M-H-C_{23}H_{36}O_{17}]^-$ 665.3885 $[C_{36}H_{57}O_{11}]^-$ 541.1741 $[C_{21}H_{33}O_{16}]^-$ 469.1550 $[C_{18}H_{29}O_{14}]^-$	[29]
16	3″-*O*-Acetylpolygalacin D	$C_{59}H_{94}O_{28}$	21.054	4.60	−0.14	1273.5780 $[M+Na]^+$ 689.3757 $[M+Na-C_{23}H_{36}O_{17}]^+$	1249.5866 $[M-H]^-$ 1117.5502 $[M-H-C_5H_8O_4]^-$ 665.3916 $[M-H-C_{23}H_{36}O_{17}]^-$ 469.1554 $[C_{18}H_{29}O_{14}]^-$	[11]
17a/17b	Platycogenic acid A/platycogenic acid B	$C_{30}H_{46}O_8$	21.166	1.60	–	535.3255 $[M+H]^+$ 517.3143 $[M+H-H_2O]^+$ 499.3056 $[M+H-(H_2O)_2]^+$ 481.2688 $[M+H-(H_2O)_3]^+$	–	[31]

Table 1 continued

No.	Compound name	Formula	RT (min)	$[M+H]^+$ mass accuracy (ppm)	$[M-H]^-$ mass accuracy (ppm)	Positive ions $[M+H]^+$ and proposed CID fragment ions	Negative ions $[M-H]^-$ and proposed CID fragment ions	Ref.
18	Platycoside C	$C_{54}H_{86}O_{25}$	21.373	4.40	1.50	1135.5480 $[M+H]^+$ 1003.5055 $[M+H-C_5H_8O_4]^+$ 841.4540 $[M+H-C_5H_8O_4-C_6H_{10}O_5]^+$ 683.3916 $[M+H-C_{18}H_{28}O_{13}]^+$ 521.3454 $[M+H-C_{18}H_{28}O_{13}-C_6H_{10}O_5]^+$	1133.5336 $[M-H]^-$ 1091.5205 $[M-H-C_2H_2O]^-$ 681.3849 $[M-H-C_{18}H_{28}O_{13}]^-$ 337.0949 $[C_{13}H_{21}O_{10}]^-$	[28]
19	16-Oxoplatycodin D	$C_{57}H_{90}O_{28}$	21.707	–	1.21	–	1221.5531 $[M-H]^-$ 811.1198 $[M-H-C_{16}H_{26}O_{12}]^-$ 635.3855 $[M-H-C_{22}H_{34}O_{18}]^-$ 541.1765 $[C_{21}H_{33}O_{16}]^-$ 409.1354 $[C_{16}H_{25}O_{12}]^-$	[14]
20	Platycodin V (2″-*O*-Acetylplatycodin D_2)	$C_{65}H_{104}O_{34}$	21.838	5.10	−0.68	1451.6213 $[M+Na]^+$ 867.4064 $[M+Na-C_{23}H_{36}O_{17}]^+$	1427.6348 $[M-H]^-$ 843.4372 $[M-H-C_{23}H_{36}O_{17}]^-$ 663.3670 $[M-H-C_{23}H_{36}O_{17}-C_6H_{12}O_6]^-$ 469.1572 $[C_{18}H_{29}O_{14}]^-$	[14]
21	Platycodin A (2″-*O*-Acetylplatycodin D)	$C_{59}H_{94}O_{29}$	22.048	–	3.17	–	1265.5750 $[M-H]^-$ 1133.5379 $[M-H-C_5H_8O_4]^-$ 681.3799 $[M-H-C_{23}H_{36}O_{17}]^-$ 469.1612 $[C_{18}H_{29}O_{14}]^-$	[11, 14]
22	2″-*O*-Acetylpolygalacin D_2	$C_{65}H_{104}O_{33}$	22.335	5.20	1.29	1435.6290 $[M+Na]^+$ 851.4097 $[M+Na-C_{23}H_{36}O_{17}]^+$	1411.6374 $[M-H]^-$ 827.4408 $[M-H-C_{23}H_{36}O_{17}]^-$ 665.3935 $[C_{36}H_{57}O_{11}]^-$ 541.1519 $[C_{21}H_{33}O_{16}]^-$ 469.1606 $[C_{18}H_{29}O_{14}]^-$	[29]
23	2″-*O*-Acetylpolygalacin D	$C_{59}H_{94}O_{28}$	23.353	–	0.24	–	1249.5861 $[M-H]^-$ 1117.5542 $[M-H-C_5H_8O_4]^-$ 665.3911 $[M-H-C_{23}H_{36}O_{17}]^-$ 469.1568 $[C_{18}H_{29}O_{14}]^-$	[11]

with product ion $[M-H-C_5H_8O_4]^-$ at *m/z* 1133.5379 and $[M-H-C_{23}H_{36}O_{17}]^-$ at *m/z* 681.3799 in negative ion mode. Comparing with literature [15], peak 21 was deduced as platycodin A (**21** in Fig. 2). The polygalacin D (peak 14) (**14** in Fig. 2) and 2″-*O*-acetyl polygalacin D (peak 23) (**23** in Fig. 2) are dehydroxylated derivatives of platycodin D and platycodin A, respectively, yielding ion difference of 16 Da between two groups. 2″-*O*-acetyl

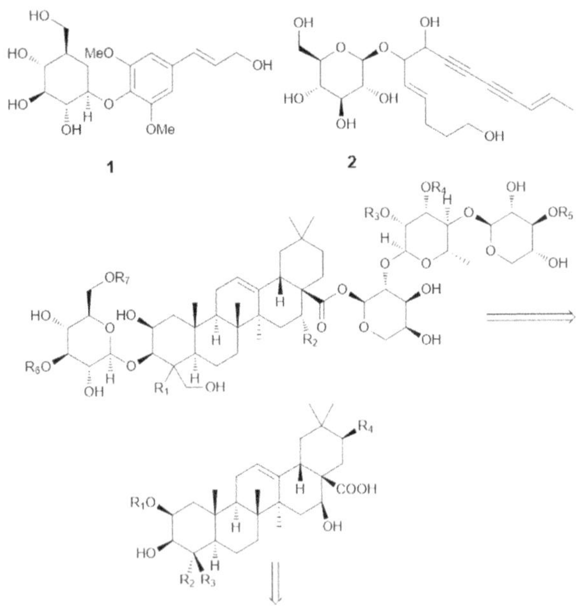

	R1	R2	R3	R4
5	β-D-Glc	CH_3	CH_3	1-0-β-D-Glc
17a	H	CH_2OH	COOH	H
17b	H	CH_3	COOH	OH

	R1	R2	R3	R4	R5	R6	R7
3	CH_2OH	OH	H	H	H	H	β-D-Glc-(1→6)-β-D-Glc
4	CH_2OH	OH	H	H	β-D-Api	H	β-D-Glc-(1→6)-β-D-Glc
6	CH_2OH	OH	H	H	H	β-D-Glc	H
7	CH_2OH	OH	H	H	β-D-Api	H	β-D-Glc
8a	CH_2OH	OH	H	H	H	H	H
9a	CH_2OH	OH	H	H	β-D-Api	β-D-Glc	H
10a	CH_2OH	OH	H	H	β-D-Api	H	H
11	CH_2OH	OH	H	Ac	β-D-Api	β-D-Glc	H
12	CH_3	OH	H	H	β-D-Api	β-D-Glc	H
13	CH_3	OH	H	H	β-D-Api	H	H
14	CH_2OH	OH	H	Ac	β-D-Api	H	H
15	CH_3	OH	H	Ac	β-D-Api	β-D-Glc	H
16	CH_3	OH	H	Ac	β-D-Api	H	H
18	CH_2OH	OH	H	Ac	H	H	H
19	CH_2OH	=O	H	H	β-D-Api	H	H
20	CH_2OH	OH	Ac	H	β-D-Api	β-D-Glc	H
21	CH_2OH	OH	Ac	H	β-D-Api	H	H
22	CH_3	OH	Ac	H	β-D-Api	β-D-Glc	H
23	CH_3	OH	Ac	H	β-D-Api	H	H

Fig. 2 Structures of components identified in sulfur-fumigated and air-dried *Jiegeng* samples

polygalacin D (peak 23) and 3″-*O*-acetyl polygalacin D (peak 16) (**16** in Fig. 2) are a pair of isomers with molecular weights of 1250 Da and produce the similar product ion spectra (Figs. 6, 7). Using LC-ESI MS/MS analysis and comparing with the chromatographic characteristics in literature [11], the two isomers were tentatively identified.

Changes of glycosides of *Jiegeng* after sulfur fumigation

Sulfur fumigation was reported to be able to cause chemical changes in herbs [16, 17]. In this study, chemical changes were observed in *Jiegeng* subjected to sulfur fumigation. Among all the compounds that showed significant changes, 23 constituents were deduced/tentatively identified. Structures of all the compounds were shown in Fig. 2. The peak heights of platycogenin A, platycodin D, platycodin D_2, platycodin D_3, polygalacin D, polygalacin D_2, deapio-platycodin D and 3″-*O*-acetyl-platycodin D_2 in sulfur-fumigated *Jiegeng* were much lower than that in the air-dried sample; peaks of compounds platycodin A, platycodin C, platycodin V, platycoside C, 16-oxoplatycodin D, 2″-*O*-acetylpolygalacin D, 2″-*O*-acetylpolygalacin D_2, 3″-*O*-acetylpolygalacin D, 3″-*O*-acetylpolygalacin D_2, and platycogenic acid B disappeared after sulfur fumigation. On the contrary, the contents of syringin, lobetyolin, platycoside E, deapio-platycodin D_2 and deapio-platycoside E slightly increased after sulfur fumigation.

Discussion

The decrease and disappearance of the glycoside compounds may be due to the hydrolysis of glycosides catalyzed by sulfurous acid (H_2SO_3) which was generated by the combination of SO_2, the product of sulfur combustion, and the water molecule in fresh *Jiegeng* [3, 15]. For instance, the partial transformation of platycodin D_2 to deapio–platycodin D_2 may be caused by H_2SO_3-catalyzed hydrolysis of platycodin D_2. On the other hand, H_2SO_3 produced during sulfur fumigation might inactivate glycoside hydrolases and then protect glycosides from hydrolysis in *Jiegeng* [3]. This would partly explain why platycoside E and deapio-platycoside E, in which there are more sugar moieties than in other glycosides of *Jiegeng*, have relatively higher content in sulfur fumigated *Jiegeng* samples than in air-dried *Jiegeng* samples.

It was reported that lobetyolin in Codonopsis Radix (*Dangshen*) could be changed to lobetyolin sulfate, which resulted in significant decrease of lobetyolin content in sulfur-fumigated *Dangshen* [16]. In this study, peak height of lobetyolin in *Jiegeng* increased by sulfur fumigation. However, no peak in the base peak chromatograms of *Jiegeng*

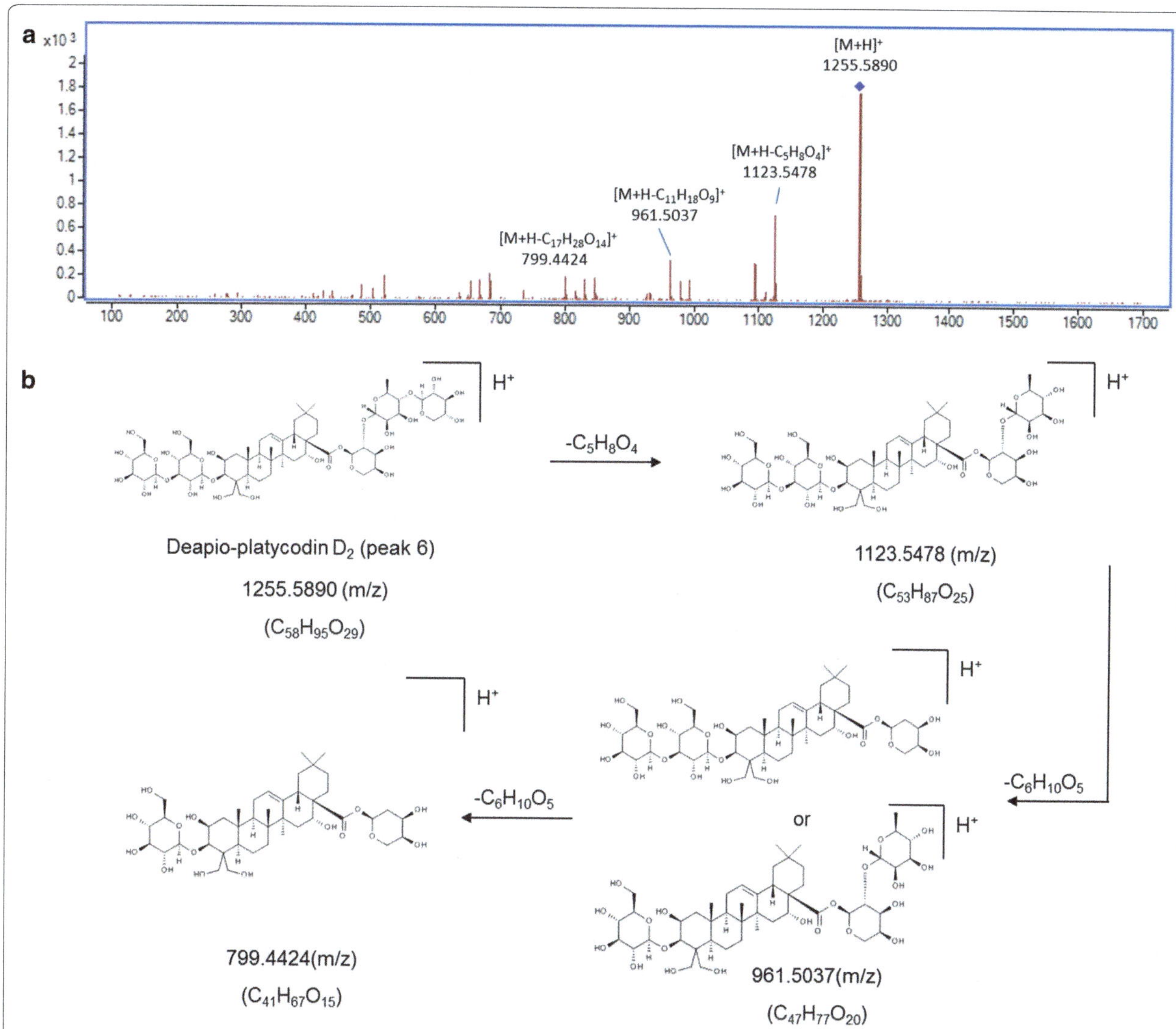

Fig. 3 Mass spectra and proposed major fragmentation pathway of deapio–platycodin D_2 in *Jiegeng* in positive ion mode. **a** Low energy CID mass spectra; **b** Proposed major fragmentation pathway

samples could be identified as a lobetyolin derivative. It has been shown that lobetyolinin could be hydrolyzed to lobetylin during sulfur fumigation [16]. To determine if this occurred during sulfur fumigation of *Jiegeng*, we extracted the quasi-molecular ion of lobetyolinin in both positive and negative ion modes. A chromatographic peak at 6.83 min in the air-dried sample (Additional file 1: Figure S1) was observed and the fragmentation patterns of this peak agreed with that of lobetyolinin [16]. In positive ion mode, quasi-molecular ion 581.2187 *(m/z)* $[M+Na]^+$ (diff = −3.18 ppm) and the corresponding product ions at 419.1494 *(m/z)* $[M+Na-C_6H_{10}O_5]^+$ and 365.0885 *(m/z)* $[M+Na-C_{14}H_{16}O_2]^+$ could be seen (Additional file 2: Figure S2). In negative ion mode, quasi-molecular ion 603.2279 *(m/z)* $[M+HCOO]^-$ (diff = −2.57 ppm) and the corresponding product ions at 467.1782 *(m/z)* $[M-H-C_7H_6]^-$ were observed (Additional file 3: Figure S3). In sulfur-fumigated sample, the content of lobetyolinin decreased significantly, which can account for the increased content of lobetyolin (Additional file 1: Figure S1). The increased content of lobetyolin might be generated by hydrolysis reaction of lobetyolinin during sulfur fumigation (Additional file 4: Figure S4). Nevertheless, the chromatographic peak of lobetyolinin was masked in the base peak chromatograms of both air-dried and sulfur-fumigated *Jiegeng* samples due to the relative low content of this compound. Figures for the tentative identification of lobetyolinin and the possible mechanism involved in the transformation were provided as Additional files 1, 2, 3 and 4.

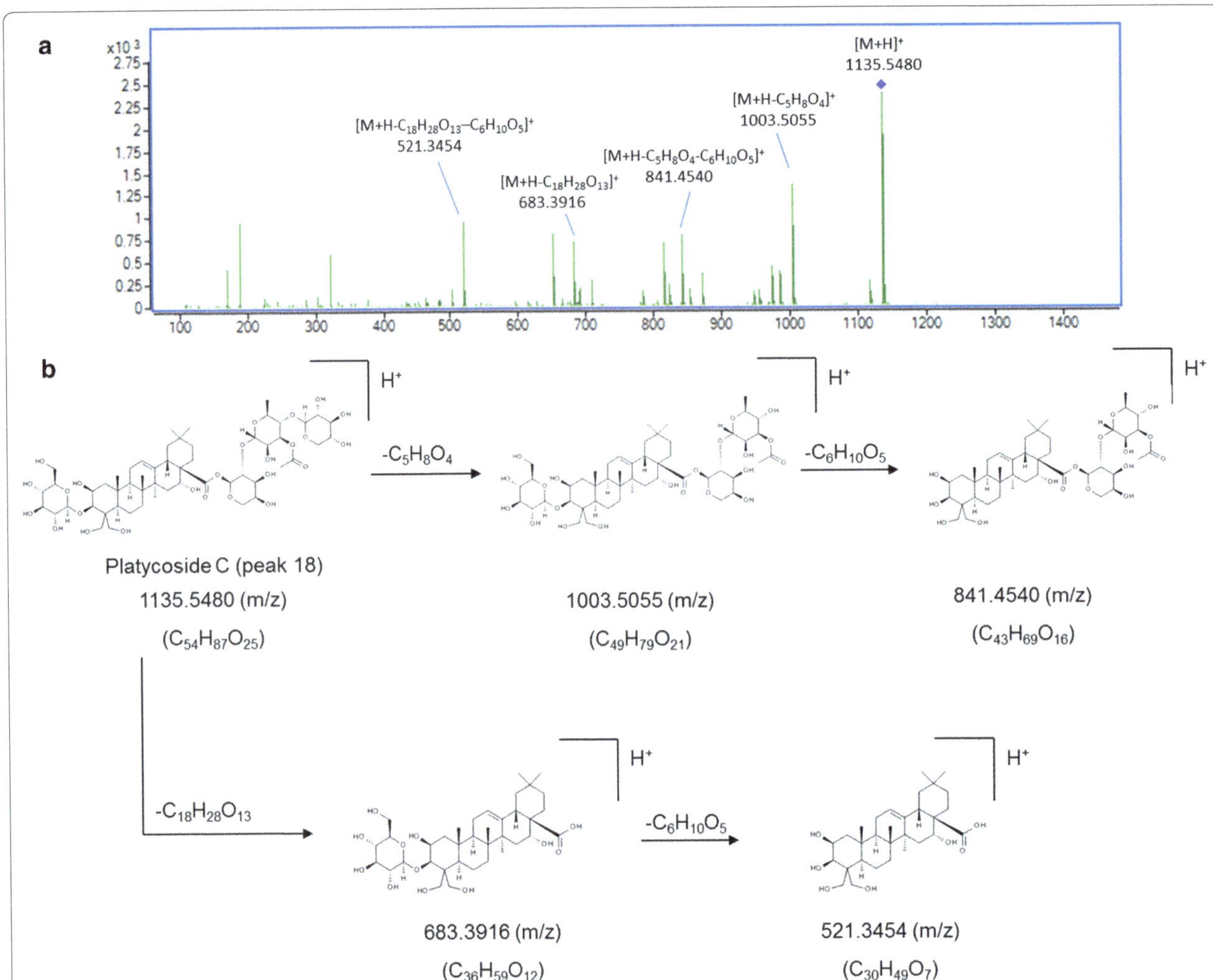

Fig. 4 Mass spectra and proposed major fragmentation pathways of platycoside C in *Jiegeng* in positive ion mode. **a** Low energy CID mass spectra; **b** Proposed major fragmentation pathway

Glycosides are the main bioactive constituents of *Jiegeng*, which have been shown to have various bioactivities. Significant decrease and/or loss of these glycosides caused by sulfur fumigation may negatively affect the bioactivities of *Jiegeng*. It has been reported that platycodin D, platycodin D_2 and platycodin D_3 have anti-HCV activity [17]; platycodin D is a potent adjuvant of specific cellular and humoral immune responses against recombinant hepatitis B antigen [13], and can reduce pancreatic lipase activity significantly [18]. Whether the decrease in contents of these glycosides during sulfur fumigation will reduce the above mentioned bioactivities of *Jiegeng* remains to be explored.

We also observed that contents of five glycosides (syringe, lobetyolin, deapio-platycodin D_2, platycoside E and deapio-platycoside E) in *Jiegeng* increased after sulfur fumigation. These glycosides also exhibit various bioactivities. Syringe has immunomodulatory [19] and anti-inflammatory properties [20], can enhance glucose utilization and lower plasma glucose level in rats of insulin deficiency [21], and can alleviate fulminant hepatic failure (FHF) induced by LPS/D-GalN [22]. Lobetyolin has significant antioxidant activity [23] and can activate NF-κB [24]. Deapio-platycodin D_2 is able to inhibit HCV activity [17]. Platycoside E and deapio-platycoside E have hemolytic activities and adjuvant potentials on the immune responses to Newcastle disease virus-based recombinant avian influenza vaccine (rL-H5) in mice [25], and both showed antioxidant activities [26]. It needs to be investigated if sulfur fumigation would enhance these bioactivities of *Jiegeng*.

Conclusions

In the present study, an UHPLC UHD Q-TOF MS/MS-based chemical profiling method was developed to reveal sulfur fumigation-caused chemical

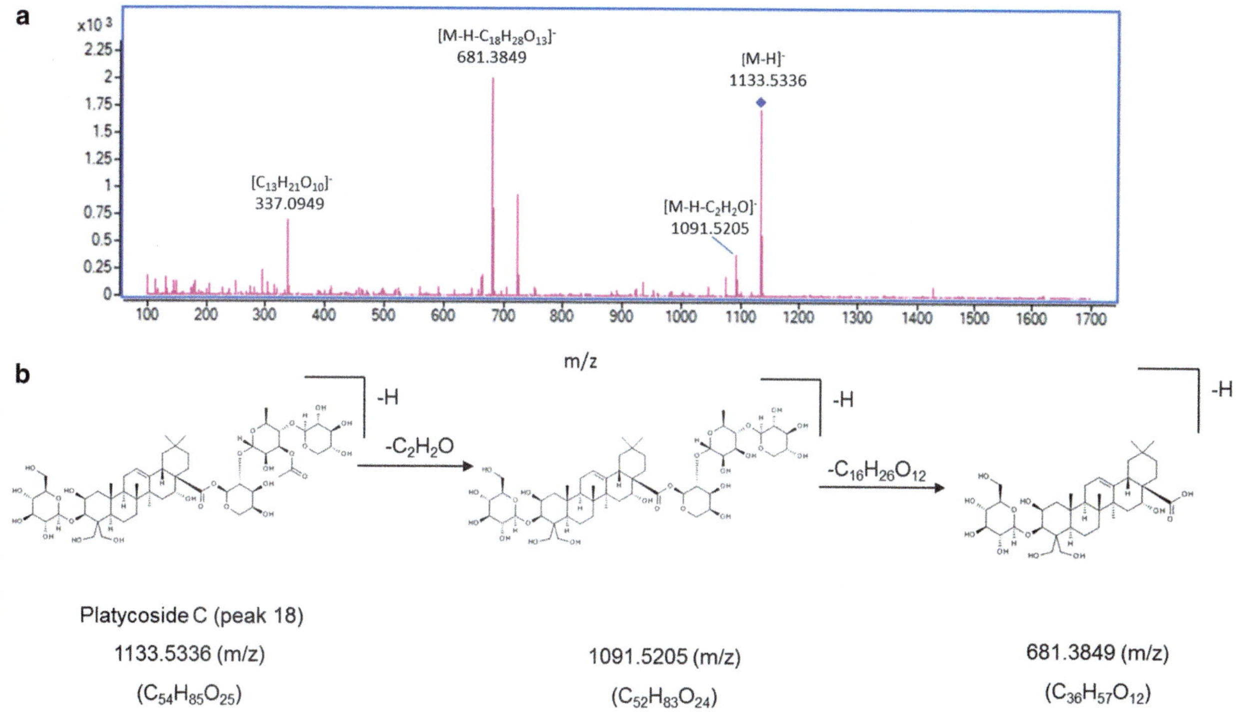

Fig. 5 Mass spectra and proposed major fragmentation pathways of platycoside C in *Jiegeng* in negative ion mode. **a** Low energy CID mass spectra; **b** Proposed major fragmentation pathway

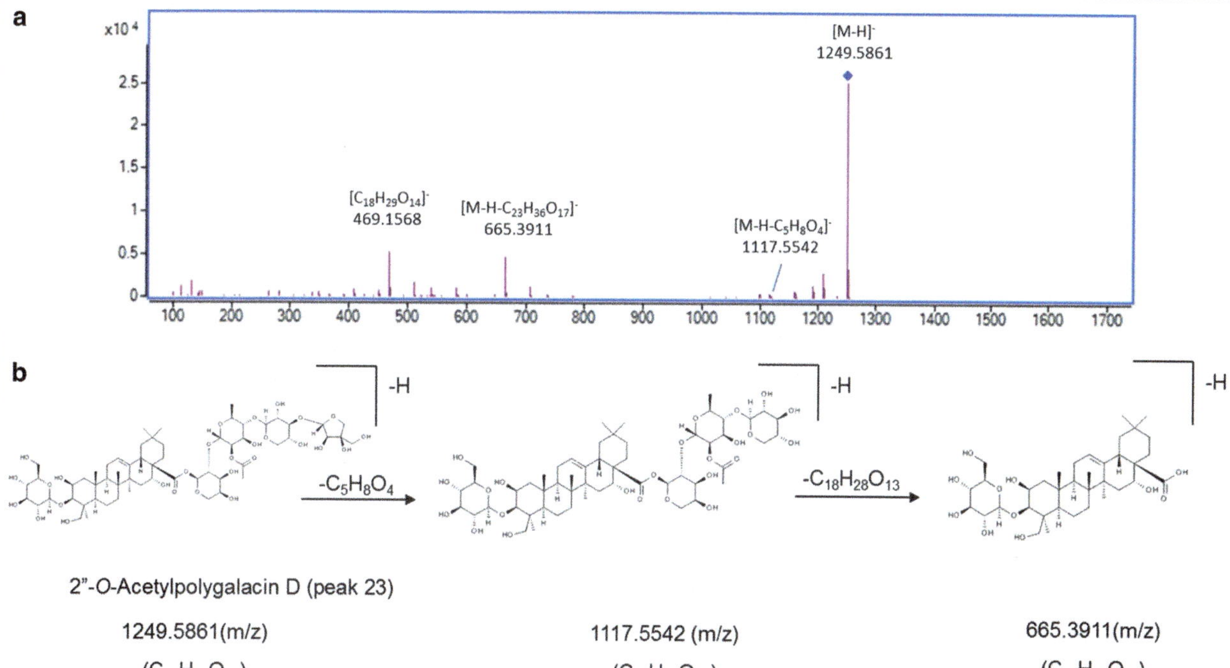

Fig. 6 Mass spectra and proposed major fragmentation pathways of 2″-*O*-acetylpolygalacin D in *Jiegeng* in negative ion mode. **a** Low energy CID mass spectra. **b** Proposed major fragmentation pathway

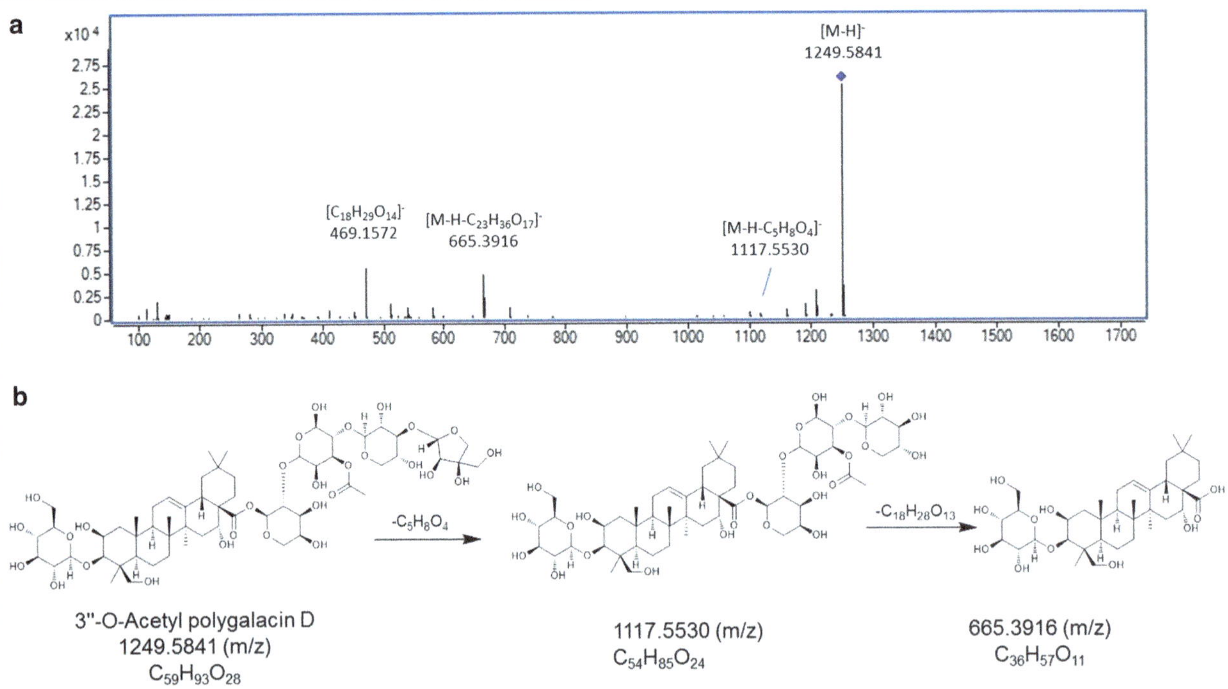

Fig. 7 Mass spectra and proposed major fragmentation pathways of 3″-*O*-acetylpolygalacin D in *Jiegeng* in negative ion mode. **a** Low energy CID mass spectra. **b** Proposed major fragmentation pathway

alterations in *Jiegeng*. We found that sulfur fumigation resulted in significant changes of glycosides, the main bioactive components of *Jiegeng*. Further studies are warranted to determine the mechanism of the transformation of glycosides during sulfur fumigation and whether sulfur fumigation will affect the efficacy and safety of *Jiegeng*.

Abbreviations

UHPLC UHD Q-TOF MS/MS: ultra-high resolution quadrupole time-of-flight mass spectrometry; CP: Pharmacopedia of the People's Republic of China; ESI: electrospray ionization; *m/z*: mass-to-charge ratio; CID: collision-induced dissociation; H_2SO_3: sulfurous acid; SO_2: sulfur dioxide.

Authors' contributions

XQM conducted the experiments and drafted the manuscript. SML carried out the identification of chemical components and drafted the manuscript. CLC participated in the optimization of liquid chromatography. TS and WDL participated in the collection of samples. HC critically reviewed the manuscript. WFF participated in the design of the study. ZLY conceived of the study, designed the experiments and finalized the manuscript. All authors read and approved the final manuscript.

Author details

[1] School of Chinese Medicine, Hong Kong Baptist University, Kowloon Tong, Hong Kong, China. [2] National Engineering Research Center for Modernization of Traditional Chinese Medicine, Zhuhai, Guangdong, China.

Acknowledgements

This work was supported by Grants FRG1/13-14/062 and FRG2/13-14/016 from the Hong Kong Baptist University, HKBU 262512 from the Research Grants Council of Hong Kong, HMRF11122521 from Food and Health Bureau of Hong Kong, and JCYJ20120829154222473 from the Science, Technology and Innovation Commission of Shenzhen, China. We thank Dr. Alexander Kai Man Leung from School of Chinese Medicine, Hong Kong Baptist University for his technical support and his help in the manuscript writing. The major equipment used in this study was substantially supported by a research Grant BCMRC/08-09/01-RDD from the Baptist Chinese Medicine Research Centre Limited.

Competing interests

The authors declared that they have no competing interests.

References

1. Wang S, Hao LJ, Zhu JJ, Zhang QW, Wang ZM, Zhang X, Song XM. Study on the effects of sulfur fumigation on chemical constituents and antioxidant activity of *Chrysanthemum morifolium* cv. Hang-ju. Phytomedicine. 2014;21(5):773–9.
2. Cao G, Li Q, Zhang J, Cai H, Cai B. A purge and trap technique to capture volatile compounds combined with comprehensive two-dimensional gas chromatography/time-of-flight mass spectrometry to investigate the effect of sulfur-fumigation on Radix Angelicae Dahuricae. Biomed Chromatogr: BMC; 2014.
3. Jiang X, Huang LF, Zheng SH, Chen SL. Sulfur fumigation, a better or worse choice in preservation of traditional Chinese medicine? Phytomedicine. 2013;20(2):97–105.
4. Duan Y, Qin KM, Zou NS, Lou YJ, Cai H, Cai BC. Sulfur-fumigation, maintenance method of Chinese herbal medicine-discard or inheritance. *Zhongguo Zhong yao za zhi = Zhongguo zhongyao zazhi =*. Chin Materia Medica. 2013;38(19):3395–9.
5. Liu X, Cai H, Ma XQ, Pei K, Cai BC. Study on HPLC fingerprints of Chrysanthemi Flos before and after sulfur-fumigation *Zhong yao cai = Zhongyaocai*. J Chin Med Materials. 2012;35(5):705–8.
6. Kan WL, Ma B, Lin G. Sulfur fumigation processing of traditional Chinese medicinal herbs: beneficial or detrimental? Front Pharmacol. 2011;2:84.
7. Wang YJ, Guo QS, Yang XW, Xu WB. GC-MS analysis of essential oil from Xiaoboju processed by aeration-desiccation and sulfur-burnin fumigation. *Zhongguo Zhong yao za zhi = Zhongguo zhongyao zazhi =*. Chin J Chin Materia Medica. 2007;32(9):808–13.
8. Farooq M, Hans RK. Metabolic effects of sulfur dioxide fumigation on *Mangifera indica* plants. Bull Environ Contam Toxicol. 1999;63(6):774–81.
9. Choi JH, Yoo KY, Park OK, Lee CH, Won MH, Hwang IK, Ryu SY, Kim YS, Yi JS, Bae YS, et al. Platycodin D and 2″-*O*-acetyl-polygalacin D_2 isolated from *Platycodon grandiflorum* protect ischemia/reperfusion injury in the gerbil hippocampus. Brain Res. 2009;1279:197–208.
10. Dzubak P, Hajduch M, Vydra D, Hustova A, Kvasnica M, Biedermann D, Markova L, Urban M, Sarek J. Pharmacological activities of natural triterpenoids and their therapeutic implications. Nat Prod Rep. 2006;23(3):394–411.
11. Ha YW, Na YC, Seo JJ, Kim SN, Linhardt RJ, Kim YS. Qualitative and quantitative determination of ten major saponins in Platycodi Radix by high performance liquid chromatography with evaporative light scattering detection and mass spectrometry. J Chromatogr A. 2006;1135(1):27–35.
12. Son H, Park YH, Lee SI, Yang HD, Moon HI. Neuroprotective activity of triterpenoid saponins from Platycodi Radix against glutamate-induced toxicity in primary cultured rat cortical cells. Molecules. 2007;12(5):1147–52.
13. Xie Y, Sun HX, Li D. Platycodin D is a potent adjuvant of specific cellular and humoral immune responses against recombinant hepatitis B antigen. Vaccine. 2009;27(5):757–64.
14. Zhan Q. Study on the guiding action of Platycodi Radix in Shengxian decotion and its chemical constituents. Shanghai: Second Military Medical University; 2012.
15. Li SL, Shen H, Zhu LY, Xu J, Jia XB, Zhang HM, Lin G, Cai H, Cai BC, Chen SL, et al. Ultra-high-performance liquid chromatography-quadrupole/time of flight mass spectrometry based chemical profiling approach to rapidly reveal chemical transformation of sulfur-fumigated medicinal herbs, a case study on white ginseng. J Chromatogr A. 2012;1231:31–45.
16. Ma XQ, Leung AK, Chan CL, Su T, Li WD, Li SM, Fong DW, Yu ZL. UHPLC UHD Q-TOF MS/MS analysis of the impact of sulfur fumigation on the chemical profile of Codonopsis Radix (Dangshen). The Analyst. 2014;139(2):505–16.
17. Kim JW, Park SJ, Lim JH, Yang JW, Shin JC, Lee SW, Suh JW, Hwang SB. Triterpenoid saponins isolated from *Platycodon grandiflorum* inhibit hepatitis C virus replication. Evid Based Complement Alternat Med. 2013;2013:560417.
18. Xu BJ, Han LK, Zheng YN, Lee JH, Sung CK. In vitro inhibitory effect of triterpenoidal saponins from Platycodi Radix on pancreatic lipase. Arch Pharmacal Res. 2005;28(2):180–5.
19. Cho JY, Nam KH, Kim AR, Park J, Yoo ES, Baik KU, Yu YH, Park MH. In-vitro and in-vivo immunomodulatory effects of syringin. J Pharm Pharmacol. 2001;53(9):1287–94.
20. Choi J, Shin KM, Park HJ, Jung HJ, Kim HJ, Lee YS, Rew JH, Lee KT. Anti-inflammatory and antinociceptive effects of sinapyl alcohol and its glucoside syringin. Planta Med. 2004;70(11):1027–32.
21. Niu HS, Liu IM, Cheng JT, Lin CL, Hsu FL. Hypoglycemic effect of syringin from *Eleutherococcus senticosus* in streptozotocin-induced diabetic rats. Planta Med. 2008;74(2):109–13.
22. Gong X, Zhang L, Jiang R, Wang CD, Yin XR, Wan JY. Hepatoprotective effects of syringin on fulminant hepatic failure induced by D-galactosamine and lipopolysaccharide in mice. J Appl Toxicol. 2014;34(3):265–71.
23. Dumlu MU, Gurkan E, Tuzlaci E. Chemical composition and antioxidant activity of *Campanula alliariifolia*. Nat Prod Res. 2008;22(6):477–82.
24. Hong S, Yong Y, Kang K, Shin SY, Lee YH, Lim Y. NF-kappa B activation by compounds found in *Platycodon grandiflorum* extract. J Microbiol Biotechn. 2009;19(6):556–9.
25. Sun HX, Chen LQ, Wang JJ, Wang KW, Zhou JY. Structure-function relationship of the saponins from the roots of *Platycodon grandiflorum* for hemolytic and adjuvant activity. Int Immunopharmacol. 2011;11(12):2047–56.
26. Ryu CS, Kim CH, Lee SY, Lee KS, Choung KJ, Song GY, Kim BH, Ryu SY, Lee HS, Kim SK. Evaluation of the total oxidant scavenging capacity of saponins isolated from *Platycodon grandiflorum*. Food Chem. 2012;132(1):333–7.
27. Guo WJAMTB. Studies on constituents and quality control of saponins in *Platycodon grandiflorum*. Peking Union Medical College. 2009.
28. Nikaido T, Koike K, Mitsunaga K, Saeki T. Triterpenoid saponins from root of *Platycodon grandiflorum*. Nat Med (Tokyo). 1998;52:54–9.
29. Yoo DS, Choi YH, Cha MR, Lee BH, Kim SJ, Yon GH, Hong KS, Jang YS, Lee HS, Kim YS, et al. HPLC-ELSD analysis of 18 platycosides from balloon flower roots (Platycodi Radix) sourced from various regions in Korea and geographical clustering of the cultivation areas. Food Chem. 2011;129(2):645–51.
30. Choi YH, Yoo DS, Choi CW, Cha MR, Kim YS, Lee HS, Lee KR, Ryu SY. Platyconic acid A, a genuine triterpenoid saponin from the roots of *Platycodon grandiflorum*. Molecules. 2008;13(11):2871–9.
31. Kubota T, Kitatani H, Hinoh H. The structure of platycogenic acids A, B, and C, further triterpenoid constituents of *Platycodon grandiflorum* A. De Candolle. J Chem Soc. 1969;22:1313–4.

5

Phytochemicals and potential health effects of *Sambucus williamsii* Hance (*Jiegumu*)

Hui-Hui Xiao[1,2], Yan Zhang[3], Raymond Cooper[2], Xin-Sheng Yao[4*] and Man-Sau Wong[1,2*]

Abstract

Sambucus williamsii Hance (*Jiegumu*) is traditionally used in Chinese medicine to treat bone and joint diseases. The major phytochemicals in *S. williamsii* are lignans, terpenoids, and phenolic acids, together with trace amounts of essential oils, minerals, amino acids, and natural pigments. In this review, a database search for studies published from 1990 to November 2015 was conducted using PubMed, the China Academic Journals Full-Text Database, and Google Scholar with the keywords "*Sambucus williamsii* Hance", "*Sambucus williamsii*", "*Sambucus williamsii* + clinic", "*Sambucus williamsii* + biology", "*Sambucus williamsii* + chemicals", and "*Jiegumu*", which covered chemical studies, cell culture studies, animal experiments, and clinical studies. This article reviewed the compounds isolated from *S. williamsii* that may reduce the risk of cancer, and exert antifungal, antioxidant, anti-inflammatory, bone fracture healing, and anti-osteoporotic effects.

Background

Sambucus williamsii Hance (*Jiegumu*) is traditionally used in Chinese medicine to treat bone fractures, rheumatoid arthritis, gout, Kaschin–Beck disease, inflammation-related gastrointestinal disorders, kidney diseases, and wounds [1]. Recent studies [2–12] identified the phytochemicals in *S. williamsii* that exhibit various biological activities, including antifungal effects [2, 3], effects on the proliferation and differentiation of osteoblastic cells [4, 5], fracture healing effects [6], antioxidant, antiglycemic, and hypolipidemic activities [7], anti-inflammatory, gastroprotective, and antinociceptive properties [8, 9], and antiviral [10], antidiabetic [11], antimalarial [12], and antitumor [10] activities. This review describes these phytochemicals and their potential health benefits.

Search strategy

A database search for studies published from 1990 to November 2015 was conducted using PubMed, the China Academic Journals Full-Text Database, and Google Scholar with the keywords "*Sambucus williamsii* Hance", "*Sambucus williamsii*", "*Sambucus williamsii* + clinic", "*Sambucus williamsii* + biology", "*Sambucus williamsii* + chemicals", and "Jiegumu", which covered chemical studies, cell culture studies, animal experiments, and clinical studies. The latest paper was published in October 2015, and the full literature search is outlined in Fig. 1. Using the key terms described above, 1087 publications were found without limiting language, type, or content. All the hits were de-duplicated, and after restricting to English and Chinese languages, research articles, books, or theses, and titles or abstracts containing "*Sambucus williamsii* Hance" or "Jiegumu", 606 papers were identified. Of these, 258 publications with full text were further extracted on the basis that they described chemical studies, in vitro activities, in vivo experiments, and clinical studies (omitting quantitative experiments, extraction and preparation methods, pharmacodynamic studies, and resource investigations). Finally, 102 papers were included in this review.

Botanical characteristics

The genus *Sambucus* was originally placed in the family *Caprifoliaceae*, but subsequently reclassified to *Adoxaceae* according to genetic evidence and morphological

*Correspondence: tyaoxs@jnu.edu.cn; bcmswong@polyu.edu.hk
[2] Department of Applied Biology and Chemical Technology, The Hong Kong Polytechnic University, Hung Hom, Kowloon, Hong Kong, China[4] Institute of Traditional Chinese Medicine & Natural Products, College of Pharmacy, Jinan University, Guangzhou 510632, China
Full list of author information is available at the end of the article

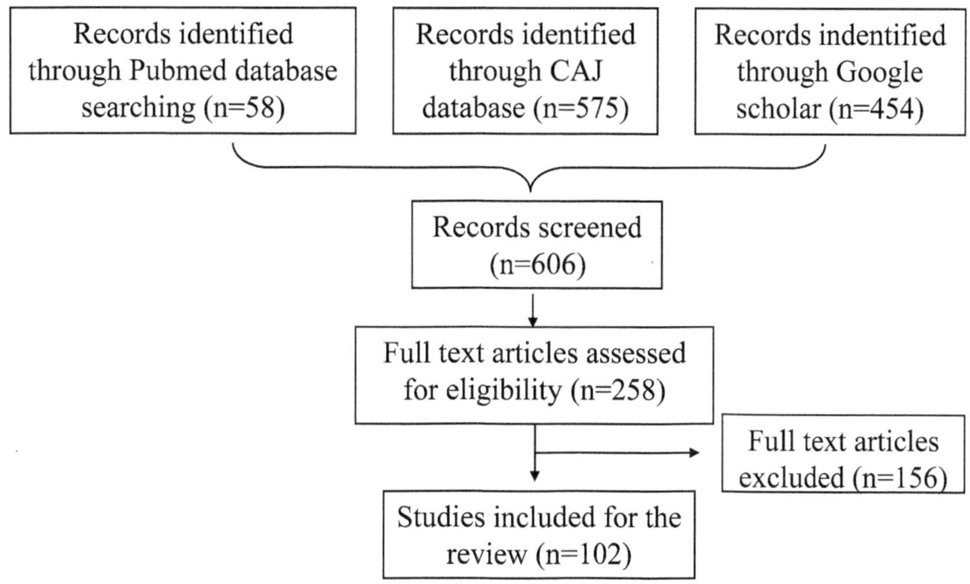

Fig. 1 Flowchart of the search strategy used in this review

comparisons, based on nucleotide sequences of the internally transcribed spacer region of nuclear ribosomal DNA, preliminary morphology, and a combination of the two data sets [13]. The family was reported to comprise at least 115 species and a large number of subspecific taxa [14, 15]. However, a recent revision by Bolli [16] recognized only nine species, with the remainder being synonymized or reduced to subspecific ranks. In China, there are five naturally occurring species within the *Sambucus Linn.* genus: *S. williamsii* and its varieties *var. williamsii* and *var. miquelii* (*Nakai*), *Sambucus adnata Wall.* (*Xuemancao*), *Sambucus sibirica Nakai* (*Xiboliya Jiegumu*) and *Sambucus chinensis Lindl.* (*Jiegucao*); and one introduced variety, *Sambucus nigra Linn.* (*Xiyang Jiegumu*) [17].

Sambucus williamsii is a shrub or small tree growing to a height of 5–6 m (Fig. 2a) that is widely distributed in northeastern China. The aging branches become reddish-brown and exhibit narrowly elliptic lenticels on their surface (Fig. 2b). The leaves are imparipinnate with 2- or 3-jugate leaflets, which are ovate–orbicular or narrowly elliptic at 5–15 × 1.2–7 cm, and irregularly serrate margins (Fig. 2c). The stems terminate in a cymose panicle of 5–11 × 4–14 cm in diameter, with numerous white or yellowish flowers (Fig. 2d). The fruit is a small glossy red berry of 3–5 mm in diameter (Fig. 2e). *Sambucus williamsii* flowers from April to May, and the seeds ripen from September to October. The plant is mostly located along mountain slopes, scrub, stream sides, and roadsides at altitudes of 540–1600 m, and has high environmental adaptability [1, 17].

Medicinal properties

The stem of *S. williamsii* has been used in Chinese medicinal formulae, in combination with other herbs, to treat bone fractures [18, 19]. Medicinal effects include relieving swelling and pain [19–21], promoting blood circulation [20, 21], and acting as an anti-inflammatory effect [21]. The other parts of *S. williamsii* such as the stem bark, root bark, fruit oil, and leaves have been investigated with various biological screening models [2–6, 22–46]. The root bark of *S. williamsii* exerted fracture healing effects [31, 34] similar to those of the stem while the other parts exhibited different effects, such as antifungal [22, 28], anti-inflammatory [33], anticancer [38], and antiaging [37] activities.

An extract of the stem prevented reductions in bone mass and bone strength induced by estrogen deficiency in ovariectomized (OVX) rats and mice [25–27], increased proliferation and differentiation of UMR-106 cells [4, 5, 30, 46], and induced differentiation of pluripotent stem cells into neurons [47]. A stem extract of *S. williamsii* exerted beneficial effects on the microarchitecture of trabecular bone and inhibitory effects on urinary calcium excretion in OVX mice by upregulating the ratio of osteoprotegerin to receptor activator of nuclear factor-κB ligand expression in bone obtained from OVX mice [26]. The stem extract exerted free radical-scavenging properties [23], reversed damage to the function of INS-1E β cells induced by alloxan, and increased insulin excretion [24], while the stem bark extract showed antifungal activities by damaging the fungal plasma membrane [2, 3, 22, 48]. The root bark extract exerted healing

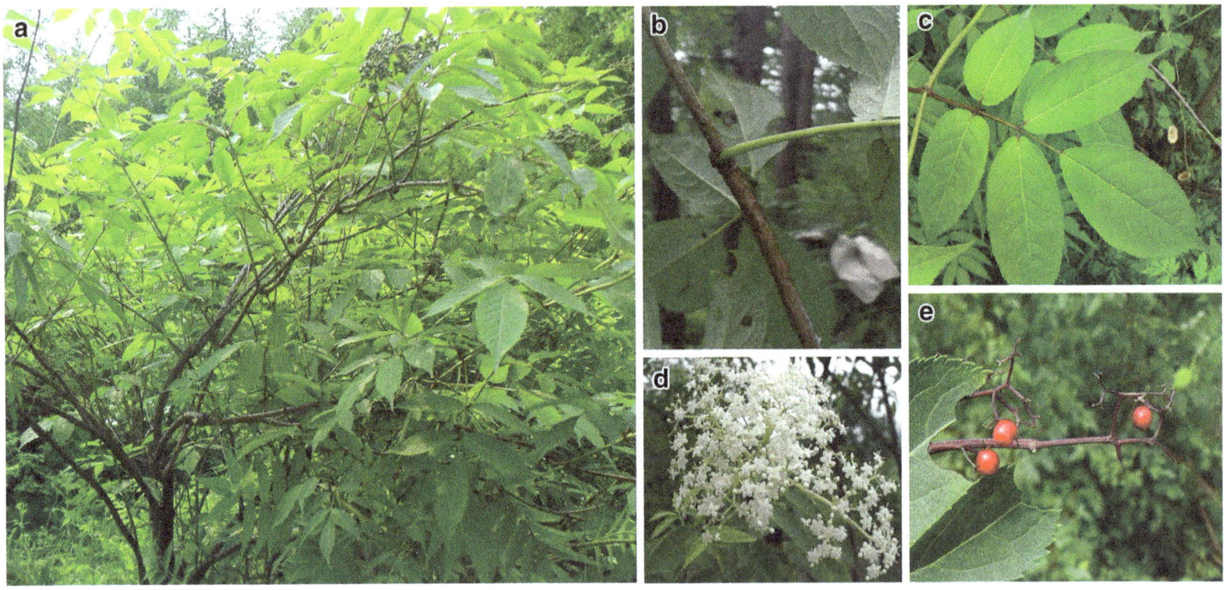

Fig. 2 *S. williamsii* Hance (*Jiegumu*) is characterized by elliptic lenticels on branches, imparipinnate leaves with irregularly serrate margins, white or yellowish flowers, and small glossy red berries. **a** *S. williamsii* Hance; **b** branch; **c** leaf; **d** flower; **e**: berry

effects on rabbit bone fractures [6, 31, 34], inhibitory effects on xylene-induced mouse ear edema and carrageenan-induced rat paw edema, and analgesic properties in rats and mice [33]. A mechanistic study showed that an ethanol extract of the root bark promoted MC3T3-E1 cell proliferation and differentiation through the bone morphogenetic protein 2/Smad/p38/c-Jun N-terminal kinase/runt-related transcription factor 2 signaling pathway [35]. The fruit oil exhibited immune-boosting [36], anticancer [38], and memory-improving [39] effects in mice, and antihyperlipidemic [37, 40] and antiaging [37] effects in rats. Furthermore, the leaves extract exhibited antibacterial [44] and anti-inflammatory [45] effects. The details of the bioactivities and chemical components in various parts of *S. williamsii* are listed in Additional file 1 [2–7, 20–34, 36–67].

Chemical composition and potential health effects

To date, publications have described chemical research on many parts of *S. williamsii*, including the stem, root bark, leaves, and berries. The chemicals discovered in these components currently include 59 lignans [2–4, 6, 22, 27, 28, 46, 49, 68], 26 terpenoids represented by 16 iridoids, two sesquiterpenoids, and eight triterpenoids [4, 6, 29, 30, 49–58], 13 phenolic acids [4, 5, 56, 58], seven aliphatic compounds [4, 7, 30, 50, 57], 50 essential oils [59, 60], and 23 other compounds [4, 6, 45, 50–52, 56, 58]. Furthermore, several minerals [61], amino acids [61], and natural pigments [62] were identified in the fruit of *S. williamsii*.

Lignans

Chemical

The lignans in *S. williamsii* include furofurans (**1**–**7**) [2, 4, 6, 28], dibenzyltyrolactones (**8**) [6], tetrahydrofurans (**9**–**15**) [4, 68], and arylnaphthalenes (**16**–**20**) [28, 63], representing the classical types of lignans, formed by oxidative coupling through a link between the β-carbons of the side chains of two phenylpropanoids (8–8′ link) [69] (Fig. 3). Benzodioxanes (**21**) [6], eupomatenoid benzofurans (**22**–**34**) [4, 6, 28, 46], and 8-*O*-4′ lignans (**35**–**43**) [6, 27, 28, 49, 63] are considered to be subtypes of neolignans, with carbon linkages between C8–*O*–C3′/C7–*O*–C4′, C8–C3′/C7–*O*–C4′, and C8–*O*–C4′, respectively (Fig. 4). Compounds **44**–**59** [4, 6, 28, 46] are oligomeric lignans composed of more than two C6–C3 units (Fig. 5). These lignans represent the most abundant compounds isolated from *S. williamsii.*

Health effects of lignans

These biphenolic compounds have similar structures to estrogens. They are the major source of phytoestrogens in the diets of Western populations and are primarily found in fiber-rich foods such as seeds, grains, vegetables, and fruits [70].

In the human gut, plant lignans are converted by intestinal bacteria into two enterolignans, enterolactone (ENL) and enterodiol (END), that exhibit biological activities and are absorbed into the bloodstream [71, 72]. Lignans also exhibit antiosteoporotic and antifungal effects [3] and can reduce the risk of cancer [73].

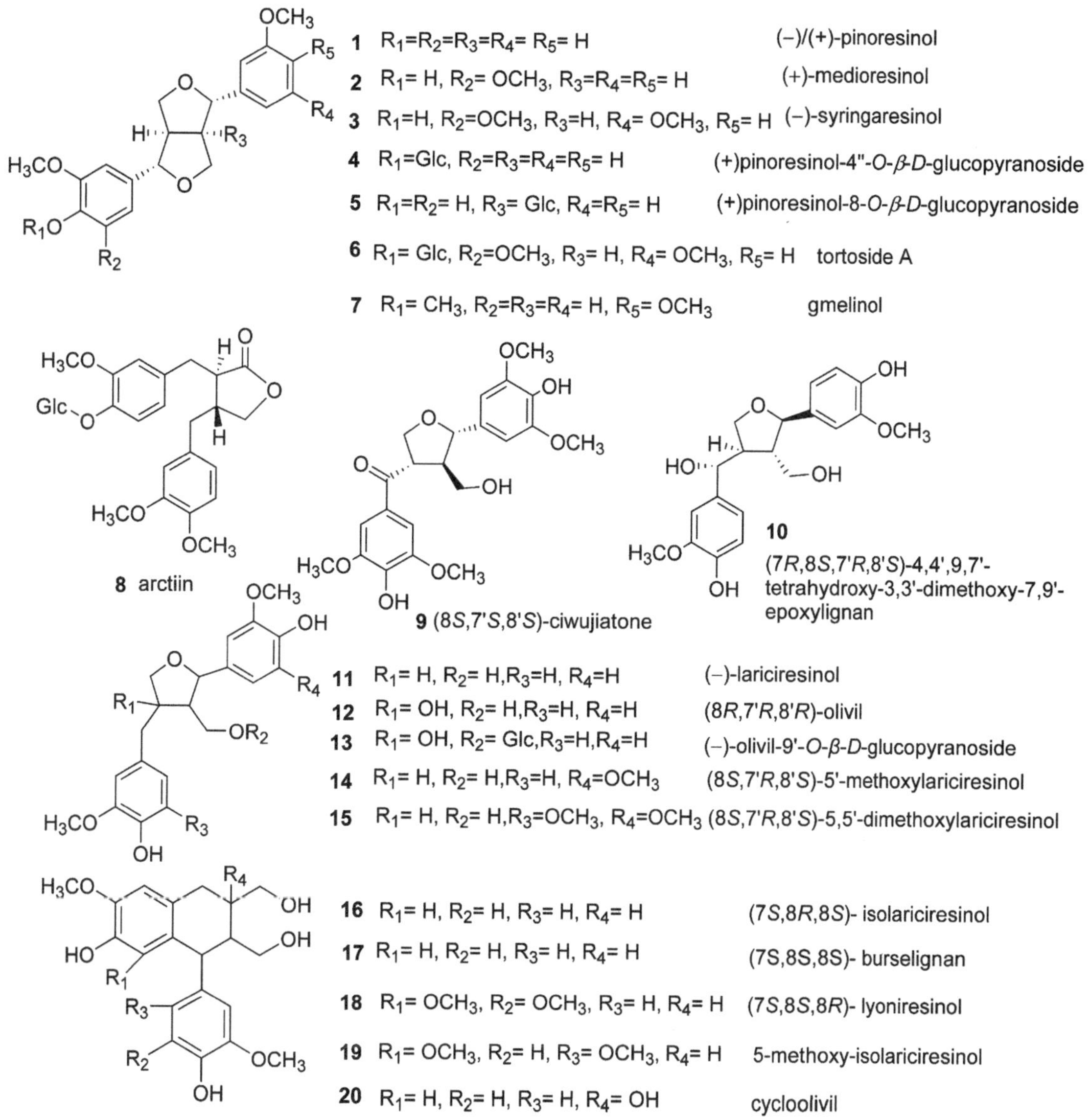

Fig. 3 Chemical structures of lignans in *S. williamsii* with representative structures: classical types of lignans with an 8–8′ link

Osteoprotective effects

The potential therapeutic effects of *S. williamsii* on postmenopausal osteoporosis in animal models and their underlying mechanisms of action [25–27] have been investigated. The active compounds with potential osteoprotective effects were identified by biological assay-guided fractionation [27, 46, 74]. Specifically, an ethanol extract of the stem of *S. williamsii* exhibited protective effects on trabecular bone mass and mechanical strength of cortical bone in OVX rats fed a normal diet and mice fed a phytoestrogen-free AIN-93M diet [25, 26]. Moreover, the chemicals including lignans, phenolic acids and triterpenoids in the ethanol extract of *S. williamsii* stem stimulated osteogenesis by promoting osteoblastic proliferation and differentiation [25, 27, 46, 68].

A combination of 50 and 95 % aqueous ethanolic fractions from a crude extract of *S. williamsii* stem purified on a reverse-phase macroporous resin column was the mixture exhibiting the most potent antiosteoporotic activity [27]. Further isolation of the *S. williamsii* active fraction by a series of chromatography steps and preparative high-performance liquid chromatography led to the separation and identification of 55 lignans [27, 28, 46, 49, 63].

In vitro experiments [75] revealed that one of these lignans, compound **38**, exhibited estrogen-like effects in osteoblast-like UMR-106 cells, MC3T3-E1 cells, and

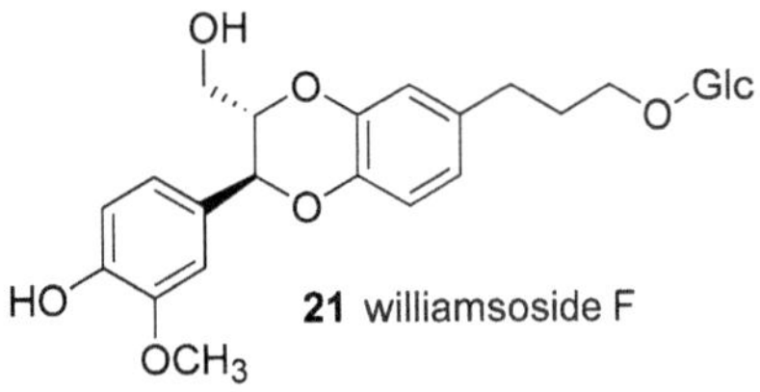

21 williamsoside F

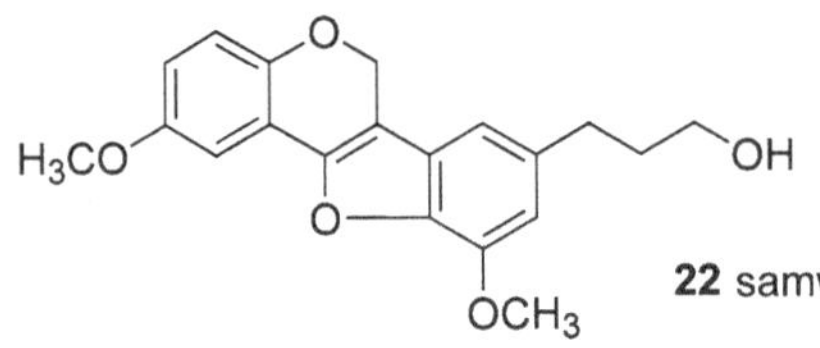

22 samwinol

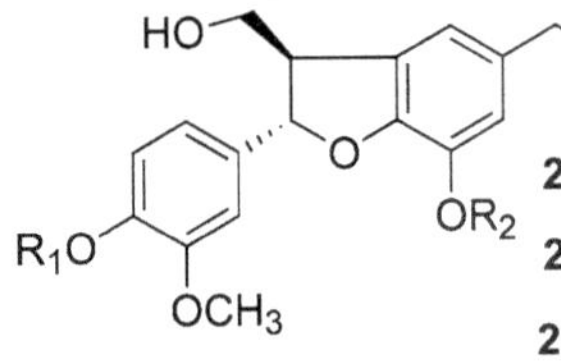

23 R_1= H, R_2= H, R_3= H (+)-cedrusin

24 R_1= H, R_2= CH_3, R_3= H dihydrodehydodiconifyl alcohol

25 R_1= H, R_2= CH_3, R_3= Glc glochidioboside

26 R_1= H, R_2= CH_3, R_3= Glc-Api samwiside

27 R_1= Glc, R_2= CH_3, R_3= H dihydrodehydrodiconiferyl alcohol-4-*O*-*β*-*D*-glucopyranoside

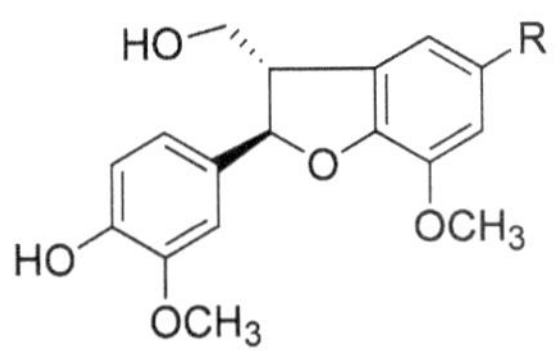

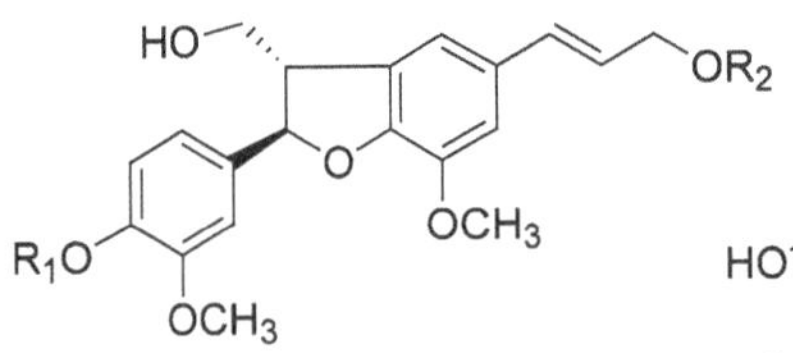

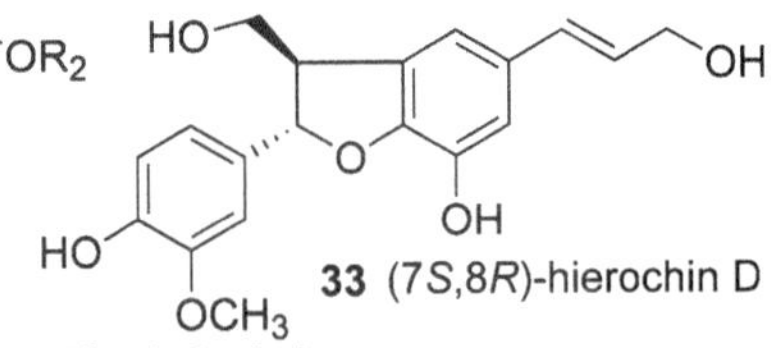

33 (7*S*,8*R*)-hierochin D

28 R= COH (7*R*,8*S*)-Ficusal

29 R= COOH (7*R*,8*S*)-Ceplignan

30 R_1= H, R_2=H (7*R*,8*S*)-dehydrodiconiferyl alcohol

31 R_1= H, R_2= CH_3 (7*R*,8*S*)-dehydrodiconiferyl alcohol-γ′-methyl ether

32 R_1=Glc, R_2= H dehydrodiconiferyl alcohol-4-*O*-*β*-*D*-glucopyranoside

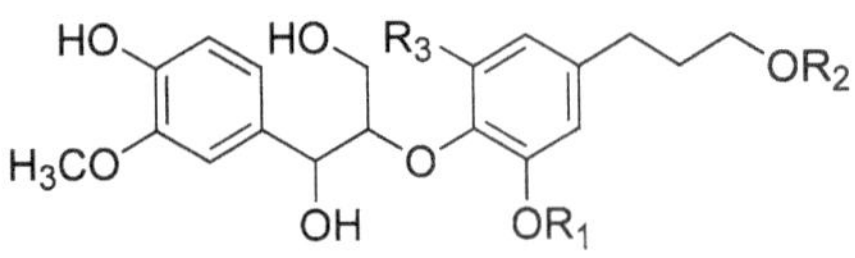

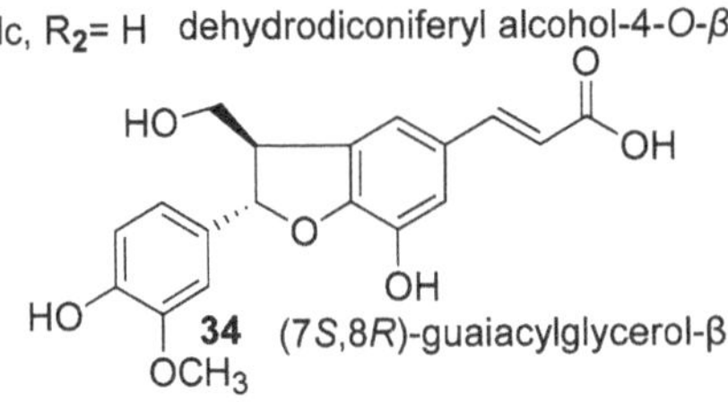

34 (7*S*,8*R*)-guaiacylglycerol-β-coniferyl aldehyde ether

35 R_1= Glc, R2= H, R_3= H 4,7,9,9'-tetrahydroxy-3-methoxy-8-*O*-4'-neolignan-3'-*O*-*β*-*D*-glucopyranoside

36 R_1= H, R_2= Glc, R_3= H williamsoside H

37 R_1= CH_3 , R_2= H, R_3= H (+/-)-*erythro*-1-(4-hydroxy-3-methoxyphenyl)-2-[4-(3-hydroxypropanyl)-2-methoxyphenoxyl]-1, 3-propanediol

38 R_1= CH_3 , R_2= H, R_3= H (+/-)-*threo*-1-(4-hydroxy-3-methoxyphenyl)-2-[4-(3-hydroxypropanyl)-2-methoxyphenoxyl]-1, 3-propanediol

39 R_1= H, R2= H, R_3= H *erythro*-3-methoxy-8,4-oxyneolignan-3,4,7,9,9 -pentol

40 R_1= H, R2= H, R_3= H *threo*-3-methoxy-8,4-oxyneolignan-3,4,7,9,9 -pentol

41 R_1= CH_3, R2= H, R_3= OCH_3 1-(4-hydroxy-3-methoxyphenyl)-2-[4-(3-hydroxypropanyl)-2,6-dimethoxyphenoxyl]-1, 3-propanediol

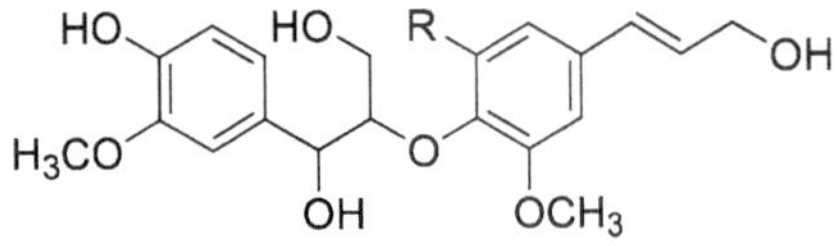

42 R= H (7*S*,8*R*)/(7*R*,8*R*)-guaiacylglycerol-*β*-*O*-4'-coniferyl ether

43 R= OCH_3 *erythro*-guaiacylglycerol-*β*-*O*-4'-sinapyl ether

Fig. 4 Chemical structures of lignans in *S. williamsii* with representative structures: neolignans with carbon linkages between C8–*O*–C3′/C7–*O*–C4′, C8–C3′/C7–*O*–C4′, and C8–*O*–C4′

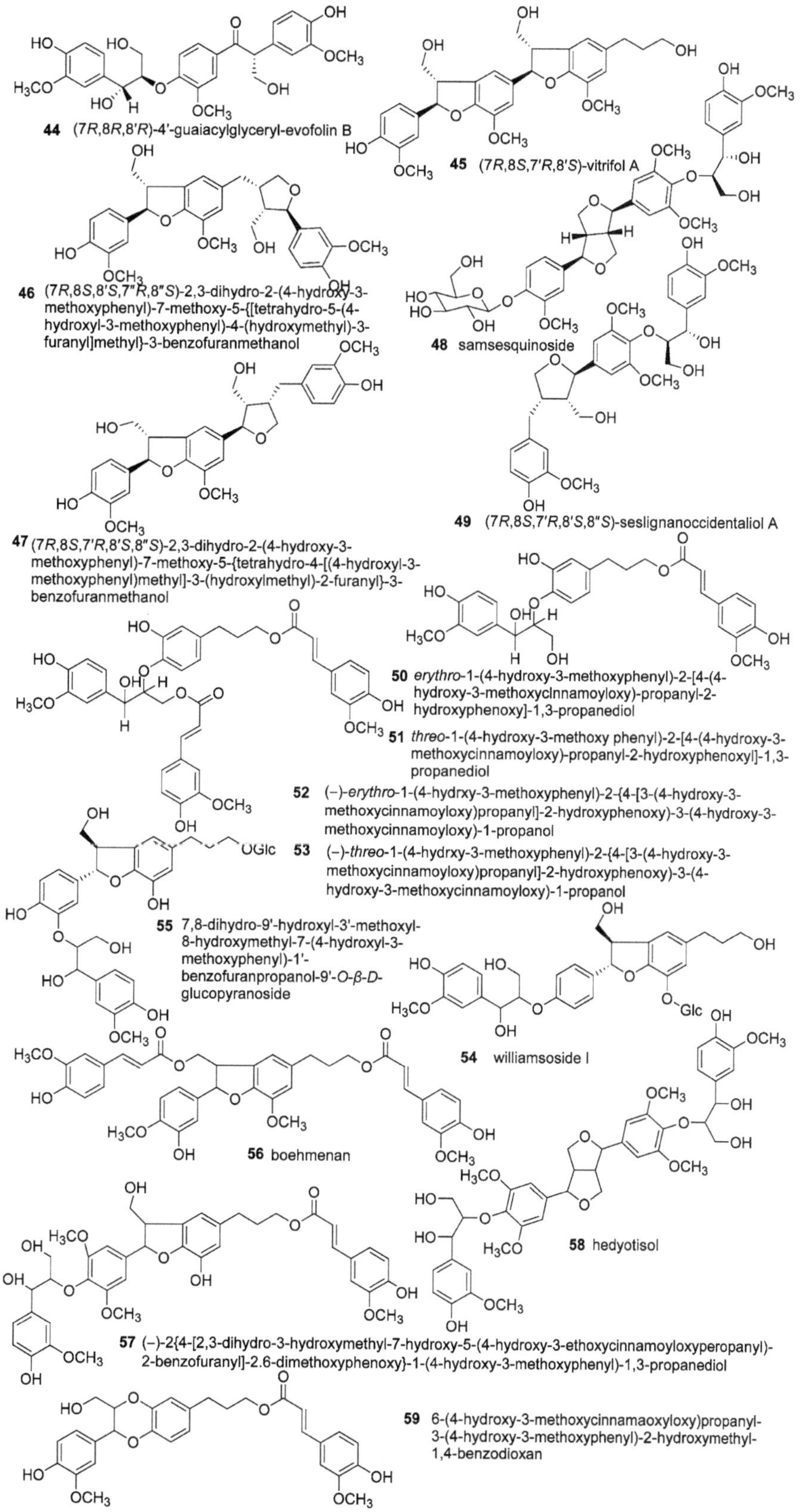

Fig. 5 Chemical structures of lignans in *S. williamsii* with representative structures: oligomeric lignans

bone mesenchymal stem cells. The results also showed that compound **38** exerted biological actions in osteoblast-like cells through ligand-independent, estrogen response element-independent, and mitogen-activated protein kinase-mediated rapid nongenomic estrogen receptor signaling pathways [75].

Antifungal activity

Pinoresinol (**1**), lariciresinol (**11**), (−)-olivil-9′-*O*-β-D-glucopyranoside (**13**), and glochidioboside (**25**) were all isolated from *S. williamsii*. They exhibited antifungal effects on human pathogenic strains through a membrane-disrupting action [2, 3, 22, 48]. (+)-Medioresinol (**2**), a furofuran-type lignan, isolated from the stem bark of *S. williamsii*, also exerted antifungal effects, but through the accumulation of reactive oxygen species in mitochondria [68].

Anticancer activity

Several studies [76, 77] showed that increased dietary lignan intake and/or increased levels of ENL and/or END might protect against or reduce the risk of breast, colon, and prostate cancers, and reduce hair loss. Lignans and their related metabolites were believed to be partly responsible for the growth inhibition of human prostate cancer cell lines [77]. ENL and END significantly inhibited the growth of prostate cancer PC-3 and LNCaP cells with 50 % inhibitive concentration at 57 and 100 μM respectively [77]. Treatment of human colon cancer SW480 cells with ENL and END, either alone or in combination, resulted in dose- and time-dependent decreases in cell number [78].

The administration of plant lignans, which were further metabolized to ENL and END, inhibited or delayed the onset of mammary cancer [71]. Although the mechanism of the anticarcinogenic action of ENL is not yet fully understood, there is intriguing evidence for ENL as a modulator of estrogen signaling [71]. Consumption of lignans such as lariciresinol (**11**) and pinoresinol (**1**) was associated with a significant reduction in breast cancer risk according to the clinical results of premenopausal women in Mexico [79].

Phenolic acids

Chemical characteristics

Thirteen phenolic compounds, vanillin (**60**), vanillic acid (**61**), acetovanillone (**62**), coniferyl aldehyde (**63**), ferulic acid (**64**), syringaldehyde (**65**), 4-hydroxybenzoic acid (**66**), 4-hydroxycinnamic acid (**67**), protocatechuic acid (**68**), indole-3-carboxylic acid (**69**), syringic acid-4-*O*-α-L-rhamnopyranoside (**70**), coniferyl alcohol (**71**), and methyl caffeate (**72**), were isolated from the stem and root bark of *S. williamsii* (Fig. 6) [5, 27, 28, 56, 58].

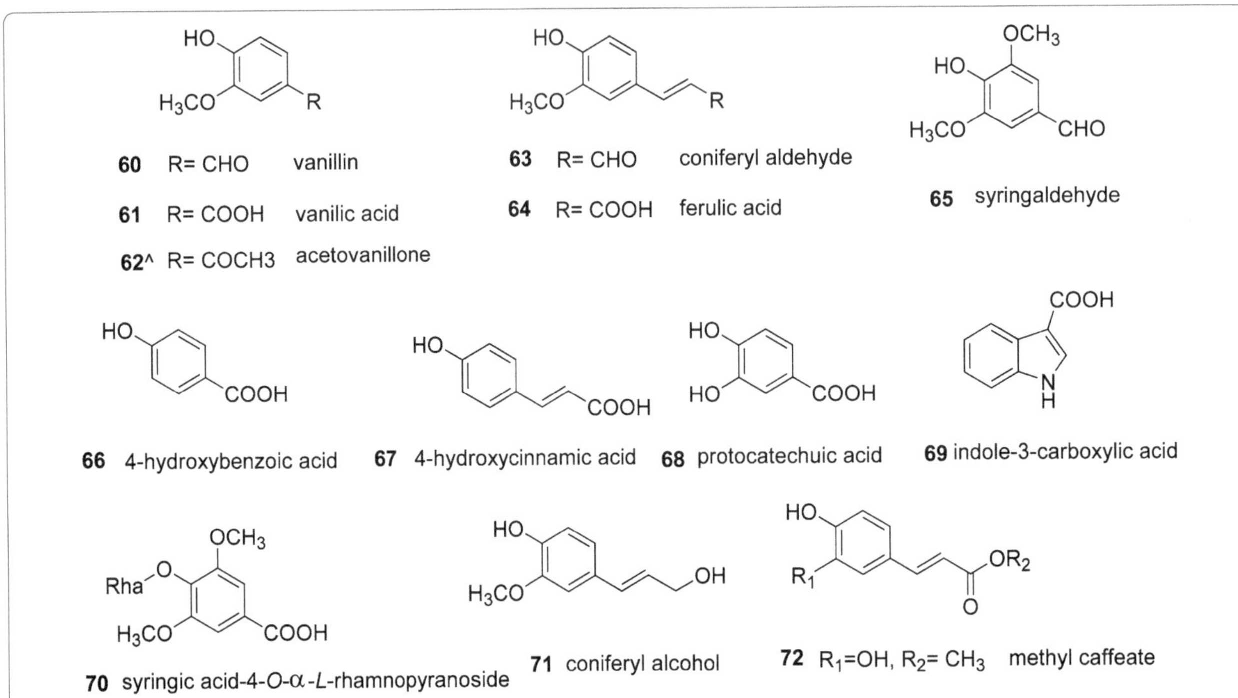

Fig. 6 Chemical structures of phenolic acids present in *S. williamsii*

Health benefits of phenolic acids

Vanillic acid (**61**) exerts estrogen-like actions in osteoblastic-like cells through a nongenomic estrogen receptor signaling pathway involving the mitogen-activated protein kinase pathway [80]. The compound also exhibits antibacterial [81] and antimicrobial [82] activities and chemopreventive effects in experimentally induced carcinogenesis [83]. The protective effects of vanillic acid on myocardial infarction were studied in isoproterenol-induced cardiotoxic rats [84]. The free radical-scavenging, antioxidant, and anti-inflammatory activities of vanillic acid reduced isoproterenol-induced oxidative stress, downregulated myocardial interleukin-1β, interleukin-6, and tumor necrosis factor-α gene expression, and inhibited inflammation, thereby preventing cell death and protecting the myocardium [84].

Ferulic acid (**64**) possesses high antioxidant capacity and exhibits a longer residence time in rats than vitamin C [85]. Ferulic acid exhibits a wide range of therapeutic effects against many chronic conditions, including inflammation, cancer, apoptosis, diabetes, cardiovascular diseases, and neurodegenerative diseases [86]. It may also assist in plant host defense against pathogens and pests [87].

Protocatechuic acid (**68**) is an effective agent in reducing the carcinogenic actions of diethyl nitrosamine in the liver [88], 4-nitroquinoline-L-oxide in the oral cavity [89], azoxymethane in the colon [90], *N*-methyl-*N*-nitrosourea in the glandular stomach tissue [91], and *N*-butyl-*N*-(4-hydroxybutyl) nitrosamine in the bladder [92]. Protocatechuic acid also exhibits protective effects against the oxidative damage induced by tert-butyl hydroperoxide in rat primary hepatocytes by quenching free radicals [93]. Syringaldehyde (**65**) has six times higher antioxidant activity than protocatechuic acid [94]. Furthermore, syringaldehyde exerts antifungal activity against *Candida guilliermondii* [95], and exhibits antioncogenic activity through its inhibitory actions on murine pulmonary and hepatic microsomes [96]. Syringaldehyde shows stimulatory effects on both proliferation and alkaline phosphatase activity in UMR-106 cells [5]. 4-Hydroxybenzoic acid (**67**) exerts a hypoglycemic effect and increases serum insulin levels and liver glycogen contents in normal rats after oral administration at 5 mg/kg [97].

Terpenoids

Chemical characteristics

Sixteen iridoids [6, 49, 51, 52, 54, 56], two sesquiterpenoids [4, 30, 58], and eight triterpenoids [4, 29, 50, 57] were identified in *S. williamsii* (Fig. 7). The iridoids are characterized by the presence of a partially hydrogenated *cis*-fused cyclopenta [c] pyran system, arising from intramolecular acetylation of a 1,5-cyclopenta dialdehyde moiety, and they are usually stabilized by acetylation or esterification. Iridoids can be subdivided into four groups: iridoid glycosides, simple iridoids or non-glycosidic iridoids, secoiridoids, and bisiridoids [98]. Compounds **73–77** were isolated as iridoid glycosides possessing a 9-carbon skeleton with glycosides linked to C1–OH. Compounds **78–88** belong to the secoiridoid subclass indicated by a bond-break between C7 and C8. Compounds **89** and **90** are the two sesquiterpenoids that have been isolated from *S. williamsii.* The eight triterpenoids are compounds **91–98** and represent three subclasses: urane (**91**, **92**), lupine (**93–95**), and oleanane (**96–98**).

Health benefits of terpenoids

Triterpenoids from plants possess a wide spectrum of pharmacological activities such as anti-inflammatory, antiulcer, antihyperlipidemic, antitumor, and hepatoprotective actions [99, 100]. α-Amyrin (**91**) possesses antimicrobial, anti-inflammatory, gastroprotective, and antinociceptive properties [8, 9], while betulinic acid (**94**) exhibits anti-inflammatory [101], antiviral [10], antidiabetic [11], antimalarial [12], and antitumor [10] activities.

Aliphatic compounds

Chemical characteristics

Seven aliphatic compounds, triacontanoic acid (**99**), tianshic acid (**100**), hexadecanoic acid (**101**), (9*E*)-8,11,12-trihydroxyoctadecenoic acid methyl ester (**102**), linoleic acid (**103**), lupeol-3-palmitate (**104**), and 1-octacosanol (**105**), were isolated and identified from the stem of *S. williamsii* (Fig. 8) [4, 7, 30, 50, 57].

Health benefits of aliphatic compounds

Linoleic acid (**103**) extracted from *S. williamsii* seed oil with a yield of 65.81 % possesses antioxidant, antiglycemic, and hypolipidemic activities [7]. It exerts free radical-scavenging activity at 61.9 mg/mL, inhibits the activity of α-glucosidase at 1.5–25 mg/mL, and significantly improves serum lipid levels in hyperlipidemic mice [7].

Lupeol-3-palmitate (**104**) significantly reduced prostaglandin E2 production in A23187-stimulated macrophages [102]. The anti-inflammatory effect of a lupeol-rich extract was similar to that exhibited by the selective cyclooxygenase inhibitor indomethacin [102, 103].

Saturated aliphatic compounds are known to have harmful effects on human health, but only trace amounts of

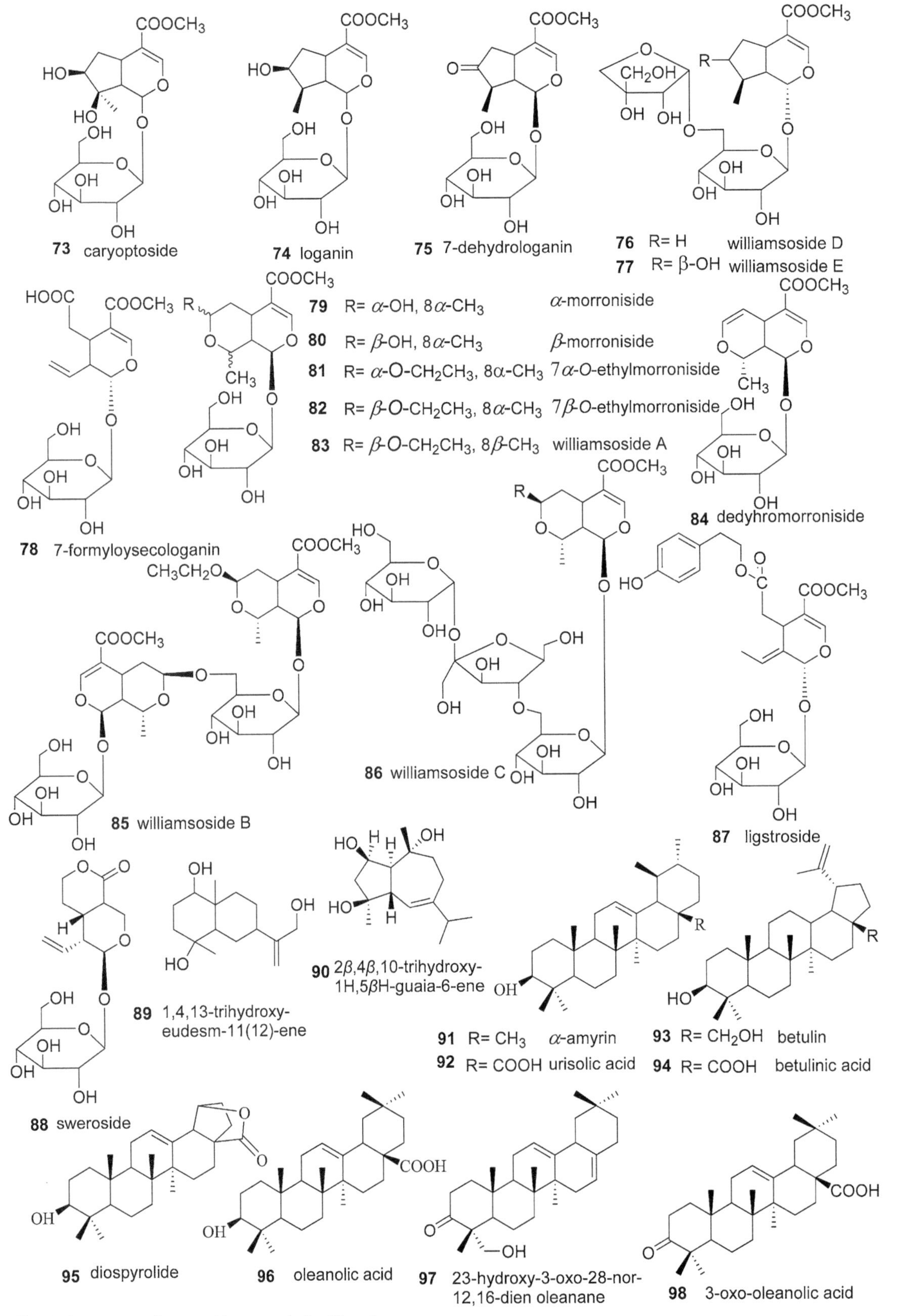

Fig. 7 Chemical structures of terpenoids present in *S. williamsii*

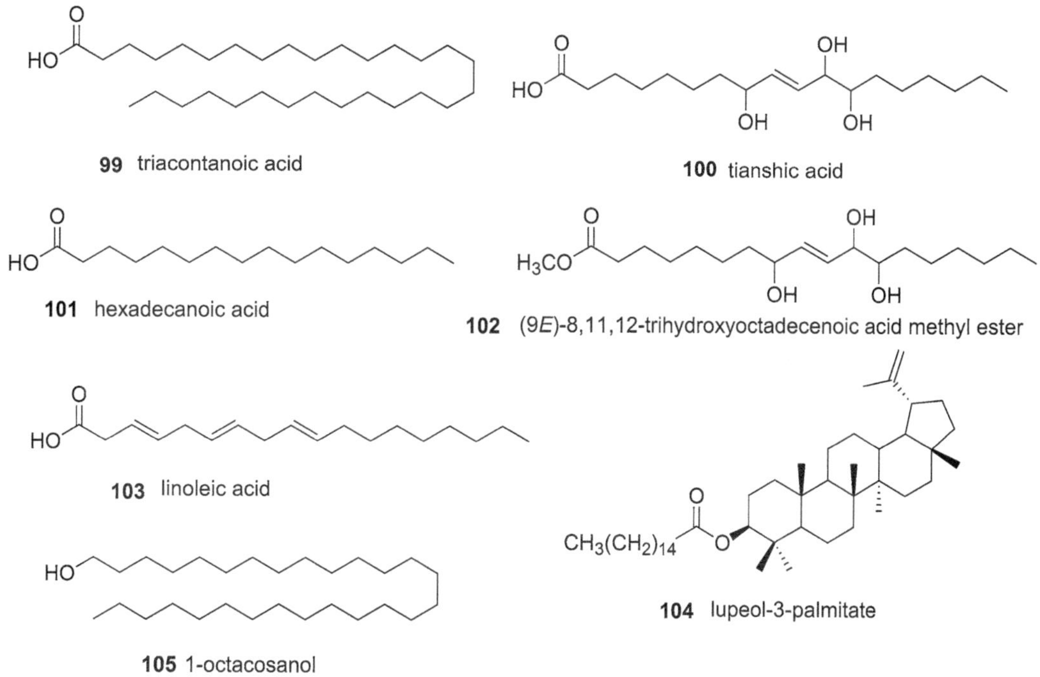

Fig. 8 Chemical structures of aliphatic compounds present in *S. williamsii*

saturated aliphatic compounds have been identified in *S. williamsii*. Hexadecanoic acid (**101**) found in *S. williamsii* induces oxidative stress and apoptosis of insulin-secreting cells [104, 105] and causes cardiac cells to undergo apoptosis [106]. It also causes insulin resistance in the brain by impairing the ability of insulin to activate intracellular signaling pathways [107], and accelerates obesity with diets containing high amounts of hexadecanoic acid [107].

Other compounds

Fifty essential oils in *S. williamsii* were extracted by steam distillation and identified by gas chromatography-mass spectrometry, as listed in Table 1. Among them, *cis*-3-hexenyl-3-methylbutanoate and salicylic acid methyl ester were the major components [60].

Several isoflavonoids, anthraquinones, steroids, alcohols, ketones, phenylpropanoids, acids, coumarins, and nitrogen-containing compounds were isolated from the stem and root bark of *S. williamsii* (Fig. 9). These compounds included puerarin (**106**), emodin (**107**), quercetin (**108**), kaempferol (**109**), 3-methoxy-4-(2-glycerol)-phenylpropanol (**110**), coniferyl alcohol 9-*O*-β-D-glucopyranoside (**111**), samwirin (**112**), samwiphenol (**113**), 8*R*-evofolin (**114**), 3-methoxy-4-(2-glycerol)-phenylpropanol (**115**), rosenonolactone (**116**), phaseic acid (**117**), umbelliferone (**118**), 3,4-dimethoxy-*N*-β-D-glucosyl pyrrole (**119**), 3-methoxyl-1*H*-pyrrole (**120**), *N*-methyl-β-alanine anhydride (**121**), β-sitosterol (**122**), β-sitosterol-β-D-glucoside (**123**), stigmasterol (**124**), 5-(1′-hydroxyethyl)-methyl nicotinate (**125**), 3-(hydroxyl-acetyl)indole (**126**), 4′-hydroxy-*N*-(4-hydroxy-3-methoxybenzoyl)-3′,5′-dimethoxy-benzamide (**127**), and (1*S*,3*S*)-1-methyl-1,2,3,4-tetrahydro-β-carboline-3-carboxylic acid (**128**) [4, 6, 29, 45, 50, 51, 56, 58]. Du et al. [61] systemically studied the berries of *S. williamsii* and identified 17 amino acids and 14 microelements (Table 2), which may account for the fruit's nutritional properties.

Conclusions

This article reviewed the phytochemicals identified from *S. williamsii*, together with their biological activities and potential health benefits. Although several biological activities were ascribed to *S. williamsii*, the most important beneficial effects identified to date, based on

Table 1 The structures and molecular formula of essential oils in *S. williamsii*

No.	Compound	Molecular formula	Relative amount (%)
1	Hexanal	$C_6H_{12}O$	0.05
2	α-Terpineol	$C_{10}H_{18}O$	0.06
3	4-Terpineol	$C_{10}H_{18}O$	0.08
4	α-Pinene	$C_{10}H_{16}$	0.09
5	Camphor	$C_{10}H_{16}O$	0.11
6	δ-Elemene	$C_{15}H_{24}$	0.11
7	Heneicosane	$C_{21}H_{44}$	0.21
8	2-Pentadecanone	$C_{15}H_{30}O$	0.24
9	3-Methyl-pentanoic acid methyl ester	$C_7H_{14}O_2$	0.26
10	6,10-Dimethyl-5,9-undecadien-2-one	$C_{13}H_{22}O3$	0.38
11	Diallyl disulphide	$C_6H_{12}S_2$	0.41
12	Eicosane	$C_{20}H_{42}$	0.42
13	3-Vinyl-1,2-dithio cyclohe-5-ene	$C_7H_{10}S_2$	0.44
14	Thymol	$C_{10}H_{14}O$	0.48
15	β-Ionone	$C_{13}H_{20}O$	0.48
16	Hexadecane	$C_{16}H_{34}$	0.64
17	Epi-bicyclosequiphellandrene	$C_{15}H_{24}$	0.69
18	Ethyl salicylate	$C_9H_{10}O_3$	0.69
19	2,4,10,14-Tetramethyl pentadecane	$C_{20}H_{42}$	0.76
20	Hexanoic acid 2-hexenyl ester	$C_{12}H_{22}O_2$	0.83
21	Heptadecane	$C_{17}H_{36}$	0.85
22	Hyacinthin	C_8H_8O	0.87
23	Dihydro-β-agarofuran	$C_{15}H_{26}O$	0.89
24	3-Methyl-pentanoic acid	$C_6H_{12}O_2$	1.10
25	1,2-Dithiolane,1,1-dioxide	$C_3H_6O_2S_2$	1.26
26	Decanal	$C_8H_{16}O$	1.30
27	1-Heptan-3-ol	$C_7H_{14}O$	1.33
28	Ethyl caproate	$C_8H_{16}O_2$	1.34
29	Isoamyl isovalerate	$C_{10}H_{20}O_2$	1.52
30	Heptanal	$C_7H_{14}O$	1.53
31	Benzaldehyde	C_7H_6O	1.85
32	Cyclotetradecane	$C_{14}H_{28}$	1.95
33	Hexanoic acid hexyl ester	$C_{12}H_{24}O_2$	1.96
34	L-Linalool	$C_{10}H_{18}O$	2.04
35	Isovaleric acid	$C_5H_{10}O_2$	2.08
36	3-Methyl-1-butanol	$C_5H_{12}O$	2.11
37	Octanal	$C_7H_{14}O$	2.11
38	*cis*-3-Hexenol	$C_6H_{12}O$	2.19
39	trans-2-Hexenyl isovalerate	$C_{11}H_{20}O_2$	2.23
40	Benzyl isovalerate	$C_{12}H_{16}O_2$	3.04
41	4-Methoxy-6-(2-propenyl)-1,3-benzodioxole	$C_{18}H_{18}O_3$	3.10
42	2-Phenylethyl-3-methylbutanoate	$C_{13}H_{18}O_2$	3.11
43	*cis*-3-Hexenyl caproate	$C_{12}H_{22}O_2$	3.24
44	3-Methyl-butanoic acid ethyl ester	$C_7H_{14}O_2$	3.68
45	2-Heptanone	$C_7H_{14}O$	3.86
46	Hexyl isovalerate	$C_{11}H_{22}O_2$	4.02
47	1-Methoxy-4-(1-propenyl)benzene	$C_{10}H_{12}O$	6.29
48	1-Methoxy-4-(2-propenyl)benzene	$C_{10}H_{12}O$	6.79
49	*cis*-3-Hexenyl-3-methylbutanoate	$C_{11}H_{20}O_2$	14.03
50	Salicylic acid methyl ester	$C_8H_8O_3$	22.89

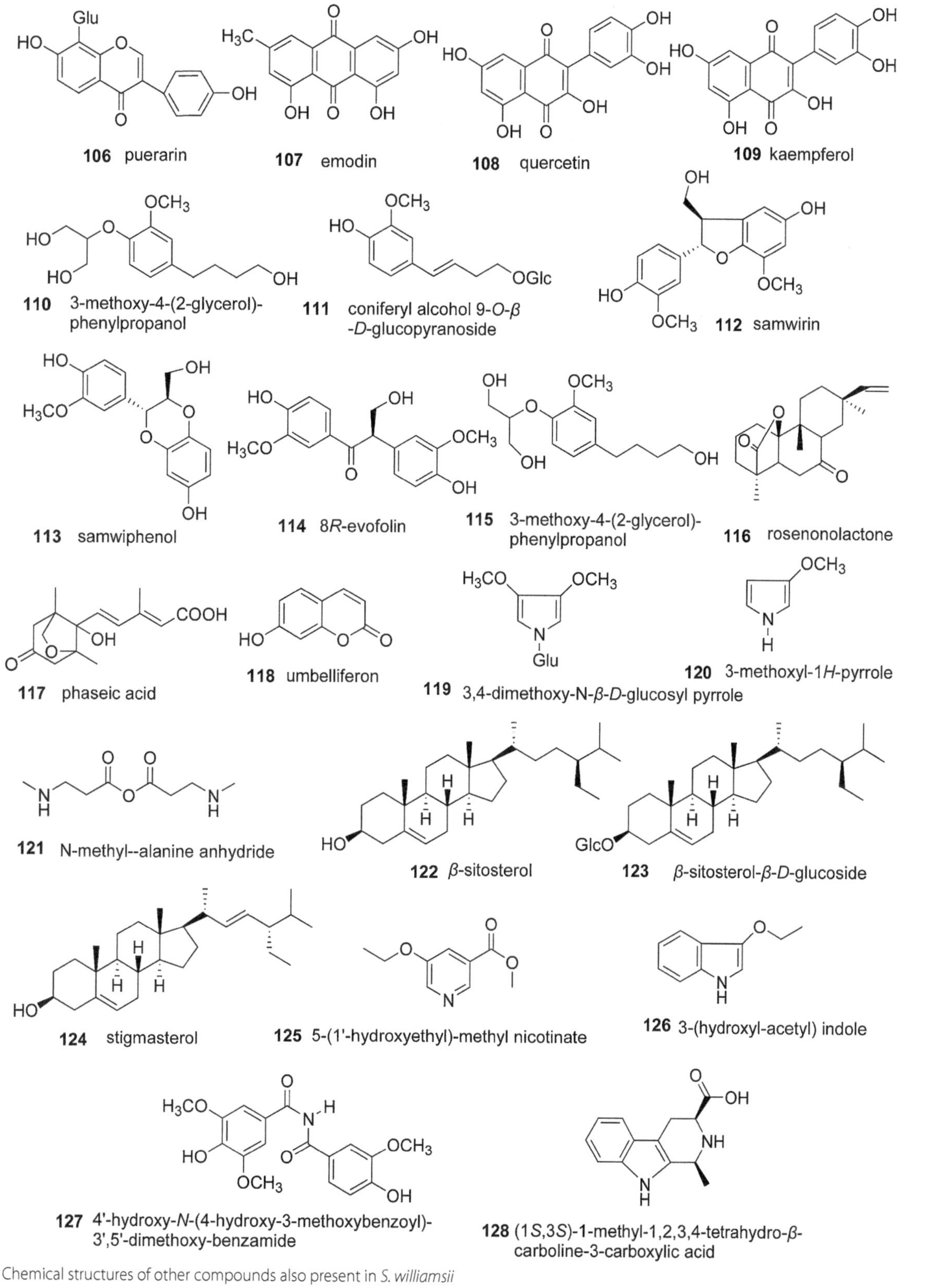

Fig. 9 Chemical structures of other compounds also present in *S. williamsii*

Table 2 The components of amino acids and microelements in *S. williamsii*

Amino acid	Content (mg/100 mL)
Aspartic acid	8.295
Threonine	2.253
Serine	3.145
Glutamic acid	9.759
Glycine	2.876
Alanine	3.152
Cysteine	0.420
Valine	2.615
Methionine	0.451
Isoleucine	2.158
Leucine	3.588
Tyrosine	1.784
Phenylalanine	2.216
Lysine	3.301
Histidine	1.279
Arginine	2.917
Proline	3.946
Microelements	**Content (μg/g)**
K	752
Ca	52.9
Zn	1.53
Fe	5.71
Cr	0.09
Cu	0.99
Mn	0.48
Ni	0.04
P	145
Sr	0.39
Ti	0.35
V	0.01
Al	10.4
Ba	0.46

the biological evidence outlined in this review, are those in the areas of osteoporosis, bone fractures, and other bone-related diseases.

Abbreviations
END: enterodiol; ENL: enterolactone; OVX: ovariectomized; *S. williamsii*: *Sambucus williamsii* Hance.

Authors' contributions
HHX and YZ searched the literature, organized materials and wrote the manuscript. RC revised the structure and polished the language. MSW and XSY designed the study and revised the manuscript. All authors read and approved the final manuscript.

Author details
[1] State Key Laboratory of Chinese Medicine and Molecular Pharmacology (Incubation), Shenzhen Research Institute of The Hong Kong Polytechnic University, Shenzhen 518057, China. [2] Department of Applied Biology and Chemical Technology, The Hong Kong Polytechnic University, Hung Hom, Kowloon, Hong Kong, China. [3] Spine Research Institute, Longhua Hospital, Shanghai University of Traditional Chinese Medicine, Shanghai 200032, China. [4] Institute of Traditional Chinese Medicine & Natural Products, College of Pharmacy, Jinan University, Guangzhou 510632, China.

Acknowledgements
We thank the State Key Laboratory of Chinese Medicine and Molecular Pharmacology (Incubation), Shenzhen for its support. This work was supported by the Central Research Fund of the Hong Kong Polytechnic University [GU324, GU256, GYM-47], the Shenzhen Basic Research Program [JCYJ20140819153305697], Longyi Innovation Team Program (LYCX-01), the National Natural Science Foundation of China [81202894, 81220108028] as well as the National Major Scientific and Program of Introducing Talents of Discipline to Universities [B13038].

Competing interests
The authors declare that they have no competing interests.

References
1. Song LR. The Editorial Committee of Chinese Herbals State Administration of Traditional Chinese Medicine. Shanghai: Shanghai Science and Technology Press; 2000. p. 544–6.
2. Choi H, Lee J, Chang YS, Woo ER, Lee DG. Isolation of (−)-olivil-9′-O-β-D-glucopyranoside from *Sambucus williamsii* and its antifungal effects with membrane-disruptive action. Biochim Biophys Acta. 2013;1828(8):2002–6.
3. Hwang B, Cho J, Hwang IS, Jin HG, Woo ER, Lee DG. Antifungal activity of lariciresinol derived from *Sambucus williamsii* and their membrane-active mechanisms in Candida albicans. Biochem Biophys Res Commun. 2011;410(3):489–93.
4. Yang XJ. The study of antiosteoporosis constituents of *Sambucus williamsii* Hance. Doctoral thesis. Shenyang Pharmaceutical University. 2005. p. 97–100.
5. Yang XJ, Wong MS, Wang NL, Chan SC, Yao XS. Effect of phenolic acids isolated from *Sambucus williamsii* on proliferation and differentiation of rat osteoblastic UMR106 cells. Chin Tradit Herb Drugs. 2005;36(11):1604–7.
6. Han H. Studies on chemical constituents and pharmacological effect of active fraction for fracture healing in *Sambucus*. Doctoral thesis. Heilongjiang University of Chinese Medicine. 2006.
7. Lv H, Chen SS, Xu XL, Zhu MM, Zhao WF, Liu KW, Liu KH. Isolation of linoleic acid from *Sambucus williamsii* seed oil extracted by high pressure fluid and its antioxidant, antiglycemic, hypolipidemic activities. Int J Food Eng. 2015;11(3):383–91.
8. Oliveira FA, Chaves MH, Almeida FRC, Lima RCP, Silva RM, Maia JL, Brito GA, Santos FA, Rao VS. Protective effect of α-and β-amyrin, a triterpene mixture from *Protium heptaphyllum* (Aubl.) March. trunk wood resin, against acetaminophen-induced liver injury in mice. J Ethnopharmacol. 2005;98(1):103–8.
9. Lima-Júnior RCP, Sousa DIM, Brito GA, Cunha GM, Chaves MH, Rao VS, Santos FA. Modulation of acute visceral nociception and bladder inflammation by plant triterpene, α, β-amyrin in a mouse model of cystitis: role of tachykinin NK1-receptors, and K(+)ATP channels. Inflamm Res. 2007;56(12):487–94.
10. Pisha E, Chai H, Lee IS, Chagwedera TE, Farnsworth NR, Cordell GA, Beecher CWW, Fong HHS, Kinghorn AS, Browh DM, Wani MC, Wall ME, Hieken TJ, Gupta TKD, Pezzuto JM. Discovery of betulinic acid as a selective inhibitor of human melanoma that functions by induction of apoptosis. Nat Med. 1995;1(10):1046–51.

11. De Melo CL, Queiroz MG, Arruda Filho ACV, Rodrigues AM, De Sousa DF, Almeida JG, Pessoa OD, Silveira ER, Menezes DB, Melo TS, Santos FA, Rao VS. Betulinic acid, a natural pentacyclic triterpenoid, prevents abdominal fat accumulation in mice fed a high-fat diet. J Agric Food Chem. 2009;57(19):8776–81.
12. Bringmann G, Saeb W, Assi LA, Francois G, Sankara NAS, Peters K, Peters KM. Betulinic acid: isolation from *Triphyophyllum peltatum* and *Ancistrocladus heyneanus*, antimalarial activity, and crystal structure of the benzyl ester. Planta Med. 1997;63(3):255–7.
13. Eriksson T, Dongohue MJ. Phylogenetic relationships of *Sambucus* and Adoxa (Adoxoideae, Adoxaceae) based on nuclear ribosomal ITS sequences and preliminary morphological data. Syst Bot. 1997;22(3):555–76.
14. von Schwerin FG. Mitteilungen der Deutschen Dendrologischen Gesellschaft. In: Monographie der gattung *Sambucus*. Nabu Press. 1909. p. 1–56.
15. von Schwerin FG. Mitteilungen der Deutschen Dendrologischen Gesellschaft. In: Revisio generis Sambucus. Nabu Press. 1920. p. 57-94.
16. Bolli R. Revision of the genus *Sambucus*. Diss Bot. 1994;223:1–256.
17. Editoral Committee of Flora Repubulicae Popularis Sinicae. Flora Repubulicae Popularis Sinicae. Beijing: Science Press; 1988. p. 4–11.
18. Lin M, Mei J, Liu X. The clinical observation of the effects of traditional chinese medicine on healing fracture. J Mod Med Health. 2009;25(6):901–2.
19. Lin M, Mei J. The clinical observation of compound JGM capsule on healing femur neck fracture. Zhongguo Zhongyi Jizheng. 2010;19(8):1306–36.
20. Song GH, Jiang B. Investigation of the major pharmacodynamic effects of compound JGM capsule. Chongqing Zhong Cao Yao Yanjiu. 2009;59:20–2.
21. Liu XW, Mei J, Lin M, Yang XD, Jiang B. Investigation of the major pharmacological effects of compound JGM capsules. Xin Zhong Yi. 2010;42(9):108–10.
22. Hwang B, Lee J, Liu QH, Woo ER, Lee DG. Antifungal effect of (+)-pinoresinol isolated from *Sambucus williamsii*. Molecules. 2010;15(5):3507–16.
23. Li AL, Xiong SL. Extraction technology and free radical scavenging properties of flavanone from *Sambucus williamsii* hance. Zhongguo Shipin Tian Jia Ji. 2010;5:113–6.
24. Song LL, Fu JN. Effects of *Sambucus* polysaccharides on rat cell proliferation and insulin secretion. Zhongguo Yao Li Xue Tong Bao. 2011;27(11):1593–6.
25. Xie F, Wu CF, Zhang Y, Yao XS, Cheung PY, Chan AS, Wong MS. Increase in bone mass and bone strength by *Sambucus williamsii* HANCE in ovariectomized rats. Biol Pharm Bull. 2005;28(10):1879–85.
26. Zhang Y, Li Q, Wan HY, Xiao HH, Lai WP, Yao XS, Wong MS. Study of the mechanisms by which *Sambucus williamsii* HANCE extract exert protective effects against ovariectomy-induced osteoporosis in vivo. Osteoporos Int. 2011;22(2):703–9.
27. Xiao HH, Dai Y, Wan HY, Wong MS, Yao XS. Bone-protective effects of bioactive fractions and ingredients in *Sambucus williamsii* HANCE. Br J Nutr. 2011;106(12):1802–9.
28. Xiao HH. Chemical constituents with antiosteoporosis effects in the bioactive fraction of *Sambucus willamsii* Hance. Doctoral thesis. Shenyang Pharmaceutical University. 2011.
29. Yang XJ, Wang NL, Wong MS, Chan SC, Yao XS. Studies of triterpenoids isolated from *Sambucus williamsii* Hance and their effects on UMR106 cell proliferation and alkaline phosphatase activity. Shenyang Yao Ke Da Xue Xuebao. 2005;22(6):449–52.
30. Yang XJ, Wong MS, Wang NL, Chan SC, Yao XS. A new eudesmane derivative and a new fatty acid ester from *Sambucus williamsii*. Chem Pharm Bull. 2006;54(5):676–8.
31. Han H, Yang BY, Xia YG, Wang QH, Kuang HX. Pharmacological Mechanism of *Sambucus williamsii* Hance in promoting fracture healing. Zhongguo Yao Shi. 2013;16(4):482–5.
32. Han H, Yang BY, Yang L, Xia YG, Wang QH, Kuang HX. Promotion of *Sambucus williamsii* root barks on fracture healing. Zhong Cao Yao. 2013;44(14):1957–61.
33. Dong PL, Yan XY, Kuang HX, Han H. Experimental study of *Sambucus williamsii* Hance on anti-inflammatory and analgesia. Zhong Yi Yao Xuebao. 2008;36(5):18–20.
34. Yang BY, He YW, Zhu XQ, Han H, Yang L, Wang QH, et al. Study on effects of *Sambucus williamsii* total glycosides tablets on fracture healing and inflammation: part I. Zhongguo Yao Shi. 2014;25(35):3269–72.
35. Yang BY, Lin XY, Yang CL, Tan JY, Li W, Kuang HX. *Sambucus williamsii* Hance promotes MC3T3-E1 cells proliferation and differentiation via BMP-2/Smad/p38/JNK/Runx2 signaling pathway. Phytother Res. 2015;29(11):1692–9.
36. Wang QY, Li TM. The study of fruit oil of *Sambucus williamsii* Hance on lymphocyte transformtion of mouse in vivo. Liaoning Da Xue Xuebao. 1995;22:105–7.
37. Liu Z, Wu JS, Wang MW. Effects of *Sambucus williamsii* Hance fruit oil on reducing plasma lipids and anti-aging. Shenyang Yao Ke Da Xue Xuebao. 1995;12(2):127–9.
38. Li XW, Shen GZ, Zhang SY, Hu R, Chen ZA, Jin ZN. Study of the anticancer effects of *Sambucus williamsii* Hance fruit oil. Zhongguo Zhong Yi Yao Ke Ji. 2000;7(2):103.
39. Shen GZ, Hu R, Zhang SY, Chen ZA, Jin ZN. The effects of *Sambucus williamsii* Hance fruit oil on the memory of mice. Zhongguo Zhong Yi Yao Ke Ji. 2000;7(2):103–4.
40. Hu R, Hong HC, Ma DB, Zheng HY. Effect of *Sambucus williamsii* Hance fruit oil on reduce plasma lipids. Beihua Da Xue Xuebao (Nat Sci). 2000;1(3):218–21.
41. Hu R, Qi JZ, Xue ZP, Jiang BW. A new medicinal and edible oil from a woody plant-*Sambucus williamsii*. Lin Ye Ke Xue. 2005;41(1):65–70.
42. Hua RZ. Five common therapy herbs forarthralgia. Zhongguo Min Jian Liao Fa. 1998;22:44.
43. Zhang HL, Han CX, Yang XJ, Wang MC, Yang QE, Bu SH. Study on chemical constituents and rat-killing activity of *Sambucus williamsii*. Xibei Zhi Wu Xuebao. 2004;24(8):1523–6.
44. Zhang T, Sun H, Wang GQ. The antibacterial effects of *Sambucus williamsii* Hance extracts to *Botrytis cinerea* Per. Ex Fr. in vitro. Liao Cheng Da Xue Xuebao. 2011;24(3):43–6.
45. Yang HM, Zheng YJ, Dai Y. Investigation of the bioactive fraction and components of *Sambucus williamsii* Hance on anti-inflammatory. Shizhen Guo Yi Guo Yao. 2012;23(2):338–9.
46. Xiao HH, Dai Y, Wong MS, Yao XS. New lignans from the bioactive fraction of *Sambucus williamsii* Hance and proliferation activities on osteoblastic-like UMR106 cells. Fitoterapia. 2014;94C:29–35.
47. Liu SP, Hsu CY, Fu RH, Huang YC, Chen SY, Lin SZ, et al. *Sambucus williamsii* induced embryonic stem cells differentiated into neurons. Biomedicine. 2015;5(1):19–23.
48. Lee H, Choi H, Ko HJ, Woo ER, Lee DG. Antifungal effect and mode of action of glochidioboside against *Candida albicans* membranes. Biochem Biophys Res Commun. 2014;444(1):30–5.
49. Ouyang F, Liu Y, Li R, Li L, Wang NL, Yao XS. Five lignans and an iridoid from *Sambucus williamsii*. Chin J Nat Med. 2011;9(1):26–9.
50. Guo XM, Zhang L, Quan JC, Hong YF, Liu MZ. Studies on the chemical constituents of *Williams elder* (*Sambucus williamsii*). Chin Tradit Herbal Drugs. 1998;29(11):727–9.
51. Lv F. Studies on the constituents of *Sambucus williamsii* Hance. Master thesis. Heilongjiang University of Chinese Medicine. 2002.
52. Han MH. Studies on the constituents of *Sambucus williamsii* Hance and on the preparation process of its compound prescription. Master Thesis. Heilongjiang University of Chinese Medicine. 2003.
53. Wang ZY, Han H, Yang BY, Xia YG, Kuang HX. Two new iridoid glycosides from the root barks of *Sambucus williamsii* Hance. Molecules. 2011;16(5):3869–74.
54. Kuang HX, Han H, Yang BY, Yang L, Jiang H, Wang QH. Two new iridoid glycosides from the root barks of *Sambucus williamsii* Hance. Molecules. 2012;17(2):1830–6.
55. Song DD, Yang BY, Yang L, Han H, Liu Y, Wang QH, et al. Chemical constituents from roots of *Sambucus williamsii* Hance. Zhong Yi Yao Xin Xi. 2014;31(3):4–6.
56. Yang BY, Song DD, Han H, Yang L, Liu Y, Wang QH, et al. Chemical constituents from roots of *Sambucus williamsii* (I). Zhong Cao Yao. 2014;45(10):1367–72.
57. Xu MM, Duan YH, Dai Y, Wang ZZ, Xiao W, Yao XS. A new nortriterpenoid from *Sambucus williamsii*. Zhong Cao Yao. 2013;44(19):2639–41.
58. Xiao HH, Dai Y, Wong MS, Yao XS. Two new phenylpropanoids and one new sesquiterpenoid from the bioactive fraction of *Sambucus williamsii*. J Asian Nat Prod Res. 2015;17(6):625–32.

59. Fu K, Fu GY, Luan FW, Bao YM, Zhang L. Study on the component of essential oil from mongolian medicine *Sambucus williamsii* Hance by GC–MS. J Inner Mong Univ Natl (Nat Sci). 2008;23(1):26–7.
60. Zhao Y, Jin J, Mao HB. Analysis of volatile oil in *Sambucus williamsii* by SPME. Guangzhou Hua Gong. 2013;41(10):165–6.
61. Du FG, Sun GR, Liu JH. Analysis on nutrient composition of *Sambucus williamsii* Hance fruits. Zi Yuan Ke Xue. 1996;4:45–8.
62. Hu R. Study on pigment extraction of *Sambucus willamsii* Hance. Econ Forest Res. 1992;10:93–4.
63. Ouyang F, Liu Y, Xiao HH, Yu HY, Wang NL, Yao XS. Lignans from stems of *Sambucus williamsii*. Zhongguo Zhong Yao Za Zhi. 2009;34(10):1225–7.
64. Chen KG, Hu R, Jiang BW. The preliminary experiment of natural pigments extraction from the peel of *Sambucus williamsii* Hance. Shipin Gong Ye Ke Ji. 1994;1(8):34–9.
65. Lou GY, Zhao Q, Chi SJ, Qin GQ. Study of the *Sambucus williamsii* Hance seed oil—a new rich source of a-linolenic acid. Zhongguo You Zhi. 1998;23(3):59.
66. Li F. Analysis on nutritional components from wild *Sambucus williamsii* Hance. Yunnan Hua Gong. 2007;34(1):50–1.
67. Zhao MJ. The clinical experience of using *Sambucus williamsii* Hance on osteoarthritis. Zhongguo Min Zu Min Jian Yi Yao. 2010;14:212.
68. Hwang JH, Hwang I, Liu QH, Woo ER, Lee DG. (+)-Medioresinol leads to intracellular ROS accumulation and mitochondria-mediated apoptotic cell death in *Candida albicans*. Biochimie. 2012;94(8):1784–93.
69. Ayres DC, Loike JD. Lignans: chemical, biological and clinical properties. New York: Press Syndicate of the University of Cambridge; 1990. p. 166–256.
70. Buck K, Zaineddin AK, Vrieling A, Heinz J, Linseisen J, Flesch-Janys D, et al. Estimated enterolignans, lignan-rich foods, and fibre in relation to survival after postmenopausal breast cancer. Br J Cancer. 2011;105(8):1151–7.
71. Saarinen NM, Wärri A, Airio M, Smeds A, Mäkelä S. Role of dietary lignans in the reduction of breast cancer risk. Mol Nutr Food Res. 2007;51:857–66.
72. Adlercreutz H. Lignans and human health. Crit Rev Clin Lab Sci. 2007;44(5–6):483–525.
73. Milder IEJ, Kuijsten A, Arts ICW, Feskens EJM, Kampman E, Hollman PCH, et al. Relation between plasma enterodiol and enterolactone and dietary intake of lignans in a Dutch endoscopy-based population. J Nutr. 2007;137(5):1266–71.
74. Yang XJ, Wong MS, Wang NL, Chan SC, Yao XS. Lignans from the stems of *Sambucus williamsii* and their effects on osteoblastic UMR106 cells. J Asian Nat Prod Res. 2007;9(7):583–91.
75. Xiao HH, Gao QG, Ho MX, Zhang Y, Wong KC, Dai Y, et al. An 8-*O*-4′ norlignan exerts oestrogen-like actions in osteoblastic cells via rapid nongenomic ER signaling pathway. J Ethnopharmacol. 2015;170:39–49.
76. Kuijsten A, Arts ICW, Vree TB, Hollman PCH. Pharmacokinetics of enterolignans in healthy men and women consuming a single dose of secoisolariciresinol diglucoside. J Nutr. 2005;135(4):795–801.
77. Lin X, Switzer BR, Demark-Wahnefried W. Effect of mammalian lignans on the growth of prostate cancer cell lines. Anticancer Res. 2000;21(6A):3995–9.
78. Qu H, Madl RL, Takemoto DJ, Baybutt RC, Wang W. Lignans are involved in the antitumor activity of wheat bran in colon cancer SW480 cells. J Nutr. 2005;135(3):598–602.
79. Torres-Sanchez L, Galvan-Portillo M, Wolff MS, Lopez-Carrillo L. Dietary consumption of phytochemicals and breast cancer risk in Mexican women. Public Health Nutr. 2009;12(6):825–31.
80. Xiao HH, Gao QG, Zhang Y, Wong KC, Dai Y, Yao XS, et al. Vanillic acid exerts oestrogen-like activities in osteoblast-like UMR 106 cells through MAP kinase (MEK/ERK)-mediated ER signaling pathway. J Steroid Biochem Mol Biol. 2014;144:382–91.
81. Rai RP, Maurya MS. Synthesis and evaluation of antibacterial activity of vanillin derivatives. J Sci Technol India. 1996;4:275–6.
82. Delaquis P, Stanich K, Toivonen P. Effect of pH on the inhibition of *Listeria* spp. by vanillin and vanillic acid. J Food Prot. 2005;68(7):1472–6.
83. Tsuda H, Uehara N, Iwahori Y, Asamoto M, Ligo M, Nagao M, et al. Chemopreventive effects of β-carotene, α-tocopherol and five naturally occurring antioxidants on initiation of hepatocarcinogenesis by 2-amino-3-methylimidazo [4,5-f] qumoline in the rat. Cancer Sci. 1994;85(12):1214–9.
84. Prince PSM, Rajakumar S, Dhanasekar K. Protective effects of vanillic acid on electrocardiogram, lipid peroxidation, antioxidants, proinflammatory markers and histopathology in isoproterenol induced cardiotoxic rats. Eur J Pharmacol. 2011;668(1):233–40.
85. Adam A, Crespy V, Levrat-Verny MA, Leenhardt F, Leuillet M, Demigné C, Rémésy C. The bioavailability of ferulic acid is governed primarily by the food matrix rather than its metabolism in intestine and liver in rats. J Nutr. 2002;132(7):1962–8.
86. Srinivasan M, Sudheer AR, Menon VP. Ferulic acid: therapeutic potential through its antioxidant property. J Clin Biochem Nutr. 2007;40(2):92–100.
87. Mckeehen JD, Busch RH, Fulcher RG. Evaluation of wheat (*Triticum aestivum* L.) phenolic acids during grain development and their contribution to *Fusarium* resistance. J Agric Food Chem. 1999;47(4):1476–82.
88. Tanaka T, Kojima T, Kawamori T, Yoshimi N, Mori H. Chemoprevention of diethylnitrosamine-induced hepatocarcinogenesis by a simple phenolic acid protocatechuic acid in rats. Cancer Res. 1993;53(12):2775–9.
89. Tanaka T, Kawamori T, Ohnishi M, Okamoto K, Mori H, Hara A. Chemoprevention of 4-nitroquinoline-1-oxide-induced oral carcinogenesis by dietary protocatechuic acid during initiation and postinitiation phases. Cancer Res. 1994;54(9):2359–65.
90. Kawamori T, Tanaka T, Kojima T, Suzui M, Ohnishi M, Mori H. Suppression of azoxymethane-induced rat colon aberrant crypt foci by dietary protocatechuic acid. Cancer Sci. 1994;85(7):686–91.
91. Tanaka T, Kojima T, Kawamori T, Mori H. Chemoprevention of digestive organs carcinogenesis by natural product protocatechuic acid. Cancer. 1995;75(S6):1433–9.
92. Hirose Y, Tanaka T, Kawamori T, Olnishi M, Makita H, Mori H, et al. Chemoprevention of urinary bladder carcinogenesis by the natural phenolic compound protocatechuic acid in rats. Carcinogenesis. 1995;16(10):2337–42.
93. Tseng TH, Wang CJ, Kao ES. *Hibiscus* protocatechuic acid protects against oxidative damage induced by tert-butylhydroperoxide in rat primary hepatocytes. Chem Biol Interact. 1996;101(2):137–48.
94. Bountagkidou OG, Ordoudi SA, Tsimidou MZ. Structure-antioxidant activity relationship study of natural hydroxybenzaldehydes using in vitro assays. Food Res Int. 2010;43(8):2014–9.
95. Gurpilhares DB, Pessoa A, Roberto IC. Glucose-6-phosphate dehydrogenase and xylitol production by *Candida guilliermondii* FTI 20037 using statistical experimental design. Process Biochem. 2006;41(3):631–7.
96. Morse MA, Kresty LA, Toburen AL. Inhibition of metabolism of 4-(methylnitrosamino)-1-(3-pyridyl)-1-butanone by dietary benzaldehydes. Cancer Lett. 1995;97(2):255–61.
97. Peungvicha P, Temsiririrkkul R, Prasain JK, Tezuka Y, Kadota S, Thirawarapan SS, et al. 4-Hydroxybenzoic acid: a hypoglycemic constituent of aqueous extract of *Pandanus odorus* root. J Ethnopharmacol. 1998;62(1):79–84.
98. Bianco A. Recent developments in iridoids chemistry. Pure Appl Chem. 1999;66(10–11):2336–8.
99. Liu J, Liu YP, Parkinson A, Klaassen CD. Effect of oleanolic acid on hepatic toxicant-activating and detoxifying systems in mice. J Pharmacol Exp Ther. 1995;275(2):768–74.
100. James LP, Mayeux PR, Hinson JA. Acetaminophen-induced hepatotoxicity. Drug Metab Dispos. 2003;31(12):1499–506.
101. Mukherjee PK, Saha K, Das J, Pal M, Saha BP. Studies on the anti-inflammatory activity of rhizomes of *Nelumbo nucifera*. Planta Med. 1997;63(4):367–9.
102. Fernández MA, Heras B, Garcia MD, Sáenz MT, Villar A. New insights into the mechanism of action of the anti-inflammatory triterpene lupeol. J Pharm Pharmacol. 2001;53(11):1533–9.

103. Fernández A, Álvarez A, GarcíA MD, Sáenz MT. Anti-inflammatory effect of *Pimenta racemosa* var. ozua and isolation of the triterpene lupeol. Il Farmaco. 2001;56(4):335–8.
104. Carlsson C, Hakan Borg LA, Welsh N. Sodium palmitate induces partial mitochondrial uncoupling and reactive oxygen species in rat pancreatic islets in vitro. Endocrinology. 1999;140(8):3422–8.
105. Maedler K, Spinas GA, Dyntar D, Moritz W, Kaiser N, Donath MY. Distinct effects of saturated and monounsaturated fatty acids on β-cell turnover and function. Diabetes. 2010;50(1):69–76.
106. Sparagna GC, Hickson-Bick DL. Cardiac fatty acid metabolism and the induction of apoptosis. Am J Med Sci. 1999;318(1):15–21.
107. Posey KA, Clegg DJ, Printz RL, Byun J, Morton GJ, Vivekanandan-Giri A, et al. Hypothalamic proinflammatory lipid accumulation, inflammation, and insulin resistance in rats fed a high-fat diet. Am J Physiol Endocrinol Metab. 2009;296(5):E1003–12.

6

Herb-partitioned moxibustion upregulated the expression of colonic epithelial tight junction-related proteins in Crohn's disease model rats

Rong Ji[1], Anqi Wang[1], Haixia Shang[1], Liu Chen[1], Chunhui Bao[1,2], Luyi Wu[1], Huangan Wu[1,2] and Yin Shi[1,2*]

Abstract

Background: Herb-partitioned moxibustion (HPM) at *Tianshu* (ST25) and *Qihai* (RN6) has been used to treat Crohn's disease (CD). Injury to intestinal epithelial tight junctions (TJs) is the leading cause of CD onset with under expression of TJ-related proteins such as occludin, claudin-1, and zonula occludens protein-1 (ZO-1). This study aimed to investigate whether HPM can change the permeability of the intestinal epithelial barrier by affecting the expression of colonic epithelial TJ-related proteins in vitro.

Methods: Forty-eight male Sprague–Dawley rats were randomly divided into four groups of twelve rats: normal control (NC) group; model control (MC) group; herb-partitioned moxibustion (HPM) group; and mesalazine control (MESA) group. The rats in the latter three groups were given trinitrobenzene sulfonic acid (TNBS) enemas to establish CD models. The HPM group was treated with HPM at *Tianshu* (ST25) and *Qihai* (RN6) once daily for 14 consecutive days, while the MESA group was given mesalazine solution (at the proportion of 0.018:1) by lavage twice daily for the same period. After the treatment period, the colon tissues from all groups were partly processed for macroscopic damage assessment and histological observation, and partly purified and cultured in vitro to examine the permeability of the intestinal epithelial cell barrier by trans-epithelial electrical resistance (TEER). Western blot and fluorescence quantitative polymerase chain reaction (FQ-PCR) analyses were performed to observe the expression of occludin, claudin-1, and ZO-1 proteins and mRNAs, respectively.

Results: In the HPM and MESA groups, the typical CD macroscopic damage, i.e., inflammatory cell infiltration in colonic mucosa and submucosa, submucosal lymphoid follicular hyperplasia, hyperemia and edema, and morphological changes were improved to different degrees in the colonic tissues (HPM, MESA vs. MC for macroscopic score of colonic damage: all $P < 0.001$). The decreasing tendencies were minor for colonic TEER values (HPM, MESA vs. MC: all $P < 0.001$), and expression of intestinal epithelial TJ-related proteins (HPM, MESA vs. MC: all $P < 0.05$) and mRNAs (HPM, MESA vs. MC: all $P < 0.05$), especially in the HPM group (HPM vs. MESA for TEER values: $P < 0.001$).

Conclusions: HPM at *Tianshu* (ST25) and *Qihai* (RN6) upregulated the expression of occludin, claudin-1, and ZO-1 in TNBS-induced CD model rats.

Background

Crohn's disease (CD) is a chronic inflammatory bowel disease (IBD) characterized by intestinal inflammatory changes induced by abnormal immune responses of the host against the intestinal tolerated commensal microflora [1, 2]. Injury to the intestinal epithelial barrier (e.g., excessive apoptosis of intestinal epithelial cells) and genetic defects in the intestinal epithelial tight junctions (TJs) (e.g., under expression of TJ-related proteins) were reported to be involved in the occurrence

*Correspondence: flysy0636@163.com
[2] Shanghai Research Institute of Acupuncture-Moxibustion and Meridian, Shanghai 200030, China
Full list of author information is available at the end of the article

and development of CD [3]. Intestinal mucosal tumor necrosis factor-alpha (TNF-α) and tumor necrosis factor receptor1 (TNFR1) were overactive in patients with mild to moderate CD [4, 5]. Malformation and dysfunction of intestinal epithelial TJs were found in patients with IBDs [6, 7], and related to under expression or abnormal distribution of intestinal epithelial TJ-related proteins [8].

Intestinal epithelial TJs are related to the permeability of the intestinal epithelial barrier [9, 10]. Changes in the permeability of the intestinal epithelial barrier are the leading pathologic alterations in CD [11, 12]. Occludin, claudin-1, and zonula occludens protein-1 (ZO-1) are major proteins for maintaining TJ permeability [8]. During active and non-active periods of CD, the expression of occludin, claudin-1, ZO-1 proteins and mRNAs were significantly reduced in the colonic mucosa, followed by increasing permeability of the intestinal epithelium and injury to the intestinal epithelial barrier [13, 14].

The goals in CD treatment are remission of inflammation, recovery of mucosa, prevention of relapse, avoidance of surgical intervention and minimization of the possibility of cancer development [15]. 5-Aminosalicylates (5-ASA) and thiopurines are clinically used in treatments for IBD [16]. 5-ASA preparations (e.g., mesalazine) are the first-line medicines for IBD treatment in mild to moderate ulcerative colitis (UC) [17]. However, they were found to be no more effective than placebo for active CD [18]. Therefore, the European Crohn's and Colitis Organization has recognized the efficiency of mesalazine as "limited" [19]. Application of thiopurines in mild to moderate CD patients is limited because of their severe side effects including abnormities in liver and renal functions, digestive intolerance and withdrawal reactions [20]. In consideration of this, alternatives that offer safe and highly effective treatment are urgently needed for patients with mild to moderate CD.

Previous clinical and experimental studies showed that herb-partitioned moxibustion (HPM) was effective in relieving abdominal pain, diarrhea and other gastrointestinal symptoms, as well as improving the Crohn's disease activity index in patients [4, 5]. HPM was able to significantly reduce the abnormal increases in TNF-α and TNFR1 in the intestinal mucosa [5]. HPM not only decreased the apoptosis of colonic epithelial cells, but also enhanced the expression of colonic epithelial TJ-related proteins in vitro [21, 22].

This study aims to investigate whether HPM would change the permeability of the intestinal epithelial barrier by affecting the expression of occludin, claudin-1,and ZO-1 in vitro.

Methods

Animals

Forty-eight male Sprague-Dawley rats (150 ± 10 g), aged 6–8 weeks, were supplied by the Experimental Animal Center, Shanghai University of Traditional Chinese Medicine (China). The experiments were approved by Ethics Committee of Shanghai University of Traditional Chinese Medicine (No. 2013025; Additional files 1 and 2). Each animal was free of any known pathogens and only used once. All rats were housed in a light-controlled room (12-h/12-h light/dark cycle with lights on at 07:00 am), with constant temperature (22 ± 1 °C) and humidity (42 ± 5 %). Prior to modeling, the rats were housed with six companions in each cage, and had free access to food and water. The animal studies were performed following the ARRIVE guideline (Additional file 3).

The 48 male rats were allocated into four groups by a randomized block design. After weighing on a scale, the rats were ranked according to their body weight, and the numbers 1 through 48 were written on the tails of the rats in ascending order. According to this order, sets off our rats with similar approximate weights comprised one block, and were simultaneously given 48 random numbers taken from the random number table (from line 6 row 8, left to right). The four rats in each block were rearranged by their random numbers into ascending order, and then allocated into four groups of twelve rats: normal control (NC) group; model control (MC) group; herb-partitioned moxibustion (HPM) group; and mesalazine control (MESA) group.

The CD models were prepared according to Morris' method [23]. Briefly, all rats were given only water for 24 h before modeling. After being weighed on the scale, the rats in all four groups were anesthetized with sodium pentobarbital (30 mg/kg 2 %; Sigma Chemical Co., USA) by intraperitoneal injection. The rats in the MC, HPM, and MESA groups were given trinitrobenzene sulfonic acid (TNBS; Sigma Chemical Co., USA) enemas(0.5 mL/100 g; formula: TNBS/50 % ethanol = 2:1), while those in the NC group were given enemas with the same dose of normal saline. The rats were fixed in the handstand position for 1 min while the rubber tubes containing the enema solution were retained in the gut cavity at 6–8 cm in depth to ensure an adequate drug action, and the tubes were then withdrawn. This procedure was repeated on days 7, 14, 21, and 28. When the CD modeling procedure was completed, two rats from each group were arbitrarily selected (by picking a number out of a box) to examine whether the modeling was sufficient by observing hematoxylin and eosinstained colonic tissues under a light microscope (Leica Microsystems GmbH, Germany).

Herbal cake and moxi cone preparation

The herbal powder formula was as follows: *Fuzi* (radix *Aconiti carmichaeli*) (10 g; Sichuan, China), *Rougui* (*Cinnamomum cassia Presl*) (2 g; Guanxi, China), *Danshen* (radix *Salviae miltiorrhizae*) (3 g; Anhui, China), *Honghua* (*Carthamus tinctorius* L.) (3 g; Henan, China), and *Muxiang* (*Saussurea costus*) (2 g; Yunnan, China). Decoction pieces of these traditional Chinese medicines were mixed, ground into a fine powder, passed through a 150-mesh sieve three times, and stored in dry and dark conditions at room temperature (25 °C). For use, 2.5 g of herbal powder was fully mixed with 3 g of *Shaoxing* wine into a thick paste, and then shaped into herbal cakes (1 cm in diameter, 0.6 cm in height) in a herbal cake mold for the experimental rats.

Moxi cones (10 mg in weight, 0.6 cm in diameter, 0.6 cm in height) were made by hand using refined mugwort floss (Huatuo, Suzhou, China).

Treatments

After excluding the rats arbitrarily selected from each group to examine whether the CD modeling was sufficient, the remaining 10 rats in each group were processed as described below.

All rats received the same fixation before treatment. The devices were adjusted until the rats felt comfortable and stopped struggling. When HPM was applied to the HPM group, the rats in the other three groups received the same fixation for the same duration.

The NC and MC groups received no treatment. For the HPM group, the fur of the lower abdomen was carefully shaved to expose the chosen acupoints, *Tianshu* (ST25) and *Qihai* (RN6). The moxa cones were ignited with an incense stick after placement on the herbal cake at *Tianshu* (ST25) and *Qihai* (RN6). Three moxa cones were used for each rat in a single treatment for 10 min. The rats received the same treatment once daily for 14 days. For the MESA group, mesalazine solution (Dr. FalkPharma, Germany) at the proportion of 0.018:1 was fed by lavage [24]. The rats received the same treatment twice daily for 14 days.

Assessment of macroscopic colonic damage

After the treatment period, all rats in the different groups were ethically euthanized with sodium pentobarbital (30 mg/kg 2 %; Sigma Chemical Co., USA) by intraperitoneal injection. Colonic tissues (2–3 cm in length; 6–8 cm away from the anus) were taken and rinsed 5–10 times with sterile phosphate-buffered saline (PBS) containing antibiotics. Assessment of macroscopic colonic damage was conducted according to previously published criteria [25], as shown in Table 1. The severity of inflammation was assessed using the same criteria.

Histological observation

Colonic tissues (1 cm) were removed for histological observation. The tissues were washed in ice-cold normal saline, fixed in 10 % formalin, embedded in paraffin, cut into 4 μm thin sections, and adhered onto plain glass slides. The sections were then baked in an oven at 58 °C for 24 h for dewaxing, stained with hematoxylin and eosin, dehydrated in 95, 90, and 70 % ethanol, cleaned up in xylene, mounted in Permount or Histoclad, and observed at 200× magnification under an Olympus CX31 optical microscope (Olympus, Japan) at 2.80 V and 2.74 A. Images were obtained with a Canon A640 camera (Canon, Japan).

Table 1 Criterion for assessment of colonic damage

	Macroscopic score	
Adhesions	None	0
	Minimal	1
	Involving several bowel loops	2
Strictures	None	0
	mild	2
	Severe, proximal dilatation	3
Ulcers	None	0
	Linear ulceration <1 cm	1
	Two linear ulcers <1 cm	2
	More sites of ulceration or one large ulcer >1 cm	3
Wall thickness	Less than 1 mm	0
	1–3 mm	1
	More than 1 mm	2
Maximum score		10

Establishment of an in vitro intestinal epithelial barrier model

The remaining tissues were cut into pieces with ophthalmic scissors, and digested with 0.4 % type IV collagenase for 2 h in an incubator at 37 °C and 5 % CO_2. The supernatants were centrifuged at 5000×*g* for 10 min. After the supernatants were discarded, the cell pellets were resuspended and seeded into culture dishes with Dulbecco's modified Eagle's medium (DMEM; Sigma-Aldrich Chemical Co., USA) containing 10 % fetal bovine serum (Sigma Chemical Co., USA) in an incubator at 37 °C and 5 % CO_2. The culture medium was changed every other day. Colonic epithelial cells were purified, digested with trypsin, and resuspended in complete medium before counting. Cells (1×10^3) were taken and placed in 48-well plates for adherence and observation. Wells with high proportions of epithelial cells were expanded in culture. The above operations were repeated until most of the epithelial cells were visible under a light microscope (Leica Microsystems GmbH, Germany). The culture was continued for 7 days [26] until a complete epithelial barrier was formed from normal colonic epithelial cells.

TEER, western blot, and fluorescence quantitative PCR (FQ-PCR) analyses of colonic epithelial cells were performed in each group.

Measurement of colonic TEER

Cultured cells in the different groups were washed once with PBS and digested with 0.25 % trypsin [27, 28]. After adding culture medium and terminating the digestion process, the cells were counted and adjusted to a density of 2.5×10^5 cells/mL. Transwell chambers for measuring transmembrane resistance were placed in 24-wellplates. Complete medium (600 μL) was added to the lower chamber, while a cell suspension (200 μL) was added to the upper chamber and cultured for 24 h at 37 °C and 5 % CO_2. The medium in the upper and lower chambers of the transwell chambers was replaced with 200 and 600 μL of medium, respectively. A small chamber with medium only was set as a negative control. The plates were measured in a Millicell ERS-2 Epithelial Volt-Ohm Meter (Millipore, USA) after vertical plug-in of an electrode into three slots on the chamber wall. The average of these three values was taken for statistical analysis. The room temperature was strictly controlled at 25 °C, because TEER values were reported to be highly sensitive to the environmental temperature [29].

Detection of occludin, claudin-1, and ZO-1 expression in the rat colonic epithelial cells cultured in vitro

Cells (2×10^6) were taken from each group, added to a celllysis buffer (100 μL) until full cleavage was achieved, and boiled (100 °C) for 5 min. The insoluble material was removed by centrifugation (5000×*g* for 5 min). The proteins in each sample (50 μL) were separated by polyacrylamide gel electrophoresis and transferred to nitrocellulose membranes. The membranes were sequentially blocked with 5 % nonfat milk in PBS for 2 h and 5 % bovine serum albumin in PBS at 4 °C overnight, and then incubated with primary antibodies for 90 min at room temperature. The primary antibodies used were rabbit polyclonal immunoglobulin (IgG) antibodies against occludin (Ab31721; Abcam, UK; 1:250 dilution), claudin-1 (Ab15098; Abcam, UK; 1:25 dilution), and ZO-1 (Sc-10804; Santa Cruz Biotechnology, USA; 1:100 dilution). Peroxidase-conjugated goat anti-rabbit IgG (A0208; Beyotime, China; 1:1000 dilution) and chemiluminescence fluids A and B (1:1) were incubated with the membranes for 1 h and 1 min, respectively. The reactive bands were detected by chemiluminescent reagents (170-5061; Bio-Rad, USA). A Tanon-5200imager (Tanon, China) was employed for image acquisition, and Image-pro plus 6.0 software (MediaCybernetics, USA) was used to analyze the gray values of the bands. All the grey values of the bands were normalized by the value for glyceraldehyde-3-phosphate dehydrogenase (GAPDH).

FQ-PCR detection of occludin, claudin-1, and ZO-1 mRNA expression in the rat colonic epithelial cells cultured in vitro

Total cellular RNA was separated from the rat colonic epithelial cell samples using Trizol reagent (1596-026; Invitrogen, USA). Three micrograms of the total RNA wasused as a template for reverse transcription of cDNAs. The cDNAs were synthesized by reverse transcription using a RevertAid cDNA Synthesis Kit (#K1622; Fermentas, USA) in accordance with the manufacturer's instructions, and then amplified, the primer sequences used for PCR amplification reaction were shown in Table 2. The following cycling conditions were used: reverse transcription at 37 °C for 1 h, inactivation of the MMLV RT enzyme at 95 °C for 5 min, and 40 cycles of 50 °C for 2 min, 95 °C for 5 min, 95 °C for 15 s, and 60 °C for 45 s. Real-time PCR was performed with a QuantiTect SYBR Green PCR Kit (#K0223; Thermo Fisher Scientific, USA) using an ABI 7500 real-time PCR system and SDS software (Applied Biosystems, USA). Data for the mRNA levels were calculated as the relative amounts normalized to that of GAPDH.

Statistical analysis

Statistical data were represented in graphs as mean ± standard deviation (SD). Statistical analyses were performed using SPSS 16.0 software (SPSS, USA). Differences within experimental groups were compared by one-way analysis of variance (ANOVA). LSD test was performed for multiple group comparison. Values of $P < 0.05$ were considered statistically significant.

Results

Colonic histopathological observations in the different groups

In the normal group (Fig. 1a), the colonic mucosa was intact, and the morphology of submucosal and muscular tissues was normal. In the MC group (Fig. 1b), there were large numbers of eosinophils with marked inflammatory cell infiltration in colonic mucosa and submucosa, and obvious submucosal lymphoid follicular hyperplasia, epithelial damage, submucosal hyperemia and edema, fibroblast proliferation, and muscle tissue damage, as well as epithelioid reactions, giant cells, and other typical pathological intestinal changes of CD. In the MESA group (Fig. 1c), there were eosinophils and inflammatory cell infiltration in colonic mucosa and submucosa, submucosal hyperemia and edema, fibroblast proliferation, small amounts of epithelioid reactions and giant cells,

Table 2 The sequence of the forward primer and reverse primer used for FQ-PCR assays

Name	Primer sense	Primer sequence (5′ → 3′)	Amplification product (bp)
GAPDH	Forward	5′-CCGAGGGCCCACTAAAGG-3′	116
	Reverse	5′-GCTGTTGAAGTCACAGGAGACAA-3′	
Occludin	Forward	5′-GGGACAGAGCCTATGGAA-3′	191
	Reverse	5′-GGAAGCGATGAAGCAAAA-3′	
Claudin-1	Forward	5′-CTGGCTTCGCTGGGATGGA -3′	100
	Reverse	5′-TGGCCTGAGCAGTCACGATGTT-3′	
ZO-1	Forward	5′-GATGAGCGGGCTACCTTA-3′	126
	Reverse	5′-ATGGGAGCGAACTGAATG-3′	

Morphological observation of colonic tissues

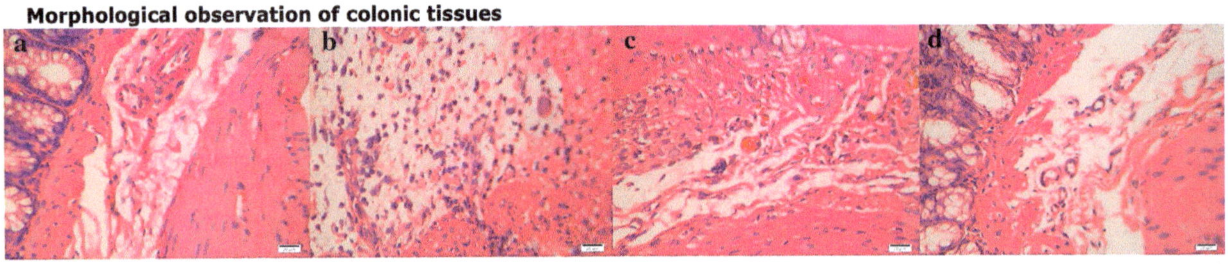

Fig. 1 Histopathological observation of the colon tissue. Hematoxylin and eosin staining method, ×200. **a** NC group; **b** MC group; **c** MESA group; **d** HPM group

and slightly disordered layers of tissue morphology. In the HPM group (Fig. 1d), there were only small amounts of inflammatory cell infiltration in colonic mucosa and submucosa, mild hyperemia, small amounts of fibroblast proliferation, and normal morphology of mucosal, submucosal, and muscular tissues.

Scores for macroscopic colonic damage in the different groups

Compared with the NC group, the MC, MESA, and HPM groups showed significant increases in the macroscopic scores for colonic damage ($P = 0.000$, $P = 0.000$, $P = 0.024$; Fig. 2). However, the macroscopic scores for colonic damage in the MESA and HPM groups were significantly lower than that in the MC group ($P = 0.000$, $P = 0.000$), although there was no significant difference between these two groups ($P = 0.075$). Both HPM and MESA therapy could significantly improve the macroscopic colonic mucosal damage in CD.

Comparison of TEER values in the different groups

As shown in Fig. 3, there was a significant decrease in the colonic TEER values in the MC group compared with the NC group ($P = 0.000$). There were significant increases in the colonic TEER values in both the HPM and MESA groups compared with the MC group ($P = 0.000$,

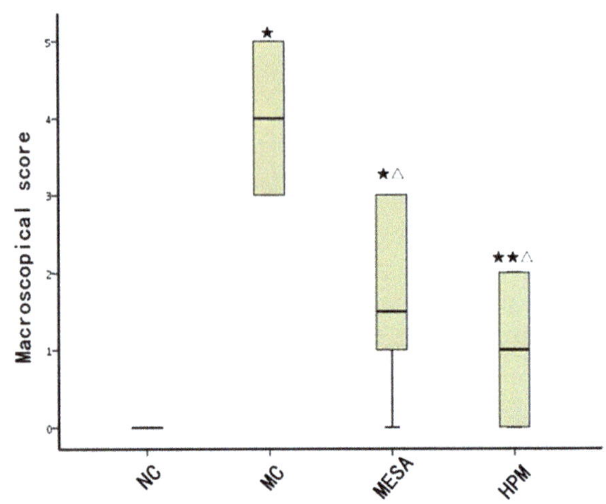

Fig. 2 Macroscopic score of colonic damage. *NC* normal control group, *MC* model control group, *MESA* mesalazine group, and *HPM* herb-partitioned moxibustion group. ★$P < 0.001$ versus NC, ★★$P < 0.05$ versus NC; △$P < 0.001$ versus MC. The data of macroscopical score do not have normal distribution, the *box-plot* is used to express, as shown below. The NC group has the same value, so the *box-plot* only have one straight line. The maximum value is equal to the upper quantile and the minimum value is equal to the lower quantile in MC group. The maximum value is equal to the upper quantile in MESA group. The maximum value is equal to the upper quantile and the minimum value is equal to the lower quantile in HPM group

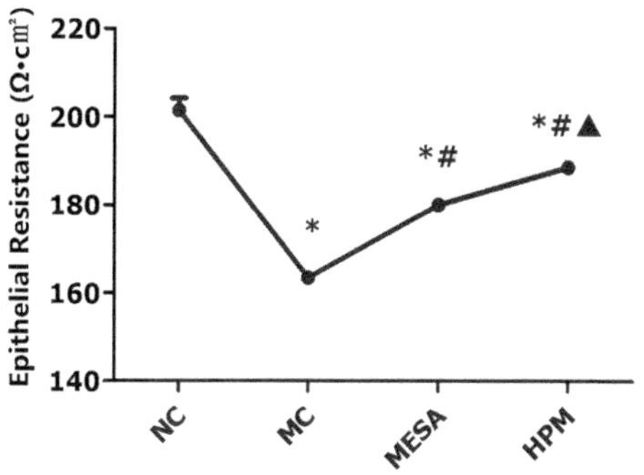

Fig. 3 Transepithelial electrical resistance values of each group. *NC* normal control group, *MC* model control group, *MESA* mesalazine group and *HPM* herb-partitioned moxibustion group. $^{*}P < 0.01$ versus NC; $^{\#}P < 0.01$ versus MC; $^{▲}P < 0.01$ versus MESA. The standard deviation in MC group (163.53 ± 0.77), MESA group (180.13 ± 1.09) and HPM group (188.60 ± 1.07) is small and not shown in the *graph*

$P = 0.000$), while the HPM group had significantly better TEER values than the MESA group ($P = 0.000$). There were also significant differences in the HPM and MESA groups compared with the NC group ($P = 0.000$, $P = 0.000$).

Expression of occludin, claudin-1, and ZO-1 proteins in the different groups

For occludin protein expression (Fig. 4a), there was a significant decrease in the MC group compared with the NC group ($P = 0.000$), significant increases in the HPM and MESA groups compared with the MC group ($P = 0.025$, $P = 0.019$), and no significant difference between the HPM group and the MESA group ($P = 0.859$), but significant differences in the HPM and MESA groups compared with the NC group ($P = 0.001$, $P = 0.000$). For claudin-1 protein expression (Fig. 4b), there was a significant decrease in the MC group compared with the NC group ($P = 0.000$), significant increases in the HPM and MESA groups compared with the MC group ($P = 0.001$, $P = 0.002$), no significant difference between the HPM group and the MESA group ($P = 0.535$), and no significant differences in the HPM and MESA groups compared with the NC group ($P = 0.196$, $P = 0.073$). For ZO-1 protein expression (Fig. 4c), there was a significant decrease in the MC group compared with the NC group ($P = 0.008$), significant increases in the HPM and MESA groups compared with the MC group ($P = 0.038$, $P = 0.046$), no significant difference between the HPM group and the MESA group ($P = 0.899$), and no significant differences in the HPM and MESA groups compared with the NC group ($P = 0.336$, $P = 0.282$).

Expression of occludin, claudin-1, and ZO-1 mRNAs in the different groups

For occludin mRNA expression (Fig. 5a), there was a significant decrease in the MC group compared with the NC group ($P = 0.000$), significant increases in the HPM and MESA groups compared with the MC group ($P = 0.028$, $P = 0.043$), and no significant difference between the HPM group and the MESA group ($P = 0.846$), but still significant differences in the HPM and MESA groups compared with the NC group ($P = 0.000$, $P = 0.000$). For claudin-1 mRNA expression (Fig. 5b), there was a significant decrease in the MC group compared with the NC group ($P = 0.000$), significant increases in the HPM and MESA groups compared with the MC group ($P = 0.035$, $P = 0.039$), and no significant difference between the HPM group and the MESA group ($P = 0.968$), but still significant differences in the HPM and MESA groups compared with the NC group ($P = 0.048$, $P = 0.044$). For ZO-1 mRNA expression (Fig. 5c), there was a significant decrease in the MC group compared with the NC group ($P = 0.000$), significant increases in the HPM and MESA groups compared with the MC group ($P = 0.017$, $P = 0.044$), and no significant difference between the HPM group and the MESA group ($P = 0.684$), but still significant differences in the HPM and MESA groups compared with the NC group ($P = 0.001$, $P = 0.000$).

Discussion

This study has demonstrated the effects of HPM on repairing the colonic epithelial barrier and upregulating the expression of occludin, claudin-1, and ZO-1 in vitro. In the study, we first observed both macroscopic and histological damage to the colonic tissues from the different groups. Immediately after the colonic tissues were removed and washed, we assessed the scores for adhesions, strictures, ulcers, and wall thickness of the colonic tissues. In the NC group, the colonic tissues showed mild hyperemia and edema, but no mucosal erosion or ulcers, which might have arisen through stimulation during the surgery process. Almost no signs of tissue adhesions and strictures were observed, and the wall thickness was normal. In the MC group, severe hyperemia and edema were generally observed in most rats, while deep and multiple ulcers were common. In several rats, we also observed slight adhesions of the adjacent colonic tissues, accompanied by loss of elasticity and smoothness of colonic tissues, and slight increases in wall thickness. This was because that our CD modeling procedure could only imitate the incipient acute colonic inflammation, which is characterized by mucosal hyperemia, edema, and ulcers. However, the symptoms of tissue adhesions, strictures,

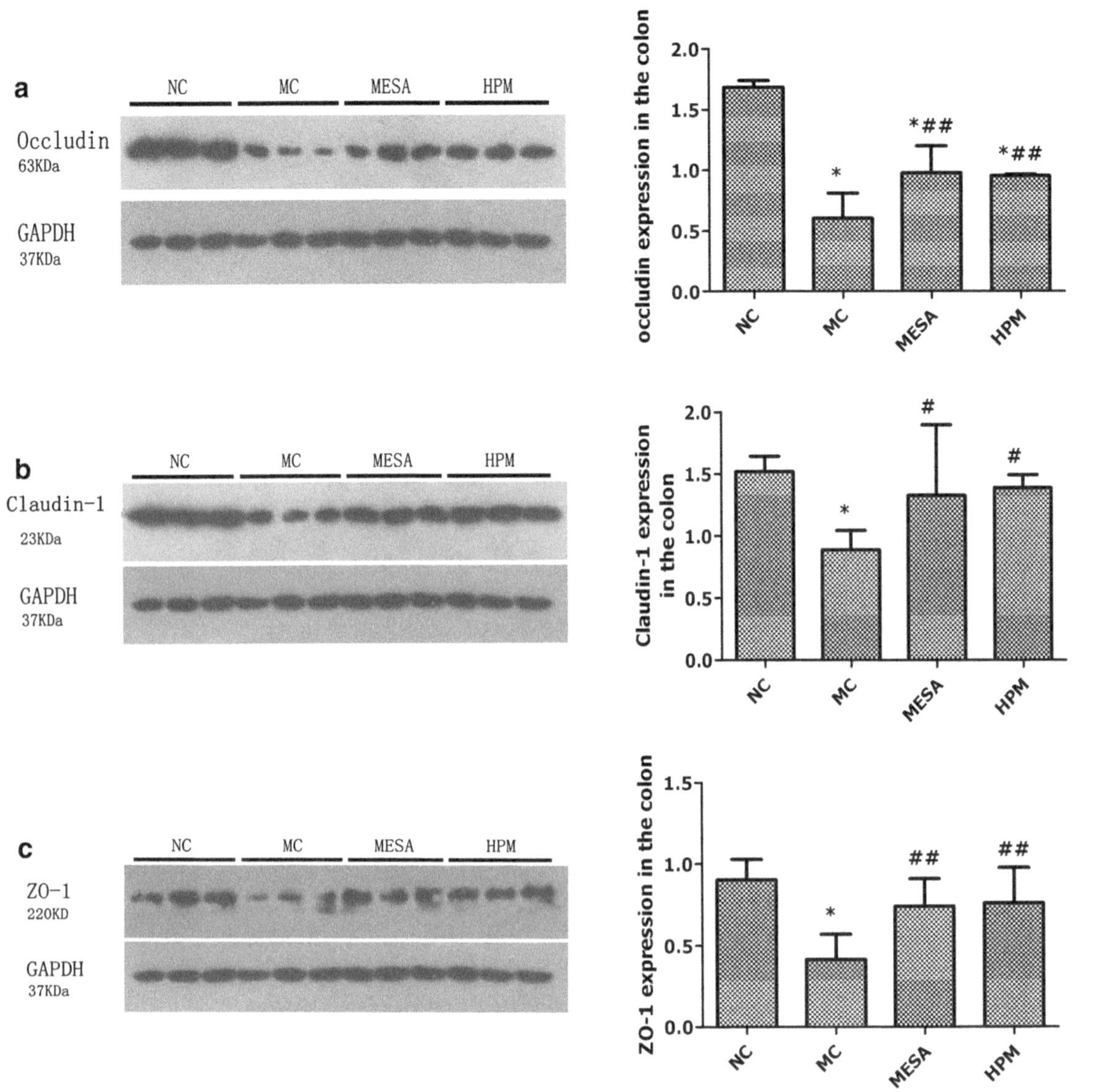

Fig. 4 Expression of colonic epithelial TJ-related proteins occludin, claudin-1 and ZO-1 in each group. **a** Expression of occludin in each group. **b** Expression of claudin-1 in each group. **c** Expression of ZO-1 in each group. *NC* normal control group, *MC* model control group, *MESA* mesalazine group, and *HPM* herb-partitioned moxibustion group. $^{*}P < 0.01$ versus NC; $^{\#}P < 0.01$ versus MC; $^{\#\#}P < 0.05$ versus MC

and intestinal wall stiffness were mainly the results of chronic recurrent inflammation. Compared with the MC group, the MESA and HPM groups showed remarkable signs of inflammation remission, as the mucosal hyperemia, edema, and ulcers were moderate and localized, and adhesions and strictures were barely observed.

By light microscopy, we observed pathological changes of the colonic tissues in the CD, HPM, and MESA groups. In tissues taken from the MC group, eosinophils and inflammatory cell infiltration in colonic mucosa and submucosa, and obvious submucosal hyperemia and edema, as well as obvious lymphoid follicles, fibroblast proliferation, and other typical CD pathological changes were observed under a light microscope. After treatment with mesalazine, these pathological changes were not improved. After treatment with HPM, there was only a small amount of inflammatory cell infiltration in colonic mucosa and submucosa, mild hyperemia, and scattered fibroblast proliferation among normal morphology of the mucosal, submucosal, and muscular tissues.

We then examined the TEER of the in vitro cultured colonic epithelial cells from the different groups. TEER determination is widely used to functionally analyze TJ dynamics in cell culture models of physiological barriers

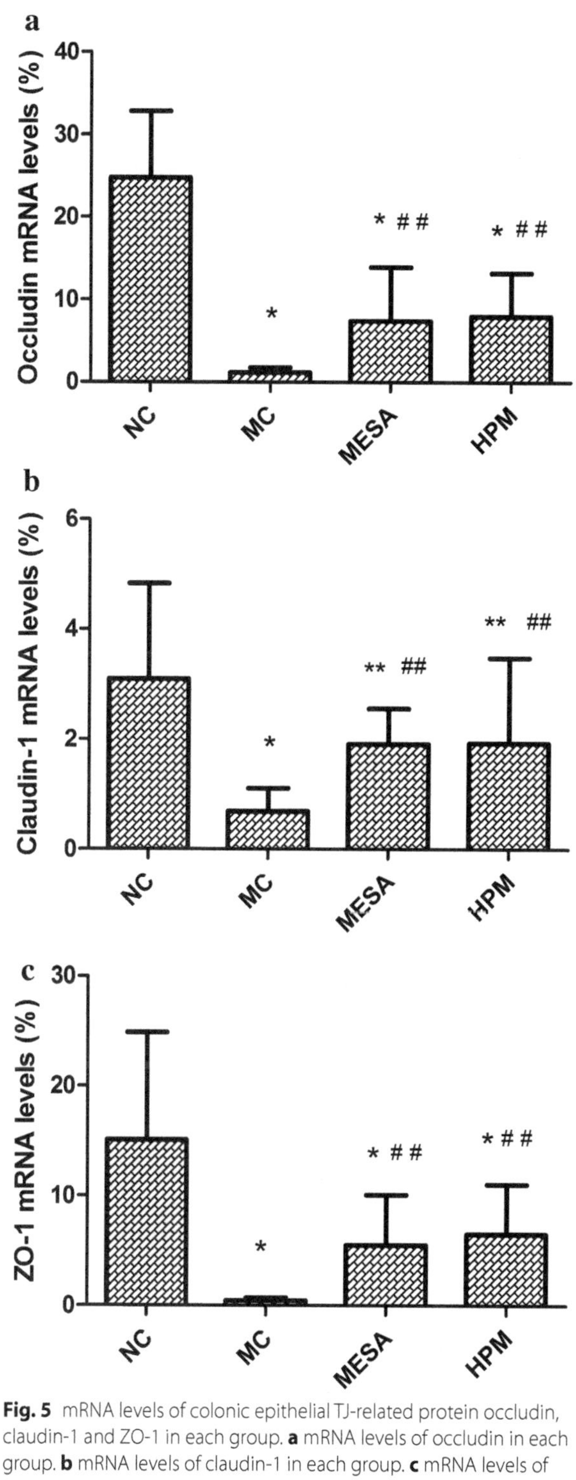

Fig. 5 mRNA levels of colonic epithelial TJ-related protein occludin, claudin-1 and ZO-1 in each group. **a** mRNA levels of occludin in each group. **b** mRNA levels of claudin-1 in each group. **c** mRNA levels of ZO-1 in each group. *NC* normal control group, *MC* model control group, *MESA* mesalazine group, and *HPM* herb-partitioned moxibustion group. **P* < 0.01 versus NC; ***P* < 0.05 versus NC; ##*P* < 0.05 versus MC

[30–32], which can be used to evaluate the paracellular permeability of epithelial monolayers. A decrease in TEER was associated with disruption of TJs and subtle changes in the cytoskeletal structure, resulting in a subsequent increase in the paracellular permeability of the epithelial monolayer [33]. In the present study, we found significant decreases in the TEER values in the MC group, but increases to different degrees in the HPM and MESA groups, with the HPM group showing larger rising trends. These findings suggested that during the pathological process of CD, the structure of TJs was impaired, leading to a subsequent decrease in the paracellular permeability of the epithelial monolayer. However, both HPM and mesalazine treatment can recover or reduce the abnormally increased colonic epithelial permeability in CD, and HPM possesses the advantages of repairing TJs and increasing the permeability of the epithelial monolayer.

The intestinal epithelium creates a chemical and mechanical barrier that separates the host from microbes [34]. The chemical barrier consists of mucus, peptides, and antimicrobial proteins secreted by goblet cells and Paneth cells, while the mechanical barrier is composed of different kinds of enterocytes and TJs to join the cells together. These barriers are responsible for permeability, i.e., selective absorption of water and nutrients in the gut lumen through either transepithelial or paracellular transport. TJs are multimolecular complexes that seal the intercellular space between adjacent epithelial cells [35] and act as a diffusion barrier to control the transportation of ions, macromolecules, and immune cells in the paracellular pathway [36], and are therefore the major determinants of epithelial permeability [37]. TJs maintain symbiosis within intestinal microflora and prevent infection or inflammation induced by bacterial translocation [38].

The TJ-related proteins of the intestinal epithelial barrier are mainly located at the top side of the enteric cavity among intestinal epithelial cells, then zonally surround the side wall and seal up the intestinal epithelial gap. TJs are composed of three transmembrane protein families [39]: claudins, junctional adhesion molecule (JAM) proteins, and TJ-associated Marvel domain proteins (TAMPs) including occludin, tricellulin, and Marvel D3. Claudins control the charge and size-selectivity of TJs, while JAMs and TAMPs stabilize TJs and maintain epithelial permeability. ZO-1 connects the multiprotein structure of TJs to peri-junctional actomyosin. These three protein families have overlapping and unique functions in the regulation of TJs [40]. In this study, occludin, claudin-1, and ZO-1 were formed into complex proteins by binding between the C-terminals of the TJ transmembrane proteins claudin-1 and occludin and the N-terminals of the cytoplasmic-attached protein ZO-1 [41], thus allowing their external parts to interact with the transmembrane junction proteins of adjacent cells. At the same time, the C-terminals of ZO-1 were connected with actin of the cytoplasmic cytoskeleton, making it possible for claudin-1 to act on these actin molecules, and thus participate in maintaining the stability and selective permeability of TJs [42]. Occludin is considered to be fundamental to the structure of TJs [43]. Knockout of the occludin gene [28] in epithelial cells can cause similar pathological intestinal changes to IBD in animals. Reduced expression of intestinal occludin protein and mRNA was observed in patients with ulcerative colitis and CD [3], suggesting the possible involvement of occludin in the pathogenesis of IBD. In the present study, in vitro experiments demonstrated radical decreases in colonic epithelial occludin protein and mRNA expression in the NC group, compared with remarkable recovery of the occludin protein and mRNA expression in the MESA and HPM groups. The same tendency was observed for the other two TJ-related proteins, claudin-1 and ZO-1.

Conclusions

HPM at *Tianshu* (ST25) and *Qihai* (RN6) upregulated the expression of occludin, claudin-1, and ZO-1 in TNBS-induced CD model rats.

Abbreviations

CD: Crohn's disease; IBD: inflammatory bowel disease; TJ: tight junction; TNF-α: tumor necrosis factor-alpha; TNFR1: tumor necrosis factor receptor-1; ZO-1: zonula occludens proteins-1; UC: ulcerative colitis; ECCO: European Crohn's and Colitis Organization; SD: Sprague–Dawley; TNBS: trinitrobenzene sulfonic acid; NC: normal control; MC: model control; HPM: herb-partitioned moxibustion; MESA: mesalazine; FQ-PCR: fluorescent quantitative polymerase chain reaction; DMEM: Dulbecco's modified Eagle's medium; PBS: phosphate buffer saline; RT: room temperature; GAPDH: glyceraldehyde-3-phosphate dehydrogenase; SD: standard deviation; ANOVA: one way analysis of variance; JAM: junctional adhesion molecule; TAMPs: TJ-associated Marvel domain proteins.

Authors' contributions

YS conceived and designed the study. RJ performed measurement of colonic TEER and cell culture. AQW performed the assessment of macroscopic colonic damage and Western blot. HXS performed FQ-PCR detection and cell culture. LC performed histological observation. HXS, LC, CHB and LYW performed data acquisition, analysis and interpretation. RJ and AQW wrote the manuscript. HGW revised the manuscript. All authors read and approved the final manuscript.

Author details

[1] College of Acumox and Tuina, Shanghai University of Traditional Chinese Medicine, Shanghai 201203, China. [2] Shanghai Research Institute of Acupuncture-Moxibustion and Meridian, Shanghai 200030, China.

Acknowledgements

The research was supported by a Grant (No. 81273844) from the National Natural Science Foundation of China. We also thank for the experimental technical support from the JRDUN Biotechnology (Shanghai) Co., Ltd.

Competing interests

The authors declare that they have no competing interests.

References

1. Kucharzik T, Lugering N, Rautenberg K, Lugering A, Schmidt MA, Stoll R, Domschke W. Role of M cells in intestinal barrier function. Ann N Y Acad Sci. 2000;915:171–83.
2. Cosnes J, Beaugerie L, Carbonnel F, Gendre JP. Smoking cessation and the course of Crohn's disease: an intervention study. Gastroenterology. 2001;120:1093–9.
3. Wu HG, Zhou LB, Shi DR, Liu SM, Liu HR, Zhang BM, Chen HP, Zhang LS. Morphological study on colonic pathology in ulcerative colitis treated by moxibustion. World J Gastroenterol. 2000;6:861–5.
4. Shi Y, Wu HG. The clinical study on herbs-partitioned moxibustion treatment of Crohn's disease. JiangXi J TCM. 2003;34:16–7.
5. Shi Y, Bao CH, Wu HG, Chen WF, Qin XD, Zhang R, Wu LY. Effect of herbs-partitioned moxibustion combined with acupuncture on the expressions of intestinal mucosa TNF-α, TNFR1, TNFR2 and apoptosis of intestinal epithelial cells in Crohn's disease patients. Shanghai J TCM. 2011;45:45–50.
6. Amasheh M, Grotjohann I, Amasheh S, Fromm A, Soderholm JD, Zeitz M, Fromm M, Schulzke JD. Regulation of mucosal structure and barrier function in rat colon exposed to tumor necrosis factor alpha and interferon gamma in vitro: a novel model for studying the pathomechanisms of inflammatory bowel disease cytokines. Scand J Gastroenterol. 2009;44:1226–35.
7. Gassler N, Rohr C, Schneider A, Kartenbeck J, Bach A, Obermuller N, Otto HF, Autschbach F. Inflammatory bowel disease is associated with changes of enterocytic junctions. Am J Physiol Gastrointest Liver Physiol. 2001;281:G216–28.
8. Poritz LS, Garver KI, Tilberg AF, Koltun WA. Tumor necrosis factor alpha disrupts tight junction assembly. J Surg Res. 2004;116:14–8.
9. McGuckin MA, Eri R, Simms LA, Florin TH, Radford-Smith G. Intestinal barrier dysfunction in inflammatory bowel diseases. Inflamm Bowel Dis. 2009;15:100–13.
10. Edelblum KL, Turner JR. The tight junction in inflammatory disease: communication breakdown. Curr Opin Pharmacol. 2009;9:715–20.
11. May GR, Sutherland LR, Meddings JB. Is small intestinal permeability really increased in relatives of patients with Crohn's disease? Gastroenterology. 1993;104:1627–32.
12. Schmitz H, Barmeyer C, Fromm M, Runkel N, Foss HD, Bentzel CJ, Riecken EO, Schulzke JD. Altered tight junction structure contributes to the impaired epithelial barrier function in ulcerative colitis. Gastroenterology. 1999;116:301–9.
13. Oshitani N, Watanabe K, Nakamura S, Fujiwara Y, Higuchi K, Arakawa T. Dislocation of tight junction proteins without F-actin disruption in inactive Crohn's disease. Int J Mol Med. 2005;15:407–10.
14. Kucharzik T, Walsh SV, Chen J, Parkos CA, Nusrat A. Neutrophil transmigration in inflammatory bowel disease is associated with differential expression of epithelial intercellular junction proteins. Am J Pathol. 2001;159:2001–9.
15. Gisbert JP, Chaparro M, Gomollon F. Common misconceptions about 5-aminosalicylates and thiopurines in inflammatory bowel disease. World J Gastroenterol. 2011;17:3467–78.
16. Iacucci M, Ghosh S. Mesalazine in inflammatory bowel disease: a trendy topic once again. Canadian J Gastroenterol. 2010;24:127–33.
17. Sutherland L, Macdonald JK. Oral 5-aminosalicylic acid for induction of remission in ulcerative colitis. The Cochrane database of systematic reviews. 2006: CD000543.
18. Feagan BG. 5-ASA therapy for active Crohn's disease: old friends, old data, and a new conclusion. Clin Gastroenterol Hepatol. 2004;2:376–8.

19. Dignass A, Van Assche G, Lindsay JO, Lemann M, Soderholm J, Colombel JF, Danese S, D'Hoore A, Gassull M, Gomollon F, et al. The second European evidence-based consensus on the diagnosis and management of Crohn's disease: current management. J Crohn's Colitis. 2010;4:28–62.
20. Terdiman JP, Gruss CB, Heidelbaugh JJ, Sultan S, Falck-Ytter YT. Practice AGAIC, Quality Management C: american Gastroenterological Association Institute guideline on the use of thiopurines, methotrexate, and anti-TNF-alpha biologic drugs for the induction and maintenance of remission in inflammatory Crohn's disease. Gastroenterology. 2013;145:1459–63.
21. Bao CH, Wu LY, Shi Y, Wu HG, Liu HR, Zhang R, Yu LQ, Wang JH. Moxibustion down-regulates colonic epithelial cell apoptosis and repairs tight junctions in rats with Crohn's disease. World J Gastroenterol. 2011;17:4960–70.
22. Shi Y, Bao CH, Wu HG, Ma XP, Yu LQ, Zhang R, Chen WF. Effect of moxibustion on colonic TNF-alpha content and influence of colonic supernatant of crohn's disease rats undergoing moxibustion on expression of occludin, claudin-1 and zonula occludens-1 proteins and genes in cultured colonic epithelial cells. Acupuncture Res. 2011;36:235–41.
23. Morris GP, Beck PL, Herridge MS, Depew WT, Szewczuk MR, Wallace JL. Hapten-induced model of chronic inflammation and ulceration in the rat colon. Gastroenterology. 1989;96:795–803.
24. Xu SY, Bian RL, Chen X: Experimental Methodology of Pharmacology. Beijing: People's Medical Publishing House; 1982 .p. 1184.
25. Vilaseca J, Salas A, Guarner F, Rodriguez R, Martinez M, Malagelada JR. Dietary fish oil reduces progression of chronic inflammatory lesions in a rat model of granulomatous colitis. Gut. 1990;31:539–44.
26. Yeh KY, Chopra DP. Epithelial cell cultures from the colon of the suckling rat. In Vitro. 1980;16:976–86.
27. Ma TY, Nguyen D, Bui V, Nguyen H, Hoa N. Ethanol modulation of intestinal epithelial tight junction barrier. Am J Physiol. 1999;276:G965–74.
28. Schmitz H, Fromm M, Bentzel CJ, Scholz P, Detjen K, Mankertz J, Bode H, Epple HJ, Riecken EO, Schulzke JD. Tumor necrosis factor-alpha (TNFalpha) regulates the epithelial barrier in the human intestinal cell line HT-29/B6. J Cell Sci. 1999;112(Pt 1):137–46.
29. Blume LF, Denker M, Gieseler F, Kunze T. Temperature corrected transepithelial electrical resistance (TEER) measurement to quantify rapid changes in paracellular permeability. Pharmazie. 2010;65:19–24.
30. Muendoerfer M, Schaefer UF, Koenig P, Walk JS, Loos P, Balbach S, Eichinger T, Lehr CM. Online monitoring of transepithelial electrical resistance (TEER) in an apparatus for combined dissolution and permeation testing. Int J Pharm. 2010;392:134–40.
31. Balda MS, Whitney JA, Flores C, Gonzalez S, Cereijido M, Matter K. Functional dissociation of paracellular permeability and transepithelial electrical resistance and disruption of the apical-basolateralintramembrane diffusion barrier by expression of a mutant tight junction membrane protein. J Cell Biol. 1996;134:1031–49.
32. Klingberg TD, Pedersen MH, Cencic A, Budde BB. Application of measurements of transepithelial electrical resistance of intestinal epithelial cell monolayers to evaluate probiotic activity. Appl Environ Microbiol. 2005;71:7528–30.
33. Narai A, Arai S, Shimizu M. Rapid decrease in transepithelial electrical resistance of human intestinal Caco-2 cell monolayers by cytotoxic membrane perturbents. Toxicol In Vitro. 1997;11:347–54.
34. Stappenbeck TS, Rioux JD, Mizoguchi A, Saitoh T, Huett A, Darfeuille-Michaud A, Wileman T, Mizushima N, Carding S, Akira S, et al. Crohn disease: a current perspective on genetics, autophagy and immunity. Autophagy. 2011;7:355–74.
35. Weber CR, Turner JR. Inflammatory bowel disease: is it really just another break in the wall? Gut. 2007;56:6–8.
36. Furuse M. Molecular basis of the core structure of tight junctions. Cold Spring Harb Perspect Biol. 2010;2:a002907.
37. Gunzel D, Yu AS. Claudins and the modulation of tight junction permeability. Physiol Rev. 2013;93:525–69.
38. Farhadi A, Banan A, Fields J, Keshavarzian A. Intestinal barrier: an interface between health and disease. J Gastroenterol Hepatol. 2003;18:479–97.
39. Rodgers LS, Beam MT, Anderson JM, Fanning AS. Epithelial barrier assembly requires coordinated activity of multiple domains of the tight junction protein ZO-1. J Cell Sci. 2013;126:1565–75.
40. Shen L. Tight junctions on the move: molecular mechanisms for epithelial barrier regulation. Ann N Y Acad Sci. 2012;1258:9–18.
41. Hermiston ML, Gordon JI. Inflammatory bowel disease and adenomas in mice expressing a dominant negative N-cadherin. Science. 1995;270:1203–7.
42. Gonzalez JE, DiGeronimo RJ, Arthur DE, King JM. Remodeling of the tight junction during recovery from exposure to hydrogen peroxide in kidney epithelial cells. Free Radic Biol Med. 2009;47:1561–9.
43. Blasig IE, Bellmann C, Cording J, Del Vecchio G, Zwanziger D, Huber O, Haseloff RF. Occludin protein family: oxidative stress and reducing conditions. Antioxid Redox Signal. 2011;15:1195–219.

7

Inhibitory effect of *trans*-ferulic acid on proliferation and migration of human lung cancer cells accompanied with increased endogenous reactive oxygen species and β-catenin instability

Yao Fong[1†], Chia-Chun Tang[2†], Huei-Ting Hu[3], Hsin-Yu Fang[4], Bing-Hung Chen[3,10], Chang-Yi Wu[3,5], Shyng-Shiou Yuan[6], Hui-Min David Wang[7], Yen-Chun Chen[3], Yen-Ni Teng[8] and Chien-Chih Chiu[3,5,6,9*]

Abstract

Background: *Trans*-ferulic (FA) acid exhibits antioxidant effects in vitro. However, the underlying mechanism of *trans*-FA activity in cellular physiology, especially cancer physiology, remains largely unknown. This study investigated the cellular physiological effects of *trans*-FA on the H1299 human lung cancer cell line.

Methods: The 2,2-diphenyl-1-picrylhydrazyl assay was used to determine free radical scavenging capability. Assessment of intracellular reactive oxygen species (ROS) was evaluated using oxidized 2′,7′-dichlorofluorescin diacetate and dihydroethidium staining. Trypan blue exclusion, colony formation, and anchorage-independent growth assays were used to determine cellular proliferation. Annexin V staining assay was used to assess cellular apoptosis by flow cytometry. Wound healing and Boyden's well assays were used to detect the migration and invasion of cells. Gelatin zymography was used to detect matrix metalloproteinase (MMP-2 and MMP-9) activity. Western blotting was used to detect expression levels of various signaling pathway proteins.

Results: DPPH assay results indicated that *trans*-FA exerted potent antioxidant effects. However, *trans*-FA increased intracellular ROS levels, including hydrogen peroxide and superoxide anion, in H1299 cells. *Trans*-FA treatment inhibited cellular proliferation and induced moderate apoptotic cell death at the highest concentration used (0.6 mM). Furthermore, *trans*-FA moderately inhibited the migration of H1299 cells at the concentrations of 0.3 and 0.6 mM and attenuated MMP-2 and MMP-9 activity. *Trans*-FA caused the phosphorylation of β-catenin, resulting in proteasomal degradation of β-catenin. Conversely, *trans*-FA treatment increased the expression of pro-apoptotic factor Bax and decreased the expression of pro-survival factor survivin.

Conclusion: Various concentrations (0.06–0.6 mM) of *trans*-FA exert both anti-proliferation and anti-migration effects in the human lung cancer cell line H1299.

Background

In 2013, the mortality rates for male and female lung cancer patients in the United States were 28 and 26 %, respectively [1]. At present, chemotherapy is the primary treatment for lung cancer [2–4], with both carboplatin and cisplatin commonly used as chemotherapy drugs [5, 6]. However, the combination of cisplatin or vinblastine with irradiation increases the level of unexpected toxicity in the body [4]. Pemetrexed (Alimta®), a next-generation antifolate drug, is used for treating malignant pleural mesothelioma and non-small cell lung cancer (NSCLC)

*Correspondence: cchiu@kmu.edu.tw
†Yao Fong and Chia-Chun Tang contributed equally to this work
[3] Department of Biotechnology, Kaohsiung Medical University, Kaohsiung 807, Taiwan
Full list of author information is available at the end of the article

but can induce scleroderma-like induration of the lower extremities [7]. It is therefore necessary to develop alternative treatment strategies for selective inhibition of lung cancer cells growth.

The carcinogenic process may be driven by mutations, leading to alterations in phenotypes, genetics, and epigenetics. The induction of oxidative stress in various cancer cells such as human pancreatic and colon adenocarcinoma cancer cell lines [8] was shown to inhibit expression of β-catenin and the matrix metalloproteinases MMP-2 and MMP-9 in colitis-associated colon carcinoma [9], induce Bax expression in urothelial cell carcinoma [10], induce apoptosis by blocking the AMPK-mTOR-survivin pathway [11], and inhibit the anchorage-independent growth (AIG) of transformed cells [12]. Chemopreventive treatment is moderate or non-cytotoxic to normal cells, but significantly inhibits cancer cell growth or metastasis. Accumulating evidence shows that anti-oxidative compounds isolated from plants exert potentially chemopreventive effects. Among these compounds are carotenoids, curcumin, and hesperidin [13, 14]. Recently, anticancer compounds derived from plants, including goniothalamin and feruloyl-L-arabinose, were shown to inhibit the growth and metastasis of human lung cancer cells [15, 16]. Additionally, moscatilin, isolated from the orchid *Dendrobrium loddigesii*, inhibited metastasis of both human breast and lung cancer cells [17, 18].

Ferulic acid (FA) is an aromatic compound, abundant in plant cell walls [19, 20]. Both isomers of FA, *cis*-FA and *trans*-FA, show a potent ability to remove reactive oxygen species (ROS) and inhibit lipid peroxidation [20, 21]. Unlike *cis*-FA, *trans*-FA is abundant in plant cells and easily isolated from various plants, thus significantly reducing the cost of its preparation [22].

Trans-FA ameliorated ionizing radiation-induced inflammation and glycerol-induced nephrotoxicity [23, 24] and modulated fluoride-induced oxidative hepatotoxicity in male Wistar rats [25]. Water-soluble *trans*-FA sugar esters protected normal rat erythrocytes against peroxyl radical 2,2′-azobis-2-amidinopropane dihydrochloride (AAPH)-induced oxidative damage [26] and exhibited protective capacity against oxidative damage caused by diabetes [27, 28]. Furthermore, *trans*-FA exhibited antiproliferative effects in colon cancer cells [29, 30], increased the radiosensitivity of cervical cancer cells [31], and exerted protective effects against chemical-induced DNA strand breaks [32, 33]. However, the effects of *trans*-FA in lung cancer have not been reported to date, and its biological mechanism remains unknown.

The study investigated the cellular and physiological effects of *trans*-FA in human lung cancer cells.

Methods

Chemicals

Trans-FA (4-hydroxy-3-methoxycinnamic acid) was purchased from Sigma-Aldrich Chemicals (#128708, St. Louis, MO, USA). *Trans*-FA was freshly dissolved in 0.01 % dimethyl sulfoxide (DMSO) and aliquoted before use.

Cell culture

The human non-small cell lung cancer (NSCLC) cell line H1299 and lung fibroblast cells HEL-299 were obtained from the American Type Culture Collection (ATCC, Manassas, VA, USA). Cells were maintained in DMEM:F-12 medium (1:1 ratio) supplemented with 8 % fetal bovine serum, 2 mM glutamine, 100 units/mL penicillin, and 100 μg/mL streptomycin (Gibco BRL, Gaithersburg, MD, USA) at 37 °C in a humidified atmosphere of 5 % CO_2 [4].

DPPH radical-scavenging activity assay

The anti-oxidant activities of *trans*-FA were measured based on the scavenging activity of 2,2-diphenyl-1-picrylhydrazyl (DPPH) (#D9132, Sigma-Aldrich) free radical [34, 35]. Briefly, vitamin C standards and various *trans*-FA concentrations were freshly prepared and diluted in methanol. Methanol (as a blank control; 10 μM) or *trans*-FA solution was added to 90 μL DPPH solution to yield a final *trans*-FA concentration of 0.15 mg/mL in a 96-well microplate. The mixture was incubated at 25 °C and protected from light. After incubation, solution absorbance was measured at 492 nm using a Multiskan Ascent 354 microplate reader (Thermo Fisher Scientific, Rockford, IL, USA). DPPH radical scavenging activity was calculated as follows:

$$\text{DPPH radical scavenging activity (\%)} = (1 - A_0/A_1) \times 100$$

where A_0 and A_1 are the absorbances of the control and *trans*-FA solutions, respectively. Each experiment was repeated three times and found to be reproducible within experimental error margins.

Cell viability and proliferation assay

Briefly, 5×10^4 cells were seeded into wells of a 12-well plate and treated with phosphate-buffered saline (PBS) (Sigma-Aldrich) as control or concentrations of *trans*-FA (0.03–0.6 mM) for 24 or 48 h. After incubation, cell viability and proliferation were analyzed by trypan blue assay and an automated cell counter (Countess™) according to the manufacturer's instructions (Invitrogen, Carlsbad, CA, USA).

Colony formation assay

Fifty cells were seeded into wells of a 6-well plate and, after 24 h of incubation, were treated with different concentrations of *trans*-FA (0.03–0.6 mM). After incubation for 11 days, cell colonies were glutaraldehyde-fixed and stained with crystal violet (0.1 % w/v) for 10 min. Colony diameter was determined using Image-Pro v3.0 software (Media Cybernetics, Silver Spring, MD, USA).

Anchorage-independent growth (AIG) assay

The assay procedure was performed as described in our previous work, with minor modifications [36]. Briefly, 1×10^3 cells were mixed with 0.75 % low melting agarose (MDBio Inc, Taipei, Taiwan). The mixtures were placed on a solidified layer of 1.5 % agarose with medium in a 12-well plate. After incubation for 13 days, cells in the upper layer were fixed with 1 % glutaraldehyde and stained with 0.1 % w/v Giemsa (Merck, Darmstadt, Germany). Colony diameter was determined using Image-Pro v3.0 software.

Cell cycle analysis

Cell cycle distribution was assessed using propidium iodide (PI; Sigma-Aldrich) staining described previously [37]. Briefly, 1×10^5 cells were treated with PBS (as vehicle control) or various *trans*-FA concentrations (0.03–0.6 mM) for 48 h. Next, cells were detached using 0.05 % trypsin (Biological Industries, Kibbutz Beit Haemek, Israel) for 5 min, harvested, and washed with PBS. Cells were then fixed with 75 % ethanol overnight. After centrifugation (Microfuge® 16, Beckman Coulter Life Sciences, Taipei, Taiwan) at 664×*g* for 15 min at 4 °C, the resulting supernatants were decanted. Cell pellets were stained with 10 μg/mL PI and 10 μg/mL RNase A (Sigma-Aldrich) in PBS buffer for 30 min at 37 °C in the dark. The samples were assayed using a FACScan flow cytometer (Becton–Dickinson, Mansfield, MA, USA) and the results were analyzed using FlowJo v7.5.5 software (Tree Star Inc., San Carlos, CA).

Assessment of apoptosis

Apoptotic cell death was assessed by annexin V and PI double staining (Pharmingen, San Diego, CA, USA) according to our previous paper [15]. Briefly, 1×10^6 cells were seeded into a 100-mm petri dish and treated with vehicle or *trans*-FA at doses of 0–0.6 mM for 48 h. Next, cells were inoculated with 10 μg/mL of annexin V-fluorescein isothiocyanate (FITC) and 20 μg/mL of PI and analyzed using a FACScan flow cytometer FlowJo v7.5.5 software.

Detection of endogenous ROS

Changes in endogenous ROS levels were assessed using the fluorescent indicators 2′,7′-dichlorofluorescin diacetate (DCFDA, Sigma-Aldrich) for hydrogen peroxide (H_2O_2) and dihydroethidium (DHE) (Invitrogen) for superoxide anion (O_2^-). A total of 1×10^5 H1299 cells were seeded into wells of a 6-well culture plate and treated with various concentrations (from 0.03 to 0.15 mM) of *trans*-FA for 24 h. Next, cells were harvested and stained with 100 nM DCFDA or 1 μM DHE for 30 min at 37 °C in PBS and then washed twice with PBS. Fluorescence was measured by flow cytometry.

Western blot assay

Western blot assays were performed as described previously [38]. Briefly, cells were harvested and lysed, lysates were centrifuged, and protein concentrations of cell pellets were determined. Next, 40 mg quantities of protein lysate were resolved by 10 % SDS–polyacrylamide gel electrophoresis and electro-transferred to polyvinylidene difluoride membranes. The membranes were blocked with 5 % nonfat milk and incubated with the following primary antibodies: Thr^{41}/Ser^{45} phosphorylated β-catenin (#2377-S, Epitomics, CA, USA), β-catenin (#sc-7963, Santa Cruz Biotech., CA, USA), Bax (#ab32503, Abcam Inc., Cambridge, MA, USA), survivin (#614701, Biolegend, CA, USA), and β-actin (#AM1021b, Abgent, San Diego, CA, USA), followed by appropriate secondary antibodies (anti-Mouse, #074-1806; anti-Rabbit, #074-1506, KPL, Gaithersburg, MD, USA). The Western-Bright™ ECL kit (Advansta, CA, USA) was used for signal detection.

Wound-healing assay

Quantities of 3×10^5 H1299 cells were seeded in wells of a 12-well plate, treated with PBS (as vehicle control) or *trans*-FA (0.03–0.6 mM), and grown to 100 % confluence. Culture monolayers were scratched using a pipette tip to create a clean 1-mm-wide wound area. After further incubation for 16 h, the wound gaps were photographed and analyzed using TScratch software (CSE Lab, Zurich, Switzerland) [39].

Transwell invasion assay

Invasion assays were performed as described in our previous work, with minor modifications [40], using 8 μm-pore Transwell® chambers (Greiner Bio-One, Frickenhausen, Germany). Control and various concentrations (from 0.03 to 0.6 mM) of *trans*-FA treated cells were cultured in triplicate at 5×10^4 cells/well in the upper inserts of 24-well Transwell® culture plates. Next, cells were fixed for 5 min and stained with 0.1 % w/v Giemsa. The cells which had invaded the lower inserts were counted by arbitrarily selecting five fields from each well. The experiments were repeated three times.

Gelatin zymography

MMP-2 and -9 activity was assessed by gelatin zymography as previously described [41], with minor modification. Briefly, 3×10^5 H1299 cells were seeded into wells of 12-well plates and cultured with various concentrations of *trans*-FA for 24 h, after which aliquots of culture medium were harvested for gelatin zymography analysis. Samples were prepared in standard SDS-PAGE loading buffer containing 0.01 % SDS without β-mercaptoethanol and were not boiled before use. Next, the samples were subjected to electrophoresis (150 V for 3 h) on 10 % SDS–polyacrylamide gels containing 1 % gelatin. After electrophoresis, the gels were thoroughly washed with distilled water containing 2.5 % Triton X-100 on a gyratory shaker for 30 min at room temperature. Gels were incubated in 100 mL reaction buffer (40 mM Tris–HCl, pH 8.0; 10 mM $CaCl_2$, and 0.02 % NaN_3) at 37 °C overnight, followed by staining with Coomassie brilliant blue R-250 (Bio basic Inc., Markham, Ontario, Canada) and de-staining with methanol-acetic acid–water (50/75/875, v/v/v). The gelatinase activities of MMP-2 and -9 were determined by analyzing signal intensity using Gel Pro v.4.0 software (Media Cybernetics, Silver Spring, MD, USA).

Statistical analysis

All data are mean ± SD from at least three experiments, with three replicates per experiment. The significance of the differences was analyzed using one-way analysis of variance (ANOVA) and SigmaPlot v12.0 software (Systat Software Inc., San Jose, CA, USA). *P* values less than 0.05 were considered statistically significant.

Results

Radical scavenging activity of *trans*-FA

The DPPH assay was used to assess the radical scavenging activity of *trans*-FA. Antioxidant activity was calculated by evaluating the capacity of *trans*-FA to scavenge DPPH. As shown in Fig. 1, *trans*-FA treatment produced significant radical-scavenging activity compared with the DMSO control. Vitamin C was serially diluted in methanol (500–7.8 μM) and used in triplicate as a positive control (Additional file 1).

The short-term effect of *trans*-FA on proliferation of NSCLC cells

H1299 cells were treated with PBS (as vehicle control) or different concentrations of *trans*-FA for 24 or 48 h before gross morphological changes were examined by light microscopy to determine the effect of *trans*-FA on cell growth (Fig. 2a). Cells exhibited no significant change in morphology compared with the vehicle control. Next, measurement of cell survival was performed by trypan blue dye exclusion assay. Low doses (>0.15 mM) of *trans*-FA exerted no significant cytotoxic effect, but moderate cytotoxicity was observed with 0.3 and 0.6 mM treatment for 48 h (Fig. 2b).

The long-term effect of *trans*-FA on colony formation and AIG assay in NSCLC cells

As shown in Fig. 3a, *trans*-FA inhibited colony formation in H1299 cells after 11 days of treatment. The calculated colony diameters for *trans*-FA concentrations of 0, 0.06, 0.15, 0.3 and 0.6 mM were 100 ± 0.00, 77.19 ± 2.70, 64.19 ± 2.75, 56.75 ± 4.23 and 4.59 ± 1.25 % (n = 3), respectively. Figure 3c shows that long-term treatment with *trans*-FA inhibited the AIG capacity of H1299 cells. Furthermore, the results of the colony formation showed the selectively inhibitory effect of *trans*-FA on cellular proliferation between lung cancer cells H1299 and lung fibroblast cells HEL-299 (Additional file 2). The calculated colony diameters for *trans*-FA at 0, 0.03, 0.06, 0.15, 0.3 and 0.6 mM were 100 ± 3.10, 95.34 ± 4.18, 85.64 ± 1.08, 75.51 ± 2.41, 70.41 ± 1.71 and 61.36 ± 2.70 % (n = 3), respectively.

Trans-FA caused moderate G_0/G_1 accumulation

The effects of 48 h *trans*-FA treatment on cell cycle progression in H1299 cells were examined. *Trans*-FA treatments caused the arrest of the cell cycle at G_0/G_1 and a decrease in the percentage of the G_2/M phase (Fig. 4a, b).

Trans-FA-induced apoptosis in lung cancer cells

We investigated whether inhibition of proliferation by *trans*-FA was achieved by apoptosis in H1299 cells. Only the highest concentration (0.6 mM) of *trans*-FA increased the proportion of Annexin V^+/PI^+ cells (from 1.81 to 5.4 %) (Fig. 5). Other concentrations of *trans*-FA used in the study did not induce a significant increase in apoptotic populations.

Trans-FA induced changes in intracellular ROS

The endogenous level of ROS can regulate a variety of cellular physiological processes, including survival, proliferation, angiogenesis, and signaling pathways [42]. Flow cytometry-based detection with DCFDA and DHE staining was used to detect endogenous H_2O_2 and O_2^-, respectively. As shown in Fig. 6, H_2O_2 concentrations of 100 ± 20, 317 ± 28, 364 ± 23 and 375 ± 20 % (n = 3) were observed in H1299 cells treated with different concentrations of *trans*-FA (0–0.15 mM) for 24 h. Furthermore, endogenous O_2^- concentrations of 100 ± 9, 100 ± 2, 241 ± 19 and 392 ± 7 % (n = 3) were observed with the same *trans*-FA concentrations (Fig. 6b).

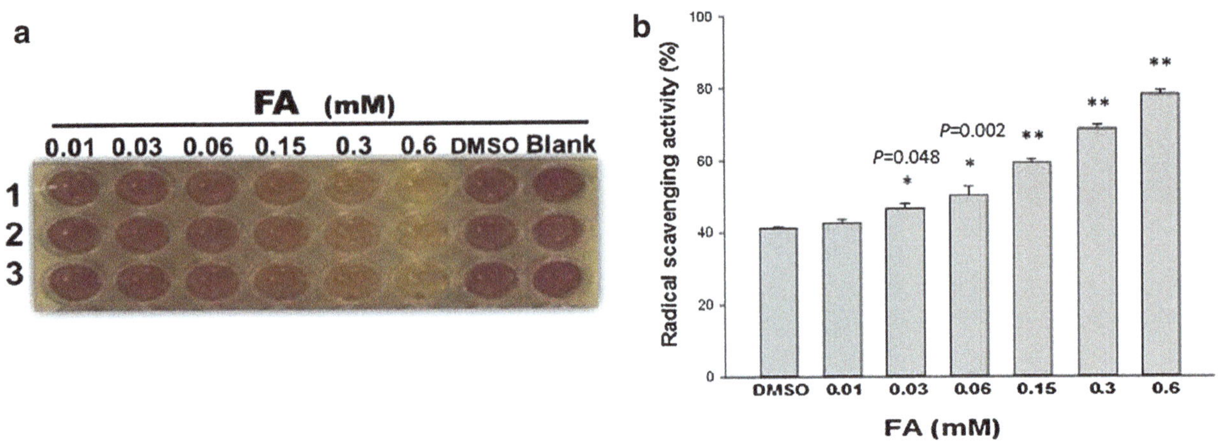

Fig. 1 DPPH radical-scavenging capacity of *trans*-FA. **a** *Trans*-FA was tested in an antioxidant assay by measuring the DPPH radical-scavenging activity. The indicated concentrations of *trans*-FA were incubated with DPPH respectively as described in the "Methods" section. **b** Quantificative analysis. The radical-scavenging capacity of *trans*-FA at indicated concentrations was quantified as the percentage decrease in absorbance at 492 nm against the DMSO control. *$P < 0.05$ and **$P < 0.001$, respectively

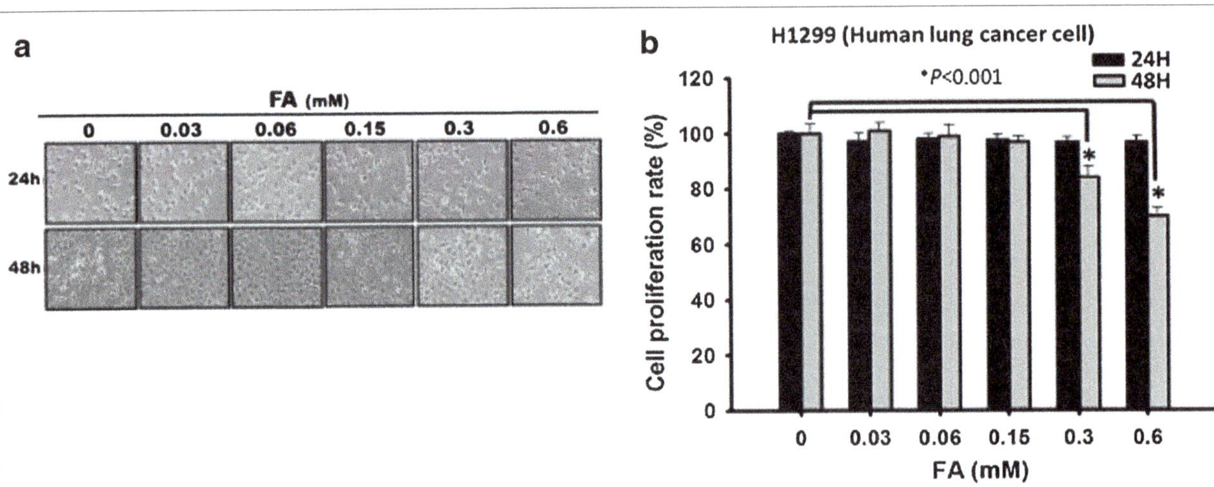

Fig. 2 Comparison of cell morphology and proliferation between of control and *trans*-FA-treated of NSCLC cells. **a** H1299 cells were treated with PBS as vehicle control or the indicated doses of *trans*-FA for 24 and 48 h, respectively. And then, morphology was examined and photographed with a light microscope. (phase contrast, X200). **b** 5×10^4 H1299 cells were seeded onto a 12-well plate, and cells were treated with indicated doses of *trans*-FA for 24 and 48 h, respectively. Cell viability was determined using the trypan blue exclusion assay described in "Methods" section. *$P < 0.001$ against vehicle control

Regulation of survival proteins by *trans*-FA

Western blotting was used to examine whether *trans*-FA treatment affected the expression of β-catenin in H1299 cells. As shown in Fig. 7, *trans*-FA treatment increased β-catenin phosphorylation at Thr^{41}/Ser^{45} but did not affect β-catenin protein levels. The anti-cancer effects of *trans*-FA might act by selective inhibition of β-catenin, a transcription factor associated with the growth and migration of H1299 cells. Anti-survival Bax protein was increased following *trans*-FA treatment in a dose-responsive manner, although the protein level of survivin was decreased.

Trans-FA attenuated the motility of lung cancer cells

Wound-healing assays were performed to investigate whether *trans*-FA affected migration of NSCLC cells. *trans*-FA treatment moderately attenuated the migration of H1299 lung cancer cells (Fig. 8). The area of the denuded zone was used as an index of the migratory ability of H1299 cells. The areas measured for *trans*-FA concentrations of 0, 0.03, 0.06, 0.15, 0.3 and 0.6 mM were 100 % ± 5.78, 96.86 % ± 2.69, 98.99 % ± 4.39, 93.95 % ± 6.77, 85.78 % ± 5.76 and 76.87 % ± 1.76 (n = 3), respectively.

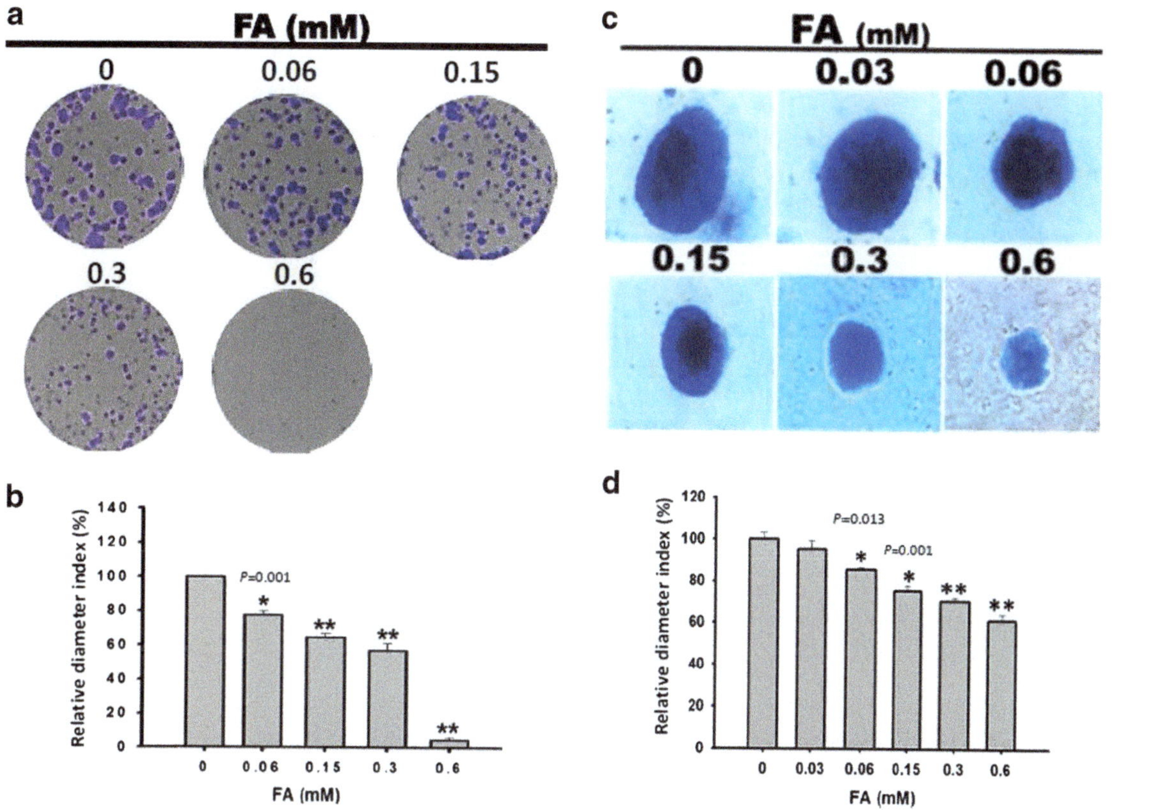

Fig. 3 The long-term effect of *trans*-FA on colony formation and anchorage-independent growth assay of NSCLC. **a** The assessment of colony formation, a 2D indicator of cell proliferation. Adherent H1299 cells were treated with indicated concentrations for 24 h. 5 × 10 cells treated with *trans*-FA were allowed to form colonies for 11 days. Afterward, colonies were fixed and stained using crystal violet. **c** Representative results showed the formation of tumor spheres, an indicator of 3D for anchorage-independent growth. H1299 cells were treated with indicated concentrations of *trans*-FA for 13 days using the soft agar assay. **b, d** Quantitative analysis of results from **a** and **c** showed the number and size of tumorspheres. *$P < 0.05$ and **$P < 0.001$, respectively

Trans-FA exerted an anti-invasion effect

A Boyden chamber assay was used to evaluate invasion ability. After treating H1299 cells with various concentrations (from 0.03 to 0.6 mM) of *trans*-FA for 16 h, the percentages of invasive cells were 100 % ± 7.49, 95.79 % ± 3.42, 95.61 % ± 5.86, 88.39 % ± 7.01, 82.57 % ± 5.87 and 68.57 % ± 4.48 (n = 3) (Fig. 9).

Trans-FA reduced the activity of MMP-2 and MMP-9

MMP-2 and MMP-9 are gelatinases which degrade extracellular matrix and thus regulate the ability of cells to migrate. Overexpression of MMP-2 and MMP-9 promotes cancer progression and is highly correlated with poor prognosis of cancer patients [43]. Therefore, targeting of MMP-2 and -9 represents a promising strategy for cancer treatment [44]. The activity of MMP-2 and MMP-9 was determined using a gelatin zymography assay (Fig. 10a). *Trans*-FA treatment (0, 0.03, 0.06, 0.15, 0.3 and 0.6 mM) significantly reduced the activity of MMP-2 [100 ± 2.95, 90.59 ± 1.96, 80.43 ± 4.46, 71.99 ± 2.9, 66.04 ± 1.59 and 55.87 ± 0.26 % (n = 3)] (Fig. 10b, c). The activity of MMP-9 [100 ± 4.44, 105.13 ± 5.29, 94.04 ± 0.99, 112.08 ± 5.24, 78.04 ± 1.86 and 53.32 ± 2.38 % (n = 3)] was also reduced.

Discussion

The radical scavenger assay findings indicated the potent anti-oxidant activity of *trans*-FA (Fig. 1). Treatment with *trans*-FA for 24 or 48 h did not affect cellular morphology and proliferation of lung cancer H1299 cells (Fig. 2). However, long-term treatment with *trans*-FA attenuated colony formation and AIG, characteristics of advanced cancer, in H1299 cells (Fig. 3). *Trans*-FA induced moderate cell proliferation at the lowest concentration tested (0.03 mM). These results were consistent with previous reports that *trans*-FA promoted proliferation of MCF7 and BT20 breast cancer cells and neural progenitor cells [45, 46]. The colony formation assay also showed the discrepant inhibitory effect of *trans*-FA on cellular proliferation of lung cancer cells H1299 and lung fibroblast cells

HEL-299 (Additional file 2), suggesting the potential of *trans*-FA for selectively inhibiting lung cancer. Furthermore, *trans*-FA significantly inhibited AIG capability in a dose-responsive manner.

Trans-FA caused an accumulation of the G_0/G_1 population and induced a moderate increase in the apoptotic population at the highest concentration (0.6 mM) (Fig. 4). G_0/G_1 cell cycle arrest is usually associated with the upregulation of cell cycle regulatory protein $p15^{INK4b}$ and $p21^{WAF1/Cip1}$ [47]. A recent study showed that perillyl alcohol, a natural compound purified from citrus fruits and herbs, causes G_1 arrest and inhibits proliferation of human immortalized keratinocyte HaCaT cells through inducing $p15^{INK4b}$ and $p21^{WAF1/Cip1}$ [47]. Annexin V staining confirmed that the anti-cancer effects of *Trans*-FA were not mediated through apoptosis (Fig. 5).

Excess endogenous ROS may inhibit cellular growth or cause cell death [48–51]. The anti-cancer effects of *trans*-FA might correlate with increased levels of ROS in H1299 cells (Fig. 6). ROS content is higher in cancer cells than in normal cells, and ROS are reported to be involved in cancer cell migration [42]. In this study, *trans*-FA treatment caused the accumulation of both H_2O_2 and $O2^-$. *Trans*-FA (0.03 mM) induced an increase in H_2O_2, but not O_2^-. Changes in endogenous ROS levels were assessed using the fluorescent indicators DCFDA for H_2O_2 and DHE for O_2^- [52]. Superoxide dismutase (SOD) converts O_2^- into H_2O_2, and is overexpressed in lung cancer compared with

a

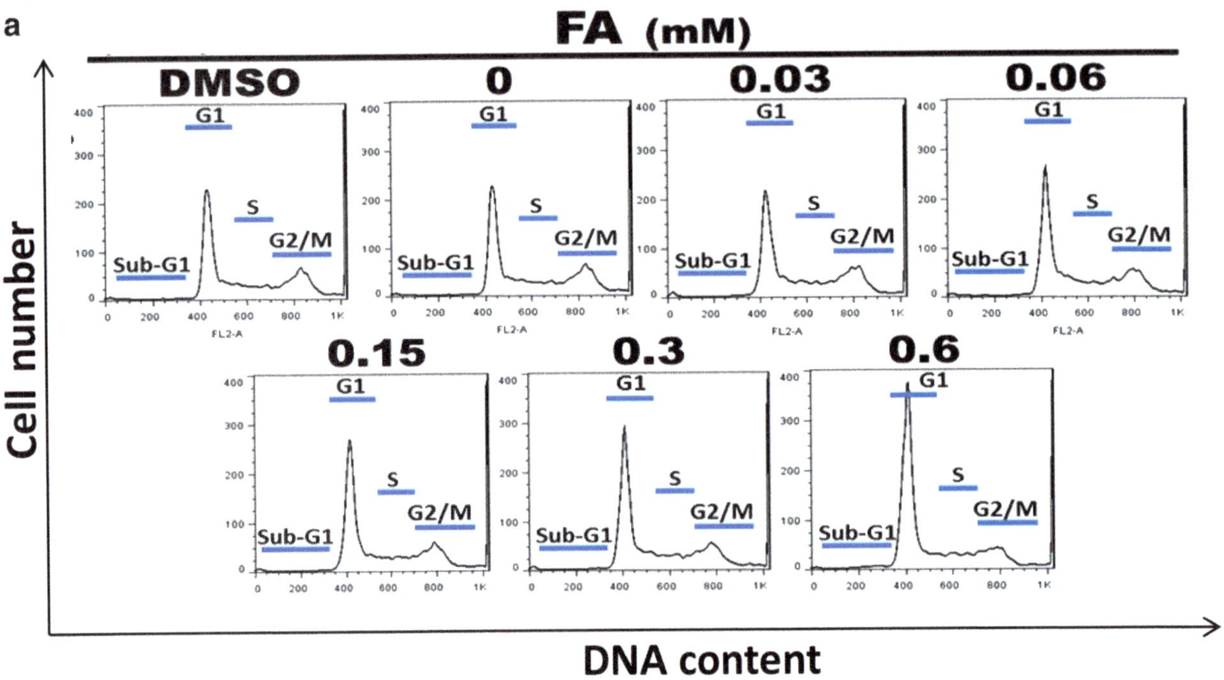

b

%phase/FA(mM)	DMSO	0	0.03	0.06	0.15	0.3	0.6
Sub-G1	2.34 ± 0.2^{a}	2.11 ± 0.3^{a}	3.7 ± 0.0^{c}	2.5 ± 0.09^{a}	1.88 ± 0.08^{b}	1.86 ± 0.21^{b}	3.24 ± 0.33^{b}
G0/G1	50.77 ± 2.4^{a}	52.89 ± 0.6^{a}	50.2 ± 0.5^{a}	54.2 ± 0.23^{b}	55.24 ± 0.85^{b}	57.26 ± 0.92^{c}	64.09 ± 0.34^{c}
S	16.47 ± 1.2^{a}	17.07 ± 0.5^{a}	17.3 ± 0.4^{a}	16.3 ± 0.21^{a}	16.66 ± 0.22^{a}	16.53 ± 0.42^{a}	14.25 ± 0.08^{b}
G2/M	30.44 ± 1.0^{a}	27.92 ± 0.7^{b}	28.7 ± 0.2^{b}	27.0 ± 0.3^{c}	26.22 ± 0.72^{c}	24.35 ± 0.46^{c}	18.42 ± 0.36^{c}

$^{a}p > 0.05$, $^{b}p < 0.05$ and $^{c}p < 0.001$ *vs.* DMSO, respectively.

Fig. 4 Effect of *trans*-FA on cell-cycle progression of H1299 cells. H1299 cells were treated with the indicated doses, 0.03, 0.06, 0.15, 0.3 and 0.6 mM of *trans*-FA for 48 h respectively. **a** An accumulation of G_0/G_1 population in *trans*-FA-treated H1299 cells and vehicle controls at 48 h. **b** The quantification analysis. Data are presented as mean ± SD (n = 3). *Different letter notations* indicate the statistical significance between control and *trans*-FA treatment groups (*a* no significance; *a* vs *b* and *a* vs *c*, statistically significant with $P < 0.05$ and 0.001, respectively)

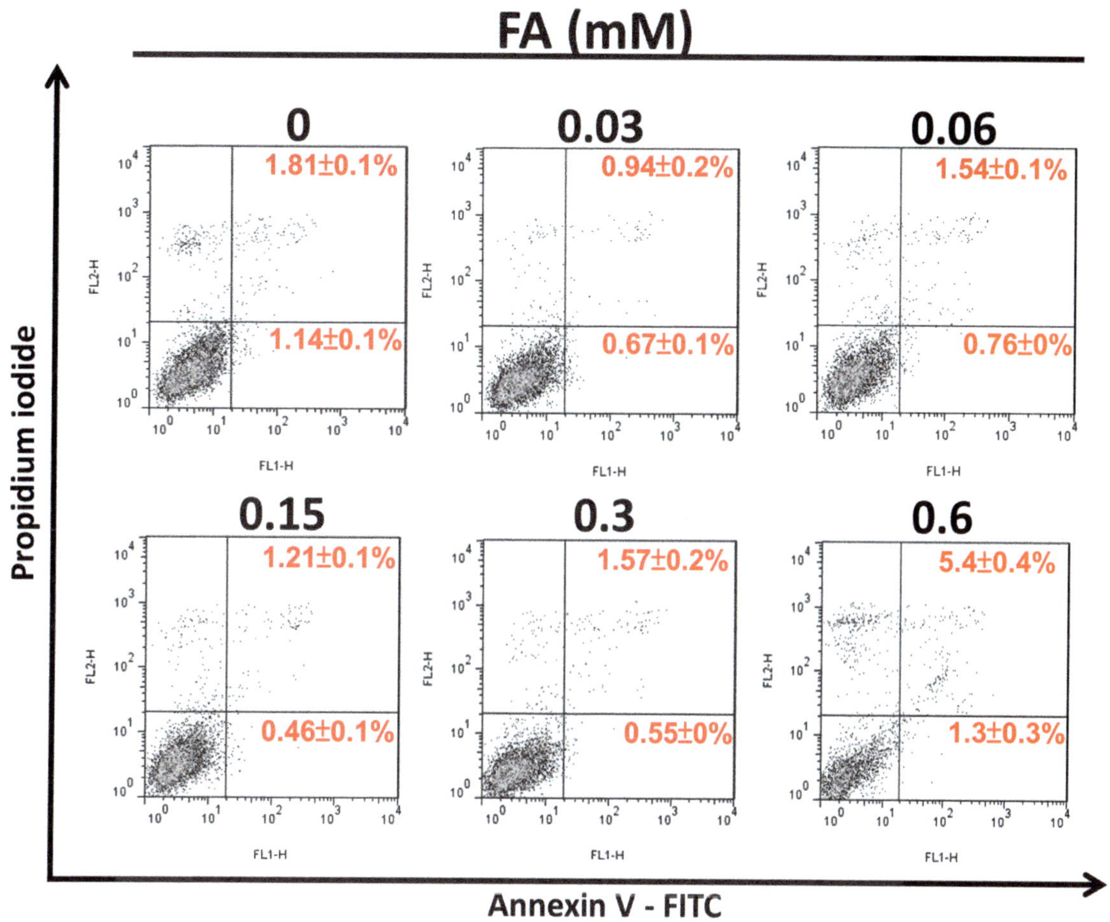

Fig. 5 Effect of *trans*-FA on apoptosis of H1299 cells. H1299 cells were treated with indicated doses, 0.03, 0.06, 0.15, 0.3 and 0.6 mM of *trans*-FA for 48 h respectively. Annexin V/PI double staining was performed to detect the apoptosis

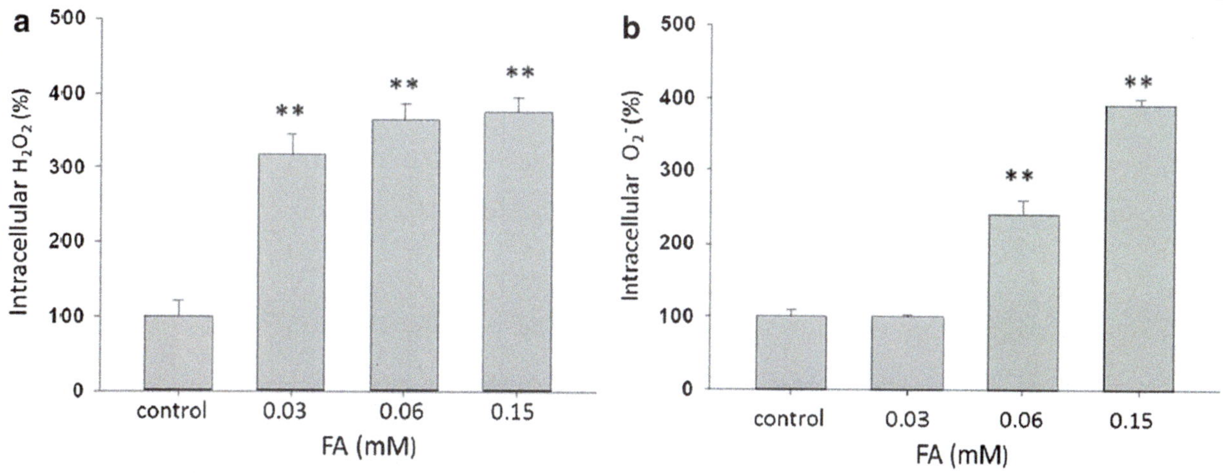

Fig. 6 *Trans*-FA up-modulates the endogenous level of ROS in H1299 cells. 1 × 10^5 H1299 cells were seeded onto a 6-well plate and treated with indicated doses of *trans*-FA (from 0.03 to 0.15 mM) 24 h respectively. Afterward, the induction of endogenous ROS was determined by **a** DCFDA or **b** DHE staining combined with a flow cytometry analysis. $^{**}P < 0.001$ against vehicle control

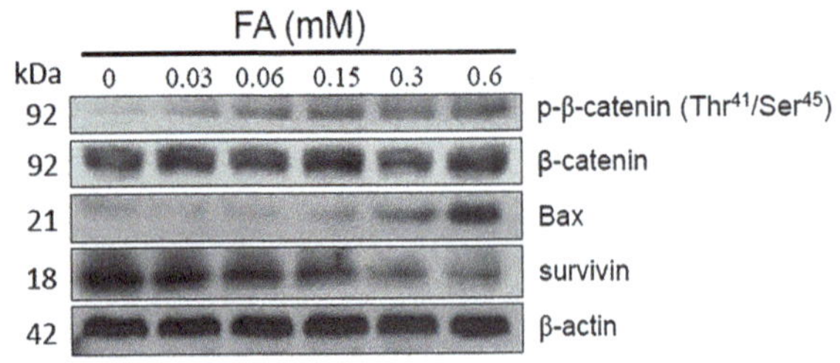

Fig. 7 Effect of *trans*-FA on survival protein of H1299 cells. H1299 cells were treated with the indicated doses, 0.03, 0.06, 0.15, 0.3 and 0.6 mM of *trans*-FA for 48 h. Western blot assay was performed

normal and non-malignant lung tissues [53]. Therefore, a moderate increase in O_2^- might be rapidly converted into H_2O_2 in lung cancer cells. However, the significant increase in endogenous O_2^- induced by *trans*-FA (>0.03 mM) may cause saturation of SOD capacity, preventing further conversion of O_2^- to H_2O_2. Accordingly, increased levels of H_2O_2 might be the product of O_2^- conversion by SOD in H1299 cells following low dose (0.03 mM) *trans*-FA treatment.

β-catenin is a transcription factor involved in cell growth and cell migration pathways. Wnt/β-catenin signaling is thus essential for the maintenance of neuronal progenitor proliferation [54]. However, phosphorylated β-catenin is inactivated and undergoes proteasomal degradation, causing the inhibition of cell growth [55].

With respect to tumorigenesis, constitutive activation or overexpression of β-catenin is frequently observed in cancers, including rectal cancer [56], colon cancer [57], breast cancer [58], prostate cancer [59], glioma [60], and lung cancer [61]. Furthermore, overexpression of

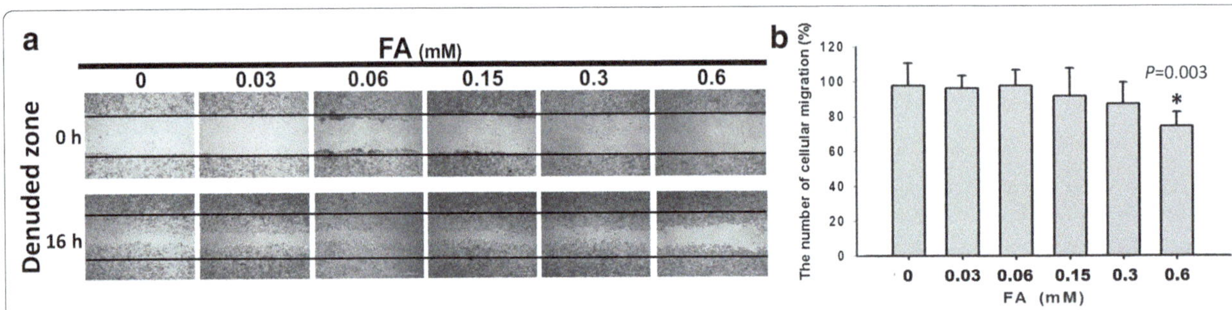

Fig. 8 Effect of *trans*-FA on the migration of H1299 cells. *Trans*-FA inhibits cell migration of NSCLC tumor H1299 cells at the highest dose (0.6 mM). **a** 3 × 10^5 cells were seeded in a 12-well plate and cells were scraped to create a clean 1-mm area within the confluent culture. Cells were treated with the indicated doses of 0.03, 0.06, 0.15, 0.3 and 0.6 mM of *trans*-FA for 16 h. Afterward, the wound gaps were photographed using an inverted phase-contrast microscopy. **b** The quantification analysis. *$P < 0.05$ for *trans*-FA treatments against vehicle control

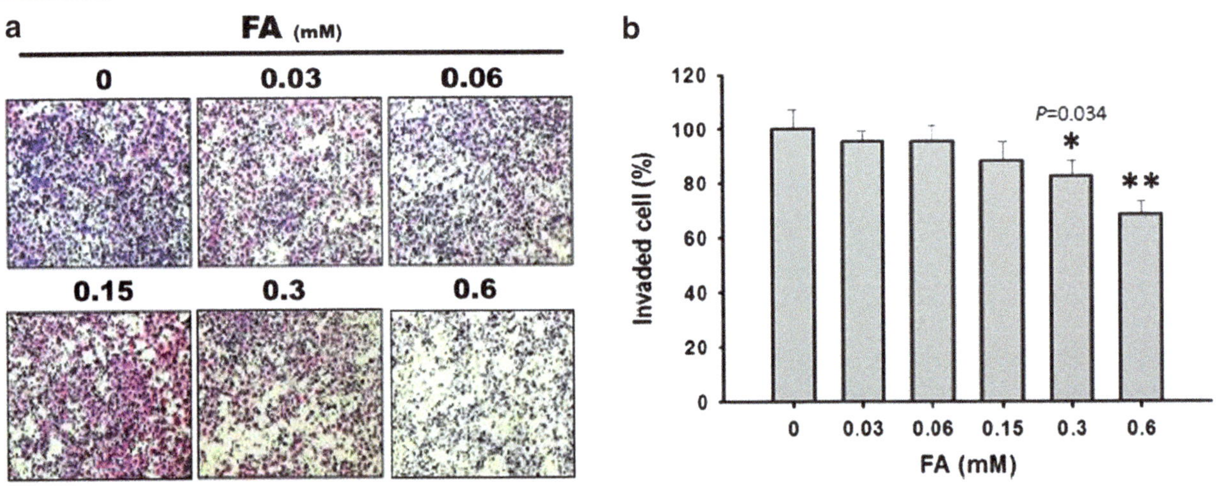

Fig. 9 Effect of *trans*-FA on the invasion of H1299 cells. **a** Cells were treated with the indicated doses of 0.03, 0.06, 0.15, 0.3 and 0.6 mM of *trans*-FA for 16 h and stained with 0.1 % w/v Giemsa stain respectively. **b** The results of the quantificative analysis. *$P < 0.05$ and **$P < 0.001$ for *trans*-FA treatments against vehicle control, respectively

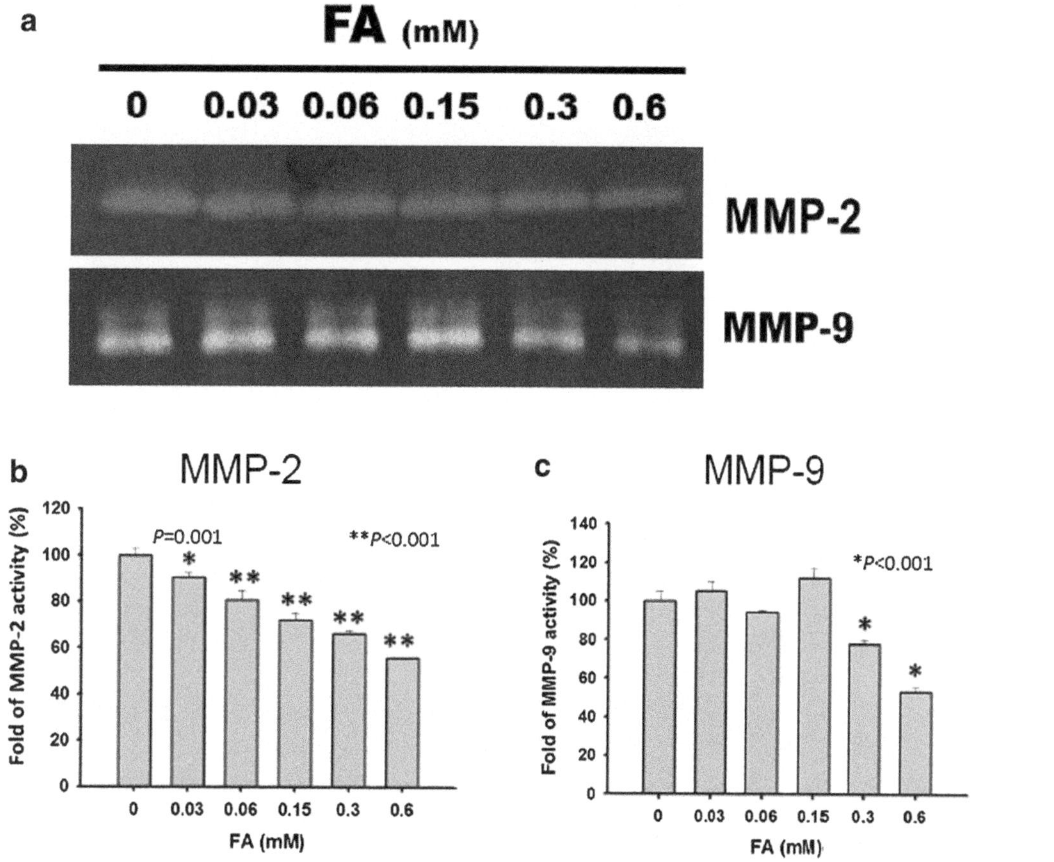

Fig. 10 Effect of *trans*-FA on activities of MMP-2 and MMP-9. H1299 cells were treated with indicated concentrations of *trans*-FA for 24 h respectively. **a** The activities of MMP-2 and MMP-9 were determined by a gelatin zymography assay (n = 3). **b**, **c** The results of the quantificative analysis. **b** $*P < 0.05$ and $**P < 0.001$ for *trans*-FA treatments against vehicle respectively. **c** $*P < 0.001$ for *trans*-FA treatments against vehicle control

β-catenin enhances the expression of cyclin D1, a critical factor for G_1/S transition during cell cycle progression in colon carcinoma cells [62]. *S*-adenosylmethionine and its metabolite, methylthioadenosine, inhibited β-catenin signaling by multiple mechanisms in colon cancer, and thus might have the potential to prevent tumorigenesis [63]. Furthermore, Wnt/β-catenin signaling was shown to be a potent activator of ROS generation, resulting in DNA damage and acceleration of cellular senescence [64]. Furthermore, Wnt/β-catenin signaling potently activated ROS generation in mesenchymal stem cells [64–66].

To clarify the underlying mechanism of *trans*-FA-induced anti-lung cancer activities, we examined whether *trans*-FA could affect the expression of cell proliferation-related transcription factor β-catenin using western blotting (Fig. 7). Our results demonstrated that *trans*-FA treatment promoted the phosphorylation of β-catenin at residues Thr^{41} and Ser^{45} [55] and led to the proteasomal degradation of cytoplasmic β-catenin, causing the downregulation of β-catenin protein levels. The Wnt pathway regulated MMP-2/-9 expression by directly targeting the MMP promoter through T-cell factor (TCF), a β-catenin interacting partner, therefore promoting cellular migration [67]. In effector T cells, endothelial cell-derived Wnt induced the expression of MMP-2/-9 through activating the Frizzled receptors to regulate the transmigration of T cells. In contrast, Wnt signaling blockade reduced the migration of effector T cells in vitro [67].

In addition to β-catenin, we also examined the role of pro-survival protein Bax, a key anti-survival factor, can promote apoptosis by binding to and antagonizing pro-survival Bcl-2 proteins such as Bcl-2 or Bcl-xL [68]. Conversely, survivin is a member of the inhibitor of apoptosis (IAP) family and acts as an inhibitor of caspase activation, thereby negatively regulating apoptosis or programmed cell death [69]. Both the Bcl-2 family and IAP proteins are critical regulators of cell proliferation and survival. In our study, the significant changes in Bax and survivin expression occurred alongside the anti-proliferation effects observed following *trans*-FA treatment (Fig. 7). As shown using colony formation and AIG assays, *trans*-FA treatment might impair cell proliferation of H1299 cells. Apart from in cells treated with higher concentrations (0.3 and 0.6 mM) of *trans*-FA, no significant increase in the population of apoptotic cells was detected. Survivin is considered an apoptosis inhibitor which promotes cellular proliferation, although decreased expression of survivin may not always cause apoptosis [69]. Ito et al. showed that both human hepatocellular carcinoma (HCC) cell lines and patient tissues expressed high levels of survivin mRNA, with detectable levels not found in normal and non-tumor areas of liver [70]. Survivin expression may be an indicator of cellular proliferation but not apoptosis in HCC tissues [70]. The degradation or expression Bax may represent a threshold for inducing apoptosis [71]. These results might explain how *trans*-FA treatment caused an increase in Bax protein expression but did not significantly induce apoptosis in H1299 cells at most concentrations tested (0.015–0.15 mM). These observations suggest that *trans*-FA treatment attenuates cellular proliferation rather than cellular survival. Therefore, the results of the proliferation assay imply that the anti-migratory effect of *trans*-FA may also be mediated by regulating the balance of pro-survival and anti-survival proteins in lung cancer cells.

Extracellular matrix-degrading MMPs, especially MMP-2 and MMP-9, are involved in the metastasis of cancer cells [72]. *Trans*-FA treatment inhibited the migration and invasion of lung cancer cells and concurrently attenuated the activities of both MMP-2 and MMP-9 (Figs. 8, 9, 10). These observations suggest a positive correlation between MMP activity and *trans*-FA-induced anti-migration in lung cancer cells.

Based on these observations, we propose that the anti-lung cancer effects of *trans*-FA might act through the modulation of endogenous ROS and β-catenin stabilization. *Trans*-FA induced the production of endogenous ROS and may cause β-catenin phosphorylation, resulting in proteasomal degradation. In addition, *trans*-FA regulated the balance between pro-survival and pro-apoptosis signals and downregulated the activities of metastasis-associated MMP-2 and MMP-9 (Fig. 11).

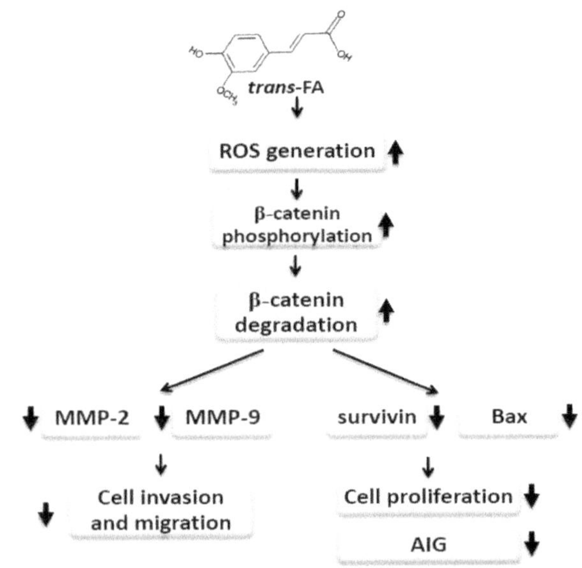

Fig. 11 Schematic diagram of hypothesized mechanism of *trans*-FA effect of lung cancer cells. *Trans*-FA induced ROS leading to degradation of phosphorylated β-catenin. *Trans*-FA induced regulation of pro-survival proteins survivin and anti-survival protein Bax caused the anti-proliferation of lung cancer H1299 cells. *Trans*-FA also reduced the activity of both MMP-2 and MMP-9, causing the down-regulation of migration of H1299 cells

Conclusion

Various concentrations (0.06–0.6 mM) of *trans*-FA exert both anti-proliferation and anti-migration effects in the human lung cancer cell line H1299.

Abbreviations

AAPH: 2,2′-azobis-2-amidinopropane dihydrochloride; AIG: anchorage-independent growth; AMPK: AMP activated protein kinase; Bax: Bcl-2-associated X protein; Bcl-2: B-cell lymphoma 2; Bcl-xL: B-cell lymphoma-extra large; DCFDA: 2′,7′-dichlorofluorescin diacetate; DHE: dihydroethidium; DMSO: dimethyl sulphoxide; DPPH: 2,2-diphenyl-1-picrylhydrazyl; ECL: enhanced chemiluminescence; FA: ferulic acid; NSCLC: non-small cell lung cancer; IAP: inhibitor of apoptosis; MMP: matrix metallopeptidase; mTOR: mammalian target of rapamycin; PBS: phosphate-buffered saline; PI: propidium iodide; RNase A: ribonuclease A; ROS: reactive oxygen species; SD: standard deviation; SDS: sodium dodecyl sulfate; SOD: superoxide dismutase; TCF: T cell factor.

Authors' contributions

YF, CCT, BHC and CCC designed the study. CCT, HTH, HYF, CYW and SSY performed the experiments. CYW, SSY, HMW and YNT analyzed and organized the data. YF, YCC and CCC wrote the manuscript. All authors read and approved the final manuscript.

Author details

[1] Department of Thoracic Surgery, Chi-Mei Medical Center, Tainan 710, Taiwan. [2] Division of Chest, Ten Chan General Hospital, Chung-Li 320, Taiwan, ROC. [3] Department of Biotechnology, Kaohsiung Medical University, Kaohsiung 807, Taiwan. [4] Department of Food Nutrition, Chung-Hwa University of Medical Technology, Tainan 701, Taiwan. [5] Department of Biological Sciences, National Sun Yat-sen University, Kaohsiung 804, Taiwan. [6] Translational Research Center, Kaohsiung Medical University Hospital, Kaohsiung 807, Taiwan. [7] Graduate Institute of Biomedical Engineering, National Chung Hsing University, Taichung 402, Taiwan. [8] Department of Biological Sciences and Technology, National University of Tainan, Tainan 700, Taiwan. [9] Research Center for Environment Medicine, Kaohsiung Medical University, Kaohsiung 807, Taiwan. [10] The Institute of Biomedical Sciences, National Sun Yat-Sen University, Kaohsiung 804, Taiwan.

Acknowledgements

The study was financially supported by Grants NSC101-2320-B-037-046-MY3, NSC102-2632-B-037-001-MY3 and MOST105-2311-B-037-001 from the Ministry of Science and Technology (MOST), Taiwan; Grants 101-CM-KMU-11, 102-CM-KMU-09 and 104-CM-KMU-006 from the ChiMei-KMU Joint Research Project, Grants NSYSU-KMU104-P031 from the NSYSU-KMU Joint Research Project, and Grant MOHW103-TD-B-111-05 from the Ministry of Health and Welfare, Taiwan; by the grants Aim for the Top Universities Grant. KMU-TP103A17, KMU-TP104A03, KMU-TP105A03 and KMU-M104008 from Kaohsiung Medical University, Taiwan; Grant Ten Chan General Hospital, Chung-Li and KMU Joint Research Project (ST102004), Taiwan.

Competing interests

The authors declare that they have no competing interests.

References

1. Siegel R, Naishadham D, Jemal A. Cancer statistics, 2013. CA Cancer J Clin. 2013;63:11–30.
2. O'Rourke N, Roque IFM, Farre Bernado N, Macbeth F. Concurrent chemoradiotherapy in non-small cell lung cancer. Cochrane Database Syst Rev. 2010;16:CD002140.
3. Pirker R, Minar W. Chemotherapy of advanced non-small cell lung cancer. Front Radiat Ther Oncol. 2010;42:157–63.
4. Wagner TD, Yang GY. The role of chemotherapy and radiation in the treatment of locally advanced non-small cell lung cancer (NSCLC). Curr Drug Targets. 2010;11:67–73.
5. Atagi S, Kawahara M, Tamura T, Noda K, Watanabe K, Yokoyama A, et al. Standard thoracic radiotherapy with or without concurrent daily low-dose carboplatin in elderly patients with locally advanced non-small cell lung cancer: a phase III trial of the Japan Clinical Oncology Group (JCOG9812). Jap J Clin Oncol. 2005;35:195–201.
6. Guo S, Liang Y, Zhou Q. Complement and correction for meta-analysis of patients with extensive-stage small cell lung cancer managed with irinotecan/cisplatin versus etoposide/cisplatin as first-line chemotherapy. J Thorac Oncol. 2011;6:406–8.
7. Corbaux C, Marie J, Meraud JP, Lacroix S, Delhoume JY, Jouary T, et al. Pemetrexed-induced scleroderma-like changes in the lower legs. Ann Dermatol Venereol. 2015;142:115–20.
8. Sun Y, Chen J, Rigas B. Chemopreventive agents induce oxidative stress in cancer cells leading to COX-2 overexpression and COX-2-independent cell death. Carcinogenesis. 2009;30:93–100.
9. Setia S, Nehru B, Sanyal SN. The PI3K/Akt pathway in colitis associated colon cancer and its chemoprevention with celecoxib, a Cox-2 selective inhibitor. Biomed Pharmacother. 2014;68:721–7.
10. Madka V, Mohammed A, Li Q, Zhang Y, Patlolla JM, Biddick L, et al. Chemoprevention of urothelial cell carcinoma growth and invasion by the dual COX-LOX inhibitor licofelone in UPII-SV40T transgenic mice. Cancer Prev Res (Phila). 2014;7:708–16.
11. Wang Y, Ma W, Zheng W. Deguelin, a novel anti-tumorigenic agent targeting apoptosis, cell cycle arrest and anti-angiogenesis for cancer chemoprevention. Mol Clin Oncol. 2013;1:215–9.
12. Zhu B, Liu GT, Wu RS, Strada SJ. Chemoprevention of bicyclol against hepatic preneoplastic lesions. Cancer Biol Ther. 2006;5:1665–73.
13. Tanaka T, Shnimizu M, Moriwaki H. Cancer chemoprevention by carotenoids. Molecules. 2012;17:3202–42.
14. Tanaka T, Makita H, Ohnishi M, Hirose Y, Wang A, Mori H, et al. Chemoprevention of 4-nitroquinoline 1-oxide-induced oral carcinogenesis by dietary curcumin and hesperidin: comparison with the protective effect of β-carotene. Cancer Res. 1994;54:4653–9.
15. Chiu CC, Liu PL, Huang KJ, Wang HM, Chang KF, Chou CK, et al. Goniothalamin inhibits growth of human lung cancer cells through DNA damage, apoptosis, and reduced migration ability. J Agric Food Chem. 2011;59:4288–93.
16. Fang HY, Wang HM, Chang KF, Hu HT, Hwang LJ, Fu TF, et al. Feruloyl-L-arabinose attenuates migration, invasion and production of reactive oxygen species in H1299 lung cancer cells. Food Chem Toxicol. 2013;58:459–66.
17. Pai HC, Chang LH, Peng CY, Chang YL, Chen CC, Shen CC, et al. Moscatilin inhibits migration and metastasis of human breast cancer MDA-MB-231 cells through inhibition of Akt and Twist signaling pathway. J Mol Med (Berl). 2013;91:347–56.
18. Kowitdamrong A, Chanvorachote P, Sritularak B, Pongrakhananon V. Moscatilin inhibits lung cancer cell motility and invasion via suppression of endogenous reactive oxygen species. Biomed Res Int. 2013;2013:765894.
19. Buanafina MM, Langdon T, Hauck B, Dalton S, Timms-Taravella E, Morris P. Targeting expression of a fungal ferulic acid esterase to the apoplast, endoplasmic reticulum or golgi can disrupt feruloylation of the growing cell wall and increase the biodegradability of tall fescue (*Festuca arundinacea*). Plant Biotechnol J. 2010;8:316–31.
20. Srinivasan M, Sudheer AR, Menon VP. Ferulic acid: therapeutic potential through its antioxidant property. J Clin Biochem Nutr. 2007;40:92–100.
21. Pan GX, Spencer L, Leary GJ. Reactivity of ferulic acid and its derivatives toward hydrogen peroxide and peracetic acid. J Agric Food Chem. 1999;47:3325–31.
22. Hartley RD, Jones EC. Phenolic components and degradability of cell walls of grass and legume species. Phytochemistry. 1977;16:1531–4.
23. Das U, Manna K, Sinha M, Datta S, Das DK, Chakraborty A, et al. Role of ferulic acid in the amelioration of ionizing radiation induced inflammation: a murine model. PLoS One. 2014;9:e97599.
24. Manikandan R, Beulaja M, Thiagarajan R, Pandi M, Arulvasu C, Prabhu NM, et al. Ameliorative effect of ferulic acid against renal injuries mediated by nuclear factor-κB during glycerol-induced nephrotoxicity in Wistar rats. Ren Fail. 2014;36:154–65.
25. Panneerselvam L, Subbiah K, Arumugam A, Senapathy JG. Ferulic acid modulates fluoride-induced oxidative hepatotoxicity in male Wistar rats. Biol Trace Elem Res. 2013;151:85–91.
26. Yuan X, Wang J, Yao H. Antioxidant activity of feruloylated oligosaccharides from wheat bran. Food Chem. 2005;90:759–64.
27. Roy S, Metya SK, Sannigrahi S, Rahaman N, Ahmed F. Treatment with ferulic acid to rats with streptozotocin-induced diabetes: effects on oxidative stress, pro-inflammatory cytokines, and apoptosis in the pancreatic beta cell. Endocrine. 2013;44:369–79.
28. Ramar M, Manikandan B, Raman T, Priyadarsini A, Palanisamy S, Velayudam M, et al. Protective effect of ferulic acid and resveratrol against alloxan-induced diabetes in mice. Eur J Pharmacol. 2012;690:226–35.

29. Janicke B, Hegardt C, Krogh M, Onning G, Akesson B, Cirenajwis HM, et al. The antiproliferative effect of dietary fiber phenolic compounds ferulic acid and p-coumaric acid on the cell cycle of Caco-2 cells. Nutr Cancer. 2011;63:611–22.
30. Jayaprakasam B, Vanisree M, Zhang Y, Dewitt DL, Nair MG. Impact of alkyl esters of caffeic and ferulic acids on tumor cell proliferation, cyclooxygenase enzyme, and lipid peroxidation. J Agric Food Chem. 2006;54:5375–81.
31. Karthikeyan S, Kanimozhi G, Prasad NR, Mahalakshmi R. Radiosensitizing effect of ferulic acid on human cervical carcinoma cells in vitro. Toxicol In Vitro. 2011;25:1366–75.
32. Stagos D, Kazantzoglou G, Magiatis P, Mitaku S, Anagnostopoulos K, Kouretas D. Effects of plant phenolics and grape extracts from Greek varieties of *Vitis vinifera* on mitomycin C and topoisomerase I-induced nicking of DNA. Int J Mol Med. 2005;15:1013–22.
33. Tanaka T, Kojima T, Kawamori T, Wang A, Suzui M, Okamoto K, et al. Inhibition of 4-nitroquinoline-1-oxide-induced rat tongue carcinogenesis by the naturally occurring plant phenolics caffeic, ellagic, chlorogenic and ferulic acids. Carcinogenesis. 1993;14:1321–5.
34. Blois MS. Antioxidant determinations by the use of a stable free radical. Nature. 1958;181:1199–200.
35. Barreto JC, Trevisan MT, Hull WE, Erben G, de Brito ES, Pfundstein B, et al. Characterization and quantitation of polyphenolic compounds in bark, kernel, leaves, and peel of mango (*Mangifera indica* L.). J Agric Food Chem. 2008;56:5599–610.
36. Tseng CN, Hong YR, Chang HW, Yu TJ, Hung TW, Hou MF, et al. Brefeldin A reduces anchorage-independent survival, cancer stem cell potential and migration of MDA-MB-231 human breast cancer cells. Molecules. 2014;19:17464–77.
37. Chiu CC, Li CH, Fuh TS, Chen WL, Huang CS, Chen LJ, et al. The suppressed proliferation and premature senescence by ganciclovir in p53-mutated human non-small-lung cancer cells acquiring herpes simplex virus-thymidine kinase cDNA. Cancer Detect Prev. 2005;29:286–93.
38. Chiu CC, Chen JY, Lin KL, Huang CJ, Lee JC, Chen BH, et al. p38 MAPK and NF-κB pathways are involved in naphtho[1,2-b] furan-4,5-dione induced anti-proliferation and apoptosis of human hepatoma cells. Cancer Lett. 2010;295:92–9.
39. Geback T, Schulz MM, Koumoutsakos P, Detmar M. TScratch: a novel and simple software tool for automated analysis of monolayer wound healing assays. Biotechniques. 2009;46:265–74.
40. Tu B, Ma TT, Peng XQ, Wang Q, Yang H, Huang XL. Targeting of COX-2 expression by recombinant adenovirus shRNA attenuates the malignant biological behavior of breast cancer cells. Asian Pac J Cancer Prev. 2014;15:8829–36.
41. Chu SC, Yang SF, Liu SJ, Kuo WH, Chang YZ, Hsieh YS. In vitro and in vivo antimetastatic effects of *Terminalia catappa* L. leaves on lung cancer cells. Food Chem Toxicol. 2007;45:1194–201.
42. Wu WS. The signaling mechanism of ROS in tumor progression. Cancer Metastasis Rev. 2006;25:695–705.
43. Liu J, Ping W, Zu Y, Sun W. Correlations of lysyl oxidase with MMP2/MMP9 expression and its prognostic value in non-small cell lung cancer. Int J Clin Exp Pathol. 2014;7:6040–7.
44. Jacob A, Prekeris R. The regulation of MMP targeting to invadopodia during cancer metastasis. Front Cell Dev Biol. 2015;3:4.
45. Chang CJ, Chiu JH, Tseng LM, Chang CH, Chien TM, Wu CW, et al. Modulation of HER2 expression by ferulic acid on human breast cancer MCF7 cells. Eur J Clin Invest. 2006;36:588–96.
46. Yabe T, Hirahara H, Harada N, Ito N, Nagai T, Sanagi T, et al. Ferulic acid induces neural progenitor cell proliferation in vitro and in vivo. Neuroscience. 2010;165:515–24.
47. Koyama M, Sowa Y, Hitomi T, Iizumi Y, Watanabe M, Taniguchi T, et al. Perillyl alcohol causes G1 arrest through p15(INK4b) and p21(WAF1/Cip1) induction. Oncol Rep. 2013;29:779–84.
48. Ushio-Fukai M, Nakamura Y. Reactive oxygen species and angiogenesis: NADPH oxidase as target for cancer therapy. Cancer Lett. 2008;266:37–52.
49. Clerkin JS, Naughton R, Quiney C, Cotter TG. Mechanisms of ROS modulated cell survival during carcinogenesis. Cancer Lett. 2008;266:30–6.
50. Wu XJ, Hua X. Targeting ROS: selective killing of cancer cells by a cruciferous vegetable derived pro-oxidant compound. Cancer Biol Ther. 2007;6:646–7.
51. Geest CR, Buitenhuis M, Groot Koerkamp MJ, Holstege FC, Vellenga E, Coffer PJ. Tight control of MEK-ERK activation is essential in regulating proliferation, survival, and cytokine production of CD34+ -derived neutrophil progenitors. Blood. 2009;114:3402–12.
52. Eruslanov E, Kusmartsev S. Identification of ROS using oxidized DCFDA and flow-cytometry. Methods Mol Biol. 2010;594:57–72.
53. Svensk AM, Soini Y, Paakko P, Hiravikoski P, Kinnula VL. Differential expression of superoxide dismutases in lung cancer. Am J Clin Pathol. 2004;122:395–404.
54. Zechner D, Fujita Y, Hulsken J, Muller T, Walther I, Taketo MM, et al. β-Catenin signals regulate cell growth and the balance between progenitor cell expansion and differentiation in the nervous system. Dev Biol. 2003;258:406–18.
55. Kim SI, Park CS, Lee MS, Kwon MS, Jho EH, Song WK. Cyclin-dependent kinase 2 regulates the interaction of axin with β-catenin. Biochem Biophys Res Commun. 2004;317:478–83.
56. Garcia-Florez LJ, Gomez-Alvarez G, Frunza AM, Barneo-Serra L, Martinez-Alonso C, Fresno-Forcelledo MF. Predictive markers of response to neoadjuvant therapy in rectal cancer. J Surg Res. 2015;194:120–6.
57. Morin PJ, Sparks AB, Korinek V, Barker N, Clevers H, Vogelstein B, et al. Activation of β-catenin-Tcf signaling in colon cancer by mutations in β-catenin or APC. Science. 1997;275:1787–90.
58. Yook JI, Li XY, Ota I, Hu C, Kim HS, Kim NH, et al. A Wnt-Axin2-GSK3β cascade regulates Snail1 activity in breast cancer cells. Nat Cell Biol. 2006;8:1398–406.
59. Verras M, Sun Z. Roles and regulation of Wnt signaling and β-catenin in prostate cancer. Cancer Lett. 2006;237:22–32.
60. Pu P, Zhang Z, Kang C, Jiang R, Jia Z, Wang G, et al. Downregulation of Wnt2 and β-catenin by siRNA suppresses malignant glioma cell growth. Cancer Gene Ther. 2009;16:351–61.
61. Stewart DJ. Wnt signaling pathway in non-small cell lung cancer. J Natl Cancer Inst. 2014;106:djt356.
62. Tetsu O, McCormick F. β-Catenin regulates expression of cyclin D1 in colon carcinoma cells. Nature. 1999;398:422–6.
63. Li TW, Peng H, Yang H, Kurniawidjaja S, Panthaki P, Zheng Y, et al. *S*-Adenosylmethionine and methylthioadenosine inhibit β-catenin signaling by multiple mechanisms in liver and colon cancer. Mol Pharmacol. 2015;87:77–86.
64. Liu H, Fergusson MM, Castilho RM, Liu J, Cao L, Chen J, et al. Augmented Wnt signaling in a mammalian model of accelerated aging. Science. 2007;317:803–6.
65. Yoon JC, Ng A, Kim BH, Bianco A, Xavier RJ, Elledge SJ. Wnt signaling regulates mitochondrial physiology and insulin sensitivity. Genes Dev. 2010;24:1507–18.
66. Zhang DY, Pan Y, Zhang C, Yan BX, Yu SS, Wu DL, et al. Wnt/β-catenin signaling induces the aging of mesenchymal stem cells through promoting the ROS production. Mol Cell Biochem. 2013;374:13–20.
67. Wu B, Crampton SP, Hughes CC. Wnt signaling induces matrix metalloproteinase expression and regulates T cell transmigration. Immunity. 2007;26:227–39.
68. Oltvai ZN, Milliman CL, Korsmeyer SJ. Bcl-2 heterodimerizes in vivo with a conserved homolog, bax, that accelerates programmed cell death. Cell. 1993;74:609–19.
69. Sah NK, Khan Z, Khan GJ, Bisen PS. Structural, functional and therapeutic biology of survivin. Cancer Lett. 2006;244:164–71.
70. Ito T, Shiraki K, Sugimoto K, Yamanaka T, Fujikawa K, Ito M, et al. Survivin promotes cell proliferation in human hepatocellular carcinoma. Hepatology. 2000;31:1080–5.
71. Bagci EZ, Vodovotz Y, Billiar TR, Ermentrout GB, Bahar I. Bistability in apoptosis: roles of bax, bcl-2, and mitochondrial permeability transition pores. Biophys J. 2006;90:1546–59.
72. Noel A, Jost M, Maquoi E. Matrix metalloproteinases at cancer tumor-host interface. Semin Cell Dev Biol. 2008;19:52–60.

Synergistic effects of melphalan and *Pinus kesiya* Royle ex Gordon (*Simaosong*) extracts on apoptosis induction in human cancer cells

Natthida Weerapreeyakul[1*], Sasipawan Machana[2] and Sahapat Barusrux[3]

Abstract

Background: This study aims to determine the synergistic effects of the chemotherapeutic drug melphalan and the phytoconstituents extracted from *Pinus kesiya* Royle ex Gordon (*Simaosong*) in human cancer cells.

Methods: *P. kesiya* twigs extracted from 50 % ethanol–water were evaluated alone (6–500 μg/mL) and in combination with melphalan (0.75–15 μg/mL). The cytotoxic effects of single extract or extract and melphalan combination were examined by a neutral red assay to investigate their antiproliferative and apoptosis induction effects in the U937 and HepG2 cell lines. Nuclei morphological change and DNA fragmentation were examined by DNA nuclei staining with 4′6-diamidino-2-phenylindole (DAPI) and agarose gel electrophoresis, respectively. The chemical constituents of the *P. kesiya* extract were assessed using gas chromatography–mass spectrometry (GC–MS) analysis. The synergistic effects of different IC_{50} ratios of the *P. kesiya* extract and melphalan combination were analyzed in each cancer cell line. The dose reduction index (DRI) was calculated to determine the extent of concentration reduction in the combination treatment compared with the concentration of each single treatment.

Results: The IC_{50} ratios for melphalan to *P. kesiya* extract that caused 75 % antiproliferation could be reduced after combination. This response was greater in the U937 cells than in the HepG2 cells (all $P < 0.001$). Melphalan and *P. kesiya* extract had a similar effect on apoptosis induction both singly and in combination. *P. kesiya* extract synergized the antiproliferation and apoptosis induction effects of melphalan.

Conclusions: Combining the *P. kesiya* extract with melphalan reduced toxicity while retaining the therapeutic efficacy of melphalan.

Background

Specific and selective apoptosis induction in targeted chemotherapy is limited due to multidrug resistance and intolerably severe side effects [1, 2]. Synergistic combinations of two or more agents could overcome the toxicity and side effects associated with the high doses of chemotherapeutic drugs in monotherapy [3]. Several herbal plant extracts are rich sources of bioactive constituents that inhibit, reverse, or retard tumorigenesis [3, 4]. Additionally, some research on herbal synergistic action indicates that the whole herb produces a better effect than any single isolated active ingredient [5, 6].

The rosin of *Pinus kesiya* Royle ex Gordon (*Simaosong*) contains szemaoenin (diterpenoid) isopimaric acid, abiet-13(14)-en-8,12-epoxy-18-oic acid, abiet-8,11,13-trien-15-hydroxy-18-oic acid, pimarol, isopimarol, abiet-8,11,13-trien-18-oic acid, and 15-hydroxyabietic acid [7]. The main compounds found in *P. kesiya* turpentine are α- and β-pinene [8]. The needle oil is rich in α- and β-pinene, citronellol, bornyl acetate, β-phellandrene, camphene, and β-caryophyllene [9]. The needles of *P. kesiya* contain dichlorobenzene isomer, 1,4-cineol,

*Correspondence: natthida@kku.ac.th
[1] Faculty of Pharmaceutical Sciences, Khon Kaen University, Khon Kaen 40002, Thailand
Full list of author information is available at the end of the article

α-terpinene, o-cimene and imonene enantiomers [10, 11], and monoterpenes [12].

P. kesiya is used to relieve flatulence, stomachache, and cough in complementary and alternative medicine [13]. The 50 % ethanol–water crude extract of the woody twigs of *P. kesiya* has an apoptotic-induction effect on both the human hepatocellular carcinoma HepG2 and the human leukemic U937 cell lines because of its cytotoxicity [14, 15]. Many studies indicate that this effect arises from the whole crude extract with its lower activity of isolated individual compounds [3–6]. The synergistic effect of the whole extract of *P. kesiya* plus the chemotherapeutic drug melphalan is of interest as it may expand the use of this herbal plant. Melphalan is an alkylating anticancer drug, leading to DNA cross-linking, DNA damage, and finally apoptosis of cancer cells [16]; however, melphalan resistance and highly toxic side effects in other tissues limit its use [17, 18]. We hypothesized that plant extracts that exhibited an anticancer activity in vitro might enhance the antiproliferative activity of melphalan, which would permit the use of a lower dosage and reduced side effects. This study aims to determine the synergistic effects of *P. kesiya* and melphalan phytoconstituents in human cancer cells.

Methods

Plant extraction

P. kesiya woody twigs were collected and taxonomically authenticated by Assistant Professor Thaweesak Thitimetharoach. The species of samples were determined using the Flora of Thailand [19] and the Thai Forest Bulletin [20]. The voucher (TT-OC-SK-910) was deposited at the Herbal Herbarium, Faculty of Pharmaceutical Sciences, Khon Kaen University, Khon Kaen Province, Thailand. The 50 % ethanol–water extract of *P. kesiya* twig was prepared as previously reported [14, 15]. Dried plants were cut and macerated with 50 % ethanol–water (1 kg:6 L) for 7 days with occasional manual shaking. The solvent was filtered, distilled by a rotary evaporator (RV 8 V, IKA, Germany) below 40°C, and freeze-dried to obtain the crude extract. The percent yield of the 50 % ethanol–water extract of *P. kesiya* was 4.3 %. Stock solution of *P. kesiya* extract was freshly prepared in dimethyl sulfoxide (DMSO) to make 100 mg/mL stock solution and further diluted with culture media to create a working solution (10 to 500 μg/mL).

Gas chromatography–mass spectrometry (GC–MS) analysis

GC–MS analysis was performed as described by Weerapreeyakul et al. [21] on an Agilent 6890 N gas chromatograph (Agilent Technologies, China) coupled to an Agilent 5973 N mass selective detector (Agilent Technologies, USA) to determine the extract composition for further standardization. Capillary GC analysis was performed using a DB-5 ms (3 m × 0.25 mm id, 0.25 μm) capillary column from Agilent Technologies (J&W Scientific, USA) with helium as the carrier gas. The column initially flowed at 80 °C for 6 min at a rate of 2 mL/min and an average velocity of 52 cm/s. The temperature was raised to 280 °C (at a rate of 5 °C/min) for 24 min. The total runtime was 70 min. The injector temperature was maintained at 250 °C and the injection volume was set at 2.0 μL in the splitless mode. The interface temperature was held at 280 °C. Mass spectra were scanned from m/z 50.0 to m/z 500.0 at a rate of 1.5 scans/s with a threshold of 150. The electron impact ionization energy was 70 eV. The chemical components of the crude extracts were identified from the chromatograms and mass spectra using the Wiley 7 N.l database (Agilent Technologies, USA).

Cell culture

The human leukemic (U937) cell line was cultured in RPMI 1640. The human hepatocellular carcinoma (HepG2) cell line and normal African green monkey kidney epithelial (Vero) cell line were cultured in DMEM (GIBCO, Invitrogen Corporation, USA). Both media were supplemented with 10 % fetal bovine serum (GIBCO, Invitrogen Corporation), 100 units/mL penicillin and 100 μg/mL streptomycin (GIBCO, Invitrogen Corporation). The cells were cultured at 37 °C in a humidified atmosphere containing 5 % CO_2.

Antiproliferative effect

The antiproliferative activity of the *P. kesiya* extract in the leukemia (U937), hepatocellular carcinoma (HepG2), and normal (Vero) cell lines was assessed by neutral red assay [14, 15]. Briefly, 100 μL of U937 cells at a density of 5×10^5 cells/mL and 100 μL of HepG2 or Vero cells at a density of 3×10^5 cells/mL were independently seeded in 96-wells plates and incubated for 24 h. After cell growth, cells were treated with various concentrations (10 to 500 μg/mL) of the *P. kesiya* crude extract or melphalan (purity 95 %, Sigma–Aldrich Chemie GmbH, Germany) dissolved in DMSO (United States Biological, USA). The maximum final concentration of the compound was 500 μg/mL to maintain 1 % v/v DMSO with a cytotoxicity <10 % compared with the untreated cells. After treated cells were exposed to the test compound for 24 h, cells were stained directly with a final concentration of 50 μg/mL neutral red dye (Sigma Chemicals Co., USA) and incubated for another 2 h. The neutral red stained viable cells were dissolved by 0.33 % hydrogen chloride in isopropanol and detected using a colorimetric-based method. The absorbance was measured at 520 and 650 nm (reference wavelength) by a spectromicroplate reader (TECAN,

Grödig, Austria). A plot of percentage cytotoxicity vs. test compound concentration was used to calculate the IC_{50}.

Apoptosis induction effect

Nuclei morphological study by 4´6-diamidino-2-phenylindole (DAPI) staining assay

The apoptosis effect of the plant crude extracts was primarily determined by fluorescent dye staining and DAPI to identify the condensation and fragmentation of nuclear DNA [14, 15]. Briefly, the cancer cells (HepG2 or U937) were treated with various concentrations of the test compounds (6 to 500 μg/mL of *P. kesiya* and 0.75 to 15 μg/mL of melphalan) for 24 h, after which the culture medium was removed and the cells were washed with fresh medium. Cells were then fixed by cold methanol. DAPI dye (Sigma–Aldrich Chemie GmbH, Germany) was then added to stain the nuclei DNA for 1 h. The excess dye was removed and 1X PBS (pH 7.4; 10 mM) was added to glycerin (at a 1:1 ratio). The DAPI staining assay was performed in triplicate in independent experiments. An inverted fluorescence microscope (Nikon eclipse 80i, Kanagawa, Japan) was used to record images of the DAPI staining. The average percentage of apoptotic cells was calculated from three independent wells with 10 eye views per well under the inverted fluorescence microscopy at a magnitude of 40×.

Analysis of DNA fragmentation

DNA fragmentation was analyzed [14, 15]. Briefly, after cancer cells were treated with various concentrations of *P. kesiya* extracts (60, 150, 300, 450, and 500 μg/mL) and melphalan (15 μg/mL) for 24 h, they were collected and washed with fresh medium. Then, the cell suspension was transferred to microcentrifuge tubes and centrifuged (Daihan Scientific, Seoul, Korea) at 300×*g* for 5 min to collect the cell pellet. The DNA in the cell pellet was extracted using a FlexiGene DNA kit (QIAGEN GmbH, Germany) then 2 μg of the DNA was analyzed using electrophoresis on 2 % agarose gels (Bio-Rad, USA) containing 0.1 mg/mL ethidium bromide (AppliChem, USA). DNA was mixed with loading dye (SibEnzyme Ltd., Russia) and the gel electrophoresed in 0.5X Tris–Borate-EDTA buffer (pH 8.3; 40 mMTris base, 45 mM boric acid, 1 mM EDTA; Sigma–Aldrich Chemie GmbH, Germany) at 250 V for 1 min and 20 V for 4 h. After electrophoresis, the DNA fragments were analyzed by In Genius L gel documentation (Syngene, USA).

Enhancement of anticancer effect of *P. kesiya* extract in vitro

The enhanced chemosensitivity of melphalan combined with *P. kesiya* on the U937 and HepG2 cell lines was determined as per Chou and Talalay [22]. The antiproliferation assay on the melphalan and *P. kesiya* extract combination treatment against the HepG2 cancer cell line after 24 h was performed using the same method as for melphalan or *P. kesiya* extract alone. The cells were treated with the *P. kesiya* extract and melphalan was added subsequently. Different concentrations of the *P. kesiya* extract and melphalan combination treatment were used (Table 1). Briefly, the melphalan concentration was fixed at 1 × IC_{50} and the *P. kesiya* concentration was varied at 0.02, 0.05, 0.1, 0.2, 0.5, 1, 1.5, and 2 × IC_{50} in the U937 and HepG2 cell lines. In another series, the *P. kesiya* extract concentration was fixed at 1 × IC_{50} and the melphalan concentration was varied at 0.05, 0.1, 0.2, 0.5, 1, 1.5, and 2 × IC_{50} in both cancer cell lines. The maximum concentration that could be used in the experiment to maintain the percentage DMSO at less than 1 % v/v was 500 μg/mL, instead of a 2 × IC_{50} concentration of *P. kesiya* (600 μg/mL), the concentration used in this study was only 500 μg/mL. After 24 h exposure, the percentage of antiproliferation for each treatment was calculated.

The combined effects were analyzed to determine whether the enhanced growth inhibitory effect was antagonistic, additive, or synergistic. The combination index (CI) was calculated (adapted from the multiple-drug effect analysis based on the median effect principle and the isobologram technique developed by Chou [22] and Eid et al. [23]). The CI took into account both the potency and shape of the dose–effect curve, which is given by Eq. (1):

$$CI = \frac{(D)_1}{(D_X)_1} + \frac{(D)_2}{(D_X)_2} \quad (1)$$

CI > 1, = 1, and <1 correspond to synergism, addition, and antagonism, respectively. The denominators $(D_x)_1$ and $(D_x)_2$ are the doses of a single treatment of the first and second compound designated as **1** and **2**, respectively. Additionally, $(D)_1$ and $(D)_2$ are the doses of the compounds **1** and **2** in the combination treatment that exhibited x % antiproliferation.

The calculated dose reduction index (DRI) was used to determine the extent of dose reduction in the combination treatment compared with the dose of each single treatment. For the combination effect, DRI was defined as $DRI_1 = (D_X)_1/(D)_1$ and $DRI_2 = (D_X)_2/(D)_2$. The relationship between DRI and CI was represented as: $CI = 1/DRI_1 + 1/DRI_2$.

The same antiproliferation experiment was performed on the normal Vero cells to provide a comparison to determine the cytotoxic effect of combining the compounds against the normal cells. The synergistic apoptotic effects of the combination of *P. kesiya* extract and melphalan were evaluated against the U937 and HepG2 cells by DAPI staining and DNA fragmentation assay.

Table 1 Concentration ratios of *P. kesiya* extract and melphalan combinations used in the combination anticancer study

IC_{50} Ratio in U937														
IC_{50} of *P. kesiya* (μg/mL)	0.02 (6)	0.05 (15)	0.1 (30)	0.2 (60)	0.5 (150)	1 (300)	1.5 (450)	2 (500[a])	1 (300)	1 (300)	1 (300)	1 (300)	1 (300)	1 (300)
IC_{50} of melphalan (μg/mL)	1 (15)	1 (15)	1 (15)	1 (15)	1 (15)	1 (15)	1 (15)	1 (15)	0.05 (0.75)	0.1 (1.5)	0.2 (3)	0.5 (7.5)	1.5 (22.5)	2 (30)
IC_{50} Ratio in HepG2														
IC_{50} of *P. kesiya* (μg/mL)	0.02 (1.1)	0.05 (2.75)	0.1 (5.5)	0.2 (11)	0.5 (27.5)	1 (55)	1.5 (83)	2 (110)	1 (55)	1 (55)	1 (55)	1 (55)	1 (55)	1 (55)
IC_{50} of melphalan (μg/mL)	1 (40)	1 (40)	1 (40)	1 (40)	1 (40)	1 (40)	1 (40)	1 (40)	0.05 (2)	0.1 (4)	0.2 (8)	0.5 (20)	1.5 (60)	2 (80)

The experimental IC_{50} concentrations of *P. kesiya* in U937 and HepG2 cells were 299.0 ± 5.2 and 52.0 ± 5.8 μg/mL, respectively

The experimental IC_{50} concentrations of melphalan in U937 and HepG2 cells were 15.0 ± 1.0 and 37.7 ± 9.8 μg/mL, respectively

[a] The maximum concentration used in the experiment to keep percentage DMSO at <1 % v/v was 500 μg/mL

Table 2 Antiproliferation of *P. kesiya* extract and melphalan combination in U937, HepG2, and Vero cell lines

IC_{50} Ratio		% Antiproliferation		
P. kesiya	Melphalan	U937	HepG2	Vero
0	1	50	50	50[a]
1	0	50	50	Inactive[b]
1	1	100 ± 7.0	95.7 ± 12.2	6.8 ± 1.9
0.02	1	46.0 ± 5.7	Nd	Nd
0.05	1	59.8 ± 5.3	Nd	Nd
0.1	1	76.6 ± 13.5	Nd	1.0 ± 3.5
0.2	1	79.3 ± 3.7	43.7 ± 2.9	4.0 ± 6.1
0.5	1	100 ± 7.0	82.1 ± 4.9	7.3 ± 1.9
1.5	1	100 ± 2.2	93.4 ± 1.6	16.4 ± 4.7
2	1	100 ± 11.3	100 ± 3.1	24.7 ± 9.1
1	0.05	46.8 ± 9.5	34.2 ± 4.4	Nd
1	0.1	51.8 ± 5.5	46.0 ± 9.1	Nd
1	0.2	73.0 ± 4.2	60.7 ± 16.4	0 ± 3.3
1	0.5	76.4 ± 3.6	65.1 ± 9.1	1.8 ± 1.2
1	1.5	100 ± 2.0	100 ± 10.5	8.6 ± 1.4
1	2	100 ± 3.4	100 ± 4.9	9.5 ± 1.9

Two-way ANOVA detected significant antiproliferative activity differences among various IC_{50} ratios ($P < 0.001$) and among various cell lines ($P < 0.001$). A significant two-way interaction was observed between IC_{50} ratio and various cell lines ($P < 0.001$)

Nd not determined

[a] IC_{50} value of melphalan in Vero cells equals 59.9 ± 3.2 μg/mL

[b] Inactive when IC_{50} of *P. kesiya* in Vero cells was >500 μg/mL

Statistical analysis

Experiments were performed in triplicate and the results were expressed as a mean ± standard deviation from three independent experiments. Statistical analysis was performed by IBM SPSS Statistics 17.0 (SPSS Inc., Chicago, IL, USA). A two-way analysis of variance (ANOVA) test followed by Fisher's least significant difference test for multiple comparisons of independent experiments were used to determine the effective enhancement of the inhibition growth by *P. kesiya* and melphalan in various cell lines. The significance level was set at $P < 0.05$. Statistical differences of percentage apoptotic cells between the *P. kesiya* treated group and the positive control group were compared by one-way ANOVA followed by Tukey's honest significant difference test with a significance level of $P < 0.05$.

Results

Antiproliferative effects of *P. kesiya* extract and melphalan singly versus in combination on U937 and HepG2 cell lines

The antiproliferative effects of *P. kesiya* extract and melphalan singly or in combination were investigated in U937 and HepG2 cell lines. The IC_{50} values of *P. kesiya* in U937 and HepG2 were 299.0 ± 5.2 μg/mL and 52.0 ± 5.8 μg/mL, respectively. The IC_{50} values of melphalan in U937 and HepG2 were 15.0 ± 1.0 μg/mL and 37.7 ± 9.8 μg/mL, respectively. Both melphalan and *P. kesiya* extract caused significantly greater antiproliferation than was observed in untreated cancer cells (control). *P. kesiya* extract exerted potent antiproliferation in the HepG2 cells at an IC_{50} value of 52.0 ± 5.8 μg/mL. *P. kesiya* extract had a stronger selectivity against the two cancer cell lines than melphalan. A significant enhanced antiproliferative effect occurred with the combination when treating human U937 and HepG2 cell lines (Table 2). A two-way ANOVA was conducted that examined the effect of IC_{50} ratio and cell types on percentage antiproliferation. There was a statistically significant interaction between the effects of IC_{50} ratio and cell types on percentage antiproliferation, $F(26, 84) = 42.654$, $P < 0.001$. A two-way ANOVA detected significant differences in the antiproliferative activity of the various IC_{50} ratios (all $P < 0.001$) and among the various cell lines ($P < 0.001$). Significantly higher antiproliferative activities were observed at *P. kesiya* to melphalan concentration ratios of 0.2:1, 0.5:1, 1:1, 1.5:1, 2:1, 1:0.2, 1:0.5, 1:1.5, and 1:2 compared with normal Vero cells ($P < 0.001$). When the concentration of melphalan was constant, an enhanced antiproliferative effect was observed at *P. kesiya* to melphalan concentration ratios of 0.05:1 and 0.5:1 in the U937 and HepG2 cell lines, respectively. Alternatively, when *P. kesiya* was constant, the enhanced antiproliferative effect was observed at melphalan to *P. kesiya* concentration ratios of 0.1:1 and 0.2:1 in the U937 and HepG2 cell lines, respectively.

Melphalan alone exhibited strong antiproliferation in normal Vero cells at an IC_{50} value of 59.9 ± 3.2 μg/mL, while *P. kesiya* extract alone was inactive in normal Vero cells. When treating the Vero cells, the antiproliferation of the combination treatment was <25 % when the concentration of melphalan was constant (Table 2). The result showed an antagonistic effect of *P. kesiya* extract on the antiproliferation of melphalan in Vero cells. In the presence of a 1 × IC_{50} concentration of *P. kesiya,* the concentration of melphalan used could be as high as 2 × IC_{50}, producing only 9.5 ± 1.9 % antiproliferation against Vero cells.

Synergistic effect of melphalan and *P. kesiya* extract combination analyzed in U937 leukemic and HepG2 hepatocellular carcinoma cell lines

The CIs of the combined effect of *P. kesiya* and melphalan in the U937 and HepG2 cell lines at IC_{75} and IC_{90} values are presented in Table 3 and Fig. 1. Our results indicated that the combination of *P. kesiya* and melphalan exhibited high synergistic effects in U937 and HepG2

Table 3 Dose reduction index (DRI) and combination index (CI)

% Antiproliferation	Cell lines	Combination treatment	DRI		CI
			P. kesiya	Melphalan	
90 % (IC_{90})	U937	Fixed [*P. kesiya*] = IC_{50}	2.3	7.8	0.56
		Fixed [melphalan] = IC_{50}	6.5	5.5	0.33
	HepG2	Fixed [*P. kesiya*] = IC_{50}	2.0	3.6	0.79
		Fixed [melphalan] = IC_{50}	2.4	3.2	0.74
75 % (IC_{75})	U937	Fixed [*P. kesiya*] = IC_{50}	1.8	8.7	0.66
		Fixed [melphalan] = IC_{50}	9.1	3.8	0.37
	HepG2	Fixed [*P. kesiya*] = IC_{50}	1.6	3.8	0.90
		Fixed [melphalan] = IC_{50}	2.7	2.4	0.79

DRI and CI of the combination treatment of *P. kesiya*/melphalan in U937 or in HepG2 cells at the concentrations that produced 90 and 75 % antiproliferation

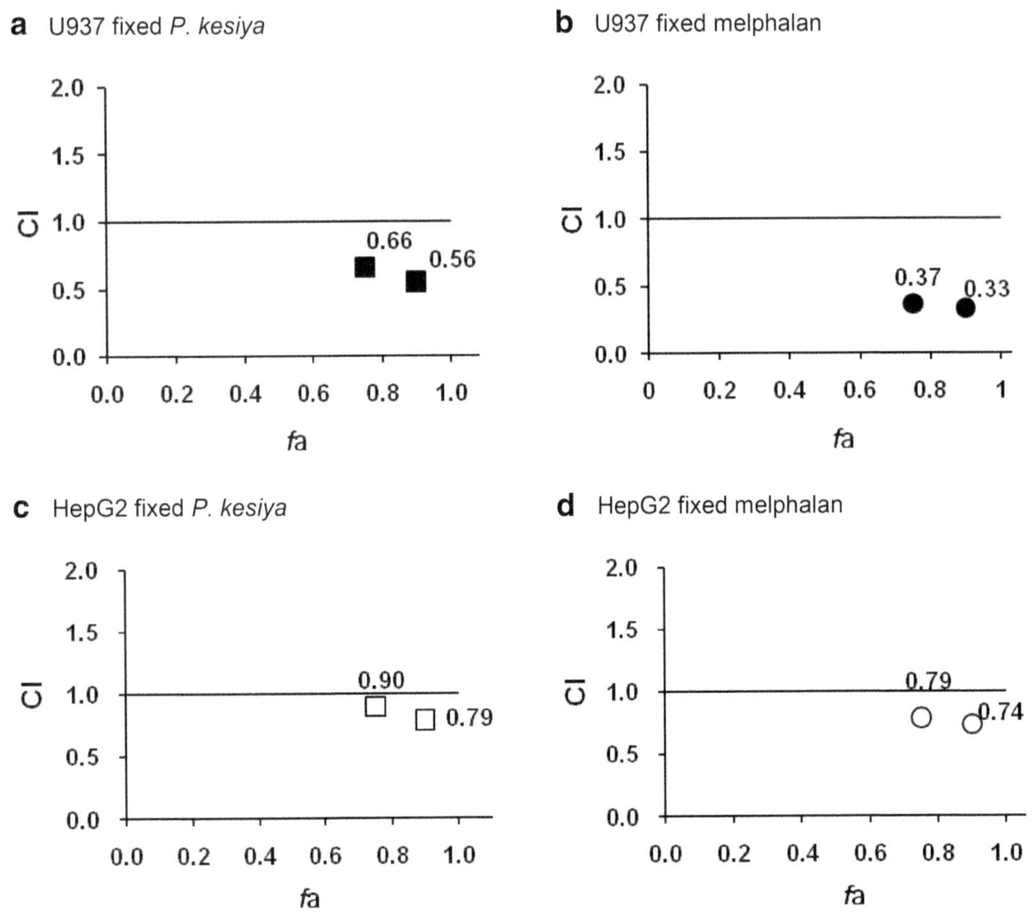

Fig. 1 Isobolograms of the plot between combination index (CI) and *fa* in U937 (*black symbol*) and HepG2 (*white symbol*). *fa* = fraction affected by D (i.e., percentage antiproliferation/100). Isobolograms of the combination of compounds when *P. kesiya* was fixed (**a**, **c**; *square*), and when melphalan was fixed (**b**, **d**; *circle*) in each cancer cell lines

cells at concentrations producing 75 and 90 % antiproliferation (IC_{75} and IC_{90}). As observed from the higher synergistic effect (low CI value), the combination therapy was more effective on the U937 cells than on the HepG2 cells.

Extent of dose reduction in the combination treatment compared with single doses of each treatment

Table 3 shows the decreased concentration of melphalan or *P. kesiya* extract in the combination therapy to produce 90 and 75 % antiproliferation in U937 cells and HepG2 cells. The concentration of melphalan (when combined with a fixed concentration of *P. kesiya* extract) necessary to inhibit cancer growth by 90 % (IC_{90}) represents a 7.8- and 3.6-fold decrease in U937 and HepG2 cells, respectively. By comparison, the concentration of *P. kesiya* extract (when combined with a fixed concentration of melphalan) needed for the IC_{90} represents a 6.5- and 2.4-fold decrease in U937 and HepG2 cells, respectively. A similar DRI trend (i.e., a greater melphalan dose reduction) for U937 cells compared with HepG2 cells was observed at 75 % antiproliferation. Dose reduction also depended on the type of cancer cells: 90 and 75 % cell death occurred when the *P. kesiya* extract concentration was fixed. The doses for melphalan per dose of *P. kesiya* extract could be reduced in the U937 cells (10.55:300 = 0.04:1 and 6.6:300 = 0.02:1) more than in the HepG2 cells (33.7:55.0 = 0.61:1 and 23.7:55.0 = 0.43:1). The synergistic effect appears to be greater for the melphalan because a greater potential dose reduction could be achieved; thus, melphalan concentrations could be significantly reduced.

Apoptotic induction effect of single treatments and of *P. kesiya* extract and melphalan combination treatment

Apoptosis induction by *P. kesiya* extract and melphalan when used singly or in combination was evaluated in HepG2 and U937 cell lines using a method based on the DAPI staining assay (Table 4) and DNA fragmentation assays (Fig. 2). In the control group, the nuclei were roundish and homogeneously stained by DAPI; in contrast, the apoptotic nuclei in the treated U937 and HepG2 cells were irregularly shaped, small, detached, and had apoptotic bodies. At a 1 × IC_{50} concentration, *P. kesiya* extract induced 42.5 ± 4.8 and 39.7 ± 2.6 % apoptosis in the U937 and HepG2 cells, respectively; melphalan induced 43.1 ± 16.3 and 53.0 ± 6.1 % apoptosis, respectively. The combination therapy of *P. kesiya* extract and melphalan was significantly more effective in inducing apoptosis against U937 and HepG2 cells.

DNA fragmentation was determined according to whether the synergistic apoptosis induction in both cancer cells occurred toward the late stage of apoptosis, as previously observed for single therapy [15]. The combined treatment of *P. kesiya* with melphalan resulted in DNA laddering in both the HepG2 and U937 cells compared with the control cells (Fig. 2).

Table 4 Effects of *P. kesiya* and melphalan on apoptosis induction in U937 and HepG2 cells

IC_{50} ratio		% Apoptotic cells	
IC_{50} of *P. kesiya*	IC_{50} of Melphalan	U937	HepG2
0	1	43.1 ± 16.3	53.0 ± 6.1
1	0	42.5 ± 4.8^b	39.7 ± 2.6^a
1	1	100^a	100^a
0.1	1	77.0 ± 1.9^a	66.7 ± 3.1^a
0.2	1	100^a	74.9 ± 12.3^a
0.5	1	100^a	92.8 ± 1.3^a
1.5	1	100^a	98.3 ± 3.0^a
2	1	100^a	100^a
1	0.05	38.6 ± 6.1^a	62.4 ± 3.2^a
1	0.1	48.4 ± 3.8^a	87.9 ± 3.3^a
1	0.2	61.3 ± 3.3^a	90.3 ± 6.0^a
1	0.5	100^a	100^a
1	1.5	100^a	100^a
1	2	100^a	100^a

One-way ANOVA of percentage apoptotic cells compared with single treatment by melphalan at 1 × IC_{50} in cancer cells

^{a} Significant difference ($P < 0.001$)

^{b} Non-significant difference ($P \geq 0.001$)

GC–MS analysis of *P. kesiya* extract

GC–MS analysis of *P. kesiya* extract was performed to obtain its characteristic fingerprint (Table 5). The GC peaks obtained were used for further chemical constituent identification and revealed several compounds:podocarpa-8,11,13-trien-15-oic acid, neopine, rosin acid, pimaric acid, oleic acid, pyrocatecol, and vanillin (Table 5).

Discussion

To our knowledge, this is the first report of a synergistic effect of *P. kesiya* extract on melphalan anticancer activity via the apoptosis induction mechanism in vitro. The U937 cells were only sensitive to melphalan, based on the lower IC_{50} value; however, the HepG2 cells were sensitive to both *P. kesiya* extract and melphalan. A wide chemopreventive index was observed in the combination treatment, probably because the cytotoxic effect was lower in the normal Vero cells. *P. kesiya* extract's potent antiproliferation effect in the HepG2 cell line and high selective antiproliferation effect in both cancer cell lines requires further investigation.

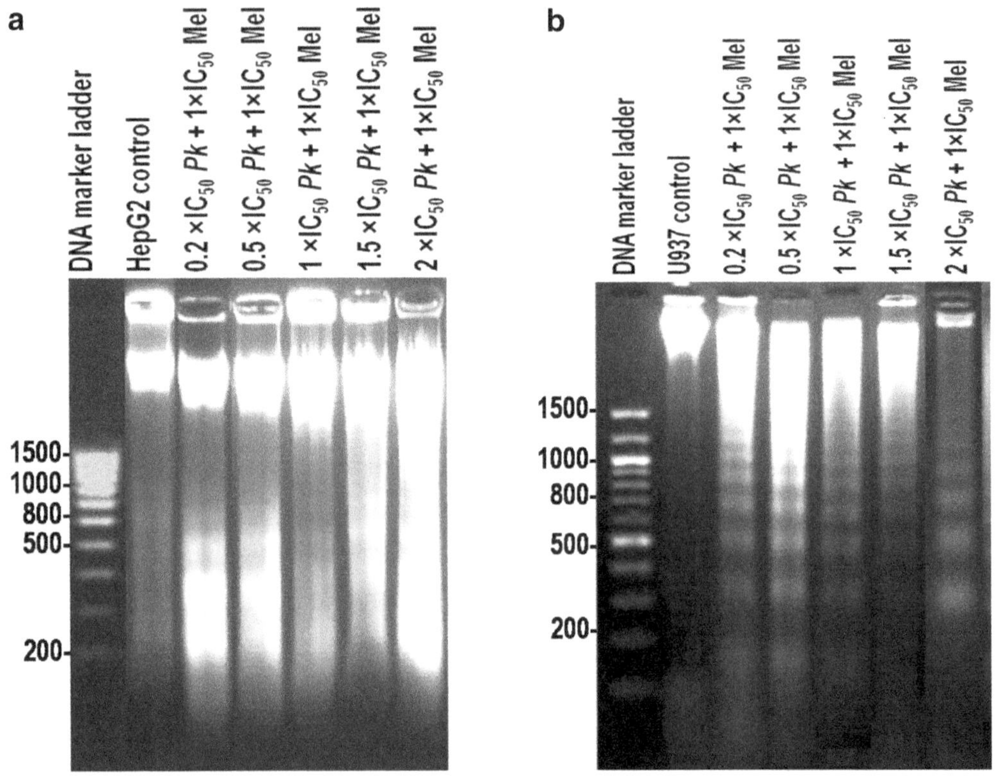

Fig. 2 DNA fragments after combination treatment of *P. kesiya* (Pk) extract with melphalan in HepG2 (**a**) and U937 (**b**) cell lines

Table 5 Identified compounds and their relative distribution in *P. kesiya*

Retention time (min)	% of Total area	Assigned compounds
11.074	2.48	Pyrocatecol (1,2-benzenediol or brenzcatechin)
16.412	2.66	trans-Sobrerol
16.703	1.88	Vanillin
29.551	1.55	Palmitic acid
32.878	4.49	Oleic acid
35.650	4.16	Benzoyl isocyanate
36.096	4.77	Pimaric acid
37.170	6.52	Rosin acid
37.907	20.16	Podocarpa-8,11,13-trien-15-oic acid, 13-isopropyl
38.525	4.31	2,3-dimethoxy-5-[2-(3-hydroxy-4-methoxyphenyl) ethenyl]phenol or Combretastatin A3
41.788	5.98	Neopine

GC–MS data of the 50 % ethanol–water crude extract of *P. kesiya*

Drug and herb combinations could significantly decrease the toxicity and chemoresistance of drugs and increase their efficacy [24, 25] i.e., increasing the efficacy of the therapeutic effect; decreasing the dosage to avoid toxicity; reducing the development of drug resistance; and providing selective synergism against a target (or efficacy synergism) vs. host (or toxicity antagonism). The ability of herbal extracts to enhance anticancer activity might also arise from the potentiation of pharmacokinetics, wherein one ingredient enhanced the therapeutic effect of another (active ingredient or drug) by modulating its pharmacokinetic properties (i.e., absorption, distribution, metabolism, and/or excretion) [24, 25]. The administration of multiple therapeutic agents is often associated with additional toxicities, which can be life threatening; however, a combination treatment with a non-toxic herbal extract like *P. kesiya* might provide superior benefits.

Previous work indicated that, in addition to the compounds identified here in *P. kesiya* extract (Table 5), gallic acid, chlorogenic acid, caffeic acid, vanillin, and coumaric acid in the 50 % ethanol–water extract of *P. kesiya* exhibited an anticancer effect [14]. The main compounds found in various parts of Pinaceae were terpenes, such as α- and β-pinene [26]. Rosin is composed of a complex mixture of different compounds, including resin acids such as abietic acid, plicatic acid, and pimaric acid. Resin acids might be derived from terpenes through partial oxidation and undergo isomerization in the presence of strong acids or with heat [27]. Hence, terpenes such as α- and β-pinene might undergo thermal conversion into resin acids under the GC–MS condition studied. One previous study reported that α-pinene expressed both apoptosis induction and anti-metastatic activity against melanoma cells [26]. A previous work has also shown that citronellol—found in the family Pinaceae—inhibited an efflux P-gp protein at an IC_{50} value of 504 μM [28].

Conclusions

Combining the *P. kesiya* extract with melphalan reduced toxicity while retaining the therapeutic efficacy (reduced approximately 4–9 fold) of melphalan.

Abbreviations

DMEM: Dulbecco's modified Eagle's medium; DMSO: dimethylsulfoxide; FBS: fetal bovine serum; HepG2: human hepatocellular carcinoma cell line; NR: neutral red; PBS: phosphate buffer solution; NCI: National Cancer Institute (USA); U937: human leukemic cell line; Vero: normal African green monkey kidney epithelial cell line.

Authors' contributions

NW designed the study. SM performed the experiments. NW and SM collected and analyzed data. SM, NW and SB analyzed and interpreted data. SM and NW wrote the manuscript. NW and SB revised manuscript. All the authors read and approved the final manuscript.

Author details

[1] Faculty of Pharmaceutical Sciences, Khon Kaen University, Khon Kaen 40002, Thailand. [2] Graduate School, Khon Kaen University, Khon Kaen 40002, Thailand. [3] Faculty of Associated Medical Sciences, Khon Kaen University, Khon Kaen 40002, Thailand.

Acknowledgements

We thank (a) The Office of the Higher Education Commission, Thailand, under the Strategic Scholarships for Thai Doctoral Degree Programs (CHE-PhD-THA-RG 3/2549), (b) Khon Kaen University for financial support, (c)The authors thank the Plant Genetics Conservation Project under the Royal Initiation of her Royal Highness Princess Maha Chakri Sirindhorn, The Bureau of The Royal Household for permission to conduct the research and Electricity Generating Authority of Thailand (EGAT) for field support and (d) Mr. Bryan Roderick Hamman and Mrs. Janice Loewen-Hamman for assistance with the English-language presentation.

Competing interests

The authors declare that they have no competing interests.

References

1. Au JLS, Panchal N, Li D, Gan Y. Apoptosis: a new pharmacodynamic endpoint. Pharm Res. 1997;14:1659–71.
2. Lee C, Raffaghello L, Longo VD. Starvation, detoxification, and multidrug resistance in cancer therapy. Drug Resist Updates. 2012;15:114–22.
3. Pinmai K, Chunlaratthanabhorn S, Ngamkitidechakul C, Soonthorn-chareon N, Hahnvajanawong C. Synergistic growth inhibitory effects of *Phyllanthus emblica* and *Terminalia bellerica* extracts with conventional cytotoxic agents: doxorubicin and cisplatin against human hepatocellular carcinoma and lung cancer cells. World J Gastroentero. 2008;14:1491–7.
4. Tang SN, Singh C, Nall D, Meeker D, Shankar S, Srivastava RK. The dietary bioflavonoid quercetin synergizes with epigallocathechin gallate (EGCG) to inhibit prostate cancer stem cell characteristics, invasion, migration and epithelial-mesenchymal transition. J Mol Signal. 2010;5:14.
5. Wagner H, Ulrich-Merzenich G. Synergy research: approaching a new generation of phytopharmaceuticals. Phytomedicine. 2009;16:97–110.
6. Machana S, Weerapreeyakul N, Barusrux S, Thumanu K, Tanthanuch W. Synergistic anticancer effect of the extracts from *Polyalthia evecta* caused apoptosis in human hepatoma (HepG2) cells. Asian Pac J Trop Biomed. 2012;2:589–96.
7. Ya C, Ming-Hua Q, Kun G, Lin Z, ZhongRong L. A new abietane diterpenoid from the rosin of *Pinus kesiya* var. *langbianensis* (Pinaceae). Acta Botanica Yunnanica (ABY). 2006;3:323–5.
8. Jingkai D, Lisheng D, Yuanfen Y, Yu W, Handong S. Chemical constituents of the turpentine of *Pinus kesiya* var. *langbianensis*. Yunnan Zhiwu Yanjiu. 1983;5:224–46.
9. Koukos PK, Papadopoulou KI, Patiaka DT, Papagiannopoulos AD. Chemical composition of essential oils from needles and twigs of balkan pine (*Pinus peuce* Grisebach) grown in Northern Greece. J Agric Food Chem. 2000;48:1266–8.
10. Mateus EP, Gomesdasilva MD, Ribeiro AB, Marriott PJ. Qualitative mass spectrometric analysis of the volatile fraction of creosote-treated railway wood sleepers by using comprehensive two-dimensional gas chromatography. J Chromatogr. 2008;1178:215–22.
11. Mateus E, Baratab RC, Zrostlíková J, Gomesdasilva MDR, Paiva MR. Characterization of the volatile fraction emitted by *Pinus* spp. by one- and two-dimensional chromatographic techniques with mass spectrometric detection. J Chromatogr. 2010;1217:1845–55.
12. Hiltunen R, Löyttyniemi K. Monoterpene composition of needle oil in *Pinus kesiya* Royle ex Gordon. Seloste: *Pinus kesiya*-männyn neulasöljyn monoterpeenikoostumus. Commun Inst For Fenn. 1978;94:1–9.
13. Hynniewta SR, Kumar Y. Herbal remedies among the Khasi traditional healers and village folk Mekhalaya. Indian J Traditional Knowl. 2008;7:581–6.
14. Machana S, Weerapreeyakul N, Barusrux S, Nonpanya A, Sripanidkulchai B, Thitimetharoch T. Cytotoxic and apoptotic effects of six herbal plants against the human hepatocarcinoma (HepG2) cell line. Chin Med. 2011;6:39.
15. Machana S, Weerapreeyakul N, Barusrux S, Thumanu K, Tanthanuch W. FTIR microspectroscopy discriminates anticancer action on human leukemic cells by extracts of *Pinus kesiya*; *Cratoxylum formosum* spp. *pruniflorum* and melphalan. Talanta. 2012;93:371–82.
16. Cloutier JF, Castonguay A, O'Connor TR, Drouin R. Alkylating agent and chromatin structure determine sequence context-dependent formation of alkylpurines. J Mol Biol. 2001;306:169–88.
17. Lialiaris T, Lyratzopoulos E, Papachristou F, Simopoulou M, Mourelatos C, Nikolettos N. Supplementation of melatonin protects human lymphocytes *in vitro* from the genotoxic activity of melphalan. Mutagenesis. 2008;23:347–54.
18. Boegsted M, Holst JM, Fogd K, Falgreen S, Sørensen S, Schmitz A, Bukh A, Johnsen HE, Nyegaard K, Dybkaer K. Generation of a predictive melphalan resistance index by drug screen of B-cell cancer cell lines. PLoS ONE. 2011;6:e19322.
19. Phengklai C. Pinaceae/Cephalotaxaceae/Cupressaceae. Flor Thail. 1972;2:193–6.
20. Phengklai C. Studies in flora of Thailand : Pinaceae. Thai For Bull. (Bot.). 1973;7:1–4.
21. Weerapreeyakul N, Nonpunya A, Barusrux S, Thitimetharoch T, Sripanidkulchai B. Evaluation of the anticancer potential of six herbs against a hepatoma cell line. Chin Med. 2012;7:15.
22. Chou TC. Theoretical basis, experimental design, and computerized simulation of synergism and antagonism in drug combination studies. Pharmacol Rev. 2006;58:621–81.
23. Eid SY, El-Readi MZ, Wink M. Synergism of three-drug combinations of sanguinarine and other plant secondary metabolites with digitonin and doxorubicin in multi-drug resistant cancer cells. Phytomedicine. 2012;19:1288–97.

24. Greco WR, Bravo G, Parsons JC. The search for synergy: a critical review from a response surface perspective. Pharmacol Rev. 1995;47:331–85.
25. Feng-Zhu JJ, Ma X, Cao ZW, Li YX, Chen YZ. Mechanisms of drug combinations from interaction and network perspectives. Nat Rev Drug Discov. 2009;8:111–28.
26. Matsuo AL, Figueiredo CR, Arruda DC, Pereira FV, Scutti JAB, Massaoka MH, Travassos LR, Sartorelli P, Lago JHG. α-Pinene isolated from *Schinus terebinthifolius* Raddi (Anacardiaceae) induces apoptosis and confers antimetastatic protection in a melanoma model. Biochem Biophys Res Commun. 2011;411:449–54.
27. Parimal K, Khale A, Pramod K. Resins from herbal origin and a focus on their applications. IJPSR. 2011;2:1077–85.
28. Yoshida N, Takagi A, Kitazawa H, Kawakami J, Adachi I. Inhibition of P-glycoprotein-mediated transport by extracts of and monoterpenoids contained in *Zanthoxyli* Fructus. Toxicol Appl Pharm. 2005;209:167–73.

9

Combination of cisplatin and bromelain exerts synergistic cytotoxic effects against breast cancer cell line MDA-MB-231 in vitro

Ahmad Zaim Mat Pauzi[1], Swee Keong Yeap[2], Nadiah Abu[1], Kian Lam Lim[3], Abdul Rahman Omar[2], Suraini Abdul Aziz[4], Adam Leow Thean Chow[1], Tamilselvan Subramani[1], Soon Guan Tan[1] and Noorjahan Banu Alitheen[1*]

Abstract

Background: Bromelain, which is a cysteine endopeptidase commonly found in pineapple stems, has been investigated as a potential anti-cancer agent for the treatment of breast cancer. However, information pertaining to the effects of combining bromelain with existing chemotherapeutic drugs remains scarce. This study aimed to investigate the possible synergistic cytotoxic effects of using bromelain in combination with cisplatin on MDA-MB-231 human breast cancer cells.

Method: MDA-MB-231 cells were treated with different concentrations (0.24–9.5 μM) of bromelain or cisplatin alone, as well as four different combinations of these two agents to assess their individual and combination effects after 24 and 48 h. Cell viability was analyzed using an MTT assay. The induction of apoptosis was assessed using cell cycle analysis and an Annexin V-FITC assay. The role of the mitochondrial membrane potential in the apoptotic process was assessed using a JC-1 staining assay. Apoptotic protein levels were assessed by western blot analysis and proteome profiling using an antibody array kit.

Results: Single-agent treatment with cisplatin or bromelain led to dose- and time-dependent decreases in the viability of the MDA-MB-231 cells at 24 and 48 h. Furthermore, most of the combinations evaluated in this study displayed synergistic effects against MDA-MB-231 cells at 48 h, with combination 1 (bromelain 2 μM + cisplatin 1.5 μM) exhibiting the greatest synergistic effect ($P = 0.000$). The results of subsequent assays indicated that combination 1 treatment induced apoptosis via mitochondria-mediated pathway. Combination 1 also resulted in significant decreases in the levels of several apoptotic proteins such as Bcl-x and HSP70, compared with bromelain ($P = 0.002$ and 0.000, respectively) or cisplatin ($P = 0.000$ and 0.001, respectively) single treatment. Notably, MDA-MB-231 cells treated with combination 1 showed increased levels of the pro-apoptotic proteins Bax compared with those treated with bromelain ($P = 0.000$) or cisplatin single treatment ($P = 0.043$).

Conclusion: Bromelain in combination with cisplatin synergistically enhanced the induction of apoptosis in MDA-MB-231 cells.

*Correspondence: noorjahan@upm.edu.my
[1] Department of Cell and Molecular Biology, Faculty of Biotechnology and Biomolecular Sciences, Universiti Putra Malaysia, 43400 Serdang, Selangor, Malaysia
Full list of author information is available at the end of the article

Background

Breast cancer is the most frequently diagnosed invasive non-skin malignancy and the leading cause of cancer-related deaths in women throughout the world [1]. In Asia, the incidence and mortality rates of breast cancer have been steadily rising for several years, with unhealthy diet, physical inactivity and obesity being identified as the main contributing factors [2]. Although there are many different strategies available for the clinical treatment of breast cancer, the effectiveness of these approaches can be limited by the occurrence of adverse side effects and the development of drug resistance.

cis-Diamminedichloroplatinum (CDDP), which is more commonly known as cisplatin, is one of the most effective anti-cancer agents currently used in clinical practice, with pronounced activity against various cancers, including breast cancer [3, 4]. Cisplatin interacts with DNA and interferes with the mechanisms responsible for its transcription and replication [5, 6]. Consequently, cisplatin treatment is associated with a number of serious side effects such as nephrotoxicity, myelosuppression, ototoxicity, anaphylactic reactions, peripheral neuropathies and hypomagnesemia [7–9]. Furthermore, the clinical application of cisplatin is limited by the development of resistance mechanisms in the cancer cells [10–12]. The combination of cisplatin with other anti-cancer agents that operate via a different mode of action could therefore be used as an effective strategy to impede the growth of human cancer cells that develop resistance to cisplatin. This strategy could also minimize the severity of the side effects associated with the individual agents, whilst maintaining or even enhancing the effectiveness of the treatment process.

Pineapple (*Ananascomosus* L.) has been used to treat a wide range of diseases in several different countries, including Thailand, Malaysia, Taiwan and China, as well as the state of Hawaii [13]. Pineapple plants are commonly used in folk medicine, especially their crown leaves, which are used to treat open wounds and inflammation. The results of a previous study demonstrated that pineapple crown leaf extract exhibited several interesting biological properties, including antimicrobial, anti-edema and anti-inflammatory activities [14].Pineapple stems have also been reported to exhibit a broad range of promising pharmacological properties. Stem bromelain is a cysteine endopeptidase, which is commonly found at a high concentration in the crude extract of pineapple stems (*Ananascomosus* L.) [15]. The results of several in vitro and in vivo studies [16–21] have demonstrated that bromelain exhibited various beneficial therapeutic effects, including anti-tumor activity. These results therefore support the potential application of stem bromelain as a therapeutic agent for the treatment of cancer. Moreover, bromelain exhibits good stability over a wide range of pH values [22, 23] and is readily adsorbed in the human intestinal tract in its functional active form when it is consumed in high concentrations (up to 12 g/day). Taken together with the fact that its consumption does not lead to any major side effects, these results further highlight the potential of bromelain as an anti-cancer agent [24, 25].

The study aimed to investigate the possible synergistic cytotoxic effects of using bromelain in combination with cisplatin for the treatment of MDA-MB-231 human breast cancer cells.

Methods

Chemicals and reagents

Unless specified otherwise, all of the chemicals used in this study, including bromelain and cisplatin, were obtained from Sigma Aldrich (St Louis, MO, USA). Stock solutions of bromelain in water were freshly prepared prior to each experiment using deionized water. The resulting aqueous solutions were filtered (0.2 μm) prior to being used in the experiments. A stock solution of cisplatin was prepared in the dark using deionized water containing 0.9% (w/w) sodium chloride. The resulting stock solution was stored at 4 °C in the absence of light prior to being used.

Cell cultures

The MDA-MB-231 cells used in this study obtained from the American Type Culture Collection (Rockville, MD, USA). The cells were cultured in Roswell Park Memorial Institute medium enriched with 10% fetal bovine serum and 100 units/mL penicillin–streptomycin antibiotic at 37 °C under a humidified atmosphere containing 5% CO_2.

MTT assay

Cell growth inhibition was determined using a colorimetric MTT assay. The assay was conducted in a 96-well plate with a cell density of 8×10^3 cells per well with an incubation period of 24 h. The medium was subsequently removed and replaced with fresh medium containing the test compound, followed by an incubation period of 24 or 48 h. The cells were then incubated with MTT solution (0.5 mg/mL) for 4 h, and the resulting formazan precipitate was dissolved in 170 μL of DMSO. The absorbance of each well was then measured at 570 nm using a microplate spectrophotometer (Bio-Tek Instruments, Winooski, VT, USA). The percentage of cell survival was calculated using the following formula: percentage (%) cell survival = [(mean absorbency in test wells)/(mean absorbency in control wells)] × 100. These experiments were conducted in triplicate. We then constructed a graph of the percentage cell viability against the concentration of the test compound. The resulting graph was used to determine the IC10, IC20, IC30, IC40 and IC50 values of bromelain and cisplatin for the single treatment of the MDA-MB-231 cells.

We also conducted a series of MTT assays using four different combinations of bromelain and cisplatin (*i.e.*, IC40 bromelain + IC10 cisplatin, IC30 bromelain + IC20 cisplatin, IC20 bromelain + IC30 cisplatin and IC10 bromelain + IC40 cisplatin) with concentrations in the range of 0.24–9.5 μM. All of these assays were conducted in a 96-well plate with a cell density of 8×10^3 cells per well with an incubation period of 24 h. The medium was subsequently removed and replaced with fresh medium containing the test compound, followed by an incubation period of 48 h. The cells were then incubated with MTT solution (0.5 mg/mL) for 4 h, and the resulting formazan precipitate was dissolved in 170 μL of DMSO. The absorbance of each well was then measured at 570 nm using a microplate spectrophotometer (Bio-Tek Instruments). All of these experiments were conducted independently in triplicate.

Annexin V-FITC assay

The cells were seeded into a 6-well plate and incubated for 24 h at 37 °C under a humidified atmosphere containing 5% CO_2. The medium in each well was subsequently replaced with fresh medium containing different concentrations of the test compounds. After an incubation period of 24 or 48 h, all of the detached/dead and viable cells were collected. The cells were then washed and resuspended with PBS. The harvested cells were stained with Annexin V for 30 min before being treated with PI and analyzed by flow cytometry using a FACScan system (Becton–Dickinson and Company, San Jose, CA, USA) equipped with version 3.3 of the CellQuest software (Becton–Dickinson and Company). This assay was conducted according to the manufacturer's protocol (BD PharmingenAnnexin V-FITC Apoptosis Detection Kit 1).

Measurement of mitochondrial membrane potential (JC-1 staining assay)

The cells were seeded into a 6-well plate and incubated for 24 h at 37 °C under a humidified atmosphere containing 5% CO_2. The medium in each well was then replaced with fresh medium containing different concentrations of the test compounds. After an incubation period of 48 h, all the detached/dead and viable cells were harvested, washed with PBS and incubated with culture medium containing JC-1 for 30 min at 37 °C in the absence of light. The cells were then washed twice with PBS, resuspended in 500 μL of PBS and immediately analyzed by flow cytometry using a FACScan system (Becton–Dickinson and Company) equipped version 3.3 of the CellQuest software.

Cell cycle analysis

The cells were seeded into a 6-well plate and incubated for 24 h at 37 °C under a humidified atmosphere containing 5% CO_2. The medium in each well was then replaced with fresh medium containing different concentrations of the test compounds. After an incubation period of 24 or 48 h, all of the detached/dead and viable cells were collected, washed with cold PBS and resuspended in 50 mL of cold PBS before being treated with 450 μL of cold ethanol. The cells were then incubated for 24 h at 4 °C. At the end of the incubation period, the cells were centrifuged (Model 5804 R, Eppendorf, Hamburg, Germany) at 200×*g* for 5 min and the resulting pellet was washed with cold PBS and resuspended in 500 μL of PBS. The cells were then incubated with 5 μL of RNase (20 μg/mL final concentration) for 30 min before being incubated with PI (50 μg/mL) on ice for 1 h in the dark. The distribution of cells was then immediately analyzed by flow cytometry using a FACScan system (Becton–Dickinson and Company) equipped with version 3.3 of the CellQuest software.

Proteome Profiler™: human apoptosis array

The cells were seeded in a 6-well plate and incubated for 24 h at 37 °C under a humidified atmosphere containing 5% CO_2. The medium in each well was then replaced with fresh medium containing different concentrations of the test compounds. After an incubation period of 48 h, the cells were washed with PBS and lysed. All of the immunodetection steps were performed using a Proteome Profiler Human Apoptosis Array Kit (R&D Systems, Minneapolis, MN, USA) in accordance with the manufacturer's instructions. Briefly, the array was washed and incubated with a mixture of biotinylated detection antibodies. Streptavidin-HRP and chemiluminescent detection reagents were used, and a signal corresponding to the amount of protein bound was produced on each capture spot. After incubation, the membranes were developed using enhanced chemiluminescence reagents and immediately viewed and analyzed using a ChemiDoc XRS + system (Bio-Rad, Hercules, CA, USA). Protein expression was normalized to a positive control, which was present in each membrane.

Western blot

The cells were seeded into a 6-well plate and incubated for 24 h at 37 °C under a humidified atmosphere containing 5% CO_2. The medium in each well was then replaced with fresh medium containing different concentrations of the test compound. Following an incubation period of 24 or 48 h, the cells were washed with PBS and lysed in RIPA lysis buffer [50 mM Hepes (pH 7.5), 150 mM NaCl, 1% deoxycholate, 1% NP-40, 0.1% sodium dodecyl sulfate

(SDS)] containing protease inhibitors (Thermo Fisher Scientific, Waltham, MA, USA). The extracted proteins (20–60 μg) were separated by electrophoresis on SDS–polyacrylamide gels, transferred to nitrocellulose membranes (Bio-Rad) and probed with respective primary antibodies against Beta-actin, Bax and Bcl-2 (Abcam, Cambridge, Massachusetts, USA). After being incubated with the corresponding secondary antibodies (Abcam, the immunoreacted proteins were detected using a chemiluminescence system (ECL Western blot substrate; Abcam, Cambridge, UK).The bands obtained were quantitated using the ImageJ software (Bio Techniques, New York, NY, USA).

Statistical analysis

All of the experiments described in this study were repeated independently for at least three times (n = 3) and measured in triplicate, unless specified otherwise. The results have been reported as the corresponding mean values ± standard deviation (SD). Statistical data for MTT assay, Annexin-V/FitC assay, JC-1 staining assay and cell cycle analysis was analyzed by the Student's *t* test and one-way analysis of variance (ANOVA), followed by Tukey's multiple comparison post hoc test. Statistical analyses were performed using version 19 of the SPSS software for Windows (IBM SPSS, Chicago, IL, USA). Differences between the experimental groups were considered significant for *P* values of less than 0.05. Data analyses to determine the CI value of the combination treatment used were performed using the CompuSyn software (Combo SynInc, City, State, USA). CI < 1 indicates synergism, CI = 1 indicates additive effect, and CI > 1 indicates antagonism.

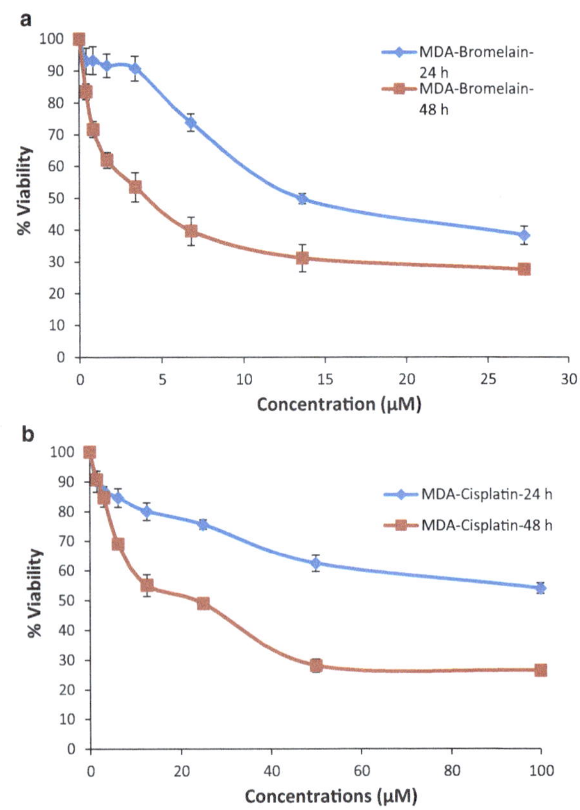

Fig. 1 Dose- and time-dependent inhibition of viability in MDA-MB-231 cells by bromelain and cisplatin single treatment. The figure shown in **a** is the MTT assay results for bromelain at 24 and 48 h, with IC50 value for bromelain at 48 h is 4.10 μM. The figure shown in **b** is the MTT assay results for cisplatin at 24 and 48 h, with IC50 value for cisplatin at 48 h is 23.0 μM. The results are expressed as mean ± SD of three separate experiments

Results

Inhibitory effects of cisplatin and bromelain (single-agent and combined treatment) on the growth of MDA-MB-231 cells

The proliferation of MDA-MB-231 cells was assessed using an MTT assay. The assay was conducted in the presence of various concentrations of cisplatin or bromelain, as well as different combinations of these two agents over 24 and 48 h to explore their effects on the MDA-MB-231 cells. The treatment of the cells with cisplatin or bromelain alone resulted in a dose-dependent and a time-dependent decrease in the viability of the MDA-MB-231 cells at 24 and 48 h, with higher concentrations and longer treatment times resulting in lower levels of cell viability (Fig. 1).

These results were used to determine the concentrations of cisplatin and bromelain required to inhibit the growth of the MDA-MB-231 cells by 50, 40, 30, 20 and 10% (*i.e.*, the IC50, IC40, IC30, IC20 and IC10 values) at 48 h. Based on these values, we were able to combine these concentrations into four different combinations of cisplatin and bromelain, which were subsequently tested against MDA-MB-231 cells for 48 h. The results of these combination studies are shown in Table 1. Combination 1 (bromelain 2 μM + cisplatin 1.5 μM) induced the greatest reduction in cell viability compared to combination 2 (*P* = 0.000), combination 3 (*P* = 0.000) and combination 4 (*P* = 0.000), indicating that it exhibited the strongest inhibitory effect of the four combinations.

Synergistic effects of combinations of cisplatin and bromelain for the treatment of MDA-MB-231 cells

The CI and DRI values, as well as the isobolograms for all of the bromelain and cisplatin combinations, are shown in Table 2. Only combinations 1, 3 and 4 gave CI values of less than 1, with combination 1 showing the lowest CI value of all of the combinations tested in the current study (CI

Table 1 Viability percentage of MDA-MB-231 at 48 h treated with bromelain and cisplatin combinations

Combination no.	Combination dosage (μM)		% viability ± SD
	Bromelain dosage (IC value)	Cisplatin dosage (IC value)	
Combination 1	2.0 μM (IC40)	1.5 μM (IC10)	50.24% ± 1.67
Combination 2	0.9 μM (IC30)	4.0 μM (IC20)	70.26% ± 2.66
Combination 3	0.5 μM (IC20)	5.9 μM (IC30)	61.30% ± 2.43
Combination 4	0.24 μM (IC10)	9.5 μM (IC40)	56.95% ± 3.61

Cytotoxicity was determined using the MTT cell viability assay. The results for MTT assay are expressed as mean ± SD of three separate experiments

Table 2 Combination index (CI) and dose reduction index (DRI) values at 48 h for bromelain and cisplatin combinations. CI < 1 indicates synergistic effect, CI = 1 indicates additive effects and CI > 1 indicates antagonistic effect

Combination no.	Combination dosage (μM)		CI value	DRI (bromelain)	DRI (cisplatin)
	Bromelain dosage (IC value)	Cisplatin dosage (IC value)			
Combination 1	2.0 μM (IC40)	1.5 μM (IC10)	0.65	1.74	12.71
Combination 2	0.9 μM (IC30)	4.0 μM (IC20)	1.36	1.27	1.73
Combination 3	0.5 μM (IC20)	5.9 μM (IC30)	0.78	3.87	1.89
Combination 4	0.24 μM (IC10)	9.5 μM (IC40)	0.75	10.59	1.50

0.65). The results of the isobolograms were consistent with those of the CI values and revealed the presence of synergistic effects for combinations 1, 3 and 4 at 48 h (Fig. 2). The DRI values also supported the presence of synergistic effects, especially for combination 1, which had the highest DRI value for cisplatin. The DRI values showed that the IC50 dose of cisplatin could be reduced 13-fold when it was used in combination with bromelain in combination 1. These results indicated that combination 1 showed the best synergistic effects of all of the combinations tested in this study at 48 h. This combination was therefore selected for the subsequent experiments.

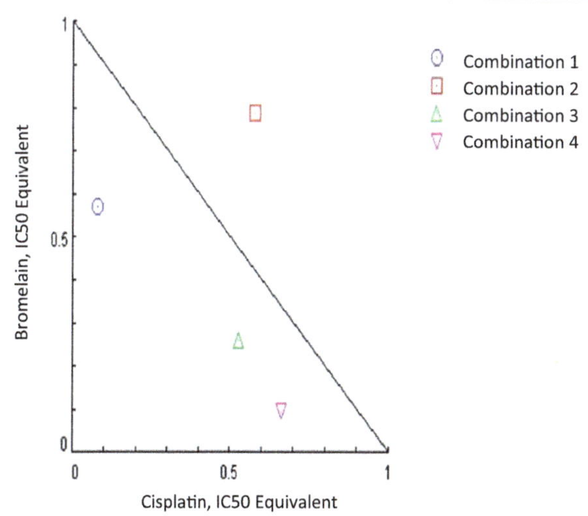

Fig. 2 Normalized isobologram plot of bromelain/cisplatin combinations treatment on MDA-MB-231 cells at 48 h

Regulation of apoptosis and cell cycle progression in MDA-MB-231 cells by bromelain, cisplatin and their combined treatment

Annexin-V/PI and cell cycle analyses were performed on the MDA-MB-231 cells treated with combination 1 to determine whether the growth inhibitory effects of this treatment could be attributed to apoptosis or cell cycle arrest. The result of the Annexin-V/PI assay showed that the single-agent treatment of the MDA-MB-231 cells with bromelain (4.1 μM) or cisplatin (23 μM) caused 31.68 and 31.07% of the cells to enter apoptosis at 48 h, respectively (Fig. 3). However, the treatment of MDA-MB-231 cells with combination 1 led to a marked increase in the population of apoptotic cells observed at 48 h to 40.69%. These results correlated well with the fraction of cells observed in sub-G0/G1 phase by cell cycle analysis (Fig. 4). The treatment of the MDA-MB-231 cells with combination 1 led to a higher level of sub-G0/G1 arrest, with 15.94% of the cells being detected in the sub-G0/G1 phase, compared with values of 13.38 and 13.83% for single-agent treatment with bromelain ($P = 0.000$) and cisplatin ($P = 0.000$), respectively. Single-agent treatment with bromelain and cisplatin, as well as combination treatment with combination 1, induced apoptosis in MDA-MB-231 cells, with the former inducing higher levels of apoptosis than either of the single-agent treatments.

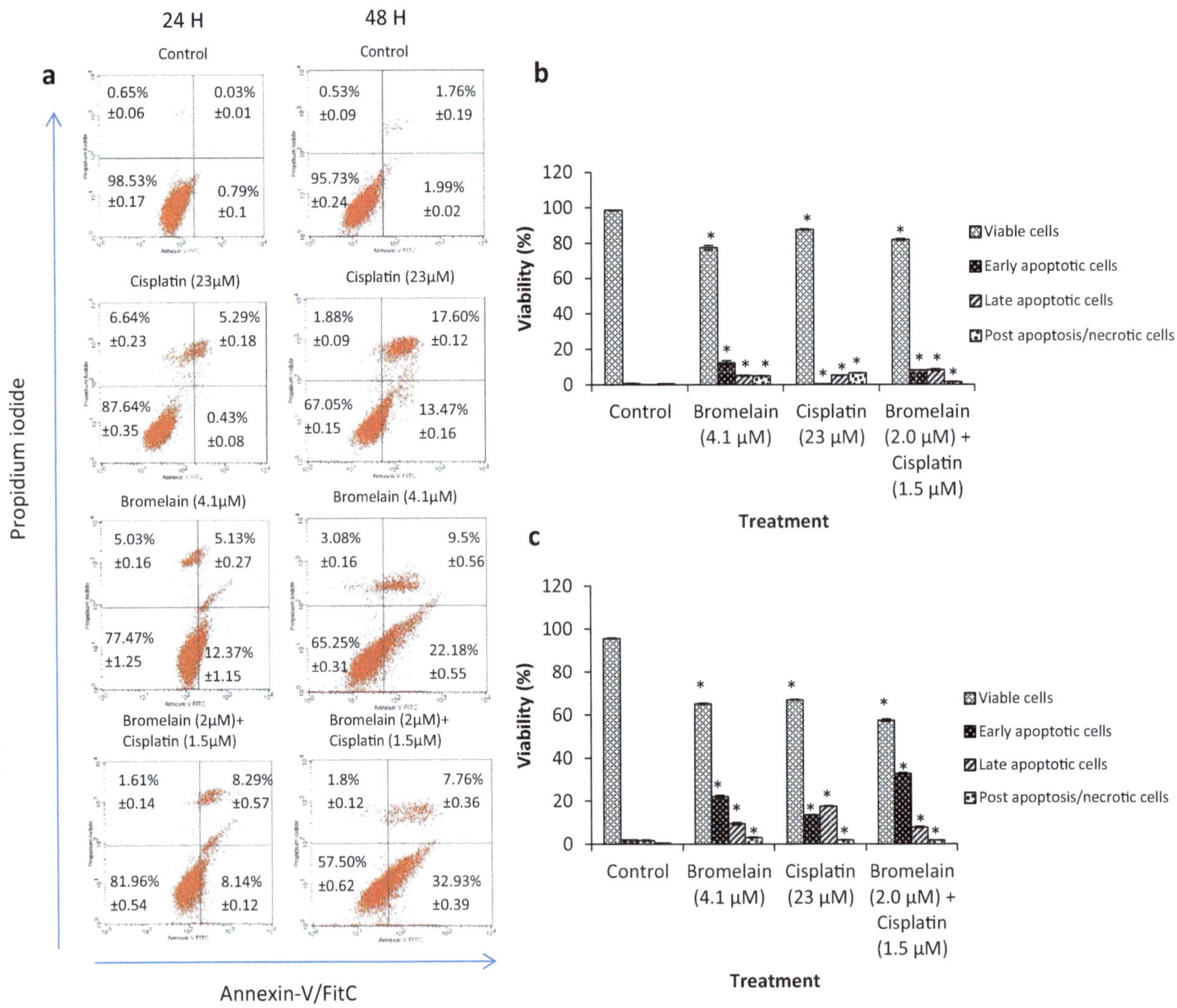

Fig. 3 FITC-Annexin V/PI and propidium iodide staining of MDA-MB-231 cells treated with bromelain, cisplatin and bromelain/cisplatin combination for 24 and 48 h. The results are expressed as mean ± SD of three separate experiments. The figures shown in **a** are results from one of the three experiments conducted. The *x-axis* (Annexin-V/FITC) and *y-axis* (propidiumiodide) represent the intensity of Annexin-V/FITC and propidium iodide staining in cells, respectively. Shown in **b** and **c** are the analyzed results for 24 and 48 h, respectively. The numerical data are presented as mean ± SD (n = 3). *$P < 0.05$ vs. Control

Activation of apoptosis via an intrinsic (mitochondrial) pathway in MDA-MB-231 cells treated with a combination of bromelain and cisplatin

A JC-1 staining assay was used to measure changes in the mitochondrial membrane potentials of the MDA-MB-231 cells subjected to the single-agent and combination treatments. As shown in Fig. 5, the percentages of cells determined to be positive for JC-1 monomers following their single-agent treatment with bromelain (4.1 μM) and cisplatin (23 μM) for 48 h were 41.82% and 51.40%, respectively. For combination 1, the percentage of cells found to be positive for JC-1 monomers was 40.58%. These values were significantly higher than that found in the untreated control, where only 9.33% of the cells tested positive for JC-1 monomers ($P = 0.000$). The mitochondrial membrane potentials of the treated cells decreased, suggesting that the treatment of the cells with either of the single agents or combination 1 triggered apoptosis via the induction of the intrinsic (mitochondrial) pathway.

Modulatory effects of bromelain and cisplatin alone, as well as a combination of these two agents on the expression levels of apoptosis-related proteins

A number of apoptotic proteins, including Bcl-2, catalase, clusterin, HO-1, livin, XIAP, HSP70, Bcl-x, Bax and HSP60 were differentially expressed in the treated and untreated MDA-MB-231 cells (Fig. 6).

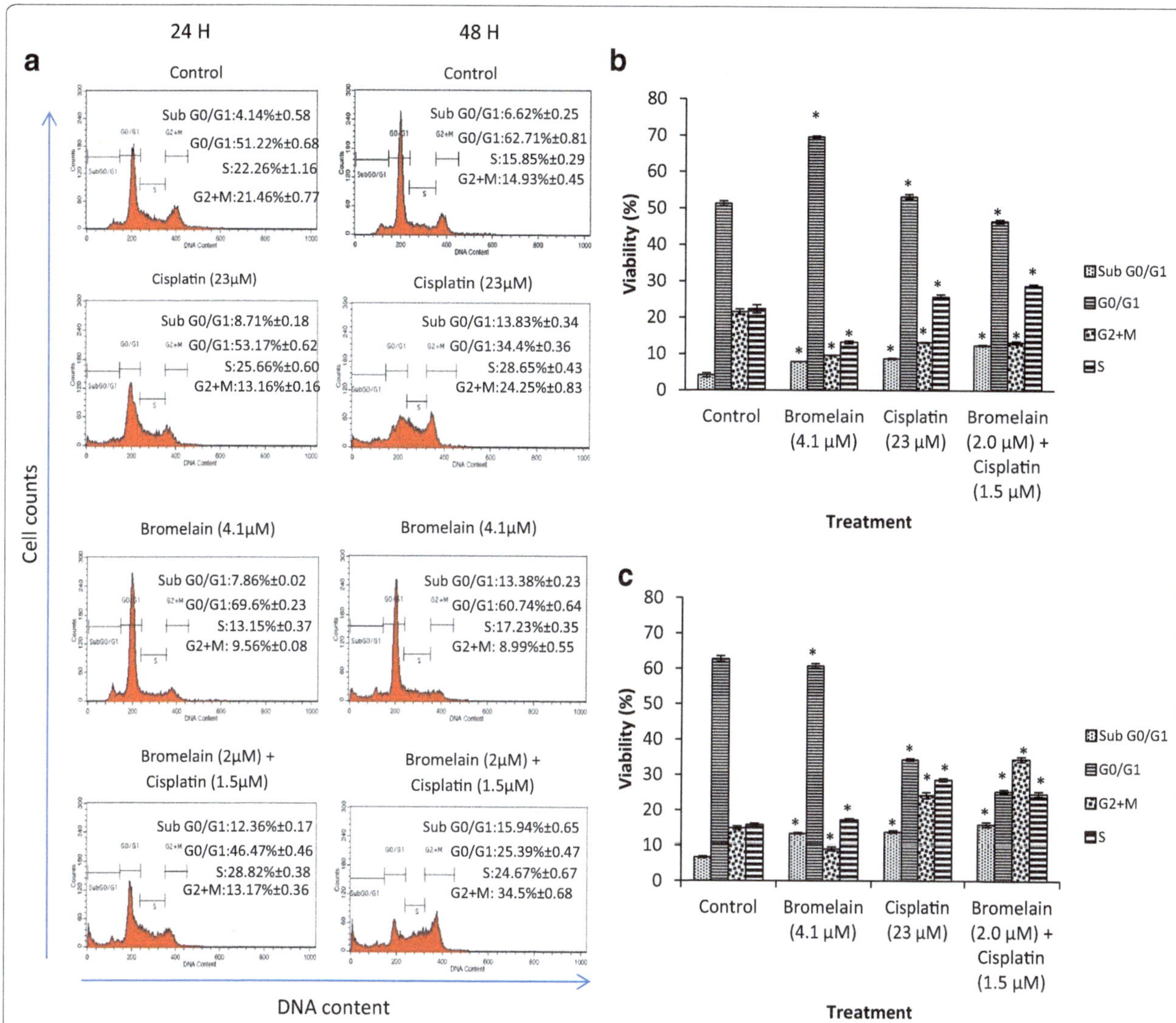

Fig. 4 Effect of bromelain, cisplatin and bromelain/cisplatin combination treatment on MDA-MB-231 cell cycle after 24 and 48 h. The figures shown in **a** are the results from one of the three experiments conducted. Data shown represent relative numbers of cells (*Y-axis*) vs. DNA content (*X-axis*). Shown in **b** and **c** are the analyzed cell cycle results for 24 and 48 h respectively. The numerical data are presented as mean ± SD (n = 3). *$P < 0.05$ vs. Control

The expression levels of Bcl-2 protein were found to be significantly reduced in the combination 1-treated cells compared with the bromelain- ($P = 0.002$) and untreated cells ($P = 0.001$). The expression level of Livin, Bax, Catalase, HO-1 and XIAP were also found to be significantly reduced in the combination 1-treated cells compared with the bromelain- ($P = 0.000$) and untreated cells ($P = 0.000$). However, the expression levels of several anti-apoptotic proteins, including HSP70 increased significantly in the MDA-MB-231 cells treated with combination 1 compared with the bromelain- ($P = 0.016$) and cisplatin-treated cells ($P = 0.001$). Moreover, the expression level of Bcl-x were also found to significantly higher in the combination 1-treated cells compared with the bromelain- ($P = 0.002$) and cisplatin-treated cells ($P = 0.000$).The expression levels of pro-apoptotic proteins HSP60 were found to be significantly reduced in the cells treated with combination 1 compared with the bromelain- ($P = 0.041$) and untreated cells ($P = 0.014$).

These results indicated that combination 1 affected the expression levels of most of the apoptotic proteins in MDA-MB-231 to a much greater extent than single-agent treatment with bromelain (4.1 μM) or cisplatin (23 μM). These results were therefore consistent with those of the JC-1 staining assay, with the fold-change values for Bax to Bcl-x and Bax to Bcl-2 suggesting the involvement of the mitochondrial pathway in the apoptosis induced by bromelain (4.1 μM), cisplatin (23 μM) and combination

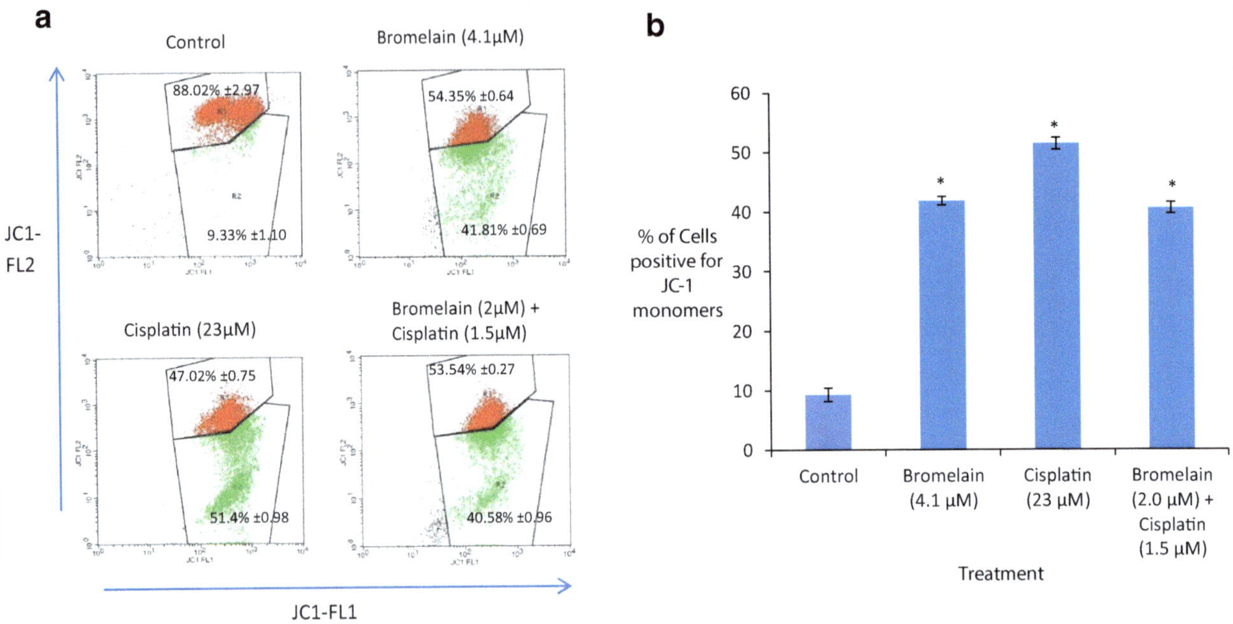

Fig. 5 Effect of bromelain, cisplatin and bromelain/cisplatin combination after 48 h treatment duration on mitochondrial membrane potential in MDA-MB-231 cells as measured by JC-1 staining. The figures shown in **a** are the results from one of the three experiments conducted. Locations of R1 region (cells population with normal mitochondrial potential) and R2 region (cells population with reduced mitochondrial potential) are marked for *each plot*. Shown in **b** are the percentages of cells positive for JC-1 monomers for the treated and untreated MDA-MB-231 cells. The numerical data are presented as mean ± SD (n = 3). **P* < 0.05 vs. Control

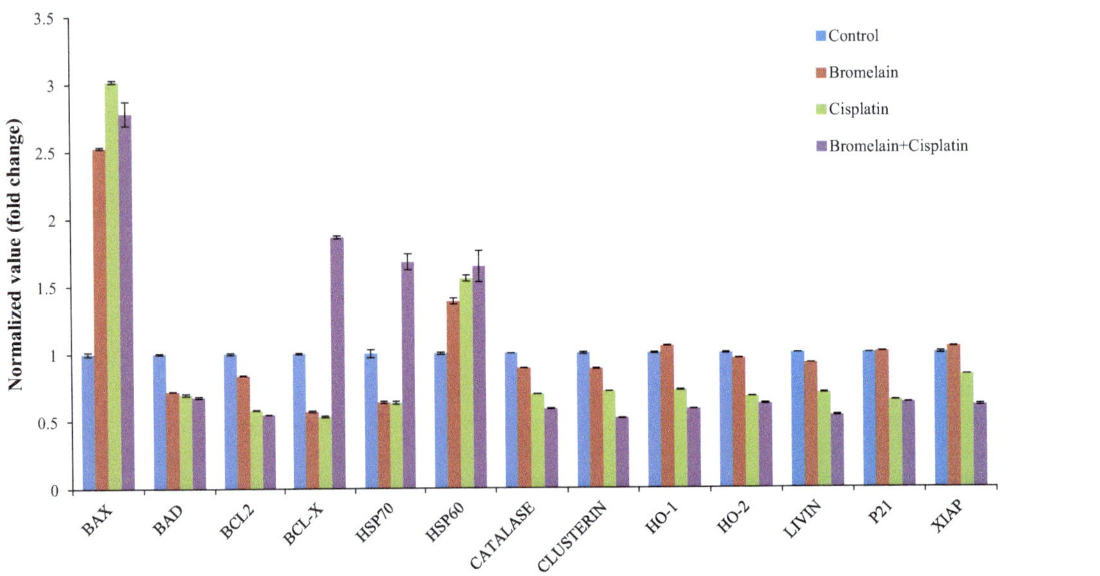

Fig. 6 Alterations of apoptosis-related proteins by bromelain, cisplatin and bromelain/cisplatin combination treatment at 48 h. Shown here are the fold-change values for the pixel density of selected apoptotic proteins of treated cells to untreated cells (control) at 48 h, obtained using Proteome Profiler: human apoptosis array (R&D System). The numerical data are presented as means of duplicate experiments (n = 3)

1. The ratios of Bax to Bcl-2 and Bax to Bcl-x were calculated and the results are shown in Fig. 7. These results revealed that was an increase in the Bax/Bcl-2 ratio following the treatment of the cells with combination 1, which was accompanied by a decrease in the Bax/Bcl-x ratio.

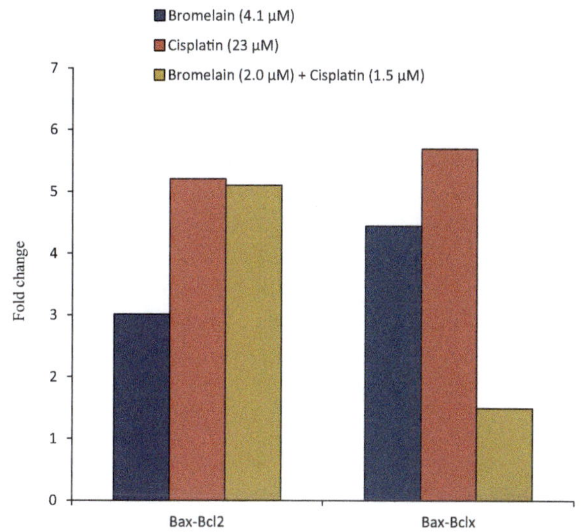

Fig. 7 Fold-change values for Bax to Bcl-x and Bax to Bcl-2 in treated cells at 48 h. The numerical data are presented as mean ± SD (n = 3)

To validate the results obtained using the Proteome Profiler Human Apoptosis Array kit, we also examined the protein extracts obtained from the MDA-MB231 cells at 48 h by western blot analysis using anti-Beta-actin, anti-Bcl-2 and anti-Bax (Fig. 8). The results of this analysis showed that the MDA-MB-231 cells treated with combination 1 contained much lower levels of the anti-apoptotic protein Bcl-2 compared with the untreated cells ($P = 0.000$), as well as the bromelain-treated ($P = 0.000$) and cisplatin-treated cells ($P = 0.000$). By contrast, we observed a higher level of the pro-apoptotic protein Bax after 48 h following the treatment of the cells with combination 1 compared with the control cells ($P = 0.009$), bromelain-treated cells ($P = 0.002$) and cisplatin-treated cells ($P = 0.043$). The results of this western blot analysis therefore suggested that the treatment of the cells with combination 1 led to a much greater decrease in the expression of Bcl-2 compared with single-agent treatment with bromelain or cisplatin. Furthermore, the observed increase in the expression of Bax highlights the importance of the role played by the mitochondrial pathway in the apoptosis of the MDA-MB-231 cells triggered by combination 1.

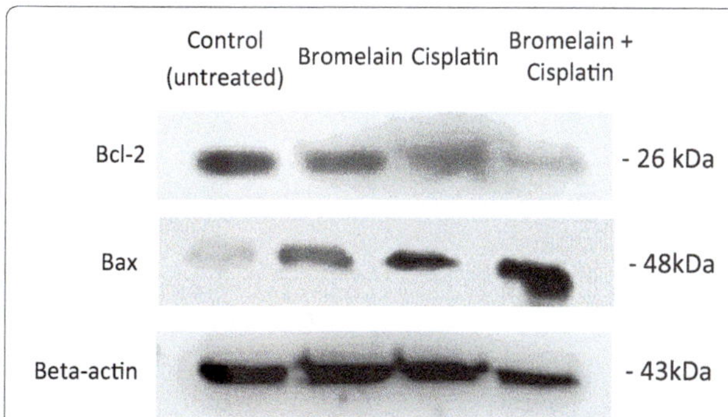

Fig. 8 Combination 1 (bromelain (2.0 μM) + cisplatin (1.5 μM)) decreased Bcl-2 protein expression and upregulated Bax protein expression. Shown here are the western blot gel images for Bcl-2, Bax and Beta-actin 35 at 48 h

Discussion

It was envisaged that the combination of bromelain and cisplatin would lead to synergistic effects, which would enhance their anti-cancer effects towards MDA-MB-231 human breast cancer cells. The CI values and isobolograms obtained using the MTT data clearly showed that the treatment of the MDA-MB-231 cells with a combination of bromelain and cisplatin resulted in a synergistic and dose-dependent increase in the inhibitory activity for combination 1 (bromelain 2 μM + cisplatin 1.5 μM) towards the growth of these cells. We also demonstrated that the IC50 dose of cisplatin was reduced almost 13-fold in combination 1. Cisplatin is a well-known anti-cancer agent, which is used in clinical practice to treat a variety of different cancers. However, despite its effectiveness and broad range of activity, the use of cisplatin is associated with several adverse side effects [3, 4, 7–9]. In contrast, the cysteine endopeptidase bromelain is a non-toxic agent with proven anti-cancer activity against various cancers [17, 24]. The concentration ratio of bromelain to cisplatin played an important role in determining the extent of the synergistic effects, as exemplified by the differences observed for different concentrations of cisplatin and bromelain in the different combinations evaluated in this study.

Annexin V-FITC and cell cycle analyses were performed on the treated and untreated MDA-MB-231 cells to determine whether the growth inhibitory effects of combination 1 could be attributed to apoptosis. The results of these assays showed that the synergistic effects of combination 1 were caused by an augmented apoptotic response. This effect could also be attributed to a different mode of action to those employed by cisplatin and bromelain. Cisplatin exerts its activity through the formation of intra- and inter-strand DNA adducts that damage the DNA and interferes with its normal functions [6, 26]. In contrast, the inhibitory effects of bromelain are dependent on its proteolytic activity, which allow it to remove certain cell surface molecules associated with cellular migration and adherence [27]. The proteolytic activity of bromelain has also been reported to promote apoptosis in a number of human cancer cells, particularly in breast cancer cells [18, 28].

Consistent with our results, previous studies have demonstrated the involvement of the mitochondrial pathway in the apoptosis induced by single-agent treatment with cisplatin or bromelain in cancer cells [28–31]. The treatment of the MDA-MB-231 cells with combination 1 resulted in a loss of mitochondrial membrane potential, which suggested that the mitochondrial pathway was involved in the apoptosis induced by combination 1.

The results obtained using the Proteome Profiler Human Apoptosis Array kit showed that combination 1 led to decreases in the expression levels of several anti-apoptotic proteins, including cIAP 1, Bcl-2, catalase, clusterin, HO-1, livin, XIAP, HSP27 and claspin. Notably, combination 1 led to considerable decreases in the expression levels of cIAP1, catalase, clusterin, HO-1, livin and XIAP compared with the cells treated with bromelain or cisplatin. Interestingly, we also observed pronounced increases in the expression levels of several anti-apoptotic proteins, including HSP70 and Bcl-x in the cells treated with combination 1 compared with the untreated cells. In contrast, we did not observe any increases in the regulation of any pro-apoptotic proteins (*e.g.*, Bax). We also observed an increase in the expression of the apoptotic protein HSP60.

Taken together with the observed decreases in the anti-apoptotic proteins Bcl-2 and HSP27, the increase observed in the pro-apoptotic protein Bax provided clear evidence that combination 1 induced mitochondria-mediated apoptosis. This result was consistent with previous studies, which established the important roles played by Bcl-2, HSP27 and Bax in the regulation of apoptosis activated through the mitochondrial pathway [32–38]. We also observed significant increases in the levels of the anti-apoptotic proteins HSP70 and Bcl-x in the cells treated with combination 1. Bcl-x and HSP70 play essential roles as anti-apoptotic proteins by preventing the release of mitochondrial apoptogenic factors such as cytochrome C and apoptosis inducing factor (AIF), and consequently inhibit apoptosis [36, 39]. The elevated levels of Bcl-x and HSP70 observed in this study would be insufficient to shut down the apoptotic process induced by combination 1 in MDA-MB-231 cells. The fold-change values shown in Fig. 6 for the pro-apoptotic protein Bax to the anti-apoptotic protein Bcl-x indicated that the increase in Bax was much greater than that of Bcl-x, suggesting that the pro-apoptotic effects of upregulated Bax would overwhelm the anti-apoptotic effects of Bcl-x. It is therefore possible that some other pathway or mechanism was being activated or inhibited by combination 1 and that this process was compensating for the interference in mitochondrial mediated-apoptosis and contributing to the synergistic effect of combination 1.

We also observed pronounced decreases in the levels of the anti-apoptotic proteins cIAP 1 and XIAP in the combination 1-treated cells. This change was attributed to an increase in the expression of HSP70. Although HSP70 is well known for its cytoprotective effects, previous studies [40, 41] have also shown that elevated levels of HSP70 may have led to an increased susceptibility to apoptosis. Elevated HSP70 levels would result in an increase in the inhibition of IkB kinase activity, which would inhibit the activity of the NF-kB pathway, leading to the inhibition of NF-kB-dependent anti-apoptotic gene induction [40–42]. Given that the expression levels of cIAP and XIAP are highly dependent on the NF-kB pathway, the inhibition of the IkB kinase by elevated levels of HSP70 would lead to a reduction in the expression levels of cIAP and XIAP. This change could therefore explain the considerable decrease observed in the levels of cIAP and XIAP in this study.

Conclusion

Bromelain in combination with cisplatin synergistically enhanced the induction of apoptosis in MDA-MB-231 cells.

Authors' contributions

SKY, NBA, TS, NA, ARO, SAA and ALTC conceived and designed the study. AZMP, SKY and KLL performed the assays. AZMP, NA and SGT wrote the manuscript. All authors read and approved to the final manuscript.

Author details

[1] Department of Cell and Molecular Biology, Faculty of Biotechnology and Biomolecular Sciences, Universiti Putra Malaysia, 43400 Serdang, Selangor, Malaysia. [2] Institute of Bioscience, Universiti Putra Malaysia, Serdang, Malaysia. [3] Faculty of Medicine and Health Sciences, Universiti Tunku Abdul Rahman, Sungai Long Campus, Jalan Sungai Long, Bandar Sungai Long, Cheras, 43000 Kajang, Selangor, Malaysia. [4] Department of Bioprocess Technology, Faculty of Biotechnology and Biomolecular Sciences, Universiti Putra Malaysia, Serdang, Selangor, Malaysia.

Acknowledgements

This research was supported by Research University Grant Scheme (Project No: 05-02-12-1718RU) provided by Universiti Putra Malaysia, Malaysia.

Competing interests

The authors declare that they have no competing interests.

References

1. Ferlay J, Shin HR, Bray F, Forman D, Mathers C, Parkin DM. Estimates of worldwide burden of cancer in 2008: GLOBOCAN 2008. Int J Cancer. 2010;127:2893–917.
2. Jemal A, Center MM, DeSantis C, Ward EM. Global patterns of cancer incidence and mortality rates and trends. Cancer Epidemiol Biomark Prev. 2010;19:1893–907.
3. Fuertes MA, Castilla J, Alonso C, Prez JM. Cisplatin biochemical mechanism of action: from cytotoxicity to induction of cell death through interconnections between apoptotic and necrotic pathways. Curr Med Chem. 2003;10:257–66.
4. Sledge GW, Loehrer PJ, Roth BJ, Einhorn LH. Cisplatin as first-line therapy for metastatic breast cancer. J Clin Oncol. 1988;6:1811–4.
5. Marchán V, Moreno V, Pedroso E, Grandas A. Towards a better understanding of the cisplatin mode of action. Chem Eur J. 2001;7:808–15.

6. Siddik ZH. Cisplatin: mode of cytotoxic action and molecular basis of resistance. Oncogene. 2003;22:7265–79.
7. Von Hoff DD, Schilsky R, Reichert CM, Reddick RL, Rozencweig M, Young RC, Muggia FM. Toxic effects of cis-dichlorodiammineplatinum (II) in man. Cancer Treat Rep. 1979;63:1527–31.
8. Laurell G, Jungnelius U. High-Dose cisplatin treatment: hearing loss and plasma concentrations. The Laryngoscope. 1990;100:724–34.
9. Gregg RW, Molepo JM, Monpetit VJ, Mikael NZ, Redmond D, Gadia M, Stewart DJ. Cisplatin neurotoxicity: the relationship between dosage, time, and platinum concentration in neurologic tissues, and morphologic evidence of toxicity. J Clin Oncol. 1992;10:795–803.
10. Galluzzi L, Senovilla L, Vitale I, Michels J, Martins I, Kepp O, Castedo M, Kroemer G. Molecular mechanisms of cisplatin resistance. Oncogene. 2012;31:1869–83.
11. Eckstein N, Servan K, Girard L, Cai D, von Jonquieres G, Jaehde U, Kassack MU, Gazdar AF, Minna JD, Royer HD. Epidermal growth factor receptor pathway analysis identifies amphiregulin as a key factor for cisplatin resistance of human breast cancer cells. J Bio Chem. 2008;283:739–50.
12. Pogribny IP, Filkowski JN, Tryndyak VP, Golubov A, Shpyleva SI, Kovalchuk O. Alterations of microRNAs and their targets are associated with acquired resistance of MCF-7 breast cancer cells to cisplatin. Int J Cancer. 2010;127:1785–94.
13. Xie W, Xing D, Sun H, Wang W, Ding Y, Du L. The effects of *Ananascomosus* L. Leaves on diabetic-dyslipidemic rats induced by alloxan and a high-fat/high-cholesterol diet. Am J Chin Med. 2005;33:95–105.
14. Dutta S, Bhattacharyya D. Enzymatic, antimicrobial and toxicity studies of the aqueous extract of *Ananascomosus* (pineapple) crown leaf. J Ethnopharmacol. 2013;150:451–7.
15. Heinecke RM, Gortner WA. Stem bromelain, a new protease preparation from pineapple plants. Econ Bot. 1957;11:225–34.
16. Taussig SJ, Batkin S. Bromelain, the enzyme complex of pineapple (*Ananascomosus*) and its clinical application. An update. J Ethnopharmacol. 1988;22:191–203.
17. Batkin S, Taussig SJ, Szekerczes J. Inhibition of tumour growth in vitro by bromelain, an extract of the pineapple (*Ananascomosus*). Plantamedica. 1985;6:538–9.
18. Dhandayuthapani S, Perez HD, Paroulek A, Chinnakkannu P, Kandalam U, Jaffe M, Rathinavelu A. Bromelain-induced apoptosis in GI-101A breast cancer cells. J Med Food. 2012;15:344–9.
19. Batkin S, Taussig S, Szekerczes J. Modulation of pulmonary metastasis (Lewis lung carcinoma) by bromelain, an extract of the pineapple stem (Ananascomosus). Cancer Invest. 1988;6:241–2.
20. Eckert K, Grabowska E, Stange R, Schneider U, Eschmann K, Maurer HR. Effects of oral bromelain administration on the impaired immunocytotoxicity of mononuclear cells from mammary tumor patients. Oncol Rep. 1999;6:1191–200.
21. Beuth J, Braun JM. Modulation of murine tumor growth and colonization by bromelaine, an extract of the pineapple plant (*Ananascomosum* L.). In Vivo. 2005;19:483–5.
22. Maurer HR. Bromelain: biochemistry, pharmacology and medical use. Cell Mol Life Sci. 2001;58:1231–45.
23. Hale LP, Greer PK, Trinh CT, James CL. Proteinase activity and stability of natural bromelain preparations. Intern Immunopharmacol. 2005;5:783–93.
24. Castell JV, Friedrich G, Kuhn CS, Poppe GE. Intestinal absorption of undegraded proteins in men: presence of bromelain in plasma after oral intake. Am J Physiol. 1997;273:139–46.
25. Seifert J, Ganser R, Brendel W. Absorption of a proteolytic enzyme originating from plants out of the gastrointestinal tract into blood and lymph of rats. Z Gastroenterol. 1979;17:1–8.
26. Jordan P, Carmo-Fonseca M. Molecular mechanisms involved in cisplatin-cytotoxicity. Cell Mol Life Sci. 2000;57:1229–35.
27. Hale LP, Greer PK, Sempowski GD. Bromelain treatment alters leukocyte expression of cell surface molecules involved in cellular adhesion and activation. Clin Immunol. 2002;104:183–90.
28. Bhui K, Tyagi S, Srivastava AK, Singh M, Roy P, Singh R, Shukla Y. Bromelain inhibits nuclear factor kappa-B translocation, driving human epidermoid carcinoma A431 and melanoma A375 cells through G2/M arrest to apoptosis. Mol Carcinog. 2012;51:231–43.
29. Park MS, De Leon M, Devarajan P. Cisplatin induces apoptosis in LLC-PK1 cells via activation of mitochondrial pathways. J Am Soc Nephrol. 2002;13:858–65.
30. Melendez-Zajgla J, Cruz E, Maldonado V, Espinoza AM. Mitochondrial changes during the apoptotic process of HeLa cells exposed to cisplatin. Biochem Mol Biol Int. 1999;47:765–71.
31. Bhui K, Prasad S, George J, Shukla Y. Bromelain inhibits COX-2 expression by blocking the activation of MAPK regulated NF-kappa B against skin tumor-initiation triggering mitochondrial death pathway. Cancer Lett. 2009;282:167–76.
32. Bruey JM, Ducasse C, Bonniaud P, Ravagnan L, Susin SA, Diaz-Latoud C, Gurbuxani S, Arrigo AP, Kroemer G, Solary E, Garrido C. Hsp27 negatively regulates cell death by interacting with cytochrome c. Nat Cell Biol. 2000;2:645–52.
33. Paul C, Manero F, Gonin S, Kretz-Remy C, Virot S, Arrigo AP. Hsp27 as a negative regulator of cytochrome C release. Mol Cell Biol. 2002;22:816–34.
34. Wei MC, Zong WX, Cheng EHY, Lindsten T, Panoutsakopoulou V, Ross AJ, Roth KA, MacGregor GR, Thompson CB, Korsmeyer SJ. Proapoptotic BAX and BAK: a requisite gateway to mitochondrial dysfunction and death. Science. 2001;292:727–30.
35. Marzo I, Brenner C, Zamzami N, Jürgensmeier JM, Susin SA, Vieira HL, Prevost MC, Xie Z, Matsuyama S, Reed JC, Kroemer G. Bax and adenine nucleotide translocator cooperate in the mitochondrial control of apoptosis. Science. 1998;281:2027–31.
36. Yang J, Liu X, Bhalla K, Kim CN, Ibrado AM, Cai J, Peng TI, Jones DP, Wang X. Prevention of apoptosis by Bcl-2: release of cytochrome c from mitochondria blocked. Science. 1997;275:1129–32.
37. Kluck RM, Bossy-Wetzel E, Green DR, Newmeyer DD. The release of cytochrome c from mitochondria: a primary site for Bcl-2 regulation of apoptosis. Science. 1997;275:1132–6.
38. Susin SA, Zamzami N, Castedo M, Hirsch T, Marchetti P, Macho A, Daugas E, Geuskens M, Kroemer G. Bcl-2 inhibits the mitochondrial release of an apoptogenic protease. J Exp Med. 1996;184:1331–41.
39. Gurbuxani S, Schmitt E, Cande C, Parcellier A, Hammann A, Daugas E, Kouranti I, Spahr C, Pance A, Kroemer G, Garrido C. Heat shock protein 70 binding inhibits the nuclear import of apoptosis-inducing factor. Oncogene. 2003;22:6669–78.
40. Ran R, Lu A, Zhang L, Tang Y, Zhu H, Xu H, Feng Y, Han C, Zhou G. Rigby Ac, Sharp FR: Hsp70 promotes TNF-mediated apoptosis by binding IKKγ and impairing NF-κB survival signaling. Genes Dev. 2004;18:1466–81.
41. Feng X, Bonni S, Riabowol K. HSP70 induction by ING proteins sensitizes cells to tumor necrosis factor alpha receptor-mediated apoptosis. Mol Cell Biol. 2006;26:9244–55.
42. Guzhova IV, Darieva ZA, Melo AR, Margulis BA. Major stress protein Hsp70 interacts with NF-kB regulatory complex in human T-lymphoma cells. Cell Stress Chaperones. 1997;2:132–9.

10

Gastrodia and Uncaria (tianma gouteng) water extract exerts antioxidative and antiapoptotic effects against cerebral ischemia in vitro and in vivo

Jia Wen Xian[1], Angus Yiu-Ting Choi[1], Clara Bik-San Lau[2,3], Wing Nang Leung[1], Chun Fai Ng[2] and Chun Wai Chan[1*]

Abstract

Background: *Gastrodia and Uncaria* decoction (tianma gouteng yin) is commonly used in Chinese medicine to treat cerebral ischemia. The aim of this study was to investigate the neuroprotective effects of a water extract (GUW) of *Gastrodia elata* (tianma; GE) and *Uncaria rhynchophylla* (gouteng; UR) against ischemic insult using oxygen-glucose-deprived neuronal differentiated PC12 cells and rats subjected to middle cerebral artery occlusion (MCAO).

Methods: GUW was prepared by boiling raw GE and UR in water, followed by the lyophilization of the resulting extract. Neuronal differentiated PC12 cells were subjected to oxygen-glucose deprivation with or without GUW. The neuroprotective effects of GUW were compared with those of the corresponding GE and UR extracts to tease apart the effects of the different herbs. The synergistic effect of GE and UR in GUW was measured using a modified version of Burgi's formulae. The neuroprotective mechanisms via *Nrf2* and anti-apoptotic pathways were investigated using real time PCR and enzyme activity assays. The neuroprotective effects of GUW were studied in vivo using a rat MCAO model. Neurofunctional outcome and brain infarct volume we assessed. H&E staining, cresyl violet staining and immunohistochemistry were performed to assess the histological outcome.

Results: The results of lactate dehydrogenase assay showed that GUW protected cells in a concentration-dependent manner ($P < 0.001$). Moreover, the neuroprotective effects of GUW were greater than those of GE + UR ($P = 0.018$). Burgi's formula showed that the herbs in GUW acted synergistically to protect cells from ischemic injury. GUW significantly upregulated *Bcl-2* expression ($P = 0.0130$) and reduced caspase-3 activity by 60 % ($P < 0.001$). GUW upregulated *Nrf-2* expression ($P = 0.0066$) and the antioxidant response element pathway genes. The infarct volume was reduced by 55 % at day 7 of reperfusion ($P < 0.001$), and significant improvements were observed in the neurological deficit score and beam-walking test at 7 days ($P < 0.001$). H&E and cresyl violet staining revealed higher tissue integrity in the GUW treatment group compared with MCAO rats.

Conclusion: GUW modulated the antioxidant system and antiapoptotic genes in oxygen-glucose deprived neuronal differentiated PC12 cells and MCAO sprague–dawley rats.

*Correspondence: fcwchan@cuhk.edu.hk
[1] School of Chinese Medicine, The Chinese University of Hong Kong, Shatin, New Territories, Hong Kong, People's Republic of China
Full list of author information is available at the end of the article

Background

Stroke is the third major cause of death in the world, with more than 80 % of strokes being caused by cerebral ischemia [1]. Recombinant plasminogen activator is currently the only FDA-approved drug for the treatment of acute stroke, but its effectiveness has been limited by its small therapeutic window and severe complications [2–4]. Moreover, the therapeutic dose of this drug is too low to affect the cellular mechanisms responsible for neuroprotection.

The reactive oxygen species (ROS) generated during ischemia are one of the major contributing factors to neuronal cell death [5]. Oxidative stress occurs when the rate at which ROS are cleared by the intracellular anti-oxidant system is slower than the rate at which they are produced. ROS can oxidize a variety of intracellular molecules such as DNA and lipids, eventually leading to apoptotic cell death [5]. Neurons are more susceptible to oxidative damage than most other cells because of their high metabolic rate and low expression levels of antioxidant enzymes [6].

The increase of antioxidant enzymes expression and activity might attenuate cellular ischemic injury. Nuclear factor erythroid 2-related factor 2 (*Nrf-2*) is a transcription factor that acts on the cis-acting antioxidant regulating element (ARE) to regulate the expression of antioxidant enzymes, including superoxide dismutase (SOD) and glutathione peroxidase (GPx) [7, 8]. The upregulation of *Nrf-2* and antioxidant enzymes effectively protected neurons from ischemic injury, improving histological outcomes and sensorimotor functioning of ischemic rats [9, 10]. Conversely, protein disulfide isomerase (PDI) activity prevents DNA fragmentation and cell death in hippocampal neurons from ischemic rats [11].

Chinese medicine has been used extensively to treat a variety of different brain diseases, and *Gastrodia Uncaria* decoction (tianma gouteng yin), in particular, is commonly used for treating cerebral ischemia and brain-related disease [12–16]. The main herbal components of *Gastrodia Uncaria* decoction include *Gastrodia elata* (*Tianma*; GE) and *Uncaria rhynchophylla* (*Gouteng*; UR). Several studies have demonstrated the prevention of ischemia-induced apoptosis by GE extracts and its active components [17–19]. Furthermore, the methanolic extracts of UR have been reported to exhibit neuroprotective effects against global cerebral ischemia in rats [20–22].

The aim of this study was to investigate the effects of the water extract of *Gastrodia elata* and *Uncaria rhynchophylla* (GUW) and its antioxidative mechanisms on oxygen-glucose deprived (OGD) neuronal differentiated PC12 cells and a rat middle cerebral artery occlusion (MCAO) model.

Methods

Materials

All the chemicals used in this study were purchased from Sigma-Aldrich (St. Louis, MO, USA) unless specified otherwise. Cell culture media and supplements were obtained from Life Technologies (Grand Island, NY, USA).

Extraction methods

Crude GE and UR were purchased from Zhixin Medicine Health Co. (Guangdong, China). The herbal extracts were authenticated by Dr. Zheng Ling at the Institute of Chinese Medicine, The Chinese University of Hong Kong, based on the methods described in the 2010 edition of the Chinese Pharmacopoeia (Additional file 1) [23]. Voucher specimens of GE (Specimen No: 2010–3294) and UR (Specimen No: 2010–3295) were kept at the Institute of Chinese Medicine Museum, The Chinese University of Hong Kong. The GUW extract was prepared based on the boiling procedure used for preparing GE and UR in *Gastrodia and Uncaria* decoction [24]. Briefly, GE (107.1 g) was immersed in distilled water (2.5 L) for 1 h and boiled for 45 min. UR (142.9 g) was then added, and the resulting mixture was heated at reflux for 15 min. The mixture was then cooled to room temperature and filtered, and the resulting filtrate was rotary evaporated and lyophilized using a BÜCHI Rotavapor R-220 (Flawil, Switzerland) to give a powder (Fig. 1a).

Individual extracts GE and UR were prepared separately by immersing the individual herbs in water in a 1:10 (w/v) ratio for 1 h, and then heating the resulting mixtures at reflux for 1 h. The mixtures were then filtered to give the water-soluble fractions, and stored at room temperature for later use. This process was repeated for the herbal residues of GE and UR. Both fractions were pooled together to make the individual GE (Fig. 1b) and UR (Fig. 1c) water-soluble fractions. These water-soluble fractions were subsequently converted into powders using the methods described above.

Cell line

PC12 cells (ATCC, Manassas, VA, USA) were grown in RPMI 1640 culture medium supplemented with 10 % horse serum, 5 % FBS and 100 U/mL penicillin G sodium. The cultures were maintained at 37 °C under 5 % CO_2. The PC12 cells were pre-treated with nerve growth factor 7S (Millipore, Billerica, MA, USA) to obtain neuron-like cells [25].

Cell viability measurements by MTT assay

Cell viability was assessed by using a 3-(4,5-dimethythiazol-2-yl)-2,5-diphenyl tetrazolium bromide (MTT) assay. Briefly, PC12 cells were seeded onto 96-well plates and

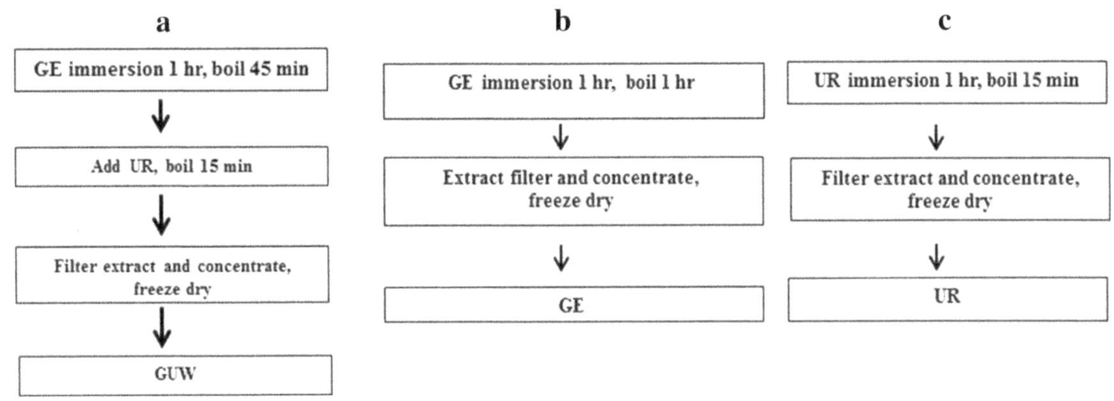

Fig. 1 Extraction protocols of **a** *Gastrodia elata* and *Uncaria rhynchophylla* water extract (GUW), **b** *Gastrodia elata* water extract (GE) and **c** *Uncaria rhynchophylla* water extract (UR)

incubated at 37 °C under 5 % CO_2 for 24 h. The cells were treated with GE, UR or GUW extracts at concentrations in the range of 0–4000 μg/mL, and the resulting mixtures were incubated for 24 h. The cells were then treated with 0.5 mg/ml MTT and incubated at 37 °C under 5 % CO_2 for 4 h. The medium was carefully aspirated and the remaining formazan crystals in each well were dissolved in dimethylsulfoxide (10 mL). The absorbance characteristics of the formazan solutions in each well were read at 490 nm using a μQuant plate reader (BioTek, Winooski, VT, USA). The relationship between the extract concentration and cell viability was visually determined. The pharmaceutical relationship between the GE and UR in GUW was calculated using a modified version of Burgi's formula [26], as follow:

$$q = \frac{E_{GE+UR}}{E_{GE} + E_{UR} - E_{GE} \times E_{UR}}$$

E_x: effectiveness of herbal extract x. For this formula, $q < 0.85$ indicates that the two drugs in question are acting in an antagonistic manner, whereas $q > 1.15$ indicates that the two drugs are acting in a synergistic manner. Values in between these limits (i.e., $0.85 < q < 1.15$) indicate that the effects of the two herbs are additive.

The effect of oxygen-glucose deprivation on PC12 cells

PC12 cells were seeded at a density of 1.5×10^4 cells/well in poly-D-lysine-coated 6-well culture plates, and grown in RPMI 1640 culture medium supplemented with 10 % horse serum, 5 % FBS and 100 U/mL penicillin G sodium. After 24 h of incubation, neural differentiation was induced by the addition of a 50 ng/mL solution of nerve growth factor 7.0S (Millipore, Billerica, MA, USA) in RPMI 1640 culture medium containing 1 % horse serum and 0.5 % FBS. The cells were differentiated for 6 days and the differentiation medium was changed on alternate days. Oxygen-glucose deprivation (OGD) was applied on neural differentiated PC12 cells, as reported previously [27]. PC12 cells were cultured with glucose-free RPMI 1640 in an air-tight hypoxia chamber (STEMCELL Technologies Inc., Vancouver, Canada). Experimental groups were defined as follows: control, OGD, GUW, GE, UR and GE + UR. GUW was added to the different groups at concentrations of 1000, 2000 and 4000 μg/mL. Unless specified otherwise, the GUW treatment group was treated with 2000 μg/mL of GUW. The chamber was filled with anoxia gas composed of 95 % N_2/5 % CO_2 for 30 min at a flow rate of 3 L/min and the cells were then incubated for 8 h at 37 °C to simulate ischemia. For the control group, the cell cultures were subjected to the experimental procedures described above using normal RPMI 1640 as the culture medium and PBS as a vehicle, followed by incubation under normoxic conditions.

Cytotoxicity assay

Cell death was measured after OGD based on the amount of lactate dehydrogenase (LDH) leaked into the culture medium using an LDH cytotoxicity detection kit (TaKaRa, Otsu, Japan), according to manufacturer's instructions.

Flow cytometry analysis of ROS

Intracellular ROS production was detected using a dichloro-dihydro-fluorescein diacetate (DCFH-DA) assay [28]. Briefly, 10 μM DCFH-DA was added to the PC12 cells after OGD, and the cells were then incubated at 37 °C for 30 min in the dark. Fluorescent signals were detected by flow cytometry using a FACSCanto™ II system (Becton–Dickinson, Franklin Lakes, NJ, USA), as reported previously [29]. The results were expressed as the relative percentage of DCF-fluorescence in the target groups compared with the cells in the control group.

Real-time polymerase chain reaction (RT-PCR)

Total mRNA was prepared using the Trizol reagent (Invitrogen Life Technologies, Carlsbad, CA, USA) according to manufacturer's instructions. cDNA was synthesized using the Promega Improm II Reverse Transcription System (Promega, Madison, Wi, USA) according to the manufacturer's instructions. RT-PCR experiments were conducted at a final volume of 10 μL containing 5 μL of 2× SYBR® Green I master mix (BIO-RAD, Hercules, CA, USA), 0.5 μL of forward and reverse primers, and 1.0 μL of cDNA diluted in 3 μL of DEPC H_2O. The nucleotide sequences of the primers used in this experiment were as follows: (1) PDI, forward 5′-TCTGGA GGAGGAGGACAAC-3′, reverse 5′- TGGAAAACACA TCGCTATT-3′; (2) *Bcl-2*, forward 5′-ATACCTGGGCC ACAAGTGAG-3′, reverse 5′-TGATTTGACCATTTGCC TGA-3′; (3) *Nrf-2*, forward 5′-GAGACGGCCATGACTG AT-3′, reverse 5′-GTGAGGGGATCGATGAGTAA-3′; and (4) β-actin, forward 5′-GAGGCCCCTCTGAACCCT AA-3′, reverse 5′-ACCAGAGGCATACAGGGACAA-3′. A comparative CT method was used to compare the fold difference in the expression of these systems relative to the control.

Superoxide dismutase (SOD) assay

The SOD activity in the PC12 cells after OGD was measured using a SOD assay kit (Cayman Chemical, Ann Arbor, MI, USA). Tetrazolium salt, xanthine oxidase and cell lysate were added to a 96-well plate. The OD540 value of the formazan produced was measured by a fluorescent microplate reader (FLUOstar OPTIMA, BMG LABTECH, Ortenberg, Germany). The results of these experiments were expressed as the relative percentage of SOD activity of each sample compared with the control.

Glutathione peroxidase assay

The GPx levels in the PC12 cells after OGD were measured using a Glutathione Peroxidase assay kit (Cayman Chemical) according to manufacturer's instructions. The activity of GPx was estimated by measuring the optical density at 340 nm (OD340) using a Quant system (BioTek).

Catalase assay

The catalase activity of the PC12 cells was measured after OGD and the subsequent drug treatment processes using a catalase fluorometric detection kit (Enzo Life Sciences, Farmingdale, NY, USA), following the manufacturer's instructions. The optical density at 595 nm (OD595) of resorufin was recorded. The results were expressed as the relative percentage of catalase activity of each sample compared with the control cells.

Caspase-3 assay

After OGD, the PC12 cells were lysed with lysis buffer (Thermo Scientific, Waltham, MA, USA). Following two freeze–thaw cycles, the cell lysates were centrifuged at 21,500×*g* (Heraeus Multifuge 1S-R with Microliter Rotor, Thermo Scientific) for 3 min at 4 °C. The supernatants were subsequently collected and stored at −80 °C prior to being analyzed. The caspase-3 activity of the lysates was measured using a caspase-3 colorimetric protease assay kit (Thermo Scientific). The results were expressed as the relative percentage of caspase-3 activity of each sample compared with the control cells.

Animals

Male Sprague–Dawley rats, weighing 260–280 g, were housed in cages (45 × 30 × 20 cm^3) on 12-h light/dark cycle with ad libitum access to chow and water. The animal studies were performed following the ARRIVE guideline (Additional file 2). All of the experimental animal procedures used in this study were conducted with the approval of the Ethics Committee of the Chinese University of Hong Kong (AEEC ref number: 11/068/MIS-5) (Additional files 3, 4, 5).

Middle cerebral artery occlusion (MCAO)

Rats were arbitrarily divided into three groups: GUW treatment, Control and Sham groups. After MCAO or a sham operation, the rats in the control and sham groups were orally administered with distilled water, whereas the rats in the GUW treatment group were administered with 288.6 mg/kg GUW once daily by oral gavage using an intragastric tube for 7 consecutive days.

Sprague–Dawley rats were intraperitoneally anesthetized with 400 mg/kg of chloral hydrate (VWR International Ltd, Poole, England). The cerebral blood flow (CBF) in these animals was intraoperatively monitored by laser Doppler flowmetery (PeriFlux System 5000, Perimed AB, Stockholm, Sweden). The probe holder (Probe holder PH07-6, Perimed AB) was located at the right cerebrum at 1 mm posterior and 2 mm lateral to the bregma above the skull. Briefly, the external carotid artery (ECA) and its branches were isolated and ligated. A round tip 4-0 nylon suture was inserted into the internal carotid artery (ICA) through the opening at the ECA and advanced to the anterior cerebral artery to occlude the middle cerebral artery (MCA). Once the MCA was occluded, the CBF was reduced by 60 %. After 2 h of occlusion-induced ischemia, reperfusion was allowed by the gentle removal of the nylon filament. For the sham rats, the left CCA and ECA were exposed without inserting the filament into the ICA.

Infarct volume assessment

Brain infarct volume was quantified by 2,3,5-triphenyltetrazolium chloride (TTC) staining [30, 31]. Rats were euthanized with an overdose of pentobarbital at 7 days post-operation. The brains of the rats were harvested and cut into slices of 2 mm in thickness. The fresh brain slices were immersed in 2 % TTC solution in PBS for 20 min at 37 °C and their images were subsequently captured using an Epson Perfection 1260 desktop scanner (Seiko Epson Corporation, Nagano, Japan) at a resolution of 600 dpi. The area of the white infarct region was then analyzed using Adobe Photoshop CS4 Extended Version 11.0.1 (Adobe Systems Inc., San Jose, CA, USA). The infarct volume of a slice was calculated using the following equation:

$$\begin{aligned}\text{Infarct volume} &= \text{Infarct area of the slice}\\ &\quad \times \text{thickness of the slice (2 mm)}\end{aligned}$$

The total infarct volume was calculated by summing up the infarct volumes of the different slices.

Cresyl violet staining

At the end of the experiment at day 7, the animals were anesthetized and their brains were perfused transcardially with phosphate buffered saline, followed by 4 % paraformaldehyde. The brains were subsequently excised, embedded with paraffin wax and cut coronally into slices of 6-μm thickness. These sections were then stained with 0.1 % cresyl violet for 10 min.

Immunohistochemistry

The expression levels of *Nrf-2* and *Bcl-2* at the penumbra of the rats were examined by immunohistochemistry. At 7 days after MCAO, the rats were euthanized and their brains were harvested and cut into slices of 6-μm thickness, as above mentioned. These sections were then blocked with FBS containing 10 % goat serum and 1 % BSA, and incubated with rabbit polyclonal anti-*Nrf-2* (1:200; Abcam, Cambridge, UK) and rabbit polyclonal anti-*Bcl-2* (1:400; Abcam) overnight at 4 °C. The slices were then washed with PBS and incubated with Alexa Fluor® 555 Goat Anti-Rabbit IgG (H + L) (Invitrogen Life Technologies) for 1 h with dilutions of 1:400 and 1:800 for binding on anti-*Nrf-2* and anti-*Bcl-2*, respectively. The slices were then washed with PBS and counterstained with DAPI. Fluorescence images were captured with ApoTome.2 system (Carl Zeiss AG, Jena, Germany).

Neurological deficit score

Neurological deficit score (NDS) was performed using a modified Bederson's scoring system to assess the diagnosis and prognosis of GUW treatment on cerebral ischemia [32]. NDS 1: Rats showing contralateral limb flexion (to the left limbs). NDS 2: Rats showing decreased resistance to lateral push to the left. NDS 3: Rats showing contralateral circling, *i.e.*, circling to the left only. NDS 4: Rats showing spontaneous circling. The NDSs were measured at 1, 2, 3, 5 and 7 days after the MCAO.

Beam-walking test

A beam-walking test was applied to assess the motor coordination and balance control of the forelimbs and hind limbs of rats treated with the different extracts to evaluate their motor functional recovery after ischemia [33, 34]. The experimental animals were trained to complete a beam-walking test 3 days before undergoing MCAO to take baseline measurements, which involved them traversing an elevated narrow beam (2.5 × 120 cm, 80 cm above the floor) [35]. During the training days (2 days), the rats required less than 10 s to cross the beam. The rats were motivated to cross the beam by placing their home cage at the opposite end of the training stage. The rats were given 90 s to cross the walkway to their home cage. Performance was assessed by recording the mean latency of three trials to walk along the beam. This beam-walking test was performed at 1, 2, 3, 5 and 7 days after MCAO.

Statistical analysis

All data have been presented as the mean values ± SD. Student's *t* test and one way ANOVA, followed by Dunnett's multiple comparison test (GraphPad Prism 5.0 software; San Diego, CA, USA), were used for the statistical analysis. Statistical significance was taken as $P < 0.05$.

Results

Cell viability measurements by MTT assay

An MTT assay was used to determine the optimal concentration of each extract to be used on the PC12 cells.

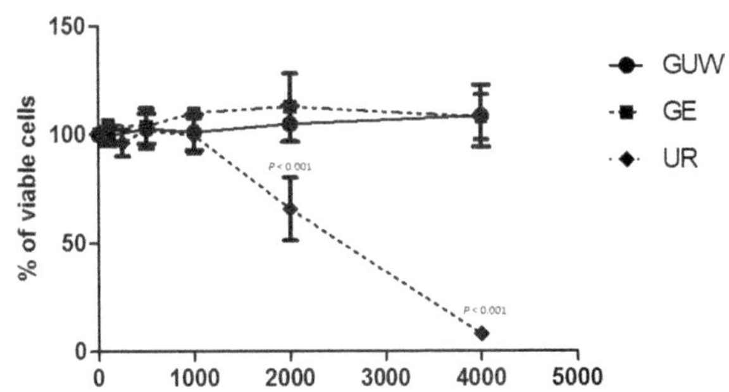

Fig. 2 Cell response curve of various *Gastrodia elata* and *Uncaria rhynchophylla* extracts. The extracts of GUW and GE did not demonstrate toxicity to PC12 cells even at high concentration of 4000 μg/mL, whereas the UR extract showed toxicity to PC12 cells at concentrations higher than 1000 μg/mL vs control by one way ANOVA, post hoc Dunnett's test (n = 4)

The GUW and GE extracts were found to be non-toxic to PC12 cells at concentrations below 4000 μg/mL (Fig. 2). However, the UR extract exhibited significant toxicity at concentrations greater than 2000 μg/mL ($P < 0.001$) and gave an IC_{50} value of 2557 μg/mL.

Effect of GUW on the morphological characteristics of PC12 cells following OGD

Neurite extensions were found in the nerve growth factor (NGF)-treated PC12 cells in the control group (Fig. 3a). In general, the cells in the OGD group become globular in shape with shorter neurite protrusions (Fig. 3b). GUW treatment did not lead to any discernible differences in the neuronal morphology and neurite branches of these cells (Fig. 3c).

GUW extracts against OGD-induced cell injury

PC12 cells showed 70 % cell death after the OGD treatment process. The treatment of the cells with GUW provided them with significant protection from OGD-induced cell death ($P < 0.001$, Fig. 3d). Moreover, GUW exhibited neuroprotective effects in a concentration-dependent manner.

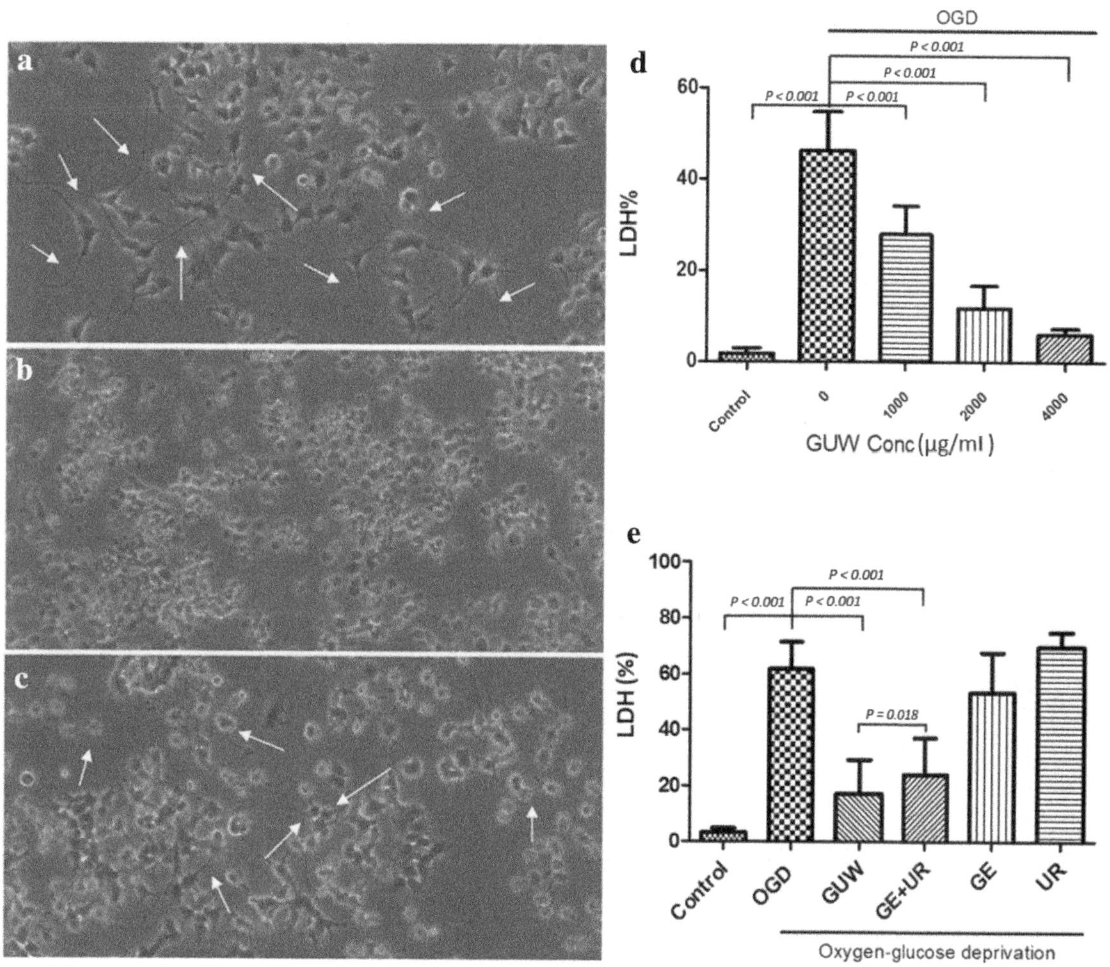

Fig. 3 Morphologies of NGF-differentiated PC12 cells under OGD with or without GUW treatment. **a** NGF-treated PC12 cells differentiated with neurite extentions without OGD treatment. **b** After OGD, cell bodies shrank with a loss of neurite outgrowth. **c** PC12 cells retained neuronal morphology with GUW treatment. (Mag. 100×). *White arrows* indicate neurite protrusions. **d** PC12 cells injury/death was quantified by LDH assay after 8 h OGD. GUW showed concentration dependent protective effects on cells. **e** PC12 cells injury/death was quantified by measuring the release of LDH from injured cells. After OGD, single extracts of GE or UR only did not exhibit significant protective effect on OGD insult on NGF-treated PC12 cell. However, both GUW and the combination of GE and UR (GE + UR) water extracts have significant protective effects. Furthermore, GUW was also found to exert significantly greater neuroprotection better than GE + UR; vs control and vs OGD by one way ANOVA, post hoc Dunnett's test (n = 4); vs GE + UR by Student's *t* test (n = 4)

Drug interaction of *Gastrodia elata* and *Uncaria rhynchophylla*

The individual GE and UR extracts (GE + UR) were mixed to form the same composition as that of GUW to investigate whether the protective effects of GUW were acting in an addictive or synergistic manner and study the pharmaceutical relationship between the two herbs in GUW. The GE- and UR-only treatments did not provide significant protection to the cells from the OGD insult (Fig. 3e). Both GUW ($P < 0.001$) and GE + UR ($P < 0.001$) significantly attenuated LDH release, while GUW exerted significantly greater neuroprotection than GE + UR ($P = 0.018$). The q value obtained in our study was 16, suggesting that the herbs in GUW were acting synergistically to protect the cells against OGD-induced cell death.

Caspase-3 activity

Caspase-3 activity increased significantly by 160 % ($P < 0.001$) compared with the control cells after exposure to OGD for 8 h (Fig. 4). However, the caspase-3 activity of the OGD groups returned to normal levels ($P < 0.001$) after they were treated with GUW (2000 μg/mL).

mRNA expression after OGD

The mRNA expression levels of *Bcl-2, PDI* and *Nrf-2* in the GUW group were 1.6-($P = 0.0130$), 2.4-($P = 0.0279$) and 1.5-fold ($P = 0.0066$) higher than those of the OGD group, whereas no significant changes were observed in these levels between the OGD and control groups (Fig. 5a). The expression of the housekeeping gene *β-actin* was measured to normalize the expression levels of the target genes.

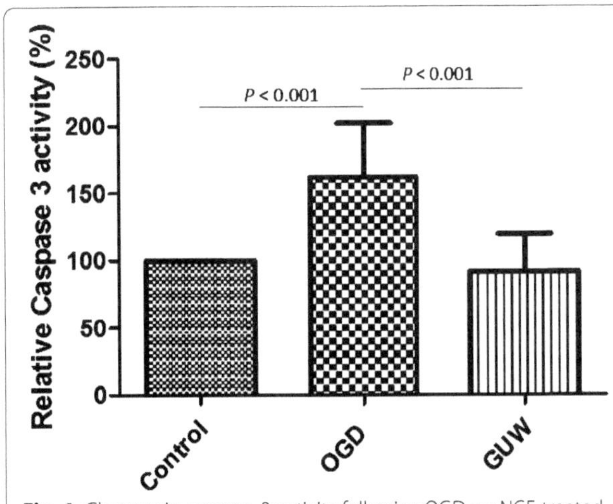

Fig. 4 Changes in caspase-3 activity following OGD on NGF-treated PC12 cells. The activity of caspase-3 in the cell lysates were measured and normalized with the control group, vs OGD by one way ANOVA, post hoc Dunnett's test (n = 4)

Flow cytometry analysis of reactive oxygen species

OGD led to a 2.5-fold increase in the quantity of intracellular ROS compared with the control group. However, we also observed a significant decrease of 40 % in the quantity of ROS in the GUW samples compared with the OGD group ($P < 0.001$; Fig. 5b).

Activity of antioxidant enzymes

The SOD activity of the NGF-treated PC12 cells exposed to OGD was 80 % lower than that of the control group ($P = 0.0174$; Fig. 5c). The treatment of these cells with GUW led to a 40 % increase in SOD activity compared with the OGD group ($P < 0.001$). The GPx and catalase activities of the NGF-treated PC12 cells decreased following their exposure to OGD ($P < 0.001$), whereas the treatment of these cells with GUW effectively restored their GPx activity ($P = 0.0385$; Fig. 5d). The catalase activity of the NGF-treated PC12 cells increased significantly by 35 % in the OGD group compared with the control group ($P < 0.001$) (Fig. 5e), but no significant difference was found in the catalase activity between the OGD and GUW treatment groups.

GUW reduced the infarct volume and improved the histological outcome after MCAO

The MCAO operation inflicted damage to different areas on the right hemisphere of the brain, including the cortex, hippocampus and basal ganglia cortex (Fig. 6a). GUW treatment led to a significant reduction in the infarct volume of brain by 55.7 % ($P < 0.001$) compared with the control group at 7 days post-operation (Fig. 6b).

Cresyl violet staining of the coronal brain sections taken from the rats in the MCAO group showed a dramatic decrease in the size of the Nissl bodies, as well as an increase in the size of the intracellular space between them (Fig. 6c). Notably, the administration of GUW rescued the neurons in the infarct region and preserved the tissue structure.

GUW led to increased expression levels of *Bcl-2* and *Nrf-2*

Immunohistochemistry was used to examine the expression levels of *Bcl-2* and *Nrf-2* 7 days after MCAO. The results revealed increases in the expression levels of *Bcl-2* (Fig. 6d) and *Nrf-2* (Fig. 6e) at the penumbra of the MCAO group. Further increases in the expression levels of these two proteins were observed in the GUW treatment group, suggesting that GUW modulated the expression levels of *Bcl-2* and *Nrf-2* in vivo.

GUW resulted in improved neurological function after MCAO

The NDS of the rats was measured on a daily basis after 2 h of ischemia and 24 h of reperfusion. The MCAO rats

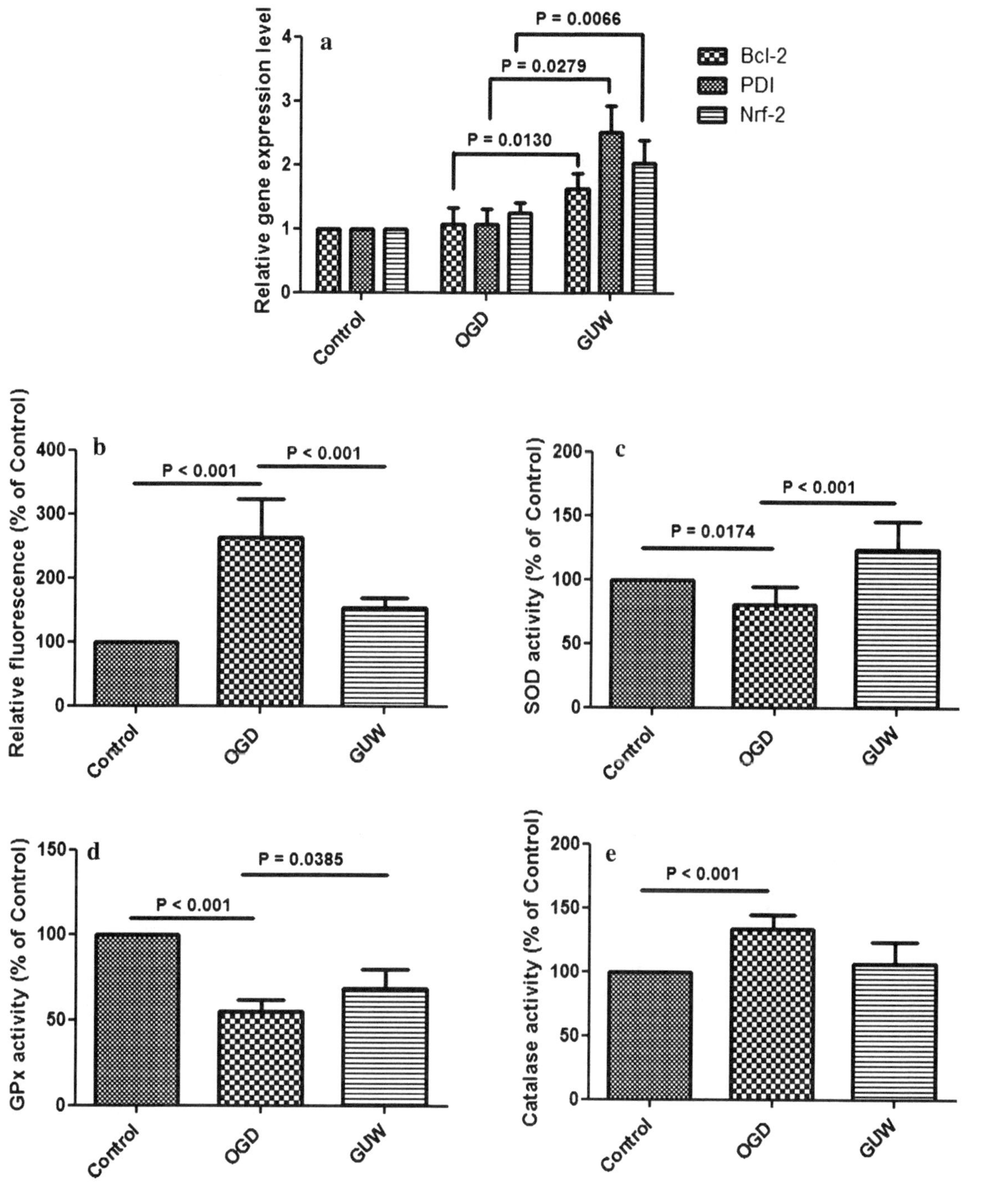

Fig. 5 **a** mRNA expression levels of antioxidant and antiapoptotic genes after OGD and GUW treatment. Ct values of the genes of interest were first normalized to intrinsic β-actin of each sample, then the fold differences among each group and control was them calculated, vs OGD by one way ANOVA, post hoc Dunnett's test (n = 4). Status of oxidative stress after OGD and GUW treatment. **b** Reactive oxygen species amount in between the control, OGD and GUW -treated group. The concentration of intracellular ROS was analyzed by flow cytometry. **c** SOD, **d** GPx and **e** Catalase activity in NGF-treated PC12 cells in different treatment groups, vs control and vs OGD by one way ANOVA, post hoc Dunnett's test (n = 4)

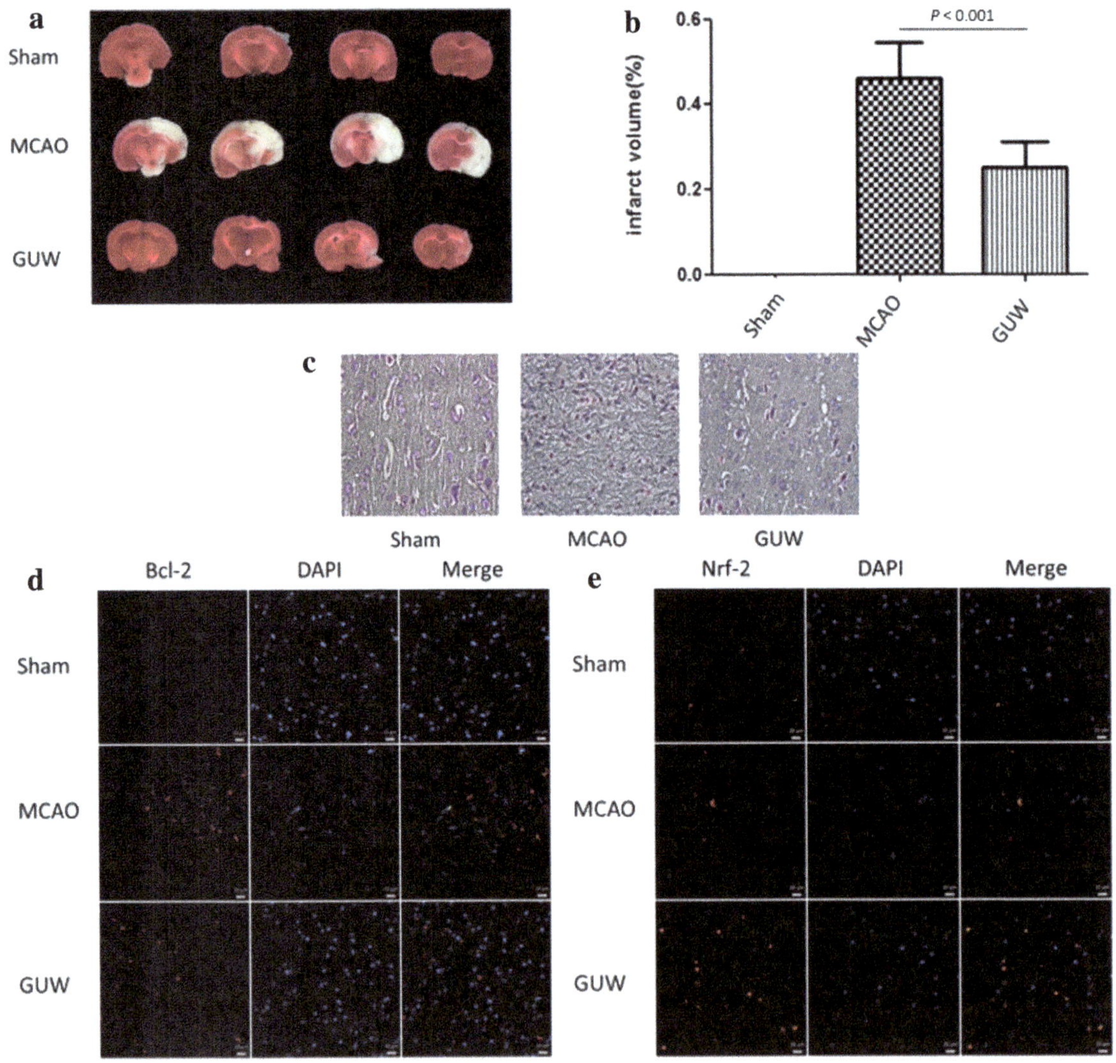

Fig. 6 GUW reduced brain infarction volume and improved histological outcome. Brains were harvested 7 days of post-operation. The brains were sliced and performed TTC staining to evaluate the infarction volume and cresyl violet staining to examine the neuronal morphology at the infarct region. **a** The percentage of brain infarction of different groups of rats at 7 days of post-operation. **b** Data are expressed as mean ± SD, vs MCAO control group by one-way ANOVA (n = 10). **c** GUW increased the number of cells with normal neuronal morphology and decreased the number of shrunken and misshapen cells in cresyl violet–stained sections (magnification factor 400×). The *Bcl-2* and *Nrf-2* expression at the penumbra was examined by immunohistochemistry. GUW showed to upregulate both proteins in the penumbra. Representative images of the expression of **d** *Bcl-2* and **e** *Nrf-2*. *Scale bar* 20 μm

scored higher than 3. Notably, GUW treatment led to a lower score after day 3 compared with the MCAO control ($P < 0.001$; Fig. 7a).

GUW led to improved behavior in the Beam-walking test after MCAO-injury

The time taken for rats to walk across the beam was recorded daily. The MCAO control rats took 31 ± 21 to 42 ± 33 s to walk along the wooden beam throughout the experimental period, which was fourfold higher than that of the sham group ($P < 0.001$). A significantly faster walking time was observed in the GUW-treated rats after 3 days of drug treatment. For example, the time taken to cross the beam in this group decreased from 39 ± 27 s at day 1 to 11 ± 6 s at day 3 ($P < 0.001$), resulting in performance comparable with that of the sham group rats (Fig. 7b).

Discussion

In this study, we investigated the protective effects of GUW on NGF-treated PC12 cells subjected to OGD by measuring LDH release. GUW protected NGF-treated

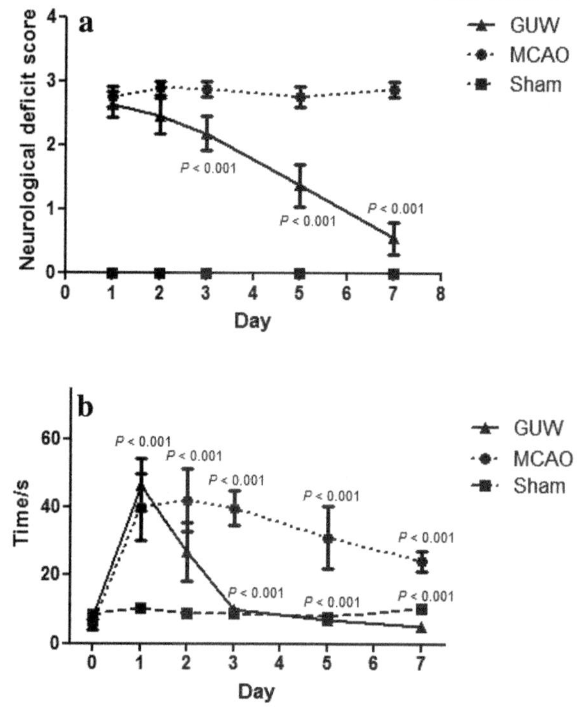

Fig. 7 Sprague Dawley rats showed recovery of neurological and locomotor function after receiving GUW treatment. **a** Daily neurological deficit score measurement of different groups. Neurological deficit score was measured and recorded on day 1, 3, 5, 7 after MCAO surgery. MCAO control group received distilled water as vehicle. Data are expressed as mean ± SD, vs control group by one way ANOVA (n = 10). **b** Results of beam walking test after brain injury. After MCAO operation, rats receiving either vehicle or GUW showed significantly longer latencies to across the beam compared to sham-injured rats. At first 3 days treatment, the time to cross beam of GUW group was shorter time than the MCAO group significantly. Data are expressed as mean ± SD, vs sham group and vs MCAO group, by one way ANOVA (n = 10)

PC12 cells against OGD-induced cell death and exhibited dose-dependent neuroprotective effects. Moreover, the neuroprotection effects of GUW were greater than those of the individual GE and UR extracts. Flow cytometry results revealed that GUW led to a significant decrease in the amount of ROS, resulting in lower caspase-3 activity. Along with the increase observed in the regulation of *Bcl-2* by RT-PCR, these findings suggest that GUW could prevent cells from undergoing apoptosis as a consequence of ischemic insults.

Oxidative stress is one of the major contributors to the pathophysiological consequences observed in cerebral ischemia [36–38]. Oxidative stress also participates in excitotoxic neuronal necrosis, leading to systemic oxidative damage and apoptosis [36, 39]. To determine whether GUW could modulate the antioxidant protective mechanism in cells, we studied its effect on the activities of several antioxidant enzymes. *Nrf-2* is a basic leucine zipper redox-sensitive transcriptional factor that regulates the expression of several cellular antioxidant and cytoprotective genes from the ARE [7, 40, 41]. The upregulation of *Nrf-2* has been reported to mitigate oxidative stress-induced tissue injury in vivo [10, 42]. In contrast, the overexpression of PDI may lead to increased resistance to hypoxic or ischemic injury in vitro and in vivo [43]. Moreover, PDI enhances chaperone activity to protect against oxidative stress injury, suggesting that PDI may participate in more than one mechanism to protect neuronal cells from ischemic injury [43, 44]. Cerebral ischemia led to decreases in GPx and SOD activity, as well as an increase in catalase activity [45]. GUW rescued the expression of GPx and SOD activity, and had no discernible impact on the catalase activity. GUW could therefore modulate the *Nrf-2*-ARE pathway and enhance the antioxidant mechanism to protect the cells from ROS-induced oxidative damage.

Although most drugs show promising in vitro results, their application in vivo has been limited by their poor blood–brain barrier permeability [46]. The active components in GUW could penetrate the blood–brain barrier in vivo [47–49]. The in vivo efficacy of GUW was investigated using a MCAO model. Although it is not possible to rescue the neurons in the infarction core, the neurons in the penumbra region may be salvaged from ischemic/reperfusion injury [50]. The results of our study showed a smaller infarct area after GUW treatment compared with the control animals, suggesting that GUW rescued the cells in the penumbra. The immunohistochemistry results showed an upregulation in the levels of *Bcl-2* and *Nrf-2* at the penumbra in the GUW treatment group. This result was consistent with the in vitro results, which showed that GUW modulated the antiapoptotic and antioxidative genes to protect the brain from cerebral ischemia. Notably, the treatment of the MCAO rats with GUW led to a reduction in their NDS, as well as a decrease in the time required to complete the beam-walking test.

The results of our interaction study for GE and UR showed that GUW was a stronger neuroprotective agent than the GE + UR mixture, suggesting that GE and UR exhibit synergistic effects in GUW capable of supporting the survival of NGF-treated PC12 cells under OGD. It is therefore likely that the decocting process for the production of GUW resulted in the formation of the active components responsible for the greater neuroprotective effect [51, 52]. This study therefore represents the first report to show that the combination of GE and UR might lead to synergistic effects. Further chemical analysis is needed in the future to determine the root cause of this synergistic effect.

Conclusion

GUW modulated the antioxidant system and antiapoptotic genes in neuronal differentiated PC12 cells at 2000 g/mL following oxygen-glucose deprivation and Sprague–Dawley rats at 288.6 mg/kg following middle cerebral artery occlusion.

Abbreviations

ARE: antioxidant response element; DCFH-DA: dichloro-dihydro-fluorescein diacetate; GE: *Gastrodia elata*; GPx: glutathione peroxidase; GUW: *Gastrodia elata* and *Uncaria rhynchophylla* water extract; LDH: lactate dehydrogenase; MCAO: middle cerebral artery occlusion; MTT: 3-[4,5-dimethylthiazol-2-yl]-2,5-diphenyltetrazolium bromide; NGF: nerve growth factor; *Nrf-2*: nuclear factor ethyroid 2-related factor 2; OGD: oxygen-glucose deprivation; *PDI*: protein disulfide isomerase; ROS: reactive oxygen species; SOD: superoxide dismutase; TTC: 2,3,5-triphenyltetrazolium chloride; UR: *Uncaria rhynchophylla*.

Authors' contributions

CWC conceived and designed the study. JWX, CFN and WNL performed the in vitro studies. JWN and AYC performed the in vivo studies. JWX and AYC collected the data. JWX, AYC, CBL and WNL analyzed the data. JWX wrote the manuscript. AYC, CWC, CBL, WNL revised the manuscript. All authors read and approved the final manuscript.

Author details

[1] School of Chinese Medicine, The Chinese University of Hong Kong, Shatin, New Territories, Hong Kong, People's Republic of China. [2] Institute of Chinese Medicine, The Chinese University of Hong Kong, Shatin, New Territories, Hong Kong, People's Republic of China. [3] State Key Laboratory of Phytochemistry and Plant Resources in West China, The Chinese University of Hong Kong, Shatin, New Territories, Hong Kong, People's Republic of China.

Acknowledgements

The project was supported by Hong Kong Health and Medical Research Fund (Ref no. 11120381), Government of the Hong Kong Special Administrative Region.

Competing interests

The authors declare that they have no competing interests.

References

1. Lloyd-Jones D, Adams RJ, Brown TM, Carnethon M, Dai S, De Simone G, Ferguson TB, Ford E, Furie K, Gillespie C, Go A, Greenlund K, Haase N, Hailpern S, Ho PM, Howard V, Kissela B, Kittner S, Lackland D, Lisabeth L, Marelli A, McDermott MM, Meigs J, Mozaffarian D, Mussolino M, Nichol G, Roger VL, Rosamond W, Sacco R, Sorlie P, Roger VL, Thom T, Wasserthiel-Smoller S, Wong ND, Wylie-Rosett J. Heart disease and stroke statistics–2010 update: a report from the American Heart Association. Circulation. 2010;121:46–215.
2. Davis S, Lees K, Donnan G. Treating the acute stroke patient as an emergency: current practices and future opportunities. Int J Clin Pract. 2006;60:399–407.
3. The National Institute of Neurological Disorders and Stroke rt-PA Stroke Study Group. Tissue plasminogen activator for acute ischemic stroke. N Engl J Med. 1995;333:1581–7.
4. Armstead WM, Ganguly K, Kiessling JW, Riley J, Chen XH, Smith DH, Stein SC, Higazi AA, Cines DB, Bdeir K, Zaitsev S, Muzykantov VR. Signaling, delivery and age as emerging issues in the benefit/risk ratio outcome of tPA For treatment of CNS ischemic disorders. J Neurochem. 2010;113:303–12.
5. Olmez I, Ozyurt H. Reactive oxygen species and ischemic cerebrovascular disease. Neurochem Int. 2012;60:208–12.
6. Bretón RR, Rodríguez JCG. Excitotoxicity and oxidative stress in acute ischemic stroke. In: Rodríguez JCG, editor. Acute ischemic stroke. Shanghai: InTech; 2012. p. 29–58.
7. Petri S, Körner S, Kiaei M. Nrf2/ARE signaling pathway: key mediator in oxidative stress and potential therapeutic target in ALS. Neurol Res Int. 2012;2012:878030.
8. Rawal AK, Muddeshwar MG, Biswas SK. *Rubia cordifolia*, *Fagonia cretica* Linn and *Tinospora cordifolia* exert neuroprotection by modulating the antioxidant system in rat hippocampal slices subjected to oxygen glucose deprivation. BMC Complement Altern Med. 2004;4:11.
9. Shih AY, Li P, Murphy TH. A small-molecule-inducible Nrf2-mediated antioxidant response provides effective prophylaxis against cerebral ischemia in vivo. J Neurosci. 2005;25:10321–35.
10. Wu QQ, Wang Y, Senitko M, Meyer C, Wigley WC, Ferguson DA, Grossman E, Chen J, Zhou XJ, Hartono J, Winterberg P, Chen B, Agarwal A, Lu CY. Bardoxolone methyl (BARD) ameliorates ischemic AKI and increases expression of protective genes Nrf2, PPARγ, and HO-1. Am J Physiol Renal Physiol. 2011;300:F1180–92.
11. Hatahet F, Ruddock LW. Protein disulfide isomerase: a critical evaluation of its function in disulfide bond formation. Antioxid Redox Signal. 2009;11:2807–50.
12. He P. Clinical efficacy of tian ma gou teng yin in the treatment of 100 cases of cerebral ischemia. Med J Chinese People's Heal. 2008;20:292.
13. Zhang HW, Tong J, Zhou G, Jia H, Jiang JY. Tianma gouteng yin formula for treating primary hypertension. Cochrane Database Syst Rev. 2012;6:008166.
14. Zhang CY, Du GY, Wang W, Ye ZG, Wang DQ, Sun XF, Zhao DZ. Effects of Tianma Gouteng Fang on transmitter amino acids in the hippocampus extracellular liquids in freely moving rats subjected to brain ischemia. Chin J Chinese Mater Medica. 2004;29:1061–5.
15. Chun HS, Kim JM, Choi EH, Chang N. Neuroprotective effects of several Korean medicinal plants traditionally used for stroke remedy. J Med Food. 2008;11:246–51.
16. Su SY, Hsieh CL. Anti-inflammatory effects of Chinese medicinal herbs on cerebral ischemia. Chin Med. 2011;6:26.
17. Kim HJ, Hwang IK, Won MH. Vanillin, 4-hydroxybenzyl aldehyde and 4-hydroxybenzyl alcohol prevent hippocampal CA1 cell death following global ischemia. Brain Res. 2007;1181:130–41.
18. Lee YS, Ha JH, Yong CS, Lee DU, Huh K, Kang YS, Lee SH, Jung MW, Kim JA. Inhibitory effects of constituents of *Gastrodia elata* Bl. on glutamate-induced apoptosis in IMR-32 human neuroblastoma cells. Arch Pharm Res. 1999;22:404–9.
19. Tsai CF, Huang CL, Lin YL, Lee YC, Yang YC, Huang NK. The neuroprotective effects of an extract of *Gastrodia elata*. J Ethnopharmacol. 2011;138:119–25.
20. Shimada Y, Goto H, Itoh T, Sakakibara I, Kubo M, Sasaki H, Terasawa K. Evaluation of the protective effects of alkaloids isolated from the hooks and stems of *Uncaria sinensis* on glutamate-induced neuronal death in cultured cerebellar granule cells from rats. J Pharm Pharmacol. 1999;51:715–22.
21. Yokoyama K, Shimada Y, Hori E, Sekiya N, Goto H, Sakakibara I, Nishijo H, Terasawa K. Protective effects of Choto-san and hooks and stems of *Uncaria sinensis* against delayed neuronal death after transient forebrain ischemia in gerbil. Phytomedicine. 2004;11:478–89.
22. Hu G. Internal chinese medicine: new treatment methods. Chengdu: Sichuan People's Publishing House; 1958.

23. Pharmacopedia Committee Pharmacopedia of the People's Republic of China. Pharmacopedia of the People's Republic of China. 20th ed. Beijing: China Medical Science and Technology Press; 2010.
24. Tabakman R, Jiang H, Shahar I, Arien-Zakay H, Levine RA, Lazarovici P. Neuroprotection by NGF in the PC12 in vitro OGD model: involvement of mitogen-activated protein kinases and gene expression. Ann NY Acad Sci. 2005;1053:84–96.
25. Williams B, Dwyer DS. Structure-based discovery of low molecular weight compounds that stimulate neurite outgrowth and substitute for nerve growth factor. J Neurochem. 2009;110:1876–84.
26. Wang H, Joseph JA. Quantifying cellular oxidative stress by dichlorofluorescein assay using microplate reader. Free Radic Biol Med. 1999;27:612–6.
27. Eruslanov E, Kusmartsev S. Identification of ROS using oxidized DCFDA and flow-cytometry. Methods Mol Biol. 2010;594:57–72.
28. Jin ZJ. About the evaluation of drug combination. Acta Pharm Sin. 2004;25:146–7.
29. Bederson JB, Pitts LH, Germano SM, Nishimura MC, Davis RL, Bartkowski HM. Evaluation of 2,3,5-triphenyltetrazolium chloride as a stain for detection and quantification of experimental cerebral infarction in rats. Stroke. 1986;17:1304–8.
30. Zhan C, Yang J. Protective effects of isoliquiritigenin in transient middle cerebral artery occlusion-induced focal cerebral ischemia in rats. Pharmacol Res. 2006;53:303–9.
31. Bederson JB, Pitts LH, Tsuji M, Nishimura MC, Davis RL, Bartkowski H. Rat middle cerebral artery occlusion: evaluation of the model and development of a neurologic examination. Stroke. 1986;17:472–6.
32. Feeney DM, Gonzalez A, Law WA. Amphetamine, haloperidol, and experience interact to affect rate of recovery after motor cortex injury. Science. 1982;217:855–7.
33. Goldstein LB, Davis JN. Beam-walking in rats: studies towards developing an animal model of functional recovery after brain injury. J Neurosci Methods. 1990;31:101–7.
34. Urakawa S, Hida H, Masuda T, Misumi S, Kim TS, Nishino H. Environmental enrichment brings a beneficial effect on beam walking and enhances the migration of doublecortin-positive cells following striatal lesions in rats. Neuroscience. 2007;144:920–33.
35. Alexandrova ML, Bochev PG. Oxidative stress during the chronic phase after stroke. Free Radic Biol Med. 2005;39:297–316.
36. Domínguez C, Delgado P, Vilches A, Martín-Gallán P, Ribó M, Santamarina E, Molina C, Corbeto N, Rodríguez-Sureda V, Rosell A, Alvarez-Sabín J, Montaner J. Oxidative stress after thrombolysis-induced reperfusion in human stroke. Stroke. 2010;41:653–60.
37. Glantz L, Avramovich A, Trembovler V, Gurvitz V, Kohen R, Eidelman LA, Shohami E. Ischemic preconditioning increases antioxidants in the brain and peripheral organs after cerebral ischemia. Exp Neurol. 2005;192:117–24.
38. Baker K, Marcus CB, Huffman K, Kruk H, Malfroy B, Doctrow SR. Synthetic combined superoxide dismutase/catalase mimetics are protective as a delayed treatment in a rat stroke model: a key role for reactive oxygen species in ischemic brain injury. J Pharmacol Exp Ther. 1998;284:215–21.
39. Nguyen T, Nioi P, Pickett CB. The Nrf2-antioxidant response element signaling pathway and its activation by oxidative stress. J Biol Chem. 2009;284:13291–5.
40. Venugopal R, Jaiswal AK. Nrf1 and Nrf2 positively and c-Fos and Fra1 negatively regulate the human antioxidant response element-mediated expression of NAD(P)H:quinone oxidoreductase1 gene. Proc Natl Acad Sci USA. 1996;93:14960–5.
41. Leonard MO, Kieran NE, Howell K, Burne MJ, Varadarajan R, Dhakshinamoorthy S, Porter AG, O'Farrelly C, Rabb H, Taylor CT. Reoxygenation-specific activation of the antioxidant transcription factor Nrf2 mediates cytoprotective gene expression in ischemia-reperfusion injury. FASEB J. 2006;20:2624–6.
42. Tanaka S, Uehara T, Nomura Y. Up-regulation of protein-disulfide isomerase in response to hypoxia/brain ischemia and its protective effect against apoptotic cell death. J Biol Chem. 2000;275:10388–93.
43. Miyata T, Takizawa S, van Ypersele de Strihou C. Hypoxia. 1. Intracellular sensors for oxygen and oxidative stress: novel therapeutic targets. Am J Physiol Cell Physiol. 2011;300:C226–31.
44. Işlekel S, Işlekel H, Güner G, Ozdamar N. Alterations in superoxide dismutase, glutathione peroxidase and catalase activities in experimental cerebral ischemia-reperfusion. Res Exp Med. 1999;199:167–76.
45. Lee JC, Won MH. Neuroprotection of antioxidant enzymes against transient global cerebral ischemia in gerbils. Anat Cell Biol. 2014;47:149–56.
46. Sanchez-Covarrubias L, Slosky LM, Thompson BJ, Davis TP, Ronaldson PT. Transporters at CNS barrier sites: obstacles or opportunities for drug delivery? Curr Pharm Des. 2014;20:1422–49.
47. Lin LC, Chen YF, Tsai TR, Tsai TH. Analysis of brain distribution and biliary excretion of a nutrient supplement, gastrodin, in rat. Anal Chim Acta. 2007;590:173–9.
48. Lin LC, Chen YF, Lee WC, Wu YT, Tsai TH. Pharmacokinetics of gastrodin and its metabolite p-hydroxybenzyl alcohol in rat blood, brain and bile by microdialysis coupled to LC-MS/MS. J Pharm Biomed Anal. 2008;8:909–17.
49. Lee CJ, Hsueh TY, Lin LC, Tsai TH. Determination of protein-unbound rhynchiphylline brain distribution by microdialysis and ultra-performance liquid chromatography with tandem mass spectrometry. Biomed Chromatogr. 2014;28:901–6.
50. Østergaard L, Jespersen SN, Mouridsen K, Mikkelsen IK, Jonsdottír KÝ, Tietze A, Blicher JU, Aamand R, Hjort N, Iversen NK, Cai C, Hougaard KD, Simonsen CZ, von Weitzel-Mudersbach P, Modrau B, Nagenthiraja K, Ribe RL, Hansen MB, Bekke SL, Dahlman MG, Puig J, Pedraza S, Serena J, Cho TH, Siemonsen S, Thomalla G, Fiehler J, Nighoghossian N, Andersen G. The role of the cerebral capillaries in acute ischemic stroke: the extended penumbra model. J Cereb Blood Flow Metab. 2013;33:635–48.
51. Jaiswal Y, Liang Z, Yong P, Chen H, Zhao Z. A comparative study on the traditional Indian Shodhana and Chinese processing methods for aconite roots by characterization and determination of the major components. Chem Cent J. 2013;7:169.
52. Liu Y, Yang J, Cai Z. Chemical investigation on Sijunzi decoction and its two major herbs Panax ginseng and *Glycyrrhiza uralensis* by LC/MS/MS. J Pharm Biomed Anal. 2006;41:1642–7.

11

Effects of intra-articular SHINBARO treatment on monosodium iodoacetate-induced osteoarthritis in rats

Won Kyung Kim[1], Hwa-Jin Chung[1,2], Yuna Pyee[1], Tae Jun Choi[1], Hyen Joo Park[1], Ji-Young Hong[1], Joon-Shik Shin[2], Jin Ho Lee[2], In-Hyuk Ha[2] and Sang Kook Lee[1*]

Abstract

Background: SHINBARO is a refined herbal formulation used to treat inflamed lesions and bone diseases. This study aimed to investigate the anti-osteoarthritic activities of intra-articular administration of SHINBARO and determine its underlying molecular mechanism in a monosodium iodoacetate (MIA)-induced osteoarthritis rat model.

Methods: Male Sprague–Dawley rats received a single intra-articular injection of MIA into the infrapatellar ligament of the right knee. Subsequently, the rats were treated with normal saline, SHINBARO, and diclofenac once daily for 21 days. Rats treated with normal saline, but not MIA, comprised the control group. Histological changes in the femur of the MIA-induced osteoarthritis rat model were observed by micro-computed tomography scanning and staining with hematoxylin and eosin, and safranin-O fast green. Serum levels of PGE_2 and anti-type II collagen antibodies in the MIA-induced osteoarthritis rat model were measured using commercial kits. Protein levels of inflammatory enzymes (iNOS, COX-2), pro-inflammatory cytokines (TNF-α, IL-1β), and inflammatory mediators (NF-κB, IκB) in cartilaginous tissues were determined by western blot analysis.

Results: Intra-articular administration of SHINBARO (IAS) at 20 mg/kg remarkably restrained the decrease in bone volume/total volume, being 28 % ($P = 0.0001$) higher than that in the vehicle-treated MIA group. IAS (2, 10, and 20 mg/kg) treatment significantly recovered the mean number of objects values with increased percentage changes of 13.5 % ($P = 0.147$), 27.5 % ($P = 0.028$), and 44.5 % ($P = 0.031$), respectively, compared with the vehicle-treated MIA group. The serum level of PGE_2 in the IAS group at 20 mg/kg was markedly inhibited by 60.6 % ($P = 0.0007$) compared with the vehicle-treated MIA group, and the anti-collagen type II antibody level in the IAS group was reduced in a dose-dependent manner. IAS (20 mg/kg) effectively suppressed the induction of inflammation-mediated enzymes (iNOS and COX-2) and pro-inflammatory cytokines (TNF-α and IL-1β). IAS treatment also downregulated the NF-κB level and increased the IκB-α level in the MIA- induced osteoarthritis rat model.

Conclusion: SHINBARO inhibited PGE_2 and anti-type II collagen antibody production and modulated the balance of inflammatory enzymes, mediators, and cytokines in the MIA-induced osteoarthritis rat model.

Keywords: SHINBARO pharmacopuncture, Monosodium iodoacetate-induced osteoarthritis, Intra-articular administration

Background

Osteoarthritis (OA) is a degenerative joint disease characterized by abrasion of articular cartilage and trabecular bone loss [1]. The chance of developing the disease increases with age, knee joint lesions, obesity, infectious diseases, and various joint inflammations [2–5]. Several previous studies suggested that abrasion of articular cartilage, subchondral bone sclerosis, and excessive formation of trabecular bone might cause OA [6–8]. Other studies highlighted the importance of prostaglandins in

*Correspondence: sklee61@snu.ac.kr
[1] College of Pharmacy, Seoul National University, Seoul 151-742, Republic of Korea
Full list of author information is available at the end of the article

OA treatment [9]. Prostaglandins are enhanced by stimuli, such as lipopolysaccharide, sodium nitroprusside, or physical injury associated with OA [10], increased macrophage migration into the synovial fluid, activated nuclear factor (NF)-κB as an inflammatory transcription factor, and both cyclooxygenase (COX)-2 and inducible nitric oxide synthase (iNOS) as inflammatory enzymes [11, 12].

Regarding alleviation of OA, although non-steroidal anti-inflammatory drugs including acetaminophen are mainly prescribed during the early stage of OA, these drugs do not effectively prevent the progression of OA [13] and there have been some problems with side effects involving the gastrointestinal tract and kidneys. In particular, the use of COX-2 inhibitors is restrictively allowed because of significant side effects on cardiovascular function [14].

Monosodium iodoacetate (MIA) is an inhibitor of glyceraldehyde-3-phosphate dehydrogenase (GAPDH) that results in a reduction of glycolysis and causes articular cartilage changes related to the histological and morphological features of OA by impeding integration of the chondral structure and inducing cell death of chondrocytes [15]. Furthermore, MIA causes a repeated progression of synovial hyperplasia and inflammatory cell infiltration, destroys articular cartilage, and induces bone loss and chondral deformation [16]. Injection of MIA into the knee joints of rats is considered a suitable model that resembles the phenomena observed in human OA and is thus applied for evaluation of chondroprotective activity [17].

SHINBARO is a purified herbal formulation containing six traditional medicines, *Ledebouriellae* Radix (*Fang Feng*), *Achyranthis* Radix (*Huai Niu Xi*), *Acanthopanacis* Cortex (*Wu Jia Pi*), *Cibotii* Rhizoma (*Gou Ji*), *Glycine* Semen (*Hei Dou*), and *Eucommiae* Cortex (*Du Zhong*), that has been used to treat inflamed lesions and bone diseases [18]. Pharmacopuncture is a new form of therapy that involves both herbal medicine administration and acupuncture to manage blood extravasation and improve blood flow. Therefore, pharmacopuncturology is considered to be a medical practice in oriental medicine that involves administration of refined herbal extracts into acupoints [19]. The anti-inflammatory activity of oral SHINBARO treatment was demonstrated in an adjuvant-induced OA rat model [18]. However, the anti-arthritic activity of SHINBARO pharmacopuncture and its underlying mechanism have not yet been determined.

This study aimed to investigate the anti-osteoarthritic activities of intra-articular administration of SHINBARO and determine its underlying molecular mechanism in an MIA-induced OA rat model.

Methods

Preparation and composition of SHINBARO

SHINBARO was prepared by Hanpoong Pharmaceutical Co. Ltd. (Jeonju, Republic of Korea). The mixture of six crude drugs, *Ledebouriellae* Radix (4.444 g), *Achyranthis* Radix (4.444 g), *Acanthopanacis* Cortex (4.444 g), *Cibotii* Rhizoma (2.778 g), *Glycine* Semen (2.778 g), and *Eucommiae* Cortex (1.389 g), was powdered and boiled for 3 h in distilled water (1 L). The mixture was then subjected to ultrafiltration through Whatman grade 2 qualitative filter paper (GE Healthcare Life Sciences, Marlborough, MA, USA) to exclude components with molecular weights above 10,000. The resulting filtrate was lyophilized to a powder using a rotary evaporator (Eyela, Miyagi, Japan), and stored at 4 °C until use. SHINBARO was administered intra-articularly at a dose of 2, 10, or 20 mg/kg in saline and orally at a dose of 20 or 200 mg/kg in saline. The same volume of saline was used as a vehicle in control rats. The validation of SHINBARO was performed by high-performance liquid chromatography (Waters™ 600 s controller, 626 pump, temperature control module, in-line degasser, 717 plus autosampler, and 996 photodiode array detector; Waters, Bedford, MA, USA) analysis of each ingredient extract using the following six indicator biological components [18]: cimifugin for *Ledebouriellae* Radix; 20-hydroxyecdysone (0.311–0.312 mg/g) for *Achyranthis* Radix; acanthoside D (0.577–0.578 mg/g) for *Acanthopanacis* Cortex; onitin-4-O-β-D-glucopyranoside for *Cibotii* Rhizoma; genistin (0.0426–0.0427 mg/g) for *Glycine* Semen; and geniposide (0.431–0.432 mg/g) for *Eucommiae* Cortex. SHINBARO was further standardized for quality control according to the regulations imposed by the Korea Food and Drug Administration.

Animals

Male Sprague–Dawley rats (200–220 g) were obtained from Central Laboratory Animal Inc. (Seoul, Korea), and housed in solid-bottom cages with free access to food and water. The temperature was maintained to 22 ± 2 °C, and a 12-h/12-h light/dark schedule was implemented. Prior to use, the animals were allowed 1 week for acclimatization within the work area environment. All animal experiments were approved by the local Animal Ethics Committee of Seoul National University (Additional file 1), and carried out in accordance with the Institutional Animal Care and Use Committee Guidelines of Seoul National University (Permission Number: SNU-120904-7) and the ARRIVE guideline (Additional files 2 and 3).

MIA-induced OA rat model

Rats were anesthetized with diethyl ether and given a single intra-articular injection of 2.5 mg MIA

(Sigma–Aldrich, St. Louis, MO, USA) into the infrapatellar ligament of the right knee [20]. MIA was dissolved in 0.9 % normal saline and administered in a 25-μL volume. The rats were arbitrarily divided into eight groups containing six rats each. Subsequently, the rats were treated with normal saline (vehicle-treated MIA group), 2, 10, or 20 mg/kg of SHINBARO by intra-articular administration (intra-articular SHINBARO group; IAS group), 20 or 200 mg/kg of SHINBARO by oral administration (oral SHINBARO group; OS group), and 5 mg/kg of diclofenac by oral administration (diclofenac group) once daily for 21 days. Rats treated with normal saline, and not MIA, were used as a control group (Table 1). The SHINBARO concentrations and MIA injection volume were selected based on previous evaluations [21]. After 21 days of treatment, the animals were euthanized and blood samples were collected for serum isolation. The femurs were dissected and stripped of soft tissue for analysis of the trabecular microarchitecture.

Morphological analysis of bone loss

The bone microarchitecture of the femur in the region at 0.6–2.1 mm from the growth plate was scanned using a micro-computed tomography (micro-CT) system (SkyScan 1076; SkyScan, Aartselaar, Belgium). The X-ray source was set at a voltage of 50 kV and a current of 200 μA and filtered with a 0.5-mm aluminum filter. The scanning angular rotation was 180° with an angular step of 0.5°. The voxel size was fixed at 8.9 μm. The morphometric indices of the bone region were determined from the micro-CT data on 3D images using CTan software (SkyScan 1076; SkyScan, Aartselaar, Belgium). The following measures characterizing the three-dimensional structure of the trabecular bone were determined: bone volume of interest (BV; μm^3); bone volume fraction (bone volume/total volume (BV/TV); %); and mean number of objects per slice (Obj.N). BV indicates the total volume of extracted cartilage from the same parts in each group. The ratio of BV/TV is the segmented trabecular bone volume to total tissue volume. Obj.N implies the connectivity of the specimens, which consisted of several cross-sectional slices of cartilage in a three-dimensional structure.

Histopathological analysis

The right knee joints from the tibia to the distal metatarsal including the tarsal joint were resected and fixed with 10 % neutral-buffered formalin for 24 h at 4 °C. The fixed specimens were decalcified with 20 % formic acid for 3 days and embedded in paraffin. Sections of the tissue specimens were acquired from the paraffin blocks at 5 μm thickness, deparaffinized, and rehydrated in the order of xylene, absolute alcohol, and 50 % alcohol. The rehydrated sections were stained with hematoxylin and eosin (H&E) for observation of morphological changes in the articular tissues and safranin-O fast green (SOFG) for evaluation of the proteoglycan (PG) contents.

Measurement of prostaglandin E_2 (PGE_2) level

The serum PGE_2 levels were measured by enzyme immunoassay (EIA) using a prostaglandin E metabolite EIA kit (Cayman Chemical Company, Ann Arbor, MI, USA). Briefly, aliquots of prepared standard solutions and sample sera were plated in 96-well plates from the PGE_2 EIA kit, and a PGE_2-acetylcholinesterase (AChE) conjugate (PGE Tracer) and PGE_2 monoclonal antibody solution were added and allowed to react at 4 °C for 24 h. Next, Ellman's reagent, which contains an AChE substrate for color formation, was added to the wells and the optical density was measured at 412 nm (VersaMax ELISA Microplate Reader; Molecular Devices, Sunnyvale, CA, USA). The PGE_2 concentrations in the serum samples were determined using a four-parameter logistic equation ($\mathrm{logit}(B/B_0) = \ln[B/B_0/(1-B/B_0)]$) by comparisons with the absorbances of the PGE_2 standard solutions at several concentrations (8, 16, 31, 62, 125, 250, 500, and 1000 pg/mL).

Table 1 Effect of SHINBARO on change in body weight of MIA-induced OA rat model

Days after treatment	Control	MIA						
		Vehicle	Intra-articular SHINBARO (mg/kg)			Oral SHINBARO (mg/kg)		Diclofenac (5 mg/kg)
			2	10	20	20	200	
0th	305.5 ± 7.9	308.1 ± 20.4	301.2 ± 17.1	305.5 ± 11.8	306.2 ± 11.8	306.2 ± 14.5	306.0 ± 16.2	288.0 ± 13.9
7th	352.9 ± 11.6	347.6 ± 14.2	335.0 ± 14.5	352.2 ± 15.0	347.2 ± 10.7	347.3 ± 11.7	351.2 ± 12.7	317.8 ± 32.0
14th	384.5 ± 9.5	378.6 ± 17.1	365.2 ± 16.1	387.8 ± 14.1	379.3 ± 11.5	376.2 ± 11.4	387.0 ± 11.7	356.0 ± 15.5
21st	411.5 ± 15.2	402.0 ± 16.3	385.5 ± 19.7	411.5 ± 15.5	401.3 ± 12.0	395.8 ± 17.3	407.8 ± 13.1	388.5 ± 9.05

SHINBARO or diclofenac was treated daily for 21 days after 2 weeks of OA induction by intra-articular injection of MIA. Body weight was measured once every 7 days after treatment of samples. Data represent as the mean ± SD (n = 6)

Measurement of anti-type II collagen antibody level

The serum anti-type II collagen antibody levels were assayed using a rat anti-type I and type II collagen IgG ELISA kit (Chondrex Inc., Redmond, WA, USA) in accordance with the manufacturer's instructions.

Ex vivo biochemical analysis of inflamed tissues

The right knee joint cartilages of the rats were removed at the end of the treatment period. The tissues were homogenized using Nuclear Extract Kit (Active Motif, Carlsbad, CA, USA) in accordance with the manufacturer's instructions. The protein levels of inflammatory enzymes (iNOS, COX-2), pro-inflammatory cytokines (tumor necrosis factor (TNF)-α, interleukin (IL)-1β), and inflammatory mediators (NF-κB, nuclear factor of κ light polypeptide gene enhancer in B-cells inhibitor (IκB)) in the cartilaginous tissues were determined by western blot analysis.

Western blot analysis

The proteins in the rat articular cartilage samples were resolved by 6–15 % sodium dodecyl sulfate–polyacrylamide gel electrophoresis (SDS-PAGE) and transferred onto PVDF membranes (Millipore, Bedford, MA, USA). The membranes were blocked with blocking buffer, comprising 5 % bovine serum albumin in phosphate-buffered saline containing 0.1 % Tween-20 (PBST), for 1 h at room temperature. After three washes with PBST, the membranes were incubated with primary antibodies against β-actin (1:1000), iNOS (1:1000), COX-2 (1:1000), IL-1β (1:1000), NF-κB (1:500), IκB-α (1:200) (Santa Cruz Biotechnology, Santa Cruz, CA, USA) and TNF-α (1:1000) (Cell Signaling, Danvers, MA, USA) diluted in 2.5 % bovine serum albumin overnight at 4 °C. The membranes were washed three times with PBST and incubated with corresponding secondary antibodies diluted in PBST (1:1000) for 2 h at room temperature. After three washes with PBST, the membranes were visualized with a WEST-ZOL plus Western Blot Detection System (Intron Biotechnology, Sungnam, Korea), and analyzed using an LAS 4000 system (Fuji Film Corp., Tokyo, Japan).

Statistical analysis

All experiments were repeated at least three times. Data were presented as means ± standard derivation for the indicated numbers of independently performed experiments. Statistical significance was assessed by one-way analysis of variance coupled with a Dunnett's *t* test. Values of $P < 0.05$ were considered statistically significant. All statistical analyses were performed using Graph Pad Prism 5.0 for Windows (GraphPad Software, La Jolla, CA, USA).

Results

Body weight changes

Changes in body weight were monitored during administration of SHINBARO or diclofenac and measured on days 0, 7, 14, and 21 as evaluation parameters for the courses of stress and toxicity in the animals. The body weight in the vehicle-treated MIA group increased at a similar rate to that in the control group (Table 1). In addition, the IAS group, OS group, and diclofenac group did not show any significant differences compared with the vehicle-treated MIA groups. No overt toxicity was observed in the IAS and OS groups compared with the vehicle-treated control groups.

Morphological analysis of bone loss

The destruction of the trabecular bone in the femur was observed by three-dimensional micro-CT to determine the effects of SHINBARO on the trabecular bone microarchitecture. As shown in Fig. 1, MIA caused significant deterioration of the trabecular bone architecture compared with the control group. However, IAS or OS treatment delayed or recovered the destruction of the trabecular bone in the MIA-induced OA model. Protective activity was also observed for oral treatment of diclofenac, a positive control, under the same experimental conditions. In addition, the bone microstructural index parameters were measured using NRrecon software (Fig. 2). The BV of the trabecular bone in the femur was clearly decreased in the vehicle-treated MIA group by 22.4 % ($P = 0.0042$) compared with the control group. However, IAS (20 mg/kg) treatment remarkably restrained the decrease in BV ($P = 0.0045$), being 40 % higher than that in the vehicle-treated MIA group. The BV of the trabecular bone in the femur was alleviated by IAS in a dose-dependent manner and recovered to almost the same level as the control group. Diclofenac treatment insignificantly increased the BV of the trabecular bone in the femur by 13.8 % in the MIA-induced OA model ($P = 0.053$). In addition, BV/TV was decreased in the vehicle-treated MIA group (22.9 %, $P = 0.0089$) compared with the control group. IAS (2, 10, and 20 mg/kg) treatment effectively recovered the BV/TV values in a dose-dependent manner with increased percentages of 9.2 % ($P = 0.015$), 19.2 % ($P = 0.001$), and 28.1 % ($P = 0.0001$), respectively, compared with the vehicle-treated MIA group, while diclofenac exhibited an increase of 7.7 % in BV/TV. Obj.N was markedly reduced in the vehicle-treated MIA group (30.4 %, $P = 0.0063$) compared with the control group, and IAS (2, 10, and 20 mg/kg) treatment significantly recovered the Obj.N values with increased percentage changes of 13.5 % ($P = 0.147$), 27.5 % ($P = 0.028$), and 44.5 % ($P = 0.031$),

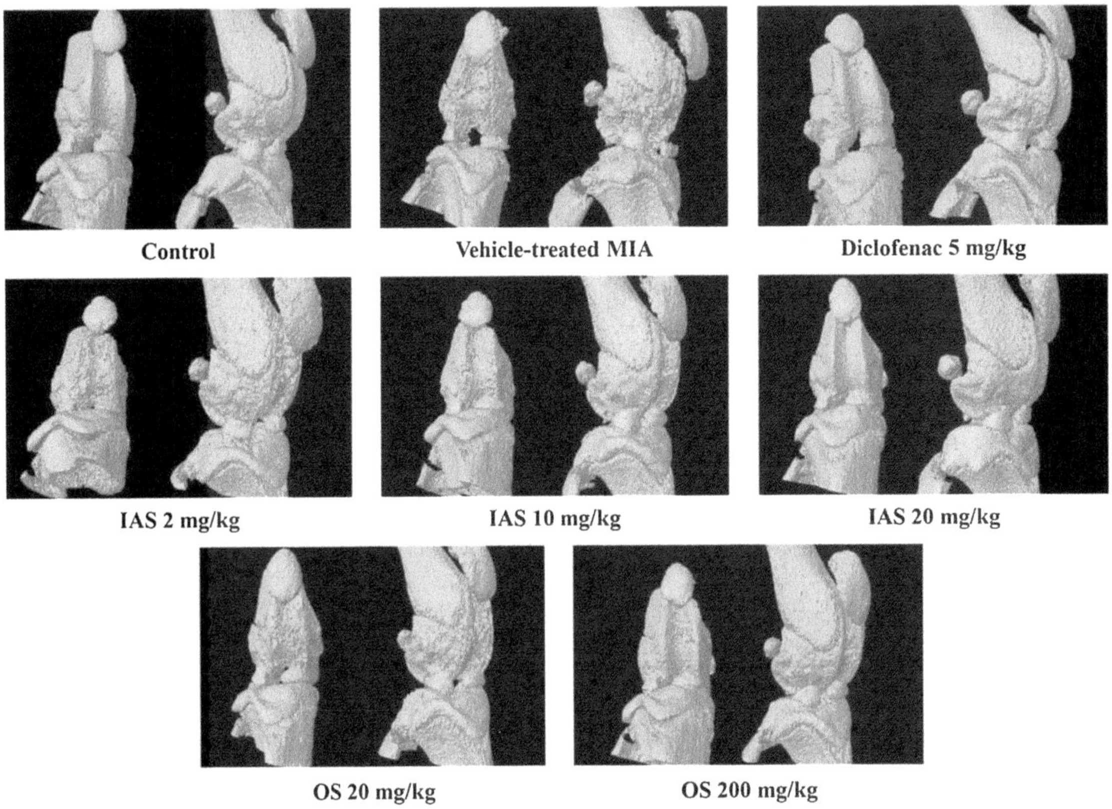

Fig. 1 Roentgenograph analysis of the knee joint after treatment of SHINBARO in MIA-induced OA rat model. Micro-cartilage and patellae of the normal and experimental animals were scanned with microCT (Skyscan1076). Data represent as the mean ± SD (n = 6). *IAS* intra-articular SHINBARO, *OS* oral SHINBARO

respectively, compared with the vehicle-treated MIA group. The diclofenac group also exhibited recovery of Obj.N with an increased percentage change of 18.0 % ($P = 0.095$) compared with the vehicle-treated MIA group. OS (20 or 200 mg/kg) treatment also improved the damage to the cartilage with increased percentage changes of 7.7 % ($P = 0.405$) and 35.3 % ($P = 0.013$), respectively, but the activity was relatively low compared with that of IAS treatment.

Histopathological analysis

We performed H&E staining for the articular cartilage surfaces of the femoral condyle and tibial plateau to determine whether IAS treatment restored the damaged surface of the knee joint toward healing. The vehicle-treated MIA group revealed severe irregular abrasions with rough edges around the femur and tibia, indicative of bone lysis, swelling, and tendency for patellar displacement (Fig. 3). This damage was significantly attenuated with the appearance of smoother articular cartilage surfaces by IAS (20 mg/kg) treatment. MIA-induced articular cartilage damage was also restored in the positive control group treated with diclofenac. SOFG staining, which stains PGs and is indicative of the degree of degeneration of cartilaginous tissue [22], was performed to observe the changes in morphology of the cartilaginous tissues. The SOFG-stained control group exhibited normal cartilage PG staining, while the vehicle-treated MIA group revealed severely damaged cartilage with marked fibrillation and PG depletion. Treatment with SHINBARO or diclofenac significantly suppressed the MIA-induced loss of PG and prevented cartilage damage (Fig. 3).

Analysis of biomarkers in serum

The effects of IAS treatment on inflammatory biomarkers were determined using serum prepared from blood samples collected in the MIA-induced OA rat model. The serum PGE_2 level in the MIA-treated group was significantly increased by 67.8 % ($P = 0.0045$) compared with the control group (Fig. 4a). IAS (20 mg/kg) treatment markedly inhibited the elevated serum PGE_2 level by 60.6 % ($P = 0.0007$) compared with the vehicle-treated MIA group. The serum PGE_2 level in the diclofenac group was inhibited by 59.5 % ($P = 0.0012$) under the same experimental conditions. Furthermore, the serum level of

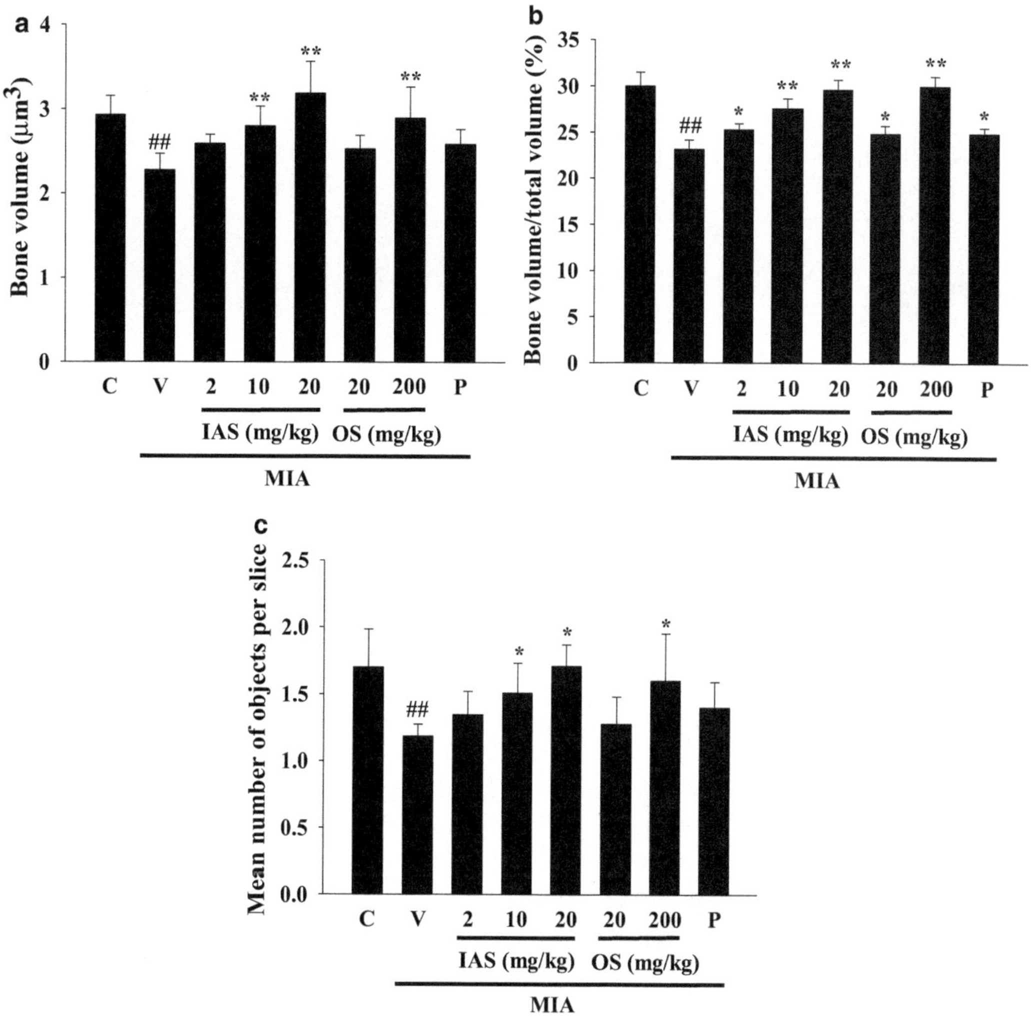

Fig. 2 Effect of SHINBARO on the bone morphometric parameters in MIA-induced OA rat model. The bone morphometric parameters including BV (**a**), BV/TV (**b**), and Obj.N (**c**) were analyzed with micro-CT SkyScan CTAN software. Data represent the mean ± SD ($n = 6$). $^{*}P < 0.05$ and $^{**}P < 0.01$ indicate statistically significant differences from the vehicle-treated MIA group. $^{\#\#}P < 0.01$ indicates statistically significant differences from the control group. *C* control group, *V* vehicle-treated MIA group, *IAS* intra-articular SHINBARO group, *OS* oral SHINBARO group, *P* positive control group (Diclofenac 5 mg/kg)

anti-type II collagen antibodies, which are responsible for activation of oxidative stress with the formation of peroxynitrite ($ONOO^-$) [7], was increased in the MIA-treated group, while IAS treatment significantly decreased the anti-type II collagen antibody level in a dose-dependent manner (Fig. 4b).

Analysis of biomarkers in cartilaginous tissue

The effects of IAS treatment on the protein expression levels of inflammation-mediated enzymes, such as iNOS and COX-2, were determined in the MIA-induced OA rat model to determine the mechanism of action of IAS treatment on the inhibition of inflammatory biomarker production. Overproduction of NO and PGE_2 is concomitant with overexpression of iNOS and COX-2, leading to swelling, irritation, and pain [23]. MIA treatment induced overexpression of iNOS and COX-2 in the cartilaginous tissues, while IAS (20 mg/kg) or OS (200 mg/kg) treatment effectively suppressed the induction of iNOS and COX-2 expression (Fig. 5).

iNOS and COX-2 expression are regulated by NF-κB [24]. NF-κB is composed of p65/p50 subunits and exists in the cytosol as inactive heterodimers bound to the inhibitory protein IκB-α. IκB-α stimulated by pro-inflammatory signals is phosphorylated by IκB kinase and degraded by a 26S proteasome-mediated pathway to facilitate translocation of NF-κB into the nucleus and regulate the transcription of iNOS and COX-2 [25]. MIA

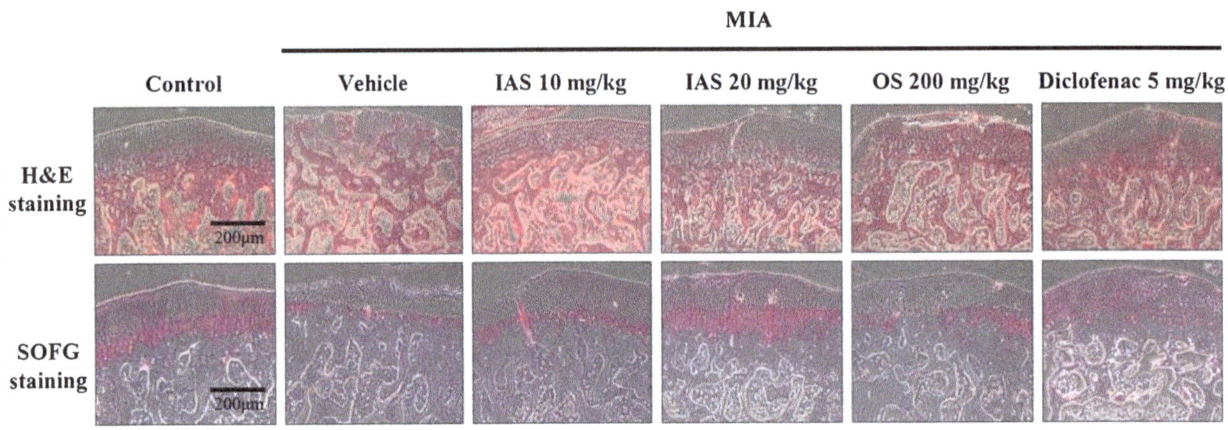

Fig. 3 Histopathological analysis of the knee joint tissues after treatment of SHINBARO in MIA-induced OA rat model. The knee joint tissues from MIA-induced OA rat model which was treated with vehicle, SHINBARO or diclofenac were stained with hematoxylin and eosin (H&E) and Safranin O-fast green (SOFG) (magnification ×100)

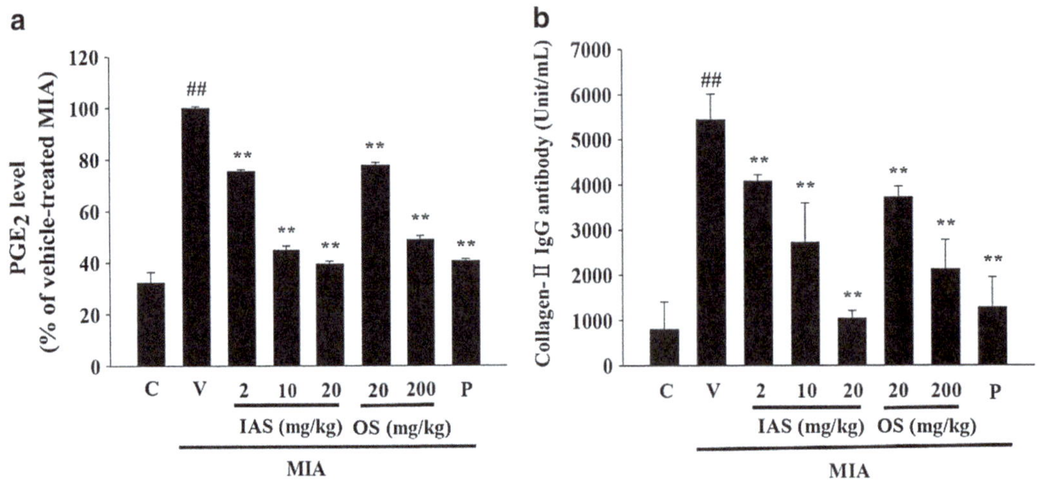

Fig. 4 Effect of SHINBARO on the serum levels of prostaglandin E_2 and collage-II antibody in MIA-induced OA rat model. Data represent the mean ± SD (n = 6). *$P < 0.05$ and **$P < 0.01$ indicate statistically significant differences from the vehicle-treated MIA group. ##$P < 0.01$ indicates statistically significant differences from the control group. *C* control group, *V* vehicle-treated MIA group, *IAS* intra-articular SHINBARO group, *OS* oral SHINBARO group, *P* positive control group (Diclofenac 5 mg/kg)

treatment upregulated the nuclear protein levels of the NF-κB subunits (p65 and p50), while IAS treatment suppressed these biomarker expression levels, especially that of the p50 subunit (Fig. 6). In addition, the protein expression of IκB-α was downregulated in the vehicle-treated MIA group compared with the control group, while IAS treatment increased the IκB-α level in the MIA-induced OA rat model. IAS treatment might inhibit the inflammatory responses through suppression of MIA-induced NF-κB activation.

Further studies were conducted to correlate the anti-inflammatory effects of IAS treatment with the regulation of expression of pro-inflammatory cytokines. The effects of IAS treatment on the expression levels of these pro-inflammatory cytokines were investigated in the MIA-induced OA rat model. The protein levels of TNF-α and IL-1β revealed overexpression in the MIA-treated group compared with the control group, while IAS treatment suppressed the elevated expression levels of TNF-α and IL-1β in the cartilaginous tissues of the MIA-induced OA rat model (Fig. 6). Therefore, IAS treatment inhibited the inflammatory response through blockade of the expression of pro-inflammatory cytokines, such as TNF-α and IL-1β.

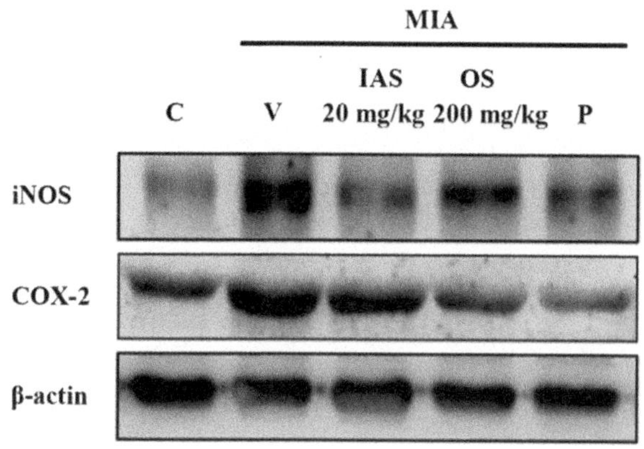

Fig. 5 Effect of SHINBARO on the protein levels of iNOS and COX-2 in cartilage from the knee joint after treatment of SHINBARO in MIA-induced OA rat model. The expressions of iNOS and COX-2 in the extracted cartilage tissues were determined by western blot analysis as described in the "Methods" section. Data were representative of three separate experiments. β-actin was used as an internal standard. *C* control group, *V* vehicle-treated MIA group, *IAS* intra-articular SHINBARO group, *OS* oral SHINBARO group, *P* positive control group (Diclofenac 5 mg/kg)

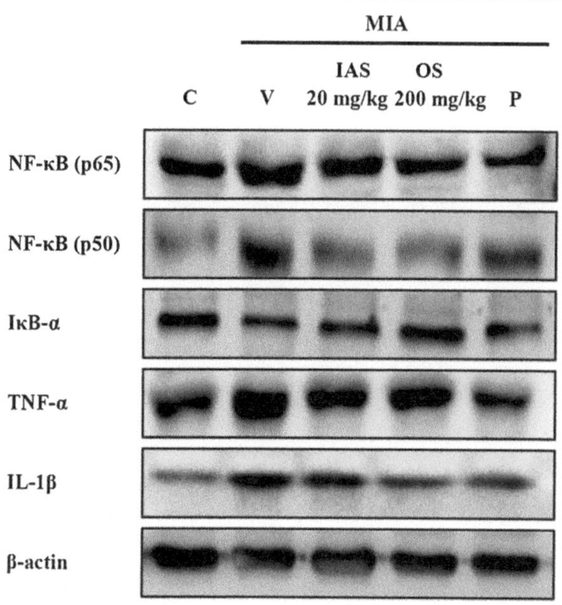

Fig. 6 Effect of SHINBARO on the protein levels of NF-κB, IκB-α, TNF-α and IL-1β in cartilage from the knee joint after treatment of SHINBARO in MIA-induced OA rat model. The expressions of NF-κB, IκB-α, TNF-α and IL-1β in the extracted cartilage tissues were determined by Western blot analysis as described in the "Methods" section. Data were representative of three separate experiments. β-actin was used as an internal standard. *C* control group, *V* vehicle-treated MIA group, *IAS* intra-articular SHINBARO group, *OS* oral SHINBARO group, *P* positive control group (Diclofenac 5 mg/kg)

Discussion

OA is a degenerative knee joint disease that causes intense pain and functional disability [26]. The disease is classified into two categories: primary or idiopathic arthritis that involves endocrinologic, genetic, and nutritional factors and secondary or subsequent arthritis that is incurred by injury, disorder, and malformation capable of causing damage to the articular cartilage [27, 28].

Although anti-inflammatory effects of OS treatment were previously reported [29], the pharmacological effects of IAS treatment, which is already practiced in clinical settings, and its underlying mechanisms of action remain to be determined. Therefore, the present study was conducted to investigate the anti-inflammatory activity of IAS treatment and its underlying mechanisms of action in the MIA-induced OA rat model.

The MIA used in the present study inhibits articular cartilage structural incorporation through suppression of GAPDH activity in the cartilage, leading to histopathological and pathomorphologic changes in the articular cartilage [30]. SHINBARO prevented the degeneration of the trabecular bone microarchitecture in the distal femur of the rat. IAS treatment also markedly restored bone loss in the MIA-induced OA model (Fig. 1). These data were supported by the protective effect of IAS treatment on the bone morphometric parameters (Fig. 2). In addition, no significant body changes or obvious toxicity were found in the IAS group (Table 1). These results indicated that IAS treatment not only preserves the bone mass, but also recovers the bone microstructural deterioration associated with MIA-induced OA without toxicity.

Healthy cartilage tends to maintain a balance between synthesis and degradation of extracellular matrix (ECM) components, such as PGs and type II collagen. However, the decomposition of the ECM becomes increased in inflamed cartilage, leading to an off-balance of matrix production and damage to the cartilaginous tissues [31]. The H&E and SOFG staining in the vehicle-treated MIA group revealed significant PG loss and lesion development, and confirmed that the cartilage injury was attenuated by IAS treatment (Fig. 3). In addition, IAS treatment markedly reduced the elevated serum level of anti-type II collagen antibodies associated with MIA in a dose-dependent manner (Fig. 4b). These findings indicate that IAS treatment might delay bone loss through decreased bone turnover.

Major biomarkers for inflammation responses were determined in serum to further confirm the effects of IAS treatment on the regulation of inflammatory responses. PGE_2 acts as an important inflammatory mediator and is a major product of COX activity, which functions pathologically in inflammatory, autoimmune, and neoplastic diseases [32]. In this study, the serum PGE_2 level was significantly higher in the vehicle-treated MIA group compared with the control group, while IAS treatment inhibited the elevation of PGE_2 production in the MIA-induced OA rat model (Fig. 4a).

Overproduction of PGE_2 is highly associated with overexpression of iNOS and COX-2 in inflammatory responses [33]. The effects of IAS on iNOS and COX-2 protein expression levels were determined to investigate the mechanism responsible for the inhibition of PGE_2 production mediated by IAS treatment. IAS suppressed the MIA-induced overexpression of iNOS and COX-2 protein levels in a dose-dependent manner (Fig. 5).

We further examined whether IAS treatment regulates the protein expression levels of upstream mediators leading to the production of iNOS and COX-2. NF-κB exists in the cytosol of cells as an inactive heterodimer bound to the inhibitory protein IκB with Rel A (p65), c-Rel, RelB, NF-κB1 (p50/150), and NF-κB2 (p52/100) [34]. However, NF-κB becomes degraded with IκB sequestration when inflammatory cytokines, TNFs, and lymphotoxins are activated by stimuli, such as mitogens, bacteria, ultraviolet light, oxidants, tetradecanoyl phorbol-13-acetate, ionizing radiation, and phosphatase inhibitors [35–37]. The activated heterodimers of NF-κB subunits p65 and p50 in the cytosol translocate into the nucleus and bind to NF-κB-binding sites in gene promoters or enhancers, thereby inducing the transcription of downstream target genes, such as cytokines, cytokine receptors, cell adhesion molecules, and growth factors. IκB is negatively regulated by phosphorylation on serine residues, which is controlled by two IκB kinases, IKKα and IKKβ [38]. In the present study, IAS treatment downregulated the protein level of NF-κB and upregulated the protein level of IκB (Fig. 6). These findings suggest that the anti-inflammatory effects of IAS treatment are associated with inhibition of NF-κB activation.

The anti-inflammatory effects of IAS treatment were also observed by measurements of the protein expression levels of pro-inflammatory cytokines, such as TNF-α and IL-1β. These cytokines promote the catabolic processes in OA, causing cartilage degradation. MIA can drive the overexpression of pro-inflammatory cytokines, but the TNF-α and IL-1β levels were effectively reduced by IAS treatment in the MIA-induced OA model (Fig. 6). These data suggest that IAS treatment inhibits inflammatory responses by suppressing the expression of pro-inflammatory cytokines, including TNF-α and IL-1β.

Conclusion

SHINBARO inhibited PGE_2 and anti-type II collagen antibody production and modulated the balance of inflammatory enzymes, mediators, and cytokines in the MIA-induced OA rat model.

Abbreviations

MIA: monosodium iodoacetate; OA: osteoarthritis; H&E: hematoxylin and eosin; SOFG: safranin-O fast green; PGE_2: prostaglandin E_2; iNOS: inducible nitric oxide synthase; COX-2: cyclooxygenase-2; TNF-α: tumor necrosis factor-α; IL-1β: interlukin-1β; NF-κB: nuclear factor-κB; IκB: inhibitory protein κB; LPS: lipopolysaccharide; GADPH: glyceraldehyde-3-phosphate dehydrogenase; IAS: intra-articular SHINBARO; OS: oral SHINBARO; BV: bone volume of interest; Obj.N: mean number of objects per slice; EIA: enzyme immunoassay; AChE: acetylcholinesterase; PG: proteoglycan; NSAIDs: non-steroidal anti-inflammatory drugs; ECM: extracellular matrix; IKK: IκB kinase.

Authors' contributions

WKK, HJC, JSS, JHL, IHH and SKL conceived and designed the study. WKK, HJC, YP and TJC performed the experiments. WKK, SKL, HJP and JYH wrote and revised the manuscript. All authors read and approved the final manuscript.

Author details

[1] College of Pharmacy, Seoul National University, Seoul 151-742, Republic of Korea. [2] Jaseng Spine and Joint Research Institute, Jaseng Medical Foundation, Seoul 135-896, Republic of Korea.

Acknowledgements

This work was supported by a Grant from the JASENG Hospital of Oriental Medicine (JS-2010-1).

Competing interests

The authors declare that they have no competing interests.

References

1. Goldring MB, Goldring SR. Osteoarthritis. J Cell Physiol. 2007;213:626–34.
2. Brook I. Microbiology and management of joint and bone infections due to anaerobic bacteria. J Orthop Sci. 2008;13:160–9.
3. Finckh A, Turesson C. The impact of obesity on the development and progression of rheumatoid arthritis. Ann Rheum Dis. 2014;73:1911–3.
4. Gladman DD, Antoni C, Mease P, Clegg DO, Nash P. Psoriatic arthritis: epidemiology, clinical features, course, and outcome. Ann Rheum Dis. 2005;64:14–7.
5. Ranganath VK, Elashoff DA, Khanna D, Park G, Peter JB, Paulus HE. Age adjustment corrects for apparent differences in erythrocyte sedimentation rate and C-reactive protein values at the onset of seropositive rheumatoid arthritis in younger and older patients. J Rheumatol. 2005;32:1040–2.
6. Roemer FW, Guermazi A, Javaid MK, Lynch JA, Niu J, Zhang Y, Felson DT, Lewis CE, Torner J, Nevitt MC. Change in MRI-detected subchondral bone marrow lesions is associated with cartilage loss: the MOST Study. A longitudinal multicentre study of knee osteoarthritis. Ann Rheum Dis. 2009;68:1461–5.
7. Deberg M, Labasse A, Christgau S, Cloos P, Bang Henriksen D, Chapelle JP, Zegels B, Reginster JY, Henrotin Y. New serum biochemical markers (Coll 2-1 and Coll 2-1 NO_2) for studying oxidative-related type II collagen network degradation in patients with osteoarthritis and rheumatoid arthritis. Osteoarthr Cartil. 2005;13:258–65.

8. Lillegraven S, van der Heijde D, Uhlig T, Kvien TK, Haavardsholm EA. What is the clinical relevance of erosions and joint space narrowing in RA? Nat Rev Rheumatol. 2012;8:117–20.
9. William GB, Justus JF, James IM, William WZ, Shawn SY, Emmett MW, Richard CH, Peter CI, Kenneth MV, Geis GS. Treatment of osteoarthritis with celecoxib, a cyclooxygenase-2 inhibitor: a randomized controlled trial. Mayo Clin Proc. 1999;74:1095–105.
10. Pelletier JP, Jovanovic D, Fernandes JC, Manning P, Connor JR, Currie MG, Di Battista JA, Martel-Pelletier J. Reduced progression of experimental osteoarthritis in vivo by selective inhibition of inducible nitric oxide synthase. Arthritis Rheum. 1998;41:1275–86.
11. Barve RA, Minnerly JC, Weiss DJ, Meyer DM, Aguiar DJ, Sullivan PM, Weinrich SL, Head RD. Transcriptional profiling and pathway analysis of monosodium iodoacetate-induced experimental osteoarthritis in rats: relevance to human disease. Osteoarthr Cartil. 2007;15:1190–8.
12. Dumond H, Presle N, Pottie P, Pacquelet S, Terlain B, Netter P, Gepstein A, Livne E, Jouzeau JY. Site specific changes in gene expression and cartilage metabolism during early experimental osteoarthritis. Osteoarthr Cartil. 2004;12:284–95.
13. Smith HS. Potential analgesic mechanisms of acetaminophen. Pain Physician. 2009;12:269–80.
14. Silverstein FE, Faich G, Goldstein JL, Simon LS, Pincus T, Whelton A, Makuch R, Eisen G, Agrawal NM, Stenson WF, Burr AM, Zhao WW, Kent JD, Lefkowith JB, Verburg KM, Geis GS. Gastrointestinal toxicity with celecoxib vs nonsteroidal anti-inflammatory drugs for osteoarthritis and rheumatoid arthritis: the CLASS study: a randomized controlled trial. Celecoxib long-term arthritis safety study. Jama. 2000;284:1247–55.
15. Kobayashi K, Imaizumi R, Sumichika H, Tanaka H, Goda M, Fukunari A, Komatsu H. Sodium iodoacetate-induced experimental osteoarthritis and associated pain model in rats. J Vet Med Sci. 2003;65:1195–9.
16. Dunham J, Hoedt-Schmidt S, Kalbhen DA. Prolonged effect of iodoacetate on articular cartilage and its modification by an anti-rheumatic drug. Int J Exp Pathol. 1993;74:283–9.
17. Kim JS, Kroin JS, Buvanendran A, Li X, van Wijnen AJ, Tuman KJ, Im HJ. Characterization of a new animal model for evaluation and treatment of back pain due to lumbar facet joint osteoarthritis. Arthritis Rheum. 2011;63:2966–73.
18. Lee SY, Kwon HK, Lee SM. SHINBARO, a new herbal medicine with multifunctional mechanism for joint disease: first therapeutic application for the treatment of osteoarthritis. Arch Pharm Res. 2011;34:1773–7.
19. Chang IA, Namgung U. Induction of regenerative responses of injured sciatic nerve by pharmacopuncture therapy in rats. J Acupunct Meridian Stud. 2013;6:89–97.
20. Bove SE, Calcaterra SL, Brooker RM, Huber CM, Guzman RE, Juneau PL, Schrier DJ, Kilqore KS. Weight bearing as a measure of disease progression and efficacy of anti-inflammatory compounds in a model of monosodium iodoacetate-induced osteoarthritis. Osteoarthr Cartil. 2003;11:821–30.
21. Kim SH, Lee CH, Lee JS, Cho KH, Kim SO, Cho SH, Cho HK, Lee SM. Anti-inflammatory activities of a herbal preparation GCSB-5 on acute and chronic inflammation. Kor J Pharmacogn. 2005;36:311–7.
22. Choi JH, Choi JH, Kim DY, Yoon JH, Youn HY, Yi JB, Rhee HI, Ryu KH, Jung K, Han CK, Kwak WJ, Cho YB. Effects of SKI 306X, a new herbal agent, on proteoglycan degradation in cartilage explant culture and collagenase-induced rabbit osteoarthritis model. Osteoarthr Cartil. 2002;10:471–8.
23. Shinmura K, Xuan YT, Tang XL, Kodani E, Han H, Zhu Y, Bolli R. Inducible nitric oxide synthase modulates cyclooxygenase-2 activity in the heart of conscious rabbits during the late phase of ischemic preconditioning. Circ Res. 2002;90:602–8.
24. Burmester GR, Stuhlmuller B, Keyszer G, Kinne RW. Mononuclear phagocytes and rheumatoid synovitis. Mastermind or workhorse in arthritis? Arthritis Rheum. 1997;40:5–18.
25. Bresnihan B. Pathogenesis of joint damage in rheumatoid arthritis. J Rheumatol. 1999;26:717–9.
26. Krasnokutsky S, Attur M, Palmer G, Samuels J, Abramson SB. Current concepts in the pathogenesis of osteoarthritis. Osteoarthr Cartil. 2008;16:1–3.
27. Siemons L, Ten Klooster PM, Vonkeman HE, van Riel PL, Glas CA, van de Laar MA. How age and sex affect the erythrocyte sedimentation rate and C-reactive protein in early rheumatoid arthritis. BMC Musculoskelet Disord. 2014;15:368.
28. Kimura Y, Seichi A, Gomi A, Kojima M, Inoue H, Kimura A. Acquired Chiari malformation secondary to atlantoaxial vertical subluxation in a patient with rheumatoid arthritis combined with atlanto-occipital assimilation. Neurol Med Chir (Tokyo). 2012;52:683–6.
29. Kim JK, Park SW, Kang JW, Kim YJ, Lee SY, Shin J, Lee S, See SM. Effect of GCSB-5, a herbal formulation, on monosodium iodoacetate-induced osteoarthritis in Rats. Evid Based Complement Alternat Med. 2012;. doi:10.1155/2012/730907.
30. Janusz MJ, Hookfin EB, Heitmeyer SA, Woessner JF, Freemont AJ, Hoyland JA, Brown KK, Hsieh LC, Almstead NG, De B, Natchus MG, Pikul S, Taiwo YO. Moderation of iodoacetate-induced experimental osteoarthritis in rats by matrix metalloproteinase inhibitors. Osteoarthr Cartil. 2001;9:751–60.
31. Sandy JD, Brown HL, Lowther DA. Degradation of proteoglycan in articular cartilage. Biochim Biophys Acta. 1978;543:536–44.
32. Steven BA, Mukundan A, Ashok RA, Robert C. The overproduction of PGE2 is highly associated with the overexpression of iNOS and COX-2 in inflammatory response. Curr Rheumatol Rep. 2001;3:535–41.
33. Jia XY, Chang Y, Sun XJ, Dai X, Wei W. The role of prostaglandin E_2 receptor signaling of dendritic cells in rheumatoid arthritis. Int Immunopharmacol. 2014;23:163–9.
34. Urban MB, Schreck R, Baeuerle PA. NF-kappa B contacts DNA by a heterodimer of the p50 and p65 subunit. EMBO J. 1991;10:1817–25.
35. Hansen SK, Nerlov C, Zabel U, Verde P, Johnsen M, Baeuerle PA, Blasi F. A novel complex between the p65 subunit of NF-kappa B and c-Rel binds to a DNA element involved in the phorbol ester induction of the human urokinase gene. EMBO J. 1992;11:205–13.
36. Sun SC, Maggirwar SB, Harhaj E. Activation of NF-kappa B by phosphatase inhibitors involves the phosphorylation of I kappa B alpha at phosphatase 2A-sensitive sites. J Biol Chem. 1995;270:18347–51.
37. Traenckner EB, Pahl HL, Henkel T, Schmidt KN, Wilk S, Baeuerle PA. Phosphorylation of human I kappa B-alpha on serines 32 and 36 controls I kappa B-alpha proteolysis and NF-kappa B activation in response to diverse stimuli. EMBO J. 1995;14:2876–83.
38. Strayhorn WD, Wadzinski BE. A novel in vitro assay for deubiquitination of I kappa B alpha. Arch Biochem Biophys. 2002;400:76–84.

12

Acupuncture as an intervention to reduce alcohol dependency

Charlotte Southern[1], Charlie Lloyd[1], Jianping Liu[2], Congcong Wang[2], Tingting Zhang[1], Martin Bland[1] and Hugh MacPherson[1*]

Abstract

Background: Acupuncture has been widely used as a treatment for alcohol dependence. An updated and rigorously conducted systematic review is needed to establish the extent and quality of the evidence on the effectiveness of acupuncture as an intervention for reducing alcohol dependence. This review aimed to ascertain the effectiveness of acupuncture for reducing alcohol dependence as assessed by changes in either craving or withdrawal symptoms.

Methods: In this systematic review, a search strategy was designed to identify randomised controlled trials (RCTs) published in either the English or Chinese literature, with a priori eligibility criteria. The following English language databases were searched from inception until June 2015: AMED, Cochrane Library, EMBASE, MEDLINE, PsycINFO, and PubMed; and the following Chinese language databases were similarly searched: CNKI, Sino-med, VIP, and WanFang. Methodological quality of identified RCTs was assessed using the Jadad Scale and the Cochrane Risk of Bias tool.

Results: Fifteen RCTs were included in this review, comprising 1378 participants. The majority of the RCTs were rated as having poor methodological rigour. A statistically significant effect was found in the two primary analyses: acupuncture reduced alcohol craving compared with all controls (SMD = −1.24, 95% CI = −1.96 to −0.51); and acupuncture reduced alcohol withdrawal symptoms compared with all controls (SMD = −0.50, 95% CI = −0.83 to −0.17). In secondary analyses: acupuncture reduced craving compared with sham acupuncture (SMD = −1.00, 95% CI = −1.79 to −0.21); acupuncture reduced craving compared with controls in RCTs conducted in Western countries (SMD = −1.15, 95% CI = −2.12 to −0.18); and acupuncture reduced craving compared with controls in RCTs with only male participants (SMD = −1.68, 95% CI = −2.62 to −0.75).

Conclusion: This study showed that acupuncture was potentially effective in reducing alcohol craving and withdrawal symptoms and could be considered as an additional treatment choice and/or referral option within national healthcare systems.

Background

Approximately 3.3 million deaths worldwide are attributed to alcohol dependency per year [1]. The prevalence of alcohol dependency in the UK in 2010 was estimated at 5.9% of the population (8.7% of men and 3.2% of women), compared with 4% in Europe [1, 2]. A dependent drinker who stops drinking will experience alcohol withdrawal syndrome; this is a distressing and life-threatening condition with symptoms that range in severity, including tremors, agitation, paroxysmal sweats, fever, nausea, and seizures [3]. These symptoms typically occur within the first 24 h of stopping drinking and can last a number of weeks [4].

In England, treatment for alcohol dependency is received by a minority (6%) of an estimated 1 million people aged 16–65 years who are alcohol dependent [2]. The UK National Institute for Health and Care Excellence (NICE) reports that non-pharmacological treatments are

*Correspondence: hugh.macpherson@york.ac.uk
[1] Department of Health Sciences, University of York, York, UK
Full list of author information is available at the end of the article

an important therapeutic option for people with alcohol-related problems, and that acupuncture is valued by service users with alcohol-related problems [2]; however, NICE acknowledges that the evidence base for the effectiveness of acupuncture is weak [2].

A preliminary search of the field identified two reviews specifically related to acupuncture as an intervention for alcohol disorders [5, 6]. The review by Kunz et al. [5] included 14 studies investigating the effectiveness of auricular acupuncture in the treatment of withdrawal from substances (opiate, cocaine, and alcohol). The authors decided not to conduct a meta-analysis owing to potential systematic and selection biases. The findings for the review were inconclusive and the effectiveness of auricular acupuncture as an intervention for withdrawal was not determined. The included studies lacked rigorous methodology, resulting in reduced internal validity. In this review, Chinese language studies were excluded.

A subsequent review by Cho and Whang [6] included 11 studies and did not limit acupuncture techniques to auricular acupuncture [6]. A meta-analysis for treatment completion rates identified no statistically significant difference between acupuncture and either sham or no acupuncture groups. The results were equivocal and the included studies lacked rigorous methodology. However, the review included languages other than English, which increased its robustness.

An updated review is needed, using rigorous review methods. In the present review, we refined the search for acupuncture as a treatment for alcohol craving and withdrawal symptoms in alcohol-dependent individuals. We included randomised controlled studies (RCTs) published in both the English and Chinese literature, and conduct meta-analyses on the main outcome measures. Therefore, the present review expands on the existing research in this area to provide fresh and relevant evidence from all RCTs to establish whether acupuncture is effective in reducing alcohol craving and withdrawal symptoms.

Methods

Eligibility of studies for this systematic review

Inclusion and exclusion criteria were pre-specified (Table 1).

Search method

The following English language databases were searched up to June 2015: AMED (OvidSP) (from 1985), the Cochrane Library, EMBASE (OVID) (from 1946), MEDLINE (OVID) (from 1946), PsycINFO (from 1987), and PubMed (from 1970); and the following Chinese language database were searched up to June 2015: CNKI (from 1994), Sino-med (from 1960), VIP (from 1989), and WanFang (from 1998). Table 2 presents the keywords used, and Appendix S1 (Additional file 1) provides the MeSH terms and keywords used in the Medline (OVID) search.

Study selection

CS screened the Western databases; titles and abstracts were analysed to exclude irrelevant and duplicate studies. CW screened the Chinese literature using the same criteria. All relevant studies were retrieved as full reports for detailed evaluation. Any study that did not satisfy the inclusion criteria was excluded.

Data extraction

Data were extracted by CS on study design, participant characteristics, results, and statistical information. Translations of the full Chinese reports were undertaken by TZ at the University of York; these translations were clarified by CS, with further clarification from CW.

Quality assessment

The included RCTs were assessed for bias and scored using the Cochrane Risk of Bias tool [7], and for methodological quality using the Jadad Scale [8].

Narrative synthesis

A narrative synthesis was performed to provide a basis for assessing each RCTs contribution to the research question in terms of interpretation, synthesis, and triangulation regarding the quantitative data.

Quantitative synthesis

Meta-analyses produced the overall effect estimates for the two primary outcomes related to craving and withdrawal symptoms. Continuous outcomes (Visual Analogue Scale and Likert-scaled options used to assess craving and Alcohol Withdrawal Syndrome Scale, the

Table 1 Defined inclusion and exclusion criteria

Population	Alcohol dependents, inpatients and outpatients. Animal studies excluded
Intervention	Acupuncture where the needle punctures the skin surface at acupuncture points; either auricular or body
Control	Sham acupuncture or treatment as usual or other treatment
Outcomes	Primary measures: alcohol craving and alcohol-withdrawal symptoms Secondary: adverse effects
Study design	RCTs comparing acupuncture to a control. Restricted to English and Chinese language publications

Table 2 Key terms (or nearest appropriate Chinese equivalent)

PICOS	Key search terms
P	Alcohol abuse; alcoholism; alcohol drinking pattern; alcohol related disorders; binge drink$; drinking behaviour; alcohol dependence; alcohol withdrawal; alcohol dependent; alcohol abstinence; alcohol addiction; alcohol misuse; alcoholism treatment; alcoholic beverage$; alcohol intoxication; alcohol withdrawal delirium; human; inpatients; outpatients; rehab$; primary care; secondary care
I	Acupuncture; electroacupuncture; meridian; ear acupuncture; auricular acupuncture; body acupuncture; traditional acupuncture; medical acupuncture; traditional Chinese medicine; alternative medicine
C	Sham acupuncture; placebo acupuncture; placebo needles; treatment as usual; conventional medicine; counselling
O	Withdrawal; alcohol withdrawal; craving$
S	Randomised control trials; RCT$; random sampling; experimental design

Mainz Alcohol Withdrawal Scale, and the Clinical Institute Withdrawal Assessment for withdrawal) were presented as the standardised mean difference (SMD) with 95% confidence intervals (CI). As each RCT did not use the same acupuncture technique, we could not assume that acupuncture in each RCT was estimating the same effect, therefore we used a random-effects model for meta-analyses. For RCTs containing either two acupuncture groups or two sham acupuncture groups, both arms were combined for the analyses. Analyses of data on craving and withdrawal outcomes at the end of the intervention phase were performed using Comprehensive Meta-Analysis Version 2 software (Biostat Inc, Englewood, NJ, USA). Forest plots were drawn using our own routines in Stata (Stata Corp, College Station, TX, USA)

Assessment of heterogeneity

Clinical heterogeneity was explored through the narrative synthesis, identifying any variations in participants and interventions. Clinical heterogeneity was present in each meta-analysis owing to differences in the acupuncture techniques used and participant status (inpatient or outpatient) in the experimental interventions. Statistical heterogeneity was investigated for I^2 statistics above 50%, i.e. demonstrative of moderate heterogeneity [9]. Secondary analyses based on variations in RCT characteristics were used to explore potential sources of heterogeneity.

Results

Description of included studies

Overview

This updated review included 15 RCTs with a total of 1378 participants; Table 3 lists the characteristics of included RCTs. Figure 1 details the PRISMA flowchart of this review.

Design

All of the studies were RCTs with a parallel study design. Most RCTs involved two arms, with the exception of three RCTs that were three-armed [10–12], and one that was four-armed [13].

Participants

Participants in 12 of the 15 RCTs satisfied one of three definitions of alcohol dependence: the Diagnostic and Statistical Manual of Mental Disorders (DSM)-III-R, the DSM-IV, the International Classification of Diseases (ICD-10), or the Chinese Classification of Mental Disorders (CCMD-3). However, three RCTs used additional selection criteria: one required participants to be inpatients of at least 14 days [13], one required participants to have been drinking within 10 days of enrolment in the outpatient alcoholism treatment programme [12], and one did not specify a definition, only stated that participants were alcohol-dependent [14]. The participants were inpatients in 11 of 15 RCTs, the exceptions were four RCTs involving outpatients [10, 12, 15, 16], and one RCT in which the setting was not specified [17]. The included RCTs were conducted in the USA (n = 3), Europe (n = 6), or East Asia (n = 6).

Description of acupuncture

The acupuncture techniques varied between RCTs. Eight RCTs used auricular acupuncture at points recommended by the UK National Acupuncture Detoxification Association (NADA); three of these eight RCTs also used body acupuncture. Seven RCTs used body acupuncture as the active treatment, either conventional needle acupuncture or electroacupuncture. All acupuncture techniques involved skin penetration.

The majority of RCTs (12 of 15) reported that the duration of needling was 30–45 min; two RCTs reported that the duration of needling was <30 min [15, 18], and one RCT did not report the duration of needling [14].

The duration of the treatment courses ranged from 5 days [19] to 12 weeks [17], or until a participant reached the withdrawal stage [11]. Six RCTs had fewer than 10 treatment sessions [10, 14, 18–21] two RCTs had 12–18 treatment sessions [13, 15], three RCTs had 24–30

Table 3 Characteristics of included RCTs investigating the effect of acupuncture on alcohol dependence

First author, (year) location	Participants (total, status, inclusion criteria)	Study design; (allocation concealment[a]); (blinding[a])	Intervention	Treatment frequency and duration	Treated acupoints	Control	Outcomes	Results reported	Adverse effects
Bullock (1987) USA [23]	N = 54 (males) Inpatients ≥20 admissions Previous treatment failure No identifiable support/group No full-time employment ≥6 months	2-arms; (B); (A)	AA + A	*Phase 1* daily (5 days) *Phase 2* 3 weekly (28 days) *Phase 3* 2 weekly (45 days)	Ear Lung, Shenmen, and either Liver, Kidney or occiput; LI4, SJ5. No manual or electro-stimulation	Non-specific ear points at "5 mml or less" from specific points	(1) Need for alcohol (2) Drinking episodes (3) Detox admissions (4) Craving (5) Completion rates	(1) p 0.003 (2) p 0.0076 (3) p 0.03 (4) p 0.015 (5) p 0.01	NR
Worner (1992) USA [12]	N = 56 (49 male) Outpatients Drinking within 10 days	3-arms; (B); (B)	AA + A	3 per week (3 months)	Ear Lung, Shenmen; LV3, ST36, SJ5, LI4, GV20	(1) Sham "transdermal stimulation" (electrocardiogram pads fixed to both forearms and to one lower leg), and TAU (2) TAU	(1) Completion rates (2) Relapse rates	No observed effects; $p > 0.05$	NR
Toteva (1996) Bulgaria [15]	N = 118 (103 male) Outpatients DSM-IV Abstinence from alcohol ≥10 days	2-arms; (B); (C)	A	Daily (12–15 sessions)	Five of six points drawn from: LI4, LI11, PC6, SJ5, SI4, GB8, GB14, HT7, Taiyang, Yintang	TAU	(1) Craving (2) Depressive symptoms (3) Participation in psycho-therapeutic programs (4) Reduction in tremor (5) Remission rate	(1) $p < 0.001$ (2) $p < 0.001$ (3) $p < 0.001$ (4) $p < 0.001$ (5) $p < 0.001$	NR
Rampes (1997) England [10]	N = 59 (46 male) Outpatients DSM-III-R	3-arms; (A); (A)	AEA; square-wave continuous electric current of 100 Hz frequency	Weekly (6 weeks)	Ear Lung (AEA), Shenmen, Sympathetic Tone	(1) Knee 2, Internal Secretion (AEA), Elbow; and TAU (2) TAU	(1) Craving (VAS) (2) Units of alcohol (3) Breathalyser (4) Anxiety (5) Completion rates	(1) p 0.64 (2) p 0.69 (3) NS (4) p 0.16 (5) p 0.49 [vs Group 2]	Drowsiness, transient bleeding on removal of needles for 1 participant
Sapir-Weise (1999) Sweden [16]	N = 72 (51 male) Outpatients DSM-III-R	2-arms; (A); (A)	AA	*Phase 1* 5 weekly (2 weeks) *Phase 2* 3 weekly (4 weeks) *Phase 3* 2 weekly (4 weeks)	Ear Lung, Shenmen, Sympathetic; and TAU	AA non-specific 3–5 mm from specific points; and TAU	(1) Successful drinking pattern (2) Craving (3) Completion rates	(1) NS (2) NS (3) p 0.071	NR

Table 3 continued

First author, (year) location	Participants (total, status, inclusion criteria)	Study design; (allocation concealment[a]); (blinding[a])	Intervention	Treatment frequency and duration	Treated acupoints	Control	Outcomes	Results reported	Adverse effects
Bullock (2002) USA [13]	N = 503 (253 male) Inpatients DSM-IV Anticipated stay ≥ 14 days	4-arms; (B); (A)	AA	Daily (excluding Sundays) for 3 weeks	Ear Liver, Lung, Shenmen, Sympathetic; TAU	(1) Symptom based, "acupuncturists were not constrained"; TAU (2) AA non-specific "within 5 mm" of specific points, TAU (3) TAU	(1) Craving (Likert Scale) (2) Completion rates	(1) *p* 0.024 (comparison of interventions) (2) *p* 0.06	NR
Karst (2002) Germany [20]	N = 34 (30 male) Inpatients ICD-10	2-arms; (B); (A)	AA + A	Daily (10 consecutive days)	Ear Kidney, Liver, Lung, Shenmen, Sympathetic; GV20, Extra 1, LI4; TAU	Sham acupuncture (Streitberger needle) at same specific points, TAU	(1) CIWA-Ar-Scale (2) BDI (3) EWL 60S (4) STAI	(1) *p* 0.045 (2) *p* 0.157 (3) NS (4) *p* 0.544	NR
Trümpler (2003) Switzerland [11]	N = 48 (28 male) Inpatients DSM-IV	3-arms; (B); (C)	AA	Daily (until end of withdrawal)	Needling "at ear points considered appropriate"; TAU	(1) Low level laser, TAU (2) Sham laser, TAU	(1) Duration of withdrawal (2) Duration of sedative prescription	(1) *p* 0.44 [vs Group 2] (2) NS	No local-side effects to acupuncture interventions
Kim (2005) Korea [14]	N = 22 (males) Inpatients Alcohol dependents	2-arms; (B); (A)	A	2 weekly (4 weeks)	Zùbin (K9)	Sham acupuncture (Park needle) at specific point	Craving (VAS)	$p < 0.05$	NR
Kunz (2007) Germany [19]	N = 109 (89 male) Inpatients ICD-10	2-arms; (B); (C)	AA	Daily (5 consecutive days)	Ear Kidney, Liver, Lung, Shenmen, Sympathetic; TAU	Aromatherapy, TAU	(1) AWS (2) Craving (VAS)	(1) NS (2) NS	Intervention: pain, mild bleeding, agitation; Control: negative thoughts, sore throat
Li (2009) China [24]	N = 100 (males) Inpatients CCMD-3	2-arms; (B); (B)	EA at a low frequency	Daily (for 6 weeks)	ST36 Nutritional supplement	TAU, nutritional supplement	(1) AWS (2) Relapse rate	(1) NS (2) $p < 0.01$	NR
Yao (2009) China [21]	N = 39 (males) Inpatients DSM-IV	2-arms; (B); (B)	A	Daily (5 consecutive days = 1 course) Total 1–3 courses	Sanyinjiao (SP-6), ST36, Insomnia	TAU, vitamins, antibiotics	(1) AWS (2) Clinical symptoms	(1) $p < 0.05$ (2) NR	Drowsiness for both groups, 1 control "addiction" to Western medicine
Zhang (2010) China [22]	N = 64 (males) Inpatients CCMD-3-R, HAMD-17	2-arms; (B); (B)	EA at a low frequency	Daily (for 4 weeks)	Baihui (DU20), Yingtang	Sham electro-acupuncture near specific points	(1) SCL-90 (2) HAM-D (3) HAM-A	(1) $p < 0.05$ (2) $p < 0.05$ (3) $p < 0.05$	NR

Table 3 continued

First author, (year) location	Participants (total, status, inclusion criteria)	Study design; (allocation concealment[a]); (blinding[a])	Intervention	Treatment frequency and duration	Treated acupoints	Control	Outcomes	Results reported	Adverse effects
Lee (2015) Korea [18]	N = 20 (males) Inpatients DSM-IV	2-arms; (B); (A)	A	Twice a week (4 weeks)	Zùbin (KI9)	Sham acupuncture (Park needle) at specific point	Craving (VAS)	$p < 0.01$	NR
Tong (2015) China [17]	N = 80 (males) ICD-10	2-arms; (B); (B)	A, herbal medicine	Every other day (for 12 weeks)	Baihui	TAU	SF-36	$p < 0.05$	NR

A acupuncture, *AA* auricular acupuncture, *AEA* auricular electroacupuncture, *AWS* alcohol withdrawal syndrome, *BDI* Beck Depression Inventory, *CCMD-3-R* Criteria for Classification and Diagnosis of Mental Diseases, *CIWA-Ar-Scale* Clinical Institute Withdrawal Assessment for Alcohol, *DSM* Diagnostic and Statistical Manual of Mental Disorders, *EA* electroacupuncture, *EWL 60S* 60-item Adjective Checklist, *HAM-A* Hamilton Rating Scale for Anxiety, *HAM-D* Hamilton Rating Scale for Depression, *ICD-10* International Classification of Diseases, *NR* not reported, *NS* not significant, *SCL-90* symptom checklist-90, *STAI* stait-trait anxiety inventory, *TAU* treatment-as-usual, *VAS* Visual Analogue Scale

[a] Allocation concealment and blinding: (A) adequate, (B) unclear, (C) inadequate

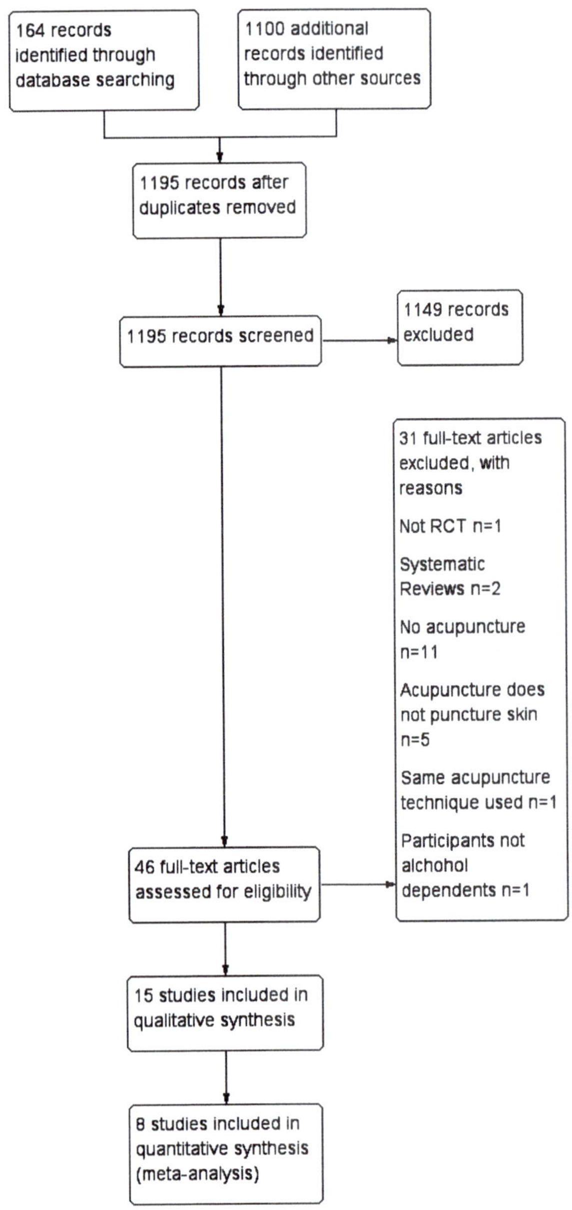

Fig. 1 PRISMA flow diagram detailing the number of studies included and/or excluded at each stage

treatment sessions [16, 22, 23], and three RCTs had 36–42 treatment sessions [12, 17, 24]. One RCT included a varying number of treatment sessions, as the sessions were continued until participants had become abstinent from alcohol [11].

Acupuncture was performed by an acupuncturist or Chinese medical practitioner (n = 7), a registered nurse-trained acupuncturist (n = 1), and NADA-trained mental health nurses (n = 1); six RCTs did not report these details. Five RCTs reported that interactions between the acupuncturist and participants were constrained by the study design; the majority (10 of 15 RCTs) did not report this information.

Description of controls

Ten RCTs used sham acupuncture as a control, with the aim of minimising differences in the treatment experience between groups, with participants blinded to the intervention. Fourteen RCTs used treatment-as-usual as an intervention, either as a control group (n = 5) or as an adjunct to the experimental treatment (n = 9). In total there were 20 control groups.

Outcomes

Alcohol craving and alcohol withdrawal symptoms were measured at key time points in the RCTs: at baseline, during intervention, and at follow-up. Visual Analogue Scale and Likert-scaled options were used to assess craving. The Alcohol Withdrawal Syndrome Scale, the Mainz Alcohol Withdrawal Scale, and the Clinical Institute Withdrawal Assessment were used to assess the severity of withdrawal symptoms. Where data on adverse events were reported, they were collected through observation by acupuncturists or self-reported by participants.

Cochrane Risk of Bias

Assessments using the Cochrane Risk of Bias tool [7] are presented in Figs. 2 and 3. Details by RCT are provided in Appendix S2 (Additional file 1).

Jadad Scale

The Jadad Scale [8] scores are presented in Table 4. Five RCTs had a high methodological quality score (≥3) and ten RCTs had a low methodological quality score (≤2). Owing to the difficulties in blinding the acupuncturist, none of the RCTs were able to score the maximum of five points; therefore a score of three, which is classified as high methodological quality, was the maximum score possible.

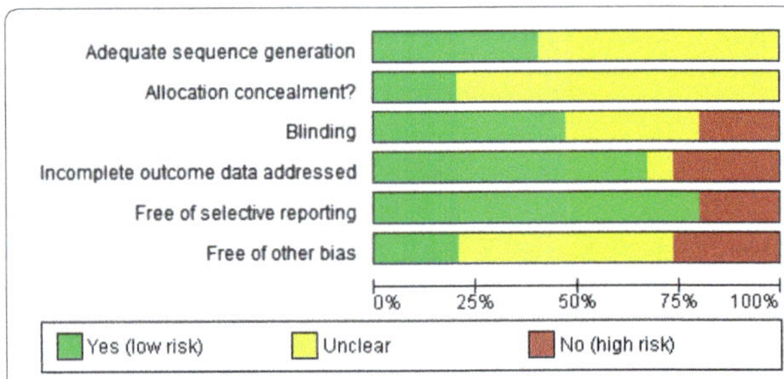

Fig. 2 Risk of Bias: review authors' judgements about each methodological quality item presented as percentage across all studies

	Adequate sequence generation	Allocation concealment?	Blinding	Incomplete outcome data addressed	Free of selective reporting	Free of other bias
Bullock 1987	?	?	+	−	+	−
Bullock 2002	+	?	+	+	−	+
Karst 2002	?	?	+	+	−	?
Kim 2005	?	?	+	+	+	?
Kunz 2007	+	?	−	+	+	−
Lee 2015	+	?	+	+	+	+
Li 2009	?	?	?	+	+	?
Rampes 1997	+	+	+	−	+	+
Sapir-Weise 1999	?	+	+	−	+	?
Tong 2015	?	?	?	+	+	?
Toteva 1996	?	?	−	−	+	−
Trumpler 2003	+	+	−	+	+	−
Worner 1992	+	?	?	?	+	?
Yao 2009	?	?	?	+	−	?
Zhang 2010	?	?	?	+	+	?

Fig. 3 Risk of bias: review authors' judgements for each domain

Primary meta-analyses

Craving Nine RCTs assessed alcohol craving. One RCT compared acupuncture with an active treatment (aromatherapy) and was therefore excluded from the analysis as it was considered an equivalent intervention [19]. Only six RCTs [10, 14–16, 18, 23] (n = 345 participants) provided sufficient statistical information to include in the meta-analysis. Five of these RCTs measured craving using a quantitative scale; however, only one RCT provided the odds ratio [23]. Therefore, the odds ratio was converted into the standardised difference, using a method suggested by Borenstein et al. [25], so that the statistical information could be included in the analysis. There was evidence of a statistically significant effect of acupuncture on self-reported experience of craving compared to all control groups (sham and treatment-as-usual) (SMD = −1.24, 95% CI = −1.96 to −0.51, Q = 30.89, df = 5, $P < 0.001$, $I^2 = 83.8\%$; Fig. 4).

Alcohol withdrawal Five RCTs assessed alcohol withdrawal symptoms. Again, the one RCT that compared acupuncture with an active treatment (aromatherapy) was excluded from the meta-analysis [19]. Two further RCTs were excluded as they provided insufficient statistical data [20, 21]. From the remaining two RCTs [11, 24] (n = 148 participants), there was evidence of a significant effect of acupuncture compared to all controls for alcohol withdrawal symptoms (SMD = −0.50, 95% CI = −0.83 to −0.17, Q = 0.11, df = 1, $P = 0.003$, $I^2 = 0\%$; Fig. 5).

Secondary subgroup and sensitivity meta-analyses

For alcohol craving, the data were split to conduct analyses that might lead to an explanation of the heterogeneity.

Acupuncture versus sham acupuncture for alcohol craving Pooling only those RCTs that compared acupuncture with sham acupuncture (n = 211 participants), acupuncture significantly reduced self-reported experience of craving (SMD = −1.00, 95% CI = −1.79 to −0.21, Q = 17.74, df = 4, $P = 0.013$, $I^2 = 77.4\%$; Fig. 6). There was a small reduction in the I^2 statistic.

Studies conducted in Western countries for alcohol craving Pooling the endpoint values for the Western-based RCTs (n = 303 participants), there was a statistically significant effect of acupuncture on self-reported experience of craving (SMD = −1.15, 95% CI = −2.12 to −0.18, Q = 27.44, df = 3, $P = 0.02$), with slightly increased heterogeneity ($I^2 = 89.07\%$; Fig. 7).

Male-only randomised controlled trials for alcohol craving Out of the 15 RCTs (n = 1378 participants), eight RCTs included females (n = 327 participants) and seven RCTs were male-only studies. An analysis was conducted on three of these male-only RCTs. Pooling the endpoint values, there was a statistically significant effect of acupuncture versus controls on self-reported experience of craving (SMD = −1.68, 95% CI = −2.62 to −0.75, Q = 4.46, df = 2, $P < 0.001$, $I^2 = 55.12\%$; Fig. 8). Excluding the RCTs containing both male and female participants considerably reduced the heterogeneity.

Adverse events

Four RCTs reported adverse effects, although data were limited. Kunz et al. [19] reported pain, mild bleeding on insertion of needles, and agitation in the acupuncture group, while the aromatherapy group experienced agitation, sneezing, negative thoughts, and sore throat. Yao [21] reported that drowsiness was experienced in both

Table 4 Jadad Scale representing scores in descending order

Study	Described as RCT?	Adequate randomisation?	Double-blind?	Details of double-blinding?	Reasons stated for withdrawals?	Total score
Bullock et al. [13]	+1	+1	+0	+0	+1	3
Kunz et al. [19]	+1	+1	+0	+0	+1	3
Lee et al. [18]	+1	+1	+0	+0	+1	3
Rampes et al. [10]	+1	+1	+0	+0	+1	3
Trümpler et al. [11]	+1	+1	+0	+0	+1	3
Worner et al. [12]	+1	+1	+0	+0	+0	2
Karst et al. [20]	+1	−1	+0	+0	+1	1
Kim et al. [14]	+1	−1	+0	+0	+1	1
Li and Guo [24]	+1	−1	+0	+0	+1	1
Yao [21]	+1	−1	+0	+0	+1	1
Zhang et al. [22]	+1	−1	+0	+0	+1	1
Bullock et al. [23]	+1	−1	+0	+0	+0	0
Sapir-Weise et al. [16]	+1	−1	+0	+0	+0	0
Toteva and Milanov [15]	+1	−1	+0	+0	+0	0
Tong et al. [17]	+1	−1	+0	+0	+0	0

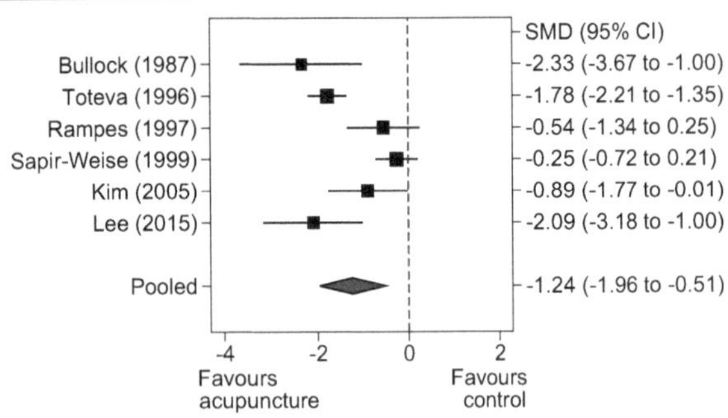

Fig. 4 *Forest plot*: acupuncture versus all controls (combined sham and treatment as usual) for alcohol craving

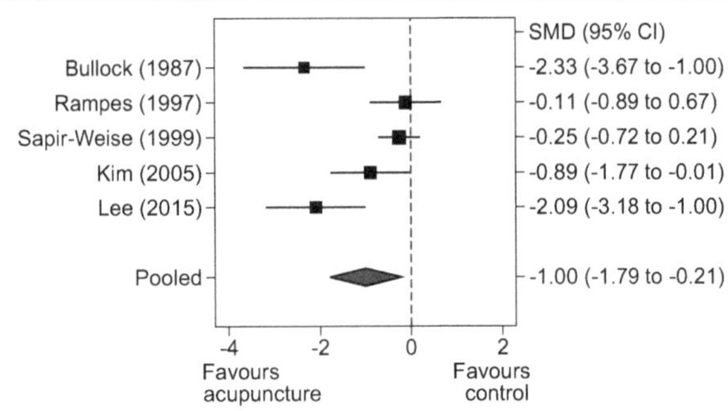

Fig. 6 *Forest plot*: acupuncture versus sham acupuncture for craving

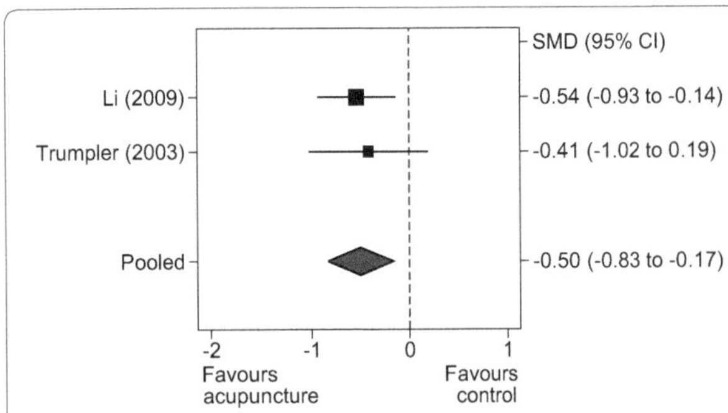

Fig. 5 *Forest plot*: acupuncture versus all controls for withdrawal symptoms

the acupuncture group (n = 1) and the control group (n = 4); however, one participant in the control group also reported an addiction to pharmaceutical medicine. Rampes et al. [10] reported drowsiness and transient bleeding on removal of needles in the electroacupuncture group at specific acupuncture points; one participant in the non-specific electroacupuncture group dropped out of the RCT owing to pain. Trümpler et al. [11] reported that no local side effects were observed. However, one participant in the acupuncture group experienced self-limiting generalised convulsions whilst sleeping on the fifth day; the convulsions lasted 5 min, and were judged to be a withdrawal-related epileptic seizure on clinical grounds.

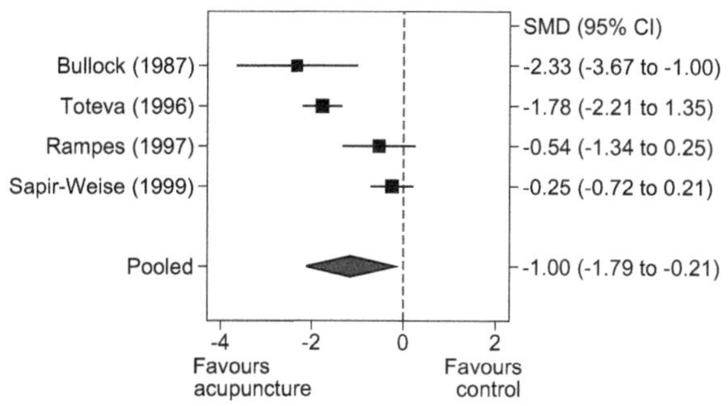

Fig. 7 *Forest plot*: acupuncture versus control groups for craving in Western studies

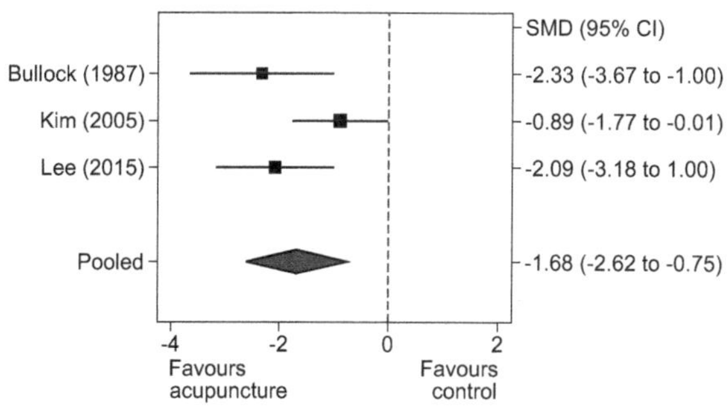

Fig. 8 *Forest plot graph*: acupuncture versus control groups for craving in male participants

Discussion

Major findings

Our review comprised 15 RCTs with 1378 patients from eight countries published in either Chinese or English. Our findings provide the first clear evidence that acupuncture might be considered an effective intervention for alcohol dependence. This evidence of significant effectiveness was observed in our two primary analyses, one showing a reduction in alcohol craving and one showing a reduction in withdrawal symptoms. In all three of our secondary analyses, we found significant reductions in alcohol craving: comparing acupuncture versus sham acupuncture; comparing acupuncture with controls in only those RCTs conducted in Western countries; and in those RCTs that recruited males only. We note that the effect size of acupuncture when all RCTs are combined is slightly larger than when compared with sham acupuncture RCTs or with Western-based RCTs, and is slightly smaller when compared with male-only RCTs. While the overall effect estimate favoured acupuncture for all analyses, some of the individual RCTs found non-significant effects of acupuncture on alcohol dependence. By pooling the data across RCTs, we increased the overall power, which led to the conclusion that acupuncture was an effective intervention.

The present review has identified pre-specified secondary analyses to explore reasons for potential heterogeneity and aid interpretation. The I^2 value for acupuncture versus all controls for alcohol craving was 83.8%; this value reduced slightly for the analysis of acupuncture versus sham acupuncture in alcohol craving (77.4%). An analysis of alcohol craving in Western-based RCTs showed increased heterogeneity (89.1%). An analysis of acupuncture for male-only participants for alcohol craving substantially reduced the heterogeneity (55.1%). Interpreting these values with reference to the 50% threshold [9] indicates that the results must be treated with caution.

Strengths and limitations

The included RCTs were rigorously assessed using two quality assessments. The included RCTs were not all of a high standard, with 10 of the 15 RCTs scoring two or less on the Jadad scale. Moreover, only eight RCTs contained sufficient statistical information on outcomes for meta-analysis; this limited the scope for comparing acupuncture with some controls. For example, because of a lack of sufficient quantitative outcome data we were unable compare acupuncture with treatment-as-usual. While we have combined changes in continuous outcomes using standardised mean differences for the purposes of conducting the meta-analyses, the individual measures of craving and withdrawal symptoms may have different measurement characteristics, which would lead to an increase in heterogeneity. Furthermore, most of the included RCTs contained a small sample size. These factors resulted in a small number of participants being included in the final analyses. The present review did not include a sufficient number of RCTs to address publication bias.

The majority of the included RCTs were conducted in a hospital setting; therefore, generalisation of the results to community settings must be done with caution. The clinical heterogeneity associated with the different acupuncture techniques limits our ability to identify which technique was more effective for treatment of alcohol disorders. Acupuncture treatments also varied in duration, frequency, and the acupuncture points used, making it difficult to assess the key characteristics that might be associated with the effectiveness of the intervention. Whilst some RCTs combined auricular acupuncture and body acupuncture as part of the same treatment, most RCTs involved either auricular or body acupuncture. Given the potential variation in modes of action, combining these two modalities (either within RCTs or between RCTs), will add to the clinical heterogeneity. Sham acupuncture also varied across RCTs. Moreover, sham acupuncture cannot be considered a physiologically inert intervention, thereby potentially leading to an underestimate of the effect of the acupuncture.

Comparisons with previous systematic reviews

The present review included an increased number of RCTs (n = 15) compared with the previous reviews of Kunz et al. [5] (n = 6) and Cho and Whang [6] (n = 11). Kunz et al. [5] did not conduct a meta-analysis, and reported that there was insufficient evidence to conclude whether auricular acupuncture is an effective intervention in the treatment of alcohol and substance abuse. Cho and Whang conducted a meta-analysis of acupuncture versus sham acupuncture for treatment completion rates, reporting no significant differences [6] but no meta-analysis was conducted by them for craving because of insufficient data. By contrast, our study found sufficient data to conduct a meta-analysis of craving with six trials included [10, 14–16, 18, 23]. Moreover, the present review is the first to provide a meta-analysis of withdrawal symptoms, albeit based on only two RCTs [11, 24]. The results we present here therefore represent an update of the evidence, with the caveat that our results are based on a small number of RCTs with variable risks of bias.

Implications for research and practice

Non-pharmacological treatments are an important therapeutic option for people with alcohol-related problems, and there is some evidence that acupuncture is valued by service users [2]. Recommendations for future studies to improve the quality and statistical power of the next review on this topic include:

- *Larger sample sizes* Further RCTs with larger sample sizes are needed. An increased sample size increases power statistically, enhancing a meta-analysis. Large sample sizes also provide the opportunity to explore potential moderators and mediators of response.
- *Relevant statistical information reported* Summary statistics on outcomes should be reported to a high standard so that these data can be included, thereby enhancing the robustness of the meta-analyses. An assessment for publication bias could also be conducted using a funnel plot.
- *Female participants* More studies should recruit female as well as male participants, so that results can be better generalised to the female population of problem drinkers.
- *Longer-term follow ups* for at least 1 year are recommended, along with parallel cost-effectiveness analyses.
- *Increase methodological quality* Future studies should follow STRICTA recommendations [26], which are guidelines specifically aimed at producing high quality reporting of acupuncture interventions, and the Consolidated Standards of Reporting Trials (CONSORT) statement [27], which are guidelines on study design and reporting to reduce potential bias and increase methodological quality.

Conclusion

This study showed that acupuncture was potentially effective in reducing alcohol craving and withdrawal symptoms and could be considered as an additional treatment choice and/or referral option within national healthcare systems.

Abbreviations

A: acupuncture; AA: auricular acupuncture; AEA: auricular electroacupuncture; AMED: allied and complementary medicine database; CCMD: Chinese Classification of Mental Disorders; CI: confidence interval; CNKI: China National Knowledge Infrastructure; CONSORT: consolidated standards of reporting trials; df: degrees of freedom; DSM: Diagnostic and Statistical Manual of Mental Disorders; EA: electroacupuncture; EMBASE: excerpta medica database; ICD: International Classification of Diseases; I^2: heterogeneity statistic; MEDLINE: national library of medicine database; MeSH: medical subject headings; NADA: national acupuncture detoxification association; NICE: national institute for health and care excellence; NR: not reported; NS: not significant; OVID: OVID database search interface; PsycINFO: psychology information database; PRISMA: preferred reporting items for systematic reviews and meta-analyses; PubMed: search engine for national library of medicine databases; Q: heterogeneity statistic; RCT: randomised controlled trial; Sino-med: Chinese biomedical literature service system; SMD: standardised mean difference; STRICTA: revised standards for reporting interventions in clinical trials of acupuncture; TAU: treatment-as-usual; VIP: Chinese science and technology periodicals database; WanFang: China medical collections database; UK: United Kingdom.

Authors' contributions

CS, CL and HM conceived the review. CCW, JPL, and CS searched, and with TTZ, extracted the data. MB performed the statistical analysis. CS and HM wrote the manuscript. All authors read and approved the final manuscript.

Author details

[1] Department of Health Sciences, University of York, York, UK. [2] Centre for Evidence-Based Chinese Medicine, Beijing University of Chinese Medicine, Beijing, China.

Acknowledgements

Acknowledgement is due to Janet Eldred for copy-editing the near final version of the manuscript.

Competing interests

The authors declare that they have no competing interests.

Availability of data and materials

All data used in this systematic review are fully available in the public domain.

Funding

The research presented in this study was not funded. Therefore no funding body influenced the design of the study, or the collection, analysis, and interpretation of data on which the manuscript is based.

References

1. World Health Organisation. WHO: Global status report on alcohol and health [Internet]. 2014. http://www.who.int/substance_abuse/publications/global_alcohol_report/en/. Accessed 24 Feb 2016.
2. National Institute for Health and Care Excellence (NICE). Alcohol-use disorders: diagnosis, assessment and management of harmful drinking and alcohol dependence | Introduction | Guidance and guidelines [Internet]. 2011. https://www.nice.org.uk/guidance/cg115/chapter/introduction. Accessed 24 Feb 2016.
3. Health and Social Care Information Centre (HSCIC). National Statistics: Statistics on Alcohol - England, 2014 [Internet]. 2014. http://www.hscic.gov.uk/catalogue/PUB14184. Accessed 24 Feb 2016.
4. Rassool GH. Alcohol and drug misuse: a handbook for students and health professionals. 1st ed. Oxford: Routledge; 2009.
5. Kunz S, Schulz M, Syrbe G, Driessen M. Acupuncture of the ear as therapeutic approach in the treatment of alcohol and substance abuse—a systematic review. Sucht. 2004;50:196–203.
6. Cho S-H, Whang W-W. Acupuncture for alcohol dependence: a systematic review. Alcohol Clin Exp Res. 2009;33:1305–13.
7. Higgins JPT, Altman DG, Gøtzsche PC, Jüni P, Moher D, Oxman AD, et al. The Cochrane collaboration's tool for assessing risk of bias in randomised trials. BMJ. 2011;343:d5928.
8. Jadad AR, Moore RA, Carroll D, Jenkinson C, Reynolds DJ, Gavaghan DJ, et al. Assessing the quality of reports of randomized clinical trials: is blinding necessary? Control Clin Trials. 1996;17:1–12.
9. Higgins JP, Thompson SG. Quantifying heterogeneity in a meta-analysis. Stat Med. 2002;21:1539–58.
10. Rampes H, Pereira S, Mortimer A, Manoharan S, Knowles M. Does electroacupuncture reduce craving for alcohol? A randomized controlled study. Complement Ther Med. 1997;5:19–26.
11. Trümpler F, Oez S, Stähli P, Brenner HD, Jüni P. Acupuncture for alcohol withdrawal: a randomized controlled trial. Alcohol Alcohol. 2003;38:369–75.
12. Worner TM, Zeller B, Schwarz H, Zwas F, Lyon D. Acupuncture fails to improve treatment outcome in alcoholics. Drug Alcohol Depend. 1992;30:169–73.
13. Bullock ML, Kiresuk TJ, Sherman RE, Lenz SK, Culliton PD, Boucher TA, et al. A large randomized placebo controlled study of auricular acupuncture for alcohol dependence. J Subst Abuse Treat. 2002;22:71–7.
14. Kim S, Kang C, Park J, Kim M, Jung T, Park J, et al. The effect of acupuncture on Zùbin (K9) in reducing alcohol craving in alcohol-dependent patients. Eur Neuropsychopharmacol. 2005;15:S580.
15. Toteva S, Milanov I. The use of body acupuncture for treatment of alcohol dependence and withdrawal syndrome: a controlled study. Am J Acupunct. 1996;24:19–26.
16. Sapir-Weise R, Berglund M, Frank A, Kristenson H. Acupuncture in alcoholism treatment: a randomized out-patient study. Alcohol Alcohol. 1999;34:629–35.
17. Tong X, Zhao F, Tong Z. Observation on Chinese herbal medicine with acupuncture therapies for alcohol dependence syndrome. JCAM. 2015;31:24–5.
18. Lee J-S, Kim S-G, Jung T-G, Jung WY, Kim S-Y. Effect of Zhubin (KI9) acupuncture in reducing alcohol craving in patients with alcohol dependence: a randomized placebo-controlled trial. Chin J Integr Med. 2015;21:307–11.
19. Kunz S, Schulz M, Lewitzky M, Driessen M, Rau H. Ear acupuncture for alcohol withdrawal in comparison with aromatherapy: a randomized-controlled trial. Alcohol Clin Exp Res. 2007;31:436–42.
20. Karst M, Passie T, Friedrich S, Wiese B, Schneider U. Acupuncture in the treatment of alcohol withdrawal symptoms: a randomized, placebo-controlled inpatient study. Addict Biol. 2002;7:415–9.
21. Yao P. Integrated traditional and western medicine treatment for alcoholic cirrhosis: compensatory period combined with alcohol dependence syndrome in 23 cases. Chin J Integr Tradit West Med Liver Disease. 2009;19:364–5.
22. Zhang Y, Zhang R, Chen Y, Wang H, Tan Q. Observation on therapeutic effect of electroacupuncture for treatment of emotional disturbance of patients with alcohol dependence syndrome in hospital. Med J Chin People's Health. 2010;22:1197–8.
23. Bullock ML, Umen AJ, Culliton PD, Olander RT. Acupuncture treatment of alcoholic recidivism: a pilot study. Alcohol Clin Exp Res. 1987;11:292–5.
24. Li G, Guo J. Studies of low frequency electroacupuncture treat for patients with alcohol dependence. World Health Digest Med Periodical. 2009;8:27–8.
25. Borenstein M, Hedges L, Higgins J, Rothstein H. Introduction to meta-analysis. Chichester: Wiley; 2009.
26. MacPherson H, Altman DG, Hammerschlag R, Youping L, Taixiang W, White A, et al. Revised standards for reporting interventions in clinical trials of acupuncture (STRICTA): extending the CONSORT statement. PLoS Med. 2010;7:e1000261.
27. Schulz KF, Altman DG, Moher D, for the CONSORT Group. CONSORT 2010 statement: updated guidelines for reporting parallel group randomised trials. BMJ. 2010;340:c332.

13

Chinese herbal medicine for constipation: *zheng*-based associations among herbs, formulae, proprietary medicines, and herb–drug interactions

Linda L. D. Zhong[1,2†], Guang Zheng[1,5†], Li Da Ge[3], Cheng Yuan Lin[1,2], Tao Huang[1,2], Ling Zhao[1,2], Cheng Lu[1,4], Ai Ping Lu[1,2,4] and Zhao Xiang Bian[1,2*]

Abstract

Background: As current symptomatic treatments of constipation are still unsatisfactory, an increasing number of patients seek help from Chinese medicine (CM), particularly Chinese herbal medicine (CHM). This study aimed to review the most frequently used CHM herbs and formulae, proprietary CHMs, and herb–drug interactions for functional constipation using *zheng* (syndrome)-based differentiation, and to determine the current practice of *zheng*-based CHM treatments for functional constipation.

Methods: We developed a search strategy to include all the related clinical studies of CHM for constipation and set inclusion and exclusion criteria as studies on subjects with constipation of all ages and both sexes, using objective measures from laboratory or imaging techniques. The interventions included single herbs, CM classical formulae, CM new formulae, and Chinese herb-derived products and combination products. The clinical study types included were quasi- or randomized controlled trials, observational clinical studies, case series or case reports, and other types of appropriate research methods. The data concerning study design, sample size, mode of recruitment, sampling and diagnostic procedure, inclusion and exclusion criteria, and participants' characteristics (including age, sex, and duration of constipation). CM patterns, CM treatment principles, treatment regimen, and CM treatment outcomes were recorded.

Results: A total of 29,832 relevant records were found, of which 8541 were duplicate records and 20,639 were excluded for reasons of irrelevance. The full text of 965 articles was retrieved for detailed assessment, following which 480 articles were excluded for various reasons. From the included articles, we retrieved 190 different CM *zheng* diagnoses from 485 individual studies. The most common *zheng* was *dual deficiency of qi and blood (N = 48)*, which was diagnosed in 948 out of 15,740 subjects. The most frequently used classical formula was *Ma-Zi-Ren-Wan* (MZRW) (N = 75) and the most frequently used proprietary CHM was *Run-Chang-Wan (N = 87)*. The most frequently used combined medication was *Da Huang* with sodium bicarbonate tablets (frequency across all studies, n = 23), followed by *Fan Xie Ye* with lactulose oral solution (n = 8), *Ma-Ren-Ruan-Jiao-Nang* with lactulose oral solution (n = 6) and *Liu-Wei-An-Xiao-Jiao-Nang* (n = 6) with mosapride citrate tablets.

*Correspondence: bzxiang@hkbu.edu.hk
†Linda LD Zhong and Guang Zheng contributed equally to this work and should be considered co-first authors
[1] School of Chinese Medicine, Hong Kong Baptist University, 7 Baptist University Road, Kowloon Tong, Hong Kong, China
Full list of author information is available at the end of the article

Conclusion: This study examined the use of CHM for constipation and summarized the herbs, formulae, proprietary medicines, and herb–drug interactions application. These data indicated there were limited information about herb-drug interactions and adverse effects of CHM and further randomized controlled trials with strict design are necessary.

Background

Constipation is a common functional bowel disorder that affects many people; 14.7 % of the United States population [1], and 15.6 % of the adult population in Hong Kong [2] experienced this problem in a large sampled cross-sectional survey published in 2014. Treatments for constipation usually include fiber supplements, osmotic and stimulant laxatives, stool softeners, and sometimes enemas for refractory constipation [3]. As current symptomatic treatments produce unsatisfactory responses [4], many patients seek help from Chinese medicine (CM), particularly Chinese herbal medicine (CHM).

Many CM interventions have been used to treat constipation. A recent review [5] listed the current clinical research findings from CM interventions for functional constipation. However, there have been no analysis of the benefits of individual interventions (or individual types of interventions) or of the qualities of individual study designs. Our research team conducted a systematic review of CHM for functional constipation [6] and showed that CHM or CHM combination therapy was more effective than some single conventional medicines [6]. However, these findings did not accurately reflect all clinical practice, as most clinical research on constipation has involved observational studies or case series, and clinical practice has mostly been limited to personal experiences and based on CM theory and *zheng* (syndrome) differentiation [7–9].

We aimed to investigate CHM applications for constipation based on *zheng* differentiation, especially the use of single herbs, CM formulae, proprietary CHMs, and herb–drug interactions. Therefore, we systematically reviewed all the available data from current databases, including clinical trials, clinical observational studies, case series, case reports, and case control studies. Because we examined large data sets from both conventional Western and CM literature, we used a data slicing algorithm for text mining [10].

This study aimed to review the most frequently used CHM herbs and formulae, proprietary CHMs, and herb–drug interactions for functional constipation using *zheng*-based differentiation, and to determine the current practice of *zheng*-based CHM treatments for functional constipation.

Methods

Literature search

The review was performed in accordance with the Preferred Reporting Items for Systematic Reviews and Meta-Analyses (PRISMA) guidelines. We used the following databases to search the conventional medicine literature: PubMed, Ovid, Evidence-Based Medicine Reviews (EBMR), and Embase. The following databases were used to search the traditional CM literature: SinoMed, Chinese National Knowledge Infrastructure (CNKI), Chinese biomedical literature (CBM) CD, and China Journals Full-text Database. From the electronic database records and bibliographic references, we identified relevant primary sources and secondary sources (such as textbooks, review articles, and meta-analyses) as follows. We selected all EBM reviews, including Cochrane DSR, ACP Journal Club, DARE, CCTR, CMR, HTA, and NHSEED from inception to April 2014; EMBASE from 1980 to April 2014; EMBASE Classic from 1947 to 1979; PubMed from inception to April 2014; Ovid MEDLINE(R) from 1950 to April 2014; Ovid OLDMEDLINE(R) from 1948 to 1965; SinoMed from 1978 to April 2014; China Journals Full-text Database from 1994 to April 2014 and CBM disc from 1979 to April 2014. The search strategy was (1) (constipation) OR (chronic constipation) OR (functional constipation); (2) (herb*) OR (herbal medicine) OR (traditional Chinese medicine) OR (Chinese medicine) OR (Complementary medicine) OR (Naturopathy); (3) (case*) OR (clinical observation*) OR (clinical trial) OR (clinical study); (1) AND (2) AND (3) (*was used for truncation).

Study selection

We included interventions using single herbs, CM classical formulae, CM new formulae, and Chinese herb-derived products and combination products. The clinical study types included were quasi- or randomized controlled trials, observational clinical studies, case series or case reports, and other types of appropriate research methods. We included studies on subjects with constipation of all ages and both sexes, studies using objective measures from laboratory or imaging techniques, and studies using measurement from nursing staff, patients, or other informants.

Data extraction

Two authors (LLDZ and GZ) independently searched the databases and selected relevant publications. If the two authors disagreed about a study's eligibility, they would check the study against the selection criteria, discuss its eligibility, and make a further decision (ZXB). One author (LLDZ) extracted the data and the other (GZ) checked the extracted data. For each study, the following information was extracted: study design, sample size, mode of recruitment, sampling and diagnostic procedure, inclusion and exclusion criteria, and participants' characteristics (including age, sex, and duration of constipation). CM patterns, CM treatment principles, treatment regimen, and CM treatment outcomes were recorded.

Quality assessment

The methodological quality of relevant studies was assessed using the Jadad scale (Additional file 1; [11]). The Jadad scale evaluates a study in terms of the description of randomization, blinding, and dropouts. The scale ranges from 1 to 5; randomized controlled trials with a score between 3 and 5 are regarded as better quality trials. Points were awarded if the study was described as randomized (1 point), had an appropriate randomization method (1 point), was described as double-blind (1 point), used an appropriate blinding method (1 point), and had a description of withdrawals and dropouts (1 point) [11].

Identification of herb-*zheng* associations

Classification based on keyword co-occurrence was conducted on the 18,272 items of constipation literature downloaded from SinoMed [12]. We also applied a dictionary-based data slicing algorithm constructed on the principle of keyword co-occurrence. We filtered the downloaded data using CM associated keywords, such as "Chinese herbal medicine," "Chinese patent medicine," and "CM syndrome/*zheng*," which were obtained from textbooks and the Internet. The keyword co-occurrence classification was a good supplement to the literature search, as it provided insights into the quantitative relationship between the individual herbs and formulae used to treat constipation. We used a wheel-shaped network to indicate the association between different types of single herbs and their *zheng* indications [10]. The wheel-shaped network was a visualized graph that showed the frequencies and correlations among the same categories [10].

Translation of terminology

All Chinese-to-English translations were deduced primarily from the *World Health Organization (WHO) Evidence-Based Complementary and Alternative Medicine International Standard Terminologies on Traditional Medicine in the Western Pacific Region* [13].

Results

We accessed 29,832 records that fit the search criteria, of which 8541 were duplicate records and 20,639 were excluded for reasons of irrelevance. The full text of 965 articles was retrieved for detailed assessment; 480 of these were excluded for various reasons (Fig. 1). Of the 485 studies that fulfilled the inclusion and exclusion criteria, 289 were on CM formulae, 91 were on proprietary CM, and 105 were on a combination of CHM and conventional treatment. The sample size of the 485 studies ranged from 35 to 250. Among all the studies, 289 (59.6 %) were case series or reports, 125 (25.8 %) were controlled trials, and 71 (14.6 %) were randomized controlled trials. For the randomized controlled trials, the mean Jadad scores were 2.06 and their average quality was quite low (Additional file 1).

CM *zheng* category and treatment criteria

From the included articles, we retrieved 190 different CM *zheng* diagnoses from 485 individual studies. The most common pattern was *dual deficiency of qi and blood (Qi Xue Liang Xu)*, which was diagnosed in 948 of the 15,740 subjects (frequency = 48, percentage among the top 10 diagnosis = 16.8 %); this was followed by *dual deficiency of qi and yin (Qi Yin Liang Xu)* (subjects = 795, frequency = 45, percentage among the top 10 diagnosis = 15.7 %), *excessive heat and qi stagnation (Qi Zhi Shi Re)* (subjects = 726, frequency = 41, percentage among the top 10 diagnosis = 14.3 %), *yang*

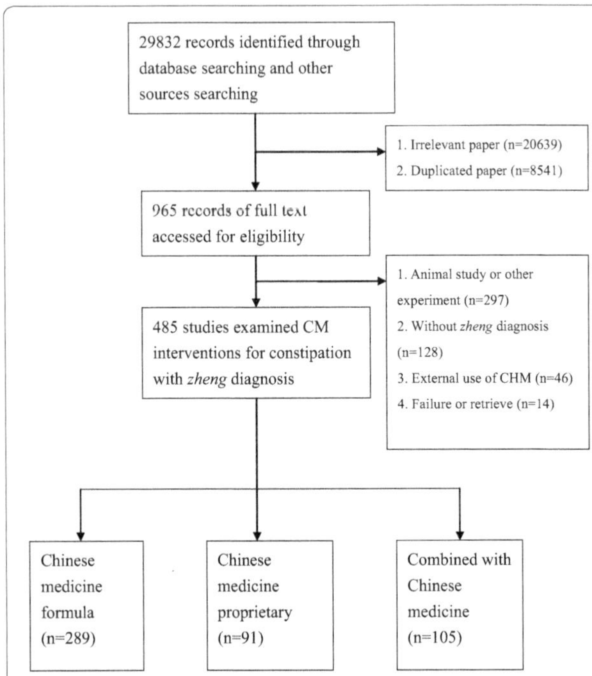

Fig. 1 Flowchart of literature selection logistics

deficiency of spleen and kidney (Pi Shen Yang Xu) (subjects = 636, frequency = 32, percentage among the top 10 diagnosis = 11.2 %), *deficiency of qi and blood (Qi Xue Liang Xu)* (subjects = 595, frequency = 26, percentage among the top 10 diagnosis = 9.1 %), *cold–heat complex (Han Re Cuo Za)* (subjects = 513, frequency = 21, percentage among the top 10 diagnosis = 7.3 %), *liver depression and spleen deficiency (Gan Yu Pi Xu)* (subjects = 495, frequency = 20, percentage among the top 10 diagnosis = 7.0 %), *deficiency–excess complex (Xu Shi Jia Za)* (subjects = 483, frequency = 20, percentage among the top 10 diagnosis = 7.0 %), *dual yin deficiency of liver and kidney (Gan Shen Yin Xu)* (subjects = 410, frequency = 17, percentage among the top 10 diagnosis = 5.9 %) and *intestinal dryness and yin deficiency (Yin Xu Chang Zao)* (subjects = 223, frequency = 16, percentage among the top 10 diagnosis = 5.6 %). Subjects diagnosed with the top 10 CM *zheng* accounted for 37 % of the 15,740 subjects (Table 1). Table 1 lists the therapeutic principles for the CM *zheng*.

CM herbs and their relationships

We identified 296 herbs from 485 clinical studies and analyzed their relationships using the wheel-shaped network (Fig. 2). In this figure, red and green nodes represent different single herbal medicines. The edges represent co-occurrence frequency in clinical studies. The edge label numbers represent the number of clinical studies demonstrating a connection between two single herbal medicines. There was a high concentration of one classical Chinese herbal formula, *Ma-Zi-Ren-Wan*, whose composition of six herbs occupied 42.5 % (1754/4127) of the total frequency of usage. Based on this, the green nodes represent CHMs in the formula *Ma-Zi-Ren-Wan* and the red nodes represent other CHMs used in clinical prescriptions [10]. Node size was calculated with the formula

$$Node\,size = LOG\left(node\_frequency\right) + Degree\,(node)$$

where *node_frequency* is the literature record number of the associated keyword calculated in text mining, *LOG* is the logarithm calculation with a base set to 10, and *Degree (node)* is the number of connections/edges each node has with other nodes. The edge line width was calculated through *LOG (edge_co-occurrent)* where *edge_co-occurrent* was the number of node/keyword pairs that co-occurred in the associated literature.

Table 2 lists the top 10 most frequently used herbs and their actions. The most frequently used herbs were further categorized and analyzed to determine their combinations in classical formulae. The most frequently used classical formulae were *Ma-Zi-Ren-Wan* [14] and *Zeng-Ye-Tang* [15].

CM *zheng*-based Chinese herbal formulae

Among the 289 studies on Chinese herbal formulae, the most frequently used formulae based on *zheng* diagnosis

Table 1 Top ten most commonly used CM *zheng* for constipation

CM *zheng*	Therapeutic principle	Number of subjects diagnosed by the diagnosis	Number of frequency among all the studies	Percentage among the total *zheng* (190)/top 10 *zheng* diagnosis (%)
Dual deficiency of qi and blood qi-xue-liang-xu	Tonify *qi* and replenish *blood*	948	48	16.8/6.2
Dual deficiency of qi and yin qi-yin-liang-xu	Tonify *qi* and replenish *yin*	795	45	15.7/5.9
Excessive heat and qi stagnation qi-zhi-shi-re	Soothe the *liver* and regulate *qi*	726	41	14.3/5.3
Yang deficiency of spleen and kidney pi-shen-yang-xu	Warm the *kidney* and fortify the spleen	636	32	11.2/4.2
Deficiency of qi and blood pi-xue-kui-xu	Tonify *qi* and engender *blood*	595	26	9.1/3.4
Cold-heat complex han-re-cuo-za	Treat *cold* with *heat* and *heat* with *cold*	513	21	7.3/2.7
Liver depression and spleen deficiency gan-yu-pi-xu	Soothe the *liver* and fortify the *spleen*	495	20	7.0/2.6
Deficiency-excess complex xu-shi-jia-za	Treat *deficiency* by tonification and excess by purgation	483	20	7.0/2.6
Dual yin deficiency of liver and kidney gan-shen-yin-xu	Enrich the *kidney* and nourish the *liver yin*	410	17	5.9/2.2
Intestinal dryness and yin deficiency yin-xu-chang-zao	Replenish *yin* and moisten dryness	223	16	5.6/2.1

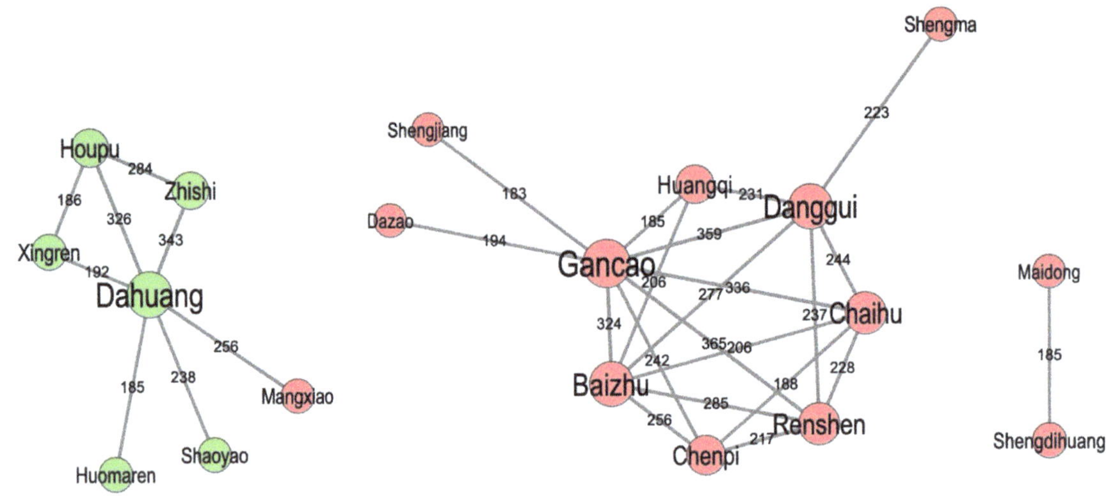

Fig. 2 Network relationship of Chinese herbal medicine in the treatment of constipation. *Red* and *green* nodes represent different single herbal medicines. The *edges* represent co-occurrence frequency in clinical studies. The *edge label numbers* represent the number of clinical studies demonstrating a connection between two single herbal medicines

were *Ma-Zi-Ren-Wan* and its modifications (frequency among all the studies, n = 75, percentage among the top 10 formulae, 33.07 %). This was followed by *Bu-Zhong-Yi-Qi-Tang* (n = 56, 22.58 %), *Ji-Chuan-Jian* (n = 51, 20.56 %), *Zeng-Ye-Tang* (n = 40, 13.84 %), and *Ba-Zhen-Tang* (n = 26, 10.48 %). The five most frequently used CM *zheng*-based Chinese herbal formulae and their indications are summarized in Table 3.

Proprietary CHMs

After the classical herbal decoctions, the next most frequently used clinical treatments for constipation were proprietary CHMs, because of their standard quality control and more convenient administration. We analyzed the most commonly used proprietary CHMs and their dosage (Table 4). The manufacturers of the proprietary CHMs are also shown, to indicate the quality and composition of the medicines. The most commonly used proprietary CHM was *Run-Chang-Wan* (frequency, n = 87), followed by *Ma-Ren-Ruan-Jiao-Nang* (n = 62), *Ma-Ren-Run-Chang-Wan* (n = 52), *Liu-Wei-An-Xiao-Jiao-Nang* (n = 50), *Fu-Fang-Lu-Hui-Jiao-Nang* (n = 35), *Si-Ni-San* (n = 32), *Liu-Wei-Neng-Xiao-Jiao-Nang* (n = 27), and *Bu-Zhong-Yi-Qi-Wan* (n = 17).

CM combined with Western medicine and adverse effects

Few clinical studies reported the combined use of CM and Western medicine for constipation. Table 5 summarized the herb–drug interactions identified. Although most studies did not mention the adverse effects associated with combined administration of herbs and drugs, or proprietary CHMs and drugs, there were 43 reported trials of the integrative use of single herbs or proprietary CHMs. Among these studies, the most frequent adjunctive use was *Da Huang* (*Radix et Rhizoma Rhei*) with *sodium bicarbonate tablets* (n = 23), followed by *Fan Xie Ye* (*Folium Sennae*) with *lactulose oral solution* (n = 8), *Ma-Ren-Ruan-Jiao-Nang* with *lactulose oral solution* (n = 6) and *Liu-Wei-An-Xiao-Jiao-Nang with mosapride citrate tablets* (n = 6).

Discussion

To our knowledge, this is the first study to examine the use of single herbs, classical CM formulae, proprietary CHMs, and the combined use of CM and Western medicine (and its adverse effects) for constipation. The classification of single herbs and CM formulae was generally based on the CM diagnostic *zheng* system. As we pointed out in our commentary paper, *zheng* diagnosis is a critical stage of CM treatment; it is the basis of CM's effectiveness and the main feature that distinguishes it from Western medicine [16]. In this review, we focused on *zheng* diagnosis, in accord with current clinical CM practice. Although we identified 190 different CM *zheng* diagnoses, only 57.9 % (281/485) of studies used the diagnosis system of *zheng* differentiation. The most commonly diagnosed *zheng* for constipation was *dual deficiency of qi and blood* (16.8 %) followed by *dual deficiency of qi and yin* (15.7 %) and *excessive heat and qi stagnation* (14.3 %). As Table 1 showed, among the top 10 CM *zheng*, five belonged to *deficiency zheng* and the others could be categorized as a combination of *deficiency* and *sufficiency* or *sufficiency* syndrome. These results are consistent with those of our previous study [16] and with other research

Table 2 Action and indication of the most ten frequently used herbs

Chinese name in pinyin	Latin name	Frequency of usage	Action	Indication
Da Huang	Radix *et Rhizoma Rhei*	428	Drains *heat* and purges accumulations; clears *heat*, transforms *dampness* and promotes urination; drains *heat* from the *blood*; invigorates the *blood* and dispels blood stasis	Intestinal *heat excess* with high fever, profuse sweating, thirst, constipation, abdominal distention and pain, delirium, a yellow tongue coat and a full pulse; blood stasis with amenorrhea, fixed abdominal masses or fixed pain
Huo Ma Ren	*Semen Cannabis*	247	Nourishes, moistens and lubricates the intestines; nourishes the *yin;* clears *heat* and promotes healing of sores; moistens dryness and benefits the hair	Constipation in the elderly; constipation after a warm febrile disease; postpartum constipation; constipation due to blood and *yin deficiency*; sores and ulcerations (auxiliary-internal and topical); promotes hair growth and treats dry hair
Fan Xie Ye	*Folium Sennae*	232	Drains downward and guides out stagnation; eliminates excess *heat* and drains *summer heat*	*Heat* in the stomach and intestines with constipation and abdominal fullness; *summer heat*
Bai Zhu	Rhizoma *Atractylodis Macrocephalae*	198	Tonifies the *spleen* and augments *qi*; dries *dampness* and promotes water metabolism; stabilizes the exterior and stops sweating	*Spleen* and *stomach deficiency* with diarrhea, fatigue; *spleen damp* or accumulation of fluids affecting the digestion; edema and reduced urination due to *spleen deficiency*; *qi deficiency* with spontaneous sweating
Dang- Gui	Radix *Angelicae Sinensis*	132	Tonifies the *blood* and regulates the menses; invigorates and harmonizes the *blood* and disperses cold; moistens the intestines and unblocks the bowels	Blood deficiency with pale, ashen complexion, lusterless nails, tinnitus; *blood deficiency* associated irregular menstruation, amenorrhea and dysmenorrhea; dry Intestines due to blood deficiency
Huang Qi	Radix *Astragali*	126	Tonifies *qi* and *blood*; strengthens the *spleen* and raises the *yang qi* of the *spleen* and *stomach*; tonifies *wei qi*, stabilizes the exterior and tonifies the *lungs*	Postpartum fever due to *qi* and *blood deficiency*; *spleen qi deficiency* with anorexia, fatigue and diarrhea; excessive sweating with *qi*, *yang* or *yin deficiency*; *dampness* in the head
Gan Cao	Radix *Glycyrrhizae*	112	Tonifies the *spleen* and augments *qi*; moistens the *lungs*, resolves phlegm and stops cough; moderates spasms and alleviates pain; clears *heat* and relieves *fire* toxicity	Spleen *qi deficiency* with shortness of breath, lassitude and loose stools; *qi* and *blood deficiency* with an irregular pulse and/or palpitations; productive or non-productive cough; raw for toxic *heat* with sore throat or carbuncles and sores
Sheng Di	Radix *Rehmanniae*	99	Clears *heat* and cools the *blood*; nourishes *yin*, generates fluids, increases saliva and treats wasting and thirsting; cools heart fire	*Ying*-stage *heat* with high fever, thirst and a scarlet tongue; hemorrhage due to *blood heat*; throat pain due to *yin deficiency*
Bai Shao	Radix *Paeoniae Alba*	94	Nourishes the *blood* and regulates menstruation; astringes *yin* and adjusts the *ying* and *wei*; calms *liver yang* and *liver wind* and alleviates pain	*Liver blood deficiency* with menstrual dysfunction, vaginal discharge and uterine bleeding; anemia; breast distention and pre-menstrual syndrome
Lu Hui	Aloe	93	Purges, drains *fire* and guides out accumulations; clears *heat* and cools the *liver*; kills parasites and strengthens the *stomach*	*Heat* accumulation with constipation, dizziness, red eyes, and irritability; chronic constipation; heat in the liver channel or liver fire with epigastric discomfort, dizziness, headache, irritability, tinnitus, constipation and fever

Table 3 Summary of top five most frequently used Chinese herbal formulae based on *zheng* diagnosis

Chinese name in pinyin	Composition in pinyin	CM *zheng*	Number of frequency among all the studies	Actions in Chinese medicine
Ma-Zi-Ren-Wan	*Huo Ma Ren* *Xing Ren* *Bai Shao* *Zhi Shi* *Hou Pu* *Da Huang*	Excessive *qi* and *heat*	75	Invigorates *Blood* Dispels *Blood* Stasis Moves *qi* Lubricates the intestines Moves the bowels Purges *heat* Alleviates pain
Bu-Zhong-Yi-Qi-Tang	*Huang Qi* *Ren Shen* *Bai Zhu* *Zhi Gan Cao* *Dang Gui* *Chen Pi* *Shen Ma* *Chai Hu*	*Qi deficiency* of *spleen* and *stomach/Sunken middle qi*	56	Tonifies *middle jiao qi* Benefits *qi* Regulates *qi* Raises *sunken yang* Lifts prolapsed organs
Ji-Chuan-Jian	*Dang Gui* *Niu Xi* *Rou Cong Rong* *Ze Xie* *Shen Ma* *Zhi Qiao*	*Yang deficiency* of *spleen* and *kidney*	51	Warms up the *kidney* Replenishes vital essence Lubricates the intestines Induces defecation
Zeng-Ye-Tang	*Xuan Shen* *Mai Dong* *Sheng Di*	*Fluid-humor deficiency*	40	Generates Fluids Moistens dryness Unblocks the bowels Nourishes *yin* Clears *heat*
Ba-Zhen-Tang	*Ren Shen* *Bai Zhu* *Fu Ling* *Zhi Gan Cao* *Shu Di* *Bai Shao* *Chuan Xiong* *Dang Gui*	*Dual deficiency* of *qi* and *blood*	26	Nourishes *qi* Benefits *blood*

on syndrome distribution among constipation patients [8, 17], which indicated that almost half of patients, especially older individuals and postpartum women, had *deficiency* syndromes [18, 19].

Of the 10 most frequently used herbs, the top three were traditional purgatives; the other herbs were *tonifying* and *replenishing* medicines, except *Lu Hui* (*Aloe vera*) [20, 21]. It is interesting that the top five CM *zheng* were *deficiency zheng*; this seemed inconsistent with the fact that the five most frequently used single herbs were purgatives. This was mainly because only 50.26 % of studies used CM *zheng* differentiation, and purgatives are mostly used for general constipation in the absence of any CM *zheng* diagnosis. Table 3 shows that the most commonly used Chinese herbal formula was *Ma-Zi-Ren-Wan*, which suggested that it formed the basis of the most commonly prescribed formulae for constipation according to both CM syndrome differentiation and Western medicine diagnosis.

Many studies of Chinese herbal formulae or proprietary CHM did not provide standard or complete criteria for syndrome diagnosis. The lack of detail and consistency in diagnosis makes these studies difficult to replicate and their findings difficult to compare with other results [22]. Most studies provided only the main composition of the formulae without any indication of dosage or quality control standards (Table 4). Although proprietary CHMs are rapidly gaining attention in the West as sources of new drugs, dietary supplements, and functional foods, the lack of consistent manufacturing processes, quality standards, scientific evidence, and validation of efficacy and safety impede worldwide acceptance of CHM [23].

Currently, herb–drug interactions are of growing concern as a clinical safety issue to clinicians and researchers [24, 25]. Proprietary CHMs are prescribed by Western medical doctors who may not fully understand the indications and actions of these medicines [26]. Although herbal medicines are natural, they are not always safe [27]. Table 5 showed the concomitant use and the adverse effects of herb–drug combinations or proprietary CHM–drug combinations based on the limited literature. These limited data showed that the incidence of adverse effects

Table 4 Summary of top ten most frequently used Chinese herbal medicine proprietary

Chinese name in pinyin (manufacturer)	Composition in pinyin	Oral dosage	Number of frequency among all the studies	Indication
Run-Chang-Wan (Shang Dong Hua Yang Pharmaceutical Co. Ltd.)	*Tao Ren* *Da Hua* *Qiang Huo* *Dang Gui* *Huo Ma Ren*	4 pills t. i. d. for oral administration	87	Constipation with CM *zheng* of *excessive qi* and *heat*, and constipation for elderly people and postpartum women
Ma-Ren-Ruan-Jiao-Nang (Actavis (Foshan) Pharmaceutical Co., Ltd.)	*Huo Ma Ren* *Xing Ren* *Bai Shao* *Zhi Shi* *Hou Pu* *Da Huang*	2 capsules t. i. d. for oral administration	62	Constipation with CM *zheng* of *excessive qi* and *heat*
Ma-Ren-Run-Chang-Wan (Bei Jing Tong Ren Tang Co., Ltd.)	*Huo Ma Ren* *Xing Ren* *Da Hua* *Bai Shao* *Mu Xiang* *Chen Pi*	1–2 big honey pills b. i. d. for oral administration	52	Constipation with CM *zheng* of *heat* in *stomach* and *intestines*
Liu-Wei-An-Xiao-Jiao-Nang (Gui Zhou Xin Bang Pharmaceutical Co., Ltd.)	*Tu Mu Xiang* *Da Huang* *Shan Nai* *Han Shui Shi* *Ke Zi* *Jian Hua*	3–6 pills b. i. d. for oral administration	50	Constipation due to indigestion and bloating; stomachache; dyspepsia
Fu-Fang-Lu-Hui-Jiao-Nang (He Bei Wan Bang & Folon Pharmaceutical Co., Ltd.)	*Lu Hui* *Qing Dai* *Zhu Sha* *Hu Po*	1–2 capsules b. i. d. for oral administration	35	Constipation with CM *zheng* of intense *fire* in *heart* and *liver*
Ma-Ren-Zi-Pi-Wan (Bao Tou Chinese Medicine Pharmaceutical Co., Ltd.)	*Huo Ma Ren* *Xing Ren* *Bai Shao* *Zhi Shi* *Hou Pu* *Da Huang* *Yu Li Ren* *Dang Gui*	1 big honey pills b. i. d. for oral administration	34	Constipation with CM *zheng* of dryness and heat in large intestine

Table 4 continued

Chinese name in pinyin (manufacturer)	Composition in pinyin	Oral dosage	Number of frequency among all the studies	Indication
Si-Ni-San (Fu Zhou Neptunus Futao Pharmaceutical Co., Ltd.)	*Chai Hu* *Zhi Shi* *Bai Shao* *Zhi Gan Cao*	6–9 g granules b. i. d. for oral administration	32	Constipation with CM *zheng* of disharmony between *spleen* and *liver*
Liu-Wei-Neng-Xiao-Jiao-Nang (Yang Zong Pharmaceutical Co., Ltd.)	*Da Hua* *Ke Zi* *Gan Jiang* *Zang Mu Xiang* *Jian Hua* *Hai Shui Shi*	2 capsules b. i. d. for oral administration	27	Constipation due to indigestion; obesity; hyperlipidemia
Bu-Zhong-Yi-Qi-Wan (Bei Jing Tong Ren Tang Co., Ltd.)	*Huang Qi* *Dang Shen* *Bai Zhu* *Dang Gui* *Shen Ma* *Chai Hu* *Chen Pi* *Zhi Gan Cao*	1–2 big honey pills b. i. d. for oral administration	17	Constipation with CM *zheng* of *qi deficiency* of *spleen* and *stomach/Sunken middle qi*

t.i.d. means ter in die, three times a day; *b.i.d.* means bis in die, twice a day

Table 5 Summary of combination of CHM and Western medicine and the reported adverse effects

	Combined used Western medicine	Frequency of reported in all the trials (n > 5)	Adverse effect (N = , percentage, %)
Single herb			
Da Huang	Sodium bicarbonate tablets	23	Symptoms of the gastrointestinal tract (N = 4, 17.3 %)
			Insomnia (N = 1, 4.3 %)
			Skin rash (N = 1, 4.3 %)
			Headache (N = 1, 4.3 %)
Fan Xie Ye	Lactulose oral solution	8	Symptoms of the gastrointestinal tract (N = 2, 25 %)
			Dizzy and anorexia (N = 1, 12.5 %)
CHM Proprietary			
Ma-Ren-Ruan-Jiao-Nang	Lactulose oral solution	6	Symptoms of the gastrointestinal tract (N = 2, 33.3 %)
			Headache (N = 1, 16.7 %)
Liu-Wei-An-Xiao-Jiao-Nang	Mosapride citrate tablets	6	Symptoms of the gastrointestinal tract (N = 3, 50 %)

was not as low as we expected, ranging from 4.3 to 50 %, although most adverse effects were symptoms of the gastrointestinal tract.

A limitation of this study was that the data were drawn from clinical studies that used several different types of design: case reports, cohort studies, and quasi- or randomized controlled trials. The quality of these studies varied and therefore it is difficult to compare them quantitatively. In addition, most studies did not provide sufficient detail regarding inclusion criteria of diseases and syndromes, quality control procedures for single herbs or proprietary CHMs, or withdrawal rates and reasons. Therefore, the analysis of the data derived from this study is limited and should be treated with caution.

Conclusion

This review examined the use of CHM for constipation and summarized the most frequently used Chinese single herbs, the 10 most frequently used CHM formulae and proprietary CHMs, and the combined use of CHM and Western medicine treatments and their reported adverse effects.

Abbreviations

CHM: Chinese herbal medicine; CM: Chinese medicine; MZRW: *Ma-Zi-Ren-Wan*; PRISMA: Preferred Reporting Items for Systematic Reviews and Meta-Analyses; EBMR: Evidence-Based Medicine Reviews; CNKI: Chinese National Knowledge Infrastructure; CBM: Chinese biomedical literature.

Authors' contributions

ZXB designed the study. LDG and CYL conducted text mining. TH and LZ retrieved the herbs and herb-drug interaction data. LLDZ and GZ searched the literature and wrote the manuscript. LDG, CYL, TH, LZ, LLDZ, GZ, CL, and APL revised the manuscript. All authors read and approved the final manuscript.

Author details

[1] School of Chinese Medicine, Hong Kong Baptist University, 7 Baptist University Road, Kowloon Tong, Hong Kong, China. [2] Hong Kong Chinese Medicine Study Centre, Hong Kong Baptist University, Hong Kong SAR, China. [3] Department of Surgery, The First People's Hospital of Xiaoshan District, Hangzhou, China. [4] Institute of Basic Research in Clinical Medicine, China Academy of Traditional Chinese Medicine, Beijing, China. [5] School of Information Science and Engineering, Lanzhou University, Lanzhou, China.

Acknowledgements

We thank Health and Health Services Research Fund (Project No. 09101501), Hong Kong SAR, and Natural Science Foundation of China Project (NSFC-81173363) for financially support this research. The funding agencies have no role in the design and execution of this project. They will not be involved to the analysis and interpretation of data, or make decision to submit the results.

Competing interests

The authors declare that they have no competing interests.

References

1. Mugie SM, Benninga MA, Di Lorenzo C. Epidemiology of constipation in children and adults: a systematic review. Best Pract Res Clin Gastroenterol. 2011;25(1):3–18.
2. Huang R, Ho SY, Lo WS, Lam TH. Physical activity and constipation in Hong Kong adolescents. PLoS ONE. 2014;9(2):e90193.
3. Pasanen ME. Evaluation and treatment of colonic symptoms. Med Clin North Am. 2014;98(3):529–47.
4. McCarberg BH. Overview and treatment of opioid-induced constipation. Postgrad Med. 2013;125(4):7–17.

5. Lin LW, Fu YT, Dunning T, Zhang AL, Ho TH, Duke M, Lo SK. Efficacy of traditional Chinese medicine for the management of constipation: a systematic review. J Altern Complement Med. 2009;15(12):1335–46.
6. Cheng CW, Bian ZX, Wu TX. Systematic review of Chinese herbal medicine for functional constipation. WJG. 2009;15(39):4886–95.
7. Suo T, Gu X, Andersson R, Ma H, Zhang W, Deng W, Zhang B, Cai D, Qin X. Oral traditional Chinese medication for adhesive small bowel obstruction. Cochrane Database Syst Rev. 2012;5:CD008836.
8. Chen CM, Lin LZ, Zhang EX. Standardized treatment of chinese medicine decoction for cancer pain patients with opioid-induced constipation: A multi-center prospective randomized controlled study. Chin J Integr Med. 2014;20(7):496–502.
9. Yao YB, Cao YQ, Guo XT, Yi J, Liang HT, Wang C, Lu JG. Biofeedback therapy combined with traditional Chinese medicine prescription improves the symptoms, surface myoelectricity, and anal canal pressure of the patients with spleen deficiency constipation. eCAM. 2013;2013:830714.
10. Zheng G, Jiang M, He X, Zhao J, Guo H, Chen G, Zha Q, Lu A. Discrete derivative: a data slicing algorithm for exploration of sharing biological networks between rheumatoid arthritis and coronary heart disease. BioData Min. 2011;4:18.
11. Moher D, Jadad AR, Tugwell P. Assessing the quality of randomized controlled trials. Current issues and future directions. Int J Technol Assess Health Care. 1996;12(2):195–208.
12. Sinomed database: http://www.sinomed.ac.cn/. Accessed 16 May 2014.
13. WHO Regional Office for the Western Pacific. WHO International Standard Terminologies on Traditional Medicine in the Western Pacific Region; 2007.
14. Zhang S. Examples for clinical use of ma zi ren wan. J Tradit Chin Med. 2002;22(3):216–7.
15. Zeng ZC, Tang ZY, Fan J, Zhou J, Qin LX, Ye SL, Sun HC, Wang BL, Li D, Wang JH, Zeng MS, Guo W, Tan YS. Consideration of the role of radiotherapy for unresectable intrahepatic cholangiocarcinoma: a retrospective analysis of 75 patients. Cancer J. 2006;12(2):113–22.
16. Bian ZX, Xu H, Lu AP, Lee MS, Cheung H. Insights of Chinese medicine syndrome study: from current status to future prospects. Chin J Integr Med. 2014;20(5):326–31.
17. Cheng CW, Kwok AO, Bian ZX, Tse DM. The quintessence of traditional Chinese medicine: syndrome and its distribution among advanced cancer patients with constipation. eCAM. 2012;2012:739642.
18. Ren Z, Wu QM, Li DD, Liu WA, Li XR, Lin XM. Post-stroke constipation treated with acupuncture therapy of regulating qi circulation of fu-organ. Zhongguo zhen jiu. 2013;33(10):893–6.
19. Cherniack EP. Use of complementary and alternative medicine to treat constipation in the elderly. Geriatr Gerontol Int. 2013;13(3):533–8.
20. Wang J, Huang JH, Cheng YF, Yang GM. Banana resistant starch and its effects on constipation model mice. J Med Food. 2014;17(8):902–7.
21. Hou ML, Chang LW, Lin CH, Lin LC, Tsai TH. Determination of bioactive components in Chinese herbal formulae and pharmacokinetics of rhein in rats by UPLC-MS/MS. Molecules. 2014;19(4):4058–75.
22. Wang J, Cui M, Jiao H, Tong Y, Xu J, Zhao Y, Han M, Liu J. Content analysis of systematic reviews on effectiveness of traditional Chinese medicine. J Tradit Chin Med. 2013;33(2):156–63.
23. Xue CC, Zhang AL, Greenwood KM, Lin V, Story DF. Traditional Chinese medicine: an update on clinical evidence. J Altern Complement Med. 2010;16(3):301–12.
24. Ge B, Zhang Z, Zuo Z. Updates on the clinical evidenced herb-warfarin interactions. eCAM. 2014;2014:957362.
25. Rahal A, Ahmad AH, Kumar A, Mahima, Verma AK, Chakraborty S, Dhama K. Clinical drug interactions: a holistic view. PJBS. 2013;16(16):751–8.
26. Chan TY. The prevalence use and harmful potential of some Chinese herbal medicines in babies and children. Vet Hum Toxicol. 1994;36(3):238–40.
27. van Andel T, de Boer HJ, Barnes J, Vandebroek I. Medicinal plants used for menstrual disorders in Latin America, the Caribbean, sub-Saharan Africa, South and Southeast Asia and their uterine properties: a review. J Ethnopharmacol. 2014;155:992.

14

Induction of apoptosis in human hepatocellular carcinoma cells by extracts of *Lannea coromandelica* (Houtt.) Merr. and *Diospyros castanea* (Craib) Fletcher

Natthida Weerapreeyakul[1], Cholpajsorn Junhom[2], Sahapat Barusrux[3*] and Thaweesak Thitimetharoch[1]

Abstract

Background: Herbal plants are a preferred source of anticancer agents. This study aims to screen the anticancer activity of a crude extract of twigs of (a) *Bombax anceps* Pierre var. *anceps* (BA); (b) *Catunaregam tomentosa* (Blume ex DC.) Tirveng. (CT); (c) *Erythrophleum succirubrum* Gagnep. (ES); (d) *Lannea coromandelica* (Houtt.) Merr. (LC); and (e) leaves and (f) twigs of *Diospyros castanea* (Craib) Fletcher (DC).

Methods: The 50 % ethanol–water extracts were prepared from each plant sample. In vitro anticancer effects of six extracts on the human hepatocellular carcinoma cell line (HepG2) in terms of cytotoxicity were investigated by neutral red assay, apoptosis induction by 4′,6-diamidino-2-phenylindole (DAPI) staining, and DNA fragmentation by agarose gel electrophoresis. Normal Vero cells were tested for comparison and to determine cancer selectivity. Gas chromatography–mass spectrometry analysis was performed to identify the compounds in the extracts.

Results: The six crude extracts had different cytotoxicities and were classified into three groups based on their IC_{50} value and selectivity index (SI). DC (twig) crude extract had both a high cytotoxicity and SI toward HepG2 cells comparable to melphalan ($P = 0.023$). The crude extracts of DC (leaves), LC (twig), and BA (twig) had moderate cytotoxicity and a lower SI. Although all crude plant extracts induced apoptosis in more than 50 % of the DAPI-positive apoptotic HepG2 cells, only DC (twig) and LC (twig) showed laddering in the DNA fragmentation assay. 2-Palmitoylglycerol was the major compound common to both. Pyrogallol and lupeol were the major compounds in DC (twig) crude extract. Hexadecanoic acid and octadecenoic acid were the major compounds in LC (twig) crude extract, which had high toxicity but low selectivity.

Conclusion: Ethanolic extracts from DC and LC twigs induced apoptosis in the HepG2 cell line. Pyrogallol and lupeol in DC (twig) might be responsible for the cytotoxicity toward the HepG2 cancer cells.

Keywords: *Diospyros castanea*, *Lannea coromandelica*, Hepatocellular carcinoma, HepG2, Cytotoxicity, Apoptosis

Background

Hepatocellular carcinoma (HCC) in men is the fifth most common malignant tumor in the world and the second most common cause of cancer death [1]. The major risk factors for HCC include infection by hepatitis B and hepatitis C viruses, both of which are endemic in northeastern Thailand [2]. Drug resistance and severe side effects on normal tissues and cells have limited the effectiveness of chemotherapy [3].

Anticancer agents have been found in natural products, such as vincristine and vinblastine from *Catharanthus roseus* [4], taxol and docetaxel from *Taxus brevifolia* [5], and camptothecins from *Camptotheca acuminata* [6–9]. The Plant Genetics Conservation Project (under the patronage of HRH Princess Maha Chakri Sirindhorn)

*Correspondence: sahapat@kku.ac.th
[3] Faculty of Associate Medical Sciences, Khon Kaen University, Khon Kaen 40002, Thailand
Full list of author information is available at the end of the article

has reported on the cytotoxic and apoptotic effects of medicinal plants against hepatoma cells [10–13]. Subsequent study was performed on the plants locally found in Thailand which were used in this study including *Lannea coromandelica* (Houtt.) Merr. (LC); *Catunaregam tomentosa* (Blume ex DC.) Tirveng. (CT); *Erythrophleum succirubrum* Gagnep (ES); *Diospyros castanea* (Craib) Fletcher (DC); and *Bombax anceps* Pierre var. *anceps* (BA).

DC belongs to the family Ebenaceae, which is widespread in the tropics and subtropics [14]. Many Diospyros species have medicinal uses in Chinese, Ayurvedic, and African traditional medicine. Almost all the major parts of these plants have been used as medicines and reported to have biological and pharmacological activities [14]. LC belongs to the family Anacardiaceae. It is a deciduous tropical tree widely distributed in Bangladesh, India, and some other tropical countries [15–18]. CT belongs to the family Rubiaceae and has been used to treat diabetes mellitus, cancer, and tuberculosis. It possesses antimicrobial, antifungal, hypotensive, analgesic, antimalaria, antioxidant, and antileukemia pharmacological properties [19]. ES belongs to the family Leguminosae (subfamily Caesalpinioideae) and is used in Thai traditional medicines for fever and skin disease. Some isolated compounds (cassaine diterpenoid dimers) from this family contribute to anticancer activity by decreasing apoptosis inhibitors or increasing apoptosis inducers; this leads to tumor necrosis factor (TNF)-related apoptosis-inducing ligand resistance in human gastric adenocarcinoma cells [20]. BA belongs to the family Bombacaceae. Plants in this family are active against many different diseases [21–24] (Table 1); however, the dichloromethane extract from the root of *B. malabaricum* is inactive in the human epidermoid carcinoma (KB) and human cervical carcinoma (HeLa) cell lines [25].

To our knowledge, the mechanism of anticancer effect of these five plants on HCC is still unknown. This study aims to screen the anticancer activity of a crude 50 % ethanol–water extract of twigs of (a) BA; (b) CT; (c) ES; (d) LC; and (e) leaves and (f) twigs of DC. The cytotoxic and apoptotic actions of the extracts were investigated with a human HCC cell line (HepG2) and compared with their effects on normal Vero cells. One advantage of using the normal Vero cell line is that Vero cell line multiplies indefinitely while primary liver cells have a limited lifetime and die after a given number of generations. Consequently, the Vero cell line is easy to handle and represents an unlimited self-replicating source with a relatively high degree of homogeneity. We then analyzed major compounds common to the different effective extracts using gas chromatography–mass spectrometry (GC–MS).

Table 1 Ethnopharmacology, pharmacological activities, and taxonomic classification of plants

Scientific name (voucher specimen no.)[a]	Part of plant	Traditional uses/pharmacological activity
Diospyros castanea (Craib) Fletcher. (TT-OC-SK-1030) Family: Ebenaceae	Leaf	*Diospyros:* lumbago, astringent, febrifuge, anti cancer activity, anti HIV activity, anti-inflammatory activity [14]
	Fruit	*Diospyros:* carminative, astringent, cure biliousness [14]
	Seed	*Diospyros:* sedative [14]
	Bark	*Diospyros:* bitter, astringent and febrifuge [14]
Lannea coromandelica (Houtt.) Merr. (TT-OC-SK-993) Family: Anacardiaceae	Stem bark	LC: elephantiasis, impotence, ulcers, halitosis, heart disease, dysentery, gout rheumatism [15]
	Bark (ethanol, acetone)	LC: wound healing, antimicrobial activity in the form of simple ointments [16]
	Root bark, stem bark (crude methanol)	LC: hypotensive activity [17], *L. velutina*: antioxidation activity [18]
Catunaregam tomentosa (Blume ex DC.) Tirveng. (TT-OC-SK-1015) Family: Rubiaceae	Crude (ethanol)	*R. cordifolia*: diabetes mellitus, cancer, TB, antimicrobial, antifungal, hypotension analgesic, anti-malarial, antioxidant, anti-leukemic, mutagenic functions [19]
Erythrophleum succirubrum Gagnep. (TT-OC-SK-1082) Family: Leguminosae-Caesalpinioideae	Bark (methanol)	ES: anticancer activity [20]
Bombax anceps Pierre var. *anceps* (TT-OC-SK-1074) Family: Bombacaceae	Crude (methanol)	*B. ceiba*: antioxidant activity [21]
	Root (H_2O/acetone)	*B. malabaricum*: demulcent, diuretic, restorative, aphrodisiac, emetic properties, astringent, antifungal activity, cytotoxicity, anti-HIV activity [22]
	Stem bark	*B. ceiba:* anticancer activity and anti-inflammation [23]
	Stem bark (methanol)	*B. ceiba:* antiangiogenic activity [24]

[a] TT-OC-SK Thaweesak Thitimetharoch, Orasa Chaichumporn, and Sureerat Kaewsaart

Methods

Chemicals and reagents

Dulbecco's modified Eagle's medium (DMEM), fetal bovine serum, penicillin, and streptomycin were purchased from GIBCO™ (Invitrogen, Grand Island, New York, USA). Acetonitrile (HPLC grade; Fisher Scientific, Leicestershire, UK), orthophosphoric acid (analytical grade; BHD, Merseyside, UK), and ultrapure water from a Milli-Q system (Millipore, Billerica, Massachusetts, USA) were used for the mobile phase preparation. Dimethylsulfoxide (DMSO), ethidium bromide, the fluorescence dye 4′,6-diamidino-2-phenylindole (DAPI), sodium bicarbonate ($NaHCO_3$), neutral red, and a standard anticancer drug (melphalan) were purchased from Sigma-Aldrich (Darmstadt, Germany). A FlexiGene DNA kit was purchased from Qiagen (Hilden, Germany), agarose (molecular grade) was purchased from Bio-Rad (Hercules, California, USA), and a DNA ladder with stain was purchased from SibEnzyme (Novosibirsk, Russia). Isopropyl alcohol (biotechnology grade) was purchased from BioBasic Inc. (Amherst, New York, USA) and 100 bp + 1.5 Kb DNA ladder with stain was purchased from SibEnzyme (Novosibirsk, Russia). All other reagents used in this study were purchased from Sigma Chemicals Co. (St. Louis, Missouri, USA). An Annexin V-FITC Apoptosis Detection Kit was purchased from Bender MedSystems GmbH (Vienna, Austria).

Preparation of plant extracts

Leaves and twigs of LC, CT, ES, BA, and DC were collected in Khon Kaen Province, Thailand. They were authenticated using taxonomic methods by Assistant Professor Thaweesak Thitimetharoch., Faculty of Pharmaceutical Sciences, Khon Kaen University. The descriptions of plant species were determined using the Flora of Thailand and the Thai Forest Bulletin [26–30]. The specimen vouchers were deposited at the medicinal herbarium of the Faculty of Pharmaceutical Sciences, Khon Kaen University, Khon Kaen province, Thailand. All plants were extracted and prepared using the following method. The crude 50 % ethanol–water extract was obtained as previously described [12]. Briefly, dried plants were cut and macerated with 50 % ethanol and water in a ratio of 1 g dried plant to 6 ml of extract solvent. This mixture was left for 7 days with occasional shaking. The solvent was filtered with Whatman filter paper No. 1, distilled in vacuo with a rotary evaporator below 40 °C, and freeze-dried to obtain the crude extracts. The percentage yields of the extracts and the plant parts from which they were obtained are shown in Table 2. Stock solution of each extract was freshly prepared in DMSO to make 100 mg/mL stock solution and further diluted with culture media to create a working solution. In all experiments, the concentrations of extracts (working solution) ranged from 10 to 500 μg/mL and the final concentration of DMSO was <1 % to retain the percentage cytotoxicity of DMSO at <10 %.

Cell culture

The HepG2 cells (human HCC cell line) and Vero cells (normal kidney epithelial cells) were grown in DMEM supplemented with 10 % fetal bovine serum, 100 U/mL penicillin, and 100 μg/mL streptomycin. The cell lines were cultured in an incubator (Procell; Jencons-PLS, USA) at 37 °C in a humidified atmosphere containing 5 % carbon dioxide (CO_2).

Cytotoxicity assay

Cell viability was measured using a neutral red (NR) assay. Cells were seeded at a density of 3×10^5 cells per well in 96-well plates (Costar 3599; Corning Inc., USA) in the medium, and incubated for 24 h. The stock solutions of plant extracts in DMSO were diluted with DMEM to the desired concentrations (10–500 μg/mL).

Table 2 Cytotoxicity of plant extracts in HepG2 and vero cells (mean ± SD) (n = 5)

Plant	Part used	% yield	IC_{50} ± SD (μg/mL)		SI
			HepG2	Vero	
L. coromandelica (LC)	Twig	6.01	307.12 ± 15.97[a]	489.37 ± 37.43	1.6[a]
C. tomentosa (CT)	Twig	6.88	316.70 ± 34.82	294.59 ± 76.25	0.9
E. succirubrum (ES)	Twig	8.94	207.89 ± 40.89	94.18 ± 29.10	0.4
D. castanea (DC)	Leaves	7.23	147.12 ± 10.34[a]	237.11 ± 43.03	1.6[a]
D. castanea (DC)	Twig	8.74	112.35 ± 18.26[b]	>500	>4.5[b, c]
B. anceps (BA)	Twig	5.96	212.74 ± 27.01[a]	>500	2.3[a]
Melphalan			39.79 ± 7.62	178.98 ± 15.25	4.5

[a] Moderate cytotoxicity with lower selectivity index (SI < 3.0)

[b] High cytotoxicity with higher selectivity index (SI > 3.0) to HepG2 cell lines

[c] Non-significant difference vs. melphalan (*P* > 0.05)

The maximum concentration of the 50 % ethanol–water extracts in each test was 500 μg/mL, such that the final concentration of DMSO did not exceed 1 % (v/v) and the cytotoxicity of DMSO was <10 %. The control wells contained only the complete medium and cells. The cells were treated with plant extracts for 24 h before the NR solution (50 μg/mL) in media was added to each well. Cells were further incubated for 1 h at 37 °C in the 5 % CO_2 incubator before being washed with buffer. The treated viable cells with NR were washed with 1X PBS buffer and were lysed with 100 μL of 0.33 % hydrochloric acid/isopropanol. The absorbance of NR that represented the viable cell was measured using a microplate spectrophotometer system (Anthos 2010; Biochrom, UK) with an absorbance of 520 nm and a reference wavelength of 650 nm [31]. The percentage cytotoxicity was calculated as previously described [32]. The extent of cytotoxicity toward HepG2 and Vero cells was presented as the average of half the maximal inhibitory concentration (IC_{50}) of the crude extract. Melphalan was used as the positive control. The selectivity of the sample against the HepG2 cancer cells was compared with the normal Vero cells and is expressed by the selectivity index (SI). The SI is the IC_{50} ratio in Vero cells versus HepG2 cells. Any sample with an SI value greater than three is considered to have high selectivity [32].

Determination of apoptotic induction

Detection of nuclear morphological changes using DAPI fluorescent dye staining assay

A DAPI staining assay was performed to identify the nuclear morphological changes in apoptotic cells as previously described [33]. Briefly, the cells were seeded at a density of 1 × 10^6 cells per well in 24-well plates in the medium and incubated for 24 h. The cells were then treated at 2 × IC50 with each plant extract or melphalan (at the highest concentration of 500 μg/mL, 0.1 % DMSO) for 24 h. The controls were the untreated wells, which contained only the complete medium and cells. After treatment, the cells were washed with 1× PBS once and harvested using centrifugation (Daihan Scientific, Seoul, Korea) at 400×*g*, at 4 °C for 5 min. The treated cells were fixed at −20 °C for 10 min with 50 μL of methanol and water (1:1). The 100 μL (1 μg/mL) of DAPI dye was added to the frozen cells and the mixture kept at 37 °C for 30 min for staining protected from light. Excess DAPI was then removed with the supernatant by centrifugation at 400×*g* at 4 °C for 5 min. A 20 μL PBS to glycerine ratio of 1:1 was added to the cells. The cells were analyzed by dropping aliquots of them onto slides and closed with the cover slip. The fluorescent dsDNA-specific dye stain showed a fragmented nuclei pattern of apoptotic cells compared with the intact nuclei of normal cells under 40× magnification using fluorescent microscope visualization (Eclipse 80i, Nikon, Kanagawa, Japan) [33–35]. The amount of apoptotic cells was counted and the percentage calculated.

DNA fragmentation detection using DNA laddering assay

A DNA ladder assay was performed to identify DNA fragmentation among apoptotic cells as previously described [12]. Briefly, 1 × 10^6 cells/well were seeded into a 24-well, flat-bottomed plate and incubated in a 5 % CO_2 incubator at 37 °C for 24 h. After treatment of cancer cells with 2 × IC_{50} of the 50 % ethanol–water extracts or melphalan for 24 h, the cells were collected and washed with medium. The DNA in the cell pellets was extracted using a FlexiGene DNA kit. Aliquots (2 μg) of the DNA were analyzed using electrophoresis at 100 V for 40 min in 1.8 % agarose gels containing 0.1 % ethidium bromide. After electrophoresis, the DNA fragments were visualized using a UV transilluminator (Vilber Lourmat Deutschland GmbH, Eberhardzell, Germany) and gel pictures were taken with a UV-illuminated camera (Syngene, UK).

GC–MS analysis

GC–MS analyses were performed on selected crude ethanolic extracts to identify the chemical components. A gas chromatography system (Model 6890 N; Agilent Technologies, Shanghai, China), coupled with a mass selective detector (Model 5973 N; Agilent Technologies, Delaware, USA) and a GC auto-sampler (Agilent 7683 Automatic Liquid Sampler, Santa Clara, California, USA), was employed for all analyses. Briefly, 2 μL of crude extracts (10.40 mg of DC, 10.74 mg of LC) were injected into the GC column equipped with a capillary column (122–5532 DB-5 ms, length 30.0 m, diameter 250 μm, film thickness 0.25 μm). The injection temperature was set to 250 °C. Helium was used as the carrier gas at a constant flow rate of 2 ml/min. The oven temperature program was 80 °C for 6 min, followed by a 5 °C min^{-1} oven temperature ramp to 280 °C within 70 min. The mass spectra were recorded with a 50–500 MHz scanning range using mass spectrometry. The chromatograms and mass spectra of constituents of the crude extracts were evaluated by comparing their mass spectra with those in the database (Wiley 7N.l database, Agilent Technology, New York, USA).

Statistical analysis

The experiments were performed in three to five replicates and data are presented as mean ± SD. The statistical significance of differences in multiple-group comparisons was evaluated with the analysis of variance (ANOVA) followed by Tukey's honestly significant difference test using SPSS version 11.5 (SPSS Inc., Chicago, IL, USA). A two-tailed Student's t test was also performed. *P* values less than 0.05 were considered statistically significant.

Results

Cytotoxic effects and SI of plant extracts on human HCC cell line

All 50 % ethanol–water crude extracts of the five plants showed a moderate to high cytotoxic effect on a human HCC cell line (HepG2). The cytotoxicity and SI values of the plant extracts for HepG2 cells are summarized in Table 2. The IC_{50} and SI of crude extract were demonstrated for the leaves of DC, twigs of DC, and LC. All of the crude 50 % ethanol–water extracts showed significantly lower cytotoxicity than melphalan (IC_{50} = 39.79 ± 7.62 μg/mL; SI = 4.5) (LC: $P < 0.001$, CT: $P < 0.001$, ES: $P < 0.001$, DC leaves: $P = 0.002$, DC twig: $P = 0.023$, and BA: $P < 0.001$, respectively). Only the crude extract of DC (twig) showed high cytotoxicity against the HepG2 cells; an effect that was significantly different to that of melphalan ($P = 0.023$).

Determination of apoptosis pattern using DAPI

Cells were stained with DAPI fluorescent dye to assess apoptosis 24 h after treatment of cell lines with plant extracts at 2 × IC_{50}. Using 40× magnification, all five plant extracts were observed to cause alterations of nuclear morphology, revealing cell shrinkage, membrane blebbing, and apoptotic bodies (Fig. 1). The percentage of apoptotic cells was determined by observation using inverted microscopy for twigs of LC, CT, ES, BA, and leaves of DC. The positive control melphalan showed the highest induction of apoptosis in HepG2 (82.5 ± 8.0 %) and twigs of DC showed the lowest (66.0 ± 11.5 %) (Table 3).

Apoptosis induction by plant extracts determined by DNA laddering assay

After treatment of HepG2 cell lines for 24 h with plant extracts, the DNA fragmentation of apoptotic cells was observed as DNA ladders using agarose gel electrophoresis. The results of DNA laddering showed that only LC and DC (twig) induced late-state apoptosis in HepG2 (Fig. 2); the other extracts did not induce late-stage apoptosis in HepG2 cells.

Major components of DC (twig) and LC (twig) extracts using GC–MS analysis

The GC–MS chromatograms of the DC (twig) and LC (twig) extracts were examined. GC peaks with retention times of 29, 32, 39 and 52 min were found for the two crude extracts and were used for further chemical constituent identification using MS database analysis (Tables 4 and 5).

2-Palmitoylglycerol was the only major compound that co-existed in both the DC (twig) and LC (twig) crude extracts. Pyrogallol (1,2,3-trihydroxybenzene or 1,2,3-benzenetriol) and lupeol (3β-Lup-20(29)-en-3-ol) were the major compounds in DC (twig) crude extract. Hexadecanoic acid (abieta-8,11,13-trien-18-oic acid) and octadecenoic acid were the major compounds in the LC (twig) crude extract.

Discussion

The five plants (LC, CT, ES, DC leaves, DC twig, and BA) used in this study are found in northeastern Thailand and were selected based on their ethnopharmacology. All the crude extracts showed significantly lower cytotoxicity than melphalan ($P < 0.001$, $P < 0.001$, $P < 0.001$, $P = 0.002$, $P = 0.023$ and $P < 0.001$, respectively). Based on their cytotoxicity and selectivity classification, the extracts could be categorized as follows: (a) potentially cytotoxic (IC_{50} < 10 μg/mL) with high selectivity (SI > 3); (b) moderately cytotoxic (IC_{50} < 100 μg/mL) with high selectivity (SI > 3); (c) moderately cytotoxic (IC_{50} < 100 μg/mL) with less selectivity (SI < 3); (d) cytotoxic to only normal cells with less selectivity; and (e) nontoxic [32]. Only the crude extract of DC (twig) could be classified as highly cytotoxic toward HepG2 cells and highly selective (SI = 4.5). The SI of this extract was not significantly different from melphalan ($P = 0.959$). DC (leaf) and other crude plant extracts had moderate cytotoxicity and less selectivity (SI < 3). The LC showed a cytotoxic effect against normal cells with low selectivity (SI < 3). To our knowledge, this study demonstrates for the first time the anticancer potential of LC extract against human HCC (HepG2) cancer cells. The extracts of CT, ES, and BA showed moderate cytotoxicity on HepG2 cells but with less selectivity.

Several chemotherapeutic compounds have been reported to induce apoptosis [36]. In apoptotic cells, specific DNA cleavage is evident on electrophoretic analysis as a characteristic ladder pattern resulting from the multiple DNA fragments of oligonucleosomal size (180–200 bp) [37]. The DNA ladder assay has a lower sensitivity for apoptosis detection [38] because ladder formation can only be clearly observed when the extent of oligonucleosomal cleavage is extensive. Although more than 50 % of the apoptotic cells were observed with the DAPI staining assay in all of the ethanolic plant extracts, only LC and DC were positive according to the DNA ladder assay.

It was necessary to standardize the two potential crude extracts for quality control experiments as 50 % ethanol–water crude extracts of DC (twig) and LC (twig) were used in the current study. We then determined which phytochemicals in the crude extracts were associated with the apoptosis effects using GC–MS analyses.

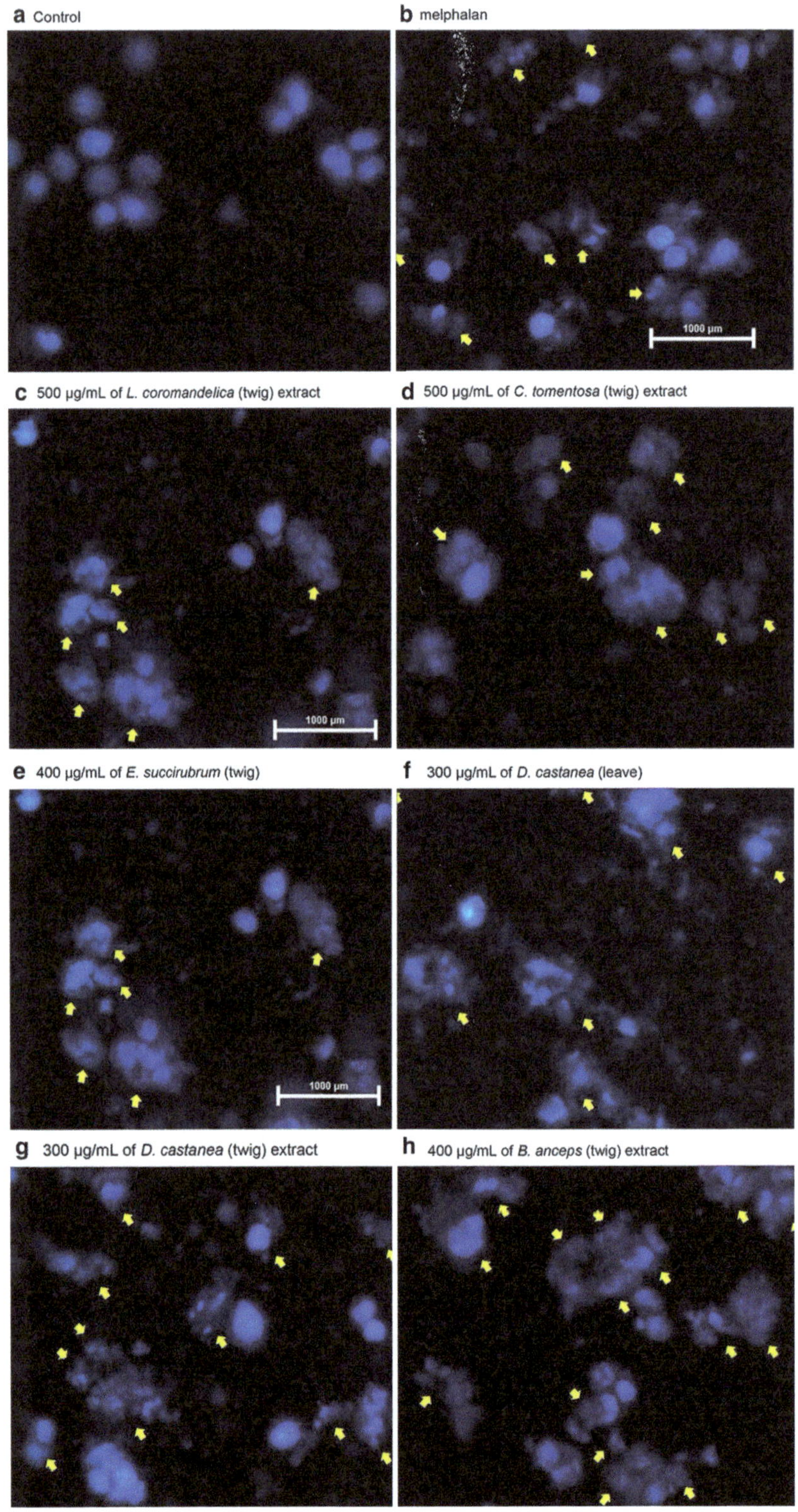

Fig. 1 Nuclei morphological change of HepG2 cells stained with DAPI fluorescent dye at 24 h. **a** Untreated HepG2 cells; **b** 80 µg/mL of melphalan; **c** 500 µg/mL of *L. coromandelica* (twig) extract; **d** 500 µg/mL of *C. tomentosa* (twig) extract; **e** 400 µg/mL of *E. succirubrum* (twig) extract; **f** 300 µg/mL of *D. castanea* (leaf) extract; **g** 300 µg/mL of *D. castanea* (twig) extract; and **h** 400 µg/mL of *B. anceps* (twig) extract. *Arrows* indicate apoptotic nuclei based on heterogeneous staining, DNA condensation, and apoptotic bodies at ×40 objective magnification

Table 3 Apoptosis induction of ethanolic plant extracts in HepG2 (mean ± SD) (n = 3)

Sample	Part	Apoptosis induction	
		% DAPI positive cell	DNA laddering
L. coromandelica (LC)	Twig	79.5 ± 5.5	Positive
C. tomentosa (CT)	Twig	69.0 ± 6.5	Negative
E. succirubrum (ES)	Twig	77.0 ± 13.5	Negative
D. castanea (DC)	Leaves	72.5 ± 12.5	Negative
D. castanea (DC)	Twig	66.0 ± 11.5	Positive
B. anceps (BA)	Twig	68.5 ± 7.5	Negative
Melphalan	–	82.5 ± 8.0	Positive

2-Palmitoylglycerol was the major compound common to the LC (twig) and DC (twig) crude extracts. 2-Palmitoylglycerol is involved in the regulation of endogenous cannabinoid receptor activity by increasing the biological activity of 2-arachidonylglycerol, and inhibition of adenyl cyclase 2-palmitoylglycerol significantly inhibits the inactivation of 2-arachidonylglycerol by neuronal and basophilic cells [39].

2-Arachidonylglycerol inhibits the production of TNF-alpha by mouse macrophages in vitro and the effect is enhanced in the presence of 2-palmitoylglycerol [40]. 2-Palmitoylglycerol is also a key component in modulating pain sensitivity as a result of its ability to interact with endocannabinoids [41]. In the present study, 2-palmitoylglycerol was the one compound found in both DC and LC extracts; however, the 2-palmitoylglycerol content was twice as low in the DC (twig) (7.5 %) than in the LC (twig) (14.0 %) and the DC extracts were more cytotoxic. It was not possible to specifically identify 2-palmitoylglycerol as the key compound; therefore, more detailed chemical identification of the plant extracts is required.

Pyrogallol was predominantly found (18.7 %) in the DC (twig) crude extract, which possessed high toxicity and selectivity against the HepG2 cells. Pyrogallol is a superoxide anion generator because it potently increases intracellular superoxide anion levels and decreases glutathione content in HeLa cells [42]. Research shows that pyrogallol-induced apoptosis resulting from the loss of mitochondrial membrane potential in calf pulmonary artery endothelial cells is accompanied by glutathione depletion [43]. In one study, the apoptosis induction of pyrogallol was indicated by a pyrogallol-type structure in a B-ring of catechins. DNA fragmentation activity was exhibited in a concentration-dependent manner in histiocytic lymphoma U937 cells after treatment with catechins containing a pyrogallol-type structure in a β-ring. Notwithstanding, catechins without a pyrogallol-type structure in any position did not show apoptosis-inducing

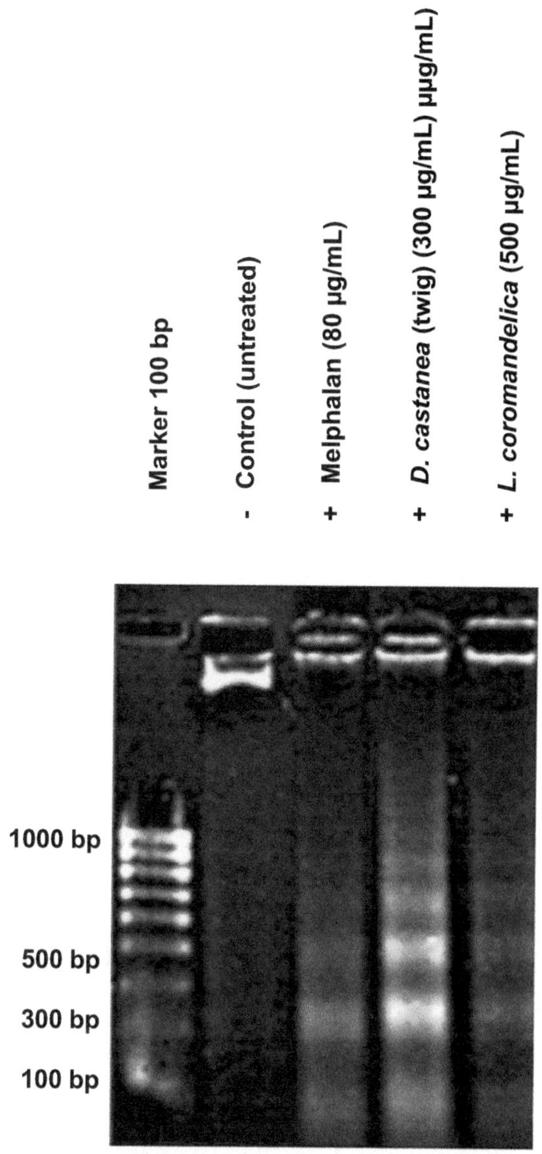

Fig. 2 DNA fragmentation in treated HepG2 cells. DNA laddering visualized in HepG2 cells after 24 h exposed to 50 % ethanol–water crude extracts of *D. castanea* and *L. coromandelica*. Untreated cells and 80 μg/mL of melphalan were used as negative and positive controls, respectively

activity [44]. A 3-*O*-gallate residue with *cis*-relationship to the β-ring enhanced the activity and the destruction of a pyrogallol-type structure by its methylation reduced this effect. By contrast, a 3-*O*-gallate residue in *trans*-relationship to the β-ring had little effect [44].

DC (twig) crude extract also contained lupeol as the third major compound (5.8 %). In a previous study, two hepatoma cell lines (SMMC7721 and HepG2) treated with lupeol decreased in a concentration-dependent manner (a) cell viability, (b) the induction of active

Table 4 Gas chromatography–mass spectrometry profile of 50 % ethanol–water crude extracts of *D. castanea* (twig)

Peak no.	Retention time (min)	% total area of prominent peak	Mass spectra	Compound
1	16.09	18.744	52, 63, 80, 97, 108, 117, 126	1,2,3-benzenetriol or pyrogallol
2	39.00	7.463	57, 74, 85, 98, 112, 123, 134, 154, 168, 182, 196, 213, 227, 239, 257, 270, 283, 299, 312, 330	2-palmitoylglycerol
3	52.73	5.824	55, 69, 81, 95, 109, 121, 135, 147, 161, 175, 189, 207, 218, 229, 243, 257, 272, 286, 297, 315, 326, 344, 357, 370, 393, 411, 426	(3β)-lup-20(29)-en-3-ol or lupeol

Table 5 Gas chromatography–mass spectrometry profile of 50 % ethanol–water crude extracts of *L. coromandelica* (twig)

Plants peak no.	RT (min)	% total area of prominent peak	Mass spectra	Compound
1	29.65	7.135	51, 60, 73, 83, 97, 107, 115, 129, 143, 157, 171, 185, 199, 213, 227, 239, 248, 256	Hexadecanoic acid or palmitic acid
2	30.05	5.013	55, 63, 73, 81, 88, 101, 108, 115, 122, 129, 136, 143, 150, 157, 167, 177, 185, 192, 199, 206, 213, 220, 227, 234, 241, 255, 263, 270, 284	Ethylhexadecanoate or ethyl palmitate
3	33.31	6.501	55, 65, 73, 83, 97, 111, 121, 129, 143, 155, 163, 171, 185, 199, 213, 222, 233, 241, 255, 264, 276, 284	Octadecanoic acid or stearic acid
4	37.77	8.621	55, 69, 81, 91, 105, 117, 129, 141, 155, 169, 183, 197, 211, 225, 239, 248, 247, 267, 276, 285, 300	Abieta-8,11,13-trien-18-oic acid or dehydroabietic acid
5	39.07	14.020	57, 74, 98, 112, 134, 154, 168, 182, 196, 213, 226, 239, 257, 270, 283, 330	2-palmitoylglycerol
6	42.14	6.166	57, 69, 84, 98, 112, 134, 154, 168, 185, 197, 210, 224, 241, 255, 267, 285, 298, 311, 327, 340, 358	Glyceryl monostearate

caspase-3 and poly (ADP-ribose) polymerase cleavage, (c) cell accumulation in the S phase, and (d) apoptosis. Treatment with lupeol three times a week also resulted in chemosensitization of hepatoma cells and significantly inhibited tumor growth in nude mice implanted with SMMC7721 cells [45]. Lupeol chemosensitized hepatoma cells synergistically with a PI3-kinase inhibitor (S14161) in both in vitro and in vivo models [46]. In the present study, the lupeol content of the DC (twig) extract (5.8 %) was higher than that of LC (twig) extract (1.0 %). Pyrogallol was the major compound in the DC (twig) extract but not in the LC (twig) extract. These two major compounds might contribute to the high cytotoxicity and high SI of DC (twig) extract as well as the high toxicity with lesser selectivity of LC (twig) extract.

Hexadecanoic acid and octadecenoic acid were also identified as the major compounds in LC (twig) crude extract in this study. The crystal structure (at a resolution of 2.5 Å) and kinetics studies have shown that n-hexadecanoic acid can act as an anti-inflammatory compound by inhibiting phospholipase A_2 in a competitive manner [47]. This fatty acid possibly contributes as the anti-hepatoma cell potential in the 50 % hydroethanolic herb extracts [13]. Pereira et al. [48] showed that the lipophilic extract from *Marthasterias glacialis* L. contained mainly palmitic acid and the sterol ergosta-7,22-dien-3-ol: these affected DNA synthesis, lipid droplets, and chromatin condensation, compatible with apoptosis in human breast cancer (MCF-7) and human neuroblastoma (SH-SY5Y) cell lines.

n-Hexadecanoic acid and 9,12-octadecadienoic acid (Z, Z) are fatty acids commonly found in the CO_2 supercritical fluid extraction that mediates apoptosis in human hepatoma SMMC-7721 cells, involving a reactive oxygen species-mediated mitochondrial signaling pathway [49]. The mixture of an octadecenoic acid extract—comprising mainly oleic and linoleic acids—from *Euphorbia kansui* resulted in a concentration-dependent reduction in the number of human gastric (SGC-7901), HCC (BEL-7402), and leukemia (HL-60) cells and significantly inhibited cell proliferation, with induced apoptosis and G_0/G_1 phase cell cycle arrest [50]. The octadecenoic acids not only caused cell apoptosis/necrosis but also functional and structural damage to the tumor cell membrane and cell ultrastructures [50]. A fraction of the dichloromethane extract of *Protaetia brevitarsis* larva (composed of at least three free fatty acids: palmitic acid, (Z)-9-octadecenoic acid, and octadecenoic acid) expresses apoptosis-inducing activity as shown by DNA laddering and caspase-3 activation in colon 26 tumor cells [51].

Conclusion

Ethanolic extracts from DC and LC twigs induced apoptosis in the HepG2 cell line. Pyrogallol and lupeol in DC (twig) might be responsible for the cytotoxicity toward the HepG2 cancer cells.

Abbreviations

BA: *Bombax anceps* Pierre var. *anceps*; CT: *Catunaregam tomentosa* (Blume ex DC.) Tirveng.; ES: *Erythrophleum succirubrum* Gagnep.; LC: *Lannea coromandelica* (Houtt.) Merr.; DC: *Diospyros castanea* (Craib) Fletcher.; HCC: hepatocellular carcinoma; DMEM: Dulbecco's modified Eagle's medium; DMSO: dimethylsulfoxide; FBS: fetal bovine serum; GC-MS: gas chromatography/mass spectrometry; NR: neutral red; DAPI: 4′,6-diamidino-2-phenylindole; PBS: phosphate buffered saline; IC_{50}: 50 % inhibitory concentration; SI: selectivity index; UV: ultraviolet.

Authors' contributions

SB designed the study. CJ performed the experiments and statistical analysis. NW wrote the manuscript. NW and SB revised the manuscript. TT performed the plant authentication, collected the plants and reviewed literature. All the authors read and approved the final version of the manuscript.

Author details

[1] Faculty of Pharmaceutical Sciences, Khon Kaen University, Khon Kaen 40002, Thailand. [2] Graduate School, Faculty of Pharmaceutical Sciences, Khon Kaen University, Khon Kaen 40002, Thailand. [3] Faculty of Associate Medical Sciences, Khon Kaen University, Khon Kaen 40002, Thailand.

Acknowledgements

Financial support is acknowledged from Khon Kaen University (KKU) through the Plant Genetics Conservation Project under the Royal Initiation of HRH Princess Maha Chakri Sirindhorn, and the Incubation Researcher Project Khon Kaen University. We thank (a) Professor Dr. David Jones for advice preparing the manuscript and (b) Mr. Bryan Roderick Hamman for assistance with the English-language presentation of the manuscript.

Competing interests

The authors declare that they have no competing interests.

References

1. Jemal A, Bray F, Center MM, Ferlay J, Ward E, Forman D. Global cancer statistics. CA Cancer J Clin. 2011;61:69–90.
2. Barusrux S, Nanok C, Puthisawas W, Pairojkul C, Poovorawan Y. Viral hepatitis B, C infection and genotype distribution among cholangiocarcinoma patients in northeast Thailand. Asian Pac J Cancer Prev. 2012;13(Suppl):83–7.
3. Liu L, Yang M, Kang R, Wang Z, Zhao Y, Yu Y, Xie M, Yin X, Livesey KM, Lotze MT, Tang D, Cao L. HMGB1-induced autophagy promotes chemotherapy resistance in leukemia cells. Leukemia. 2011;25:23–31.
4. Johnson IS, Armstrong JG, Gorman M, Jr Burnett JP. The vinca alkaloids: a new class of oncolytic agents. Cancer Res. 1963;23:1390–427.
5. Wani MC, Taylor H, Wall ME, Coggon P, McPhail A. Plant antitumor agents VI. The isolation and structure of taxol, a novel antileukemic and antitumor agent from *Taxus brevifolia*. J Amer Chem Soc. 1971;93:2325–7.
6. Wall ME, Wani MC, Cook CE, Palmer KH, McPhail AA, Sim GA. Plant antitumor agents I. The isolation and structure of camptothecin, a novel alkaloidal leukemia and tumor inhibitor from *Camptotheca acuminata*. J Amer Chem Soc. 1966;88:3888–90.
7. Li S, Han Q, Qiao C, Song J, Lung Cheng C, Xu H. Chemical markers for the quality control of herbal medicines: an overview. Chin Med. 2008;3:7.
8. Cragg GM, Newman DJ. Plants as a source of anti-cancer agents. J Ethnopharmacol. 2005;100:72–9.
9. Kinghorn AD, Su BN, Jang DS, Chang LC, Lee D, Gu JQ, Carcache-Blanco EJ, Pawlus AD, Lee SK, Park EJ, Cuendet M, Gills JJ, Bhat K, Park HS, Mata-Greenwood E, Song LL, Jang M, Pezzuto JM. Natural inhibitors of carcinogenesis. Planta Med. 2004;70:691–705.
10. Machana S, Weerapreeyakul N, Barusrux S. Anticancer effect of the extracts from *Polyalthia evecta* against human hepatoma cell line (HepG2). Asian Pac J Trop Biomed. 2012;2:368–74.
11. Machana S, Weerapreeyakul N, Barusrux S, Nonpunya A, Sripanidkulchai B, Thitimetharoch T. Cytotoxic and apoptotic effects of six herbal plants against the human hepatocarcinoma (HepG2) cell line. Chin Med. 2011;6:39.
12. Nonpunya A, Weerapreeyakul N, Barusrux S. *Cratoxylum formosum* (Jack) Dyer ssp. *pruniflorum* (Kurz) Gogel. (Hóng ya mù) extract induces apoptosis in human hepatocellular carcinoma HepG2 cells through caspase-dependent pathways. Chin Med. 2014;9:12.
13. Weerapreeyakul N, Nonpunya A, Barusrux S, Thitimetharoch T, Sripanidkulchai B. Evaluation of the anticancer potential of six herbs against a hepatoma cell line. Chin Med. 2012;7:15.
14. Mallavadhani UV, Panda AK, Rao YR. Pharmacology and chemotaxonomy of Diospyros. Phytochemistry. 1998;49:901–51.
15. Islam MT, Tahara S. Dihydroflavonols from *Lannea coromandelica*. Phytochemistry. 2000;54:901–7.
16. Sathish R, Ahmed M, Natarajan K, Lalitha KG. Evaluation of wound healing and antimicrobial activity of *Lannea coromandelica* (Houtt) Merr. J Pharm Res. 2010;3:1225–8.
17. Singh S, Sing GB. Hypotensive activity of *Lannea coromandelica* bark extract. Phytother Res. 1996;10:429–30.
18. Maiga A, Malterud KE, Diallo D, Paulsen BS. Antioxidant and 15-lipoxygenase inhibitory activities of the Malian medicinal plants *Diospyros abyssinica* (Hiern) F. White (Ebenaceae), *Lannea velutina* A. Rich (Anacardiaceae) and *Crossopteryx febrifuga* (Afzel) Benth. (Rubiaceae). J Ethnopharmacol. 2006;104:132–7.
19. Kannan M, Singh R, Narayanan M. Phytochemistry and immunopharmacological investigation of *Rubia cordifolia* Linn. (Rubiaceae). Pharmacology. 2009;3:653–62.
20. Miyagawa T, Ohtsuki T, Koyano T, Kowithayakorn T, Ishibashi M. Cassaine diterpenoid dimers isolated from *Erythrophleum succirubrum* with TRAIL-resistance overcoming activity. Tetrahedron Lett. 2009;50:4658–62.
21. Vieira TO, Said A, Aboutabl E, Azzam M, Creczynski-Pasa TB. Antioxidant activity of methanolic extract of *Bombax ceiba*. Redox Rep. 2009;14:41–6.
22. Zhang X, Zhu H, Zhang S, Yu Q, Xuan L. Sesquiterpenoids from *Bombax malabaricum*. J Nat Prod. 2007;70:1526–8.
23. Saleem M. Lupeol, a novel anti-inflammatory and anti-cancer dietary triterpene. Cancer Lett. 2009;285:109–15.
24. You YJ, Nam NH, Kim Y, Bae KH, Ahn BZ. Antiangiogenic activity of lupeol from *Bombax ceiba*. Phytother Res. 2003;17:341–4.
25. Sichaem J, Surapinit S, Siripong P, Khumkratok S, Jong-aramruang J, Tippyang S. Two new cytotoxic isomeric indole alkaloids from the roots of Nauclea orientalis. Fitoterapia. 2010;81:830–3.
26. Ebenaceae Phengklai C. In: Smitinand T, Larsen K, editors. Flora of Thailand volume 2 part 4. Bangkok: The Tistr Press Co., Ltd.; 1981. p. 281–392.
27. Chamayarit K, Staples GW, Santisuk T, Larsen K. Anacardiaceae and Convolvulaceae. In: Smitinand T, Larsen K, editors. Flora of Thailand Volume 10 Part 3. Bangkok: The Forest Herbarium, National Park, Wildlife and plant Conservation Department; 2010. p. 204.
28. Larsen K, Larsen SS, Vidal E. Leguminosae-Caesalpinioideae. In: Smitinand T, Larsen K, editors. Flora of Thailand Volume 4 Part 1. Bangkok: The Tistr Press; 1984. p. 1–129.
29. Puff C, Chamchumroon V. Thai Rubiaceae with hooks and thorns. Thai For Bull. 2003;31:65–74.
30. Phengklai C. Studies on Bombacaceae of Thailand. Thai For Bull. 1997;25:81–101.
31. Fotakis G, Timbrell JA. *In vitro* cytotoxicity assays: comparison of LDH, neutral red, MTT and protein assay in hepatoma cell lines following exposure to cadmium chloride. Toxicol Lett. 2006;160:171–7.
32. Prayong P, Barusrux S, Weerapreeyakul N. Cytotoxic activity screening of some indigenous Thai plants. Fitoterapia. 2008;79:598–601.

33. Pocasap P, Weerapreeyakul N, Barusrux S. Cancer preventive effect of Thai rat-tailed radish (*Raphanus sativus* L. var. caudatus Alef). J Funct Foods. 2014;5:1372–81.
34. Plaimee P, Weerapreeyakul N, Thumanu K, Tanthanuch W, Barusrux S. Melatonin induces apoptosis through biomolecular changes, in SK-LU-1 human lung adenocarcinoma cells. Cell Prolif. 2014;47:564–77.
35. Atale N, Gupta S, Yadav UCS, Rani V. Cell-death assessment by fluorescent and nonfluorescent cytosolic and nuclear staining techniques. J Microsc. 2014;255:7–19.
36. Gunji H, Kharbanda S, Kufe D. Induction of internucleosomal DNA fragmentation in human myeloid leukemia cells by 1-beta-D-arabinofuranosylcytosine. Cancer Res. 1991;51:741–3.
37. Collins JA, Schandi CA, Young KK, Vesely J, Willingham MC. Major DNA fragmentation is a late event in apoptosis. J Histochem Cytochem. 1997;45:923–34.
38. Yasuhara S, Zhu Y, Matsui T, Tipirneni N, Yasuhara Y, Kaneki M, Rosenzweig A, Martyn JA. Comparison of comet assay, electron microscopy, and flow cytometry for detection of apoptosis. J Histochem Cytochem. 2003;51:873–85.
39. Ben-Shabat S, Fride E, Sheskin T, Tamiri T, Rhee MH, Vogel Z, Bisogno T, De Petrocellis L, Di Marzo V, Mechoulam R. An entourage effect: inactive endogenous fatty acid glycerol esters enhance 2-arachidonoyl-glycerol cannabinoid activity. Eur J Pharmacol. 1998;353:23–31.
40. Gallily R, Breuer A, Mechoulam R. 2-Arachidonylglycerol, an endogenous cannabinoid, inhibits tumor necrosis factor-alpha production in murine macrophages, and in mice. Eur J Pharmacol. 2000;406:R5–7.
41. Walker JM, Krey JF, Chu CJ, Huang SM. Endocannabinoids and related fatty acid derivatives in pain modulation. Chem Phys Lipids. 2002;121:159–72.
42. Han YH, Kim SZ, Kim SH, Park WH. Pyrogallol as a glutathione depletor induces apoptosis in HeLa cells. Int J Mol Med. 2008;21:721–30.
43. Han YH, Moon HJ, You BR, Kim SZ, Kim SH, Park WH. JNK and p38 inhibitors increase and decrease apoptosis, respectively, in pyrogallol-treated calf pulmonary arterial endothelial cells. Int J Mol Med. 2009;24:717–22.
44. Saeki K, Hayakawa S, Isemura M, Miyase T. Importance of a pyrogallol-type structure in catechin compounds for apoptosis-inducing activity. Phytochemistry. 2000;53:391–4.
45. He Y, Liu F, Zhang L, Wu Y, Hu B, Zhang Y, Li Y, Liu H. Growth inhibition and apoptosis induced by lupeol, a dietary triterpene, in human hepatocellular carcinoma cells. Biol Pharm Bull. 2011;34:517–22.
46. Liu F, He Y, Liang Y, Wen L, Zhu Y, Wu Y, Zhao L, Li Y, Mao X, Liu H. PI3-kinase inhibition synergistically promoted the anti-tumor effect of lupeol in hepatocellular carcinoma. Cancer Cell Int. 2013;13:108.
47. Aparna V, Dileep KV, Mandal PK, Karthe P, Sadasivan C, Haridas M. Anti-inflammatory property of n-hexadecanoic acid: structural evidence and kinetic assessment. Chem Biol Drug Des. 2012;80:434–9.
48. Pereira DM, Correia-da-Silva G, Valentao P, Teixeira N, Andrade PB. Palmitic acid and ergosta-7,22-dien-3-ol contribute to the apoptotic effect and cell cycle arrest of an extract from *Marthasterias glacialis* L. in neuroblastoma cells. Mar Drugs. 2014;12:54–68.
49. Li Q, Jiang C, Zu Y, Song Z, Zhang B, Meng X, Qiu W, Zhang L. SFE-CO_2 extract from *Typhonium giganteum* Engl. tubers, induces apoptosis in human hepatoma SMMC-7721 cells involvement of a ROS-mediated mitochondrial pathway. Molecules. 2011;16:8228–42.
50. Yu F, Lu S, Shi J, McGuire PM, Wang R. Cytotoxic activity of an octadecenoic acid extract from *Euphorbia kansui* (Euphorbiaceae) on human tumour cell strains. J Pharm Pharmacol. 2008;60:253–9.
51. Yoo YC, Shin BH, Hong JH, Lee J, Chee HY, Song KS, Lee KB. Isolation of fatty acids with anticancer activity from *Protaetia brevitarsis* larva. Arch Pharm Res. 2007;30:361–5.

15

Conservation and sustainable use of medicinal plants: problems, progress, and prospects

Shi-Lin Chen[1*], Hua Yu[2,3*], Hong-Mei Luo[2], Qiong Wu[2,4], Chun-Fang Li[2] and André Steinmetz[5]

Abstract

Medicinal plants are globally valuable sources of herbal products, and they are disappearing at a high speed. This article reviews global trends, developments and prospects for the strategies and methodologies concerning the conservation and sustainable use of medicinal plant resources to provide a reliable reference for the conservation and sustainable use of medicinal plants. We emphasized that both conservation strategies (e.g. in situ and ex situ conservation and cultivation practices) and resource management (e.g. good agricultural practices and sustainable use solutions) should be adequately taken into account for the sustainable use of medicinal plant resources. We recommend that biotechnical approaches (e.g. tissue culture, micropropagation, synthetic seed technology, and molecular marker-based approaches) should be applied to improve yield and modify the potency of medicinal plants.

Background

Medicinal plants are globally valuable sources of new drugs [1–4]. There are over 1300 medicinal plants used in Europe, of which 90 % are harvested from wild resources; in the United States, about 118 of the top 150 prescription drugs are based on natural sources [5]. Furthermore, up to 80 % of people in developing countries are totally dependent on herbal drugs for their primary healthcare, and over 25 % of prescribed medicines in developed countries are derived from wild plant species [4]. With the increasing demand for herbal drugs, natural health products, and secondary metabolites of medicinal plants, the use of medicinal plants is growing rapidly throughout the world [1, 6].

A highly conservative estimate states that the current loss of plant species is between 100 and 1000 times higher than the expected natural extinction rate and that the Earth is losing at least one potential major drug every 2 years [7]. According to the International Union for Conservation of Nature and the World Wildlife Fund, there are between 50,000 and 80,000 flowering plant species used for medicinal purposes worldwide. Among these, about 15,000 species are threatened with extinction from overharvesting and habitat destruction [8] and 20 % of their wild resources have already been nearly exhausted with the increasing human population and plant consumption [9]. Although this threat has been known for decades, the accelerated loss of species and habitat destruction worldwide has increased the risk of extinction of medicinal plants, especially in China [1, 10], India [10, 11], Kenya [11], Nepal [11], Tanzania [12] and Uganda [12].

The conservation and sustainable use of medicinal plants have been studied extensively [13, 14]. Various sets of recommendations have been compiled regarding their conservation, including the establishment of systems for species inventorying and status monitoring, and the need for coordinated conservation practices based on both in situ and ex situ strategies [4]. For medicinal plants with increasingly limited supplies, sustainable use of wild resources can be an effective conservation alternative. In China and South Africa, the situation is particularly critical because of the high demands of large populations.

This article reviews global trends, developments and prospects of the strategies and methodologies concerning

*Correspondence: slchen@icmm.ac.cn; yh_2003@126.com
[1] Institute of Chinese Materia Medica, China Academy of Chinese Medical Sciences, Beijing 100700, China
[3] Shandong Center of Crop Germplasm Resources, Jinan 250100, China
Full list of author information is available at the end of the article

the conservation and sustainable use of medicinal plant resources.

Review

Literature search

We conducted systematic literature searches in the ISI Web of Science, PubMed and CNKI databases using search terms (e.g. "medicinal plant", "herbal drug", "herbal medicine", "aromatic plant", and "Chinese medicine") and keyword combinations (e.g. "in situ conservation", "ex situ conservation", "sustainable use", and "cultivation practice") to retrieve the abstracts of relevant articles (Fig. 1). The literature search spanned the period from January 2000 to December 2014, and the languages were limited to English and Chinese. We carefully reviewed all retrieved abstracts to find articles that were suitable according to the inclusion criteria (Table 1). For literature focusing on the conservation and/or sustainable use of medicinal plants, we retrieved full articles from full-text databases (ScienceDirect, Wiley, Biomed, Springer, Medline, Scopus, Elsevier, Highwire, Mcgill, Cogprints, Emedicine, Nature and Science online). From the initial search, a total of 673 abstracts were collected, including research articles, reviews, commentaries and letters. After systematic screening, 231 met the inclusion criteria. From these, full copies of 106 articles were retrieved for further evaluation. In addition, we retrieved 25 non-indexed but relevant citations from the reference lists of retrieved articles to supplement the above searches and provide a complete literature retrieval.

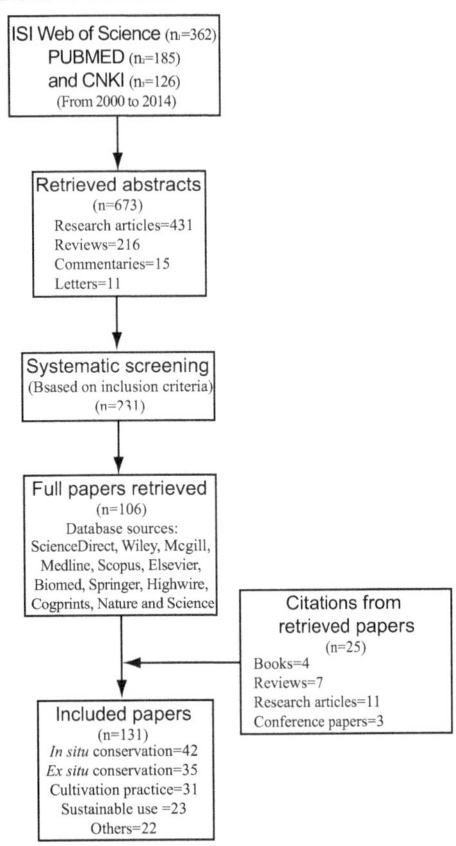

Fig. 1 Diagram for literature selection

Diversity of medicinal plants used worldwide

More than one-tenth of plant species are used in drugs and health products, with more than 50,000 species being used. However, the distribution of medicinal plants is not uniform across the world [15, 16]. For example, China and India have the highest numbers of medicinal plants used, with 11,146 and 7500 species, respectively, followed by Colombia, South Africa, the United States, and another 16 countries with percentages of medicinal plants ranging from 7 % in Malaysia to 44 % in India versus their total numbers of plant species [16–19] (Fig. 2). Certain plant families not only have higher numbers of medicinal plants, but also have higher proportions of threatened species than others [15]. Only a portion of medicinal plants that suffer from genetic erosion and resource destruction have been listed as threatened [20, 21].

Factors related to species rarity of medicinal plants

Species rarity is used to assess the extinction risk of medicinal plants, and to identify those species most at risk of extinction, prior to commencement of conservation efforts [22]. It is necessary to determine how rare each species is and in which ways rare species differ from one another. Not all medicinal plants are affected in the same way by harvesting pressures [23, 24]. Overexploitation, indiscriminate collection, uncontrolled deforestation, and habitat destruction all affect species rarity, but are insufficient to explain individual species susceptibility or resilience to harvest pressure. Multiple biological characters correlate with extinction risk, such as habitat specificity, distribution range, population size, species diversity, growth rate, and reproductive system (Table 2; Fig. 3).

Conservation strategies

Medicinal plant resources are being harvested in increasing volumes, largely from wild populations. Indeed, demand for wild resources has increased by 8–15 % per year in Europe, North America, and Asia in recent decades [8, 9]. There is a threshold below which species reproductive capacity becomes irreversibly reduced [25, 26]. Various sets of recommendations relating to the conservation of medicinal plants have been developed, such as providing both in situ and ex situ conservation

Table 1 The inclusion and exclusion criteria for study selection

Subjects	Criteria description
Inclusion criteria	The subject is about medicinal plants
	The purpose is to conserve or sustainably use
	It has a detailed description of the strategy of conservation, sustainable use or resource management
	Consistent to the three items simultaneously
Exclusion criteria	The subject is not related to medicinal plants (e.g. animals or mineral substances)
	The purpose is not for conservation or sustainable use of medicinal plants (e.g. herb extraction, drug discovery, chemical constituent or pharmacological property)
	It has no description of the strategy of conservation, sustainable use or resource management of medicinal plants

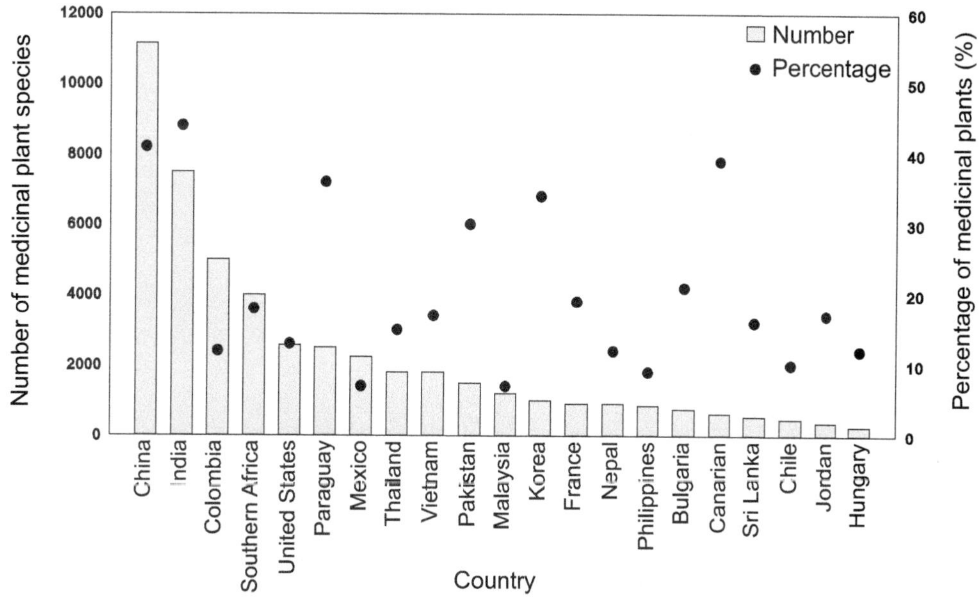

Fig. 2 Number and percentage of medicinal plant species in different countries. The *light bars* indicate the number of medicinal plant species, and the *dark dots* indicate the percentage of medicinal plants compared with the total number of plant species. Data sources from Rafieian-Kopaei [16], Hamilton [17], Marcy et al. [18], and Srujana et al. [19]

(Table 2) [15, 27]. Natural reserves and wild nurseries are typical examples to retain the medical efficacy of plants in their natural habitats, while botanic gardens and seed banks are important paradigms for ex situ conservation and future replanting [28, 29] (Fig. 4). The geographic distribution and biological characteristics of medicinal plants must be known to guide conservation activities, e.g. to assess whether species conservation should take place in nature or in a nursery.

In situ conservation

Most medicinal plants are endemic species, and their medicinal properties are mainly because of the presence of secondary metabolites that respond to stimuli in natural environments, and that may not be expressed under culture conditions [22, 29]. In situ conservation of whole communities allows us to protect indigenous plants and maintain natural communities, along with their intricate network of relationships [30]. Additionally, in situ conservation increases the amount of diversity that can be conserved [31], and strengthens the link between resource conservation and sustainable use [32]. In situ conservation efforts worldwide have focused on establishing protected areas and taking an approach that is ecosystem-oriented, rather than species-oriented [33]. Successful in situ conservation depends on rules, regulations, and potential compliance of medicinal plants within growth habitats [25, 34].

Natural reserves The degradation and destruction of habitats is a major cause of the loss of medicinal plant resources [35]. Natural reserves are protected areas of

Table 2 Summary of original investigations into the conservation and sustainable use of medicinal plants

Sources	Objectives	Features and study design	Findings and conclusions
Andel and Havinga [24]	249 medicinal plants in Suriname	Carried out a market survey to look for signs of over-harvesting by analyzing the market, harvesters and post-harvest survival of the medicinal plants	Less than half of the medicinal plants were harvested exclusively from the wild, and leaves were the main products. Most medicinal plants were harvested from secondary forest or man-made vegetation. It didn't invariably lead to the resource decline or species loss
Semwal et al. [26]	Ten rare and endangered medicinal plants	Based on the density, occurrence habitats and pressure level to evaluate the distribution pattern, population structure and conservation status of medicinal plants	It grouped the medicinal plants into restricted distribution with high pressure and well distributed with low pressure, providing insights for the conservation and management strategies of medicinal plants
Long et al. [32]	*Amorphophallus*, *Paris*, *Musella lasiocarpa*, and *Camellia sinensis*	Dealt with strategies for agrobiodiversity conservation and promotion based on studies of the medicinal plants in the Yunnan Province of China	Strategies (e.g. in situ and ex situ conservation, as well as the promotion and conservation of agrobiodiversity through sustainable uses) should be adopted to conserve and promote agrobiodiversity
Strandby and Olsen [41]	*Abies guatemalensis*	From December 2004 to August 2007 conducted a nation-wide survey with plantation owners ($n = 26$), retailers ($n = 67$) and urban consumers ($n = 993$)	It emphasized the importance of increasing legal supplies through decreasing plantation production costs and involving local communities in managing in situ resources
Yu et al. [44]	*Rheum tanguticum*	Employed a GIS-based program TCMGIS-II to integrate geographic, climate and soil type databases of China to predict the potential distribution of *R. tanguticum*	It found the potential habitats sharing similar ecological factors with native habitats appropriate for *R. tanguticum* growth. It is useful in the conservation planning and regional management of medicinal plants
Yuan et al. [47]	*Scutellaria baicalensis*	Estimated the genetic diversity and structure of 28 wild and 22 cultivated populations of *S. baicalensis* using three polymorphic chloroplast fragments	The conservation-by-cultivation is effective in protecting genetic resources, while the wild resources still need to be protected in situ. The evolutionary consequences of extensive seed exchange should be monitored carefully
Maunder et al. [49]	27 threatened medicinal plants	Surveyed 119 botanic gardens in 29 European countries, and 25 botanic gardens in 14 countries undertaking 51 conservation projects	Most medicinal plants were in a small number of collections and out of the range countries, without being included in any specific conservation project. Botanic garden collections were skewed towards ornamental species, and did not fully reflect conservation priorities

GIS geography information systems, *TCMGIS-II* the second version of GIS based program for the distribution prediction of traditional Chinese medicine

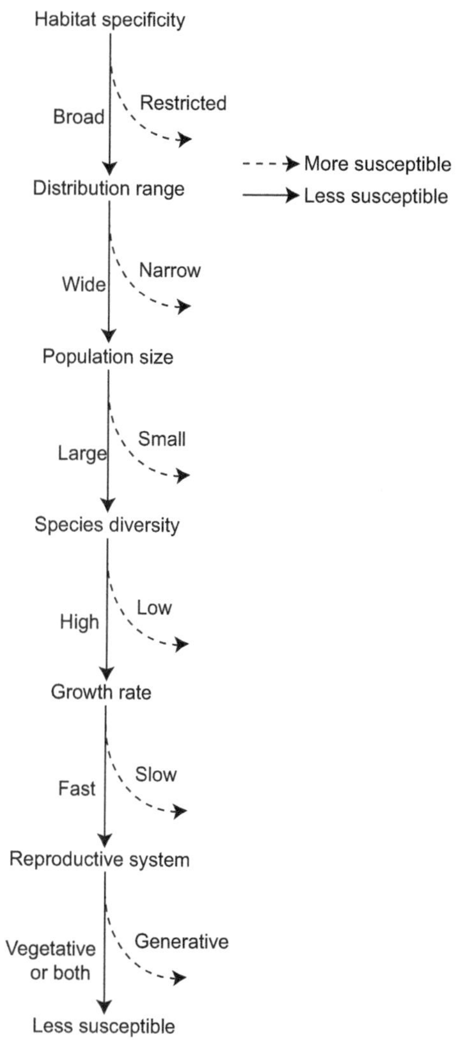

Fig. 3 Factors contributing to the susceptibility or resilience of medicinal plants in response to collection pressure. Factors include distribution range, habitat specificity, population size, species diversity, growth rate, and reproductive system. The *dark line* indicates less susceptible characteristics of medicinal plants, while the *dashed line* indicates more susceptible characteristics contributing to the rarity of medicinal plants

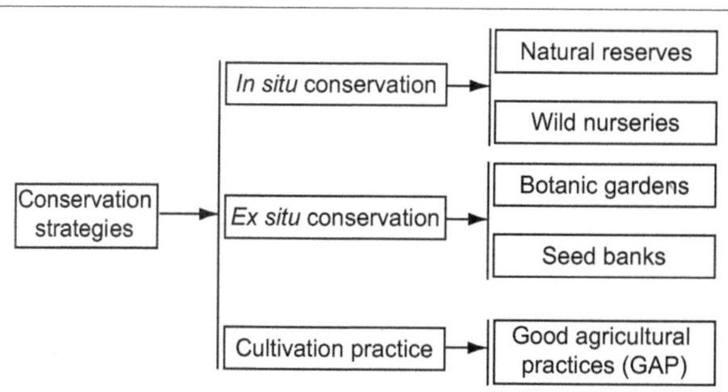

Fig. 4 Diagram of methodological systems involved in the conservation of medicinal plants

important wild resources created to preserve and restore biodiversity [36, 37]. Around the world, more than 12,700 protected areas have been established, accounting for 13.2 million km^2, or 8.81 % of the Earth's land surface [38]. Conserving medicinal plants by protecting key natural habitats requires assessing the contributions and ecosystem functions of individual habitats [39].

Wild nurseries It is impossible to designate every natural wild plant habitat as a protected area, owing to cost considerations and competing land uses [25, 40]. A wild nursery is established for species-oriented cultivating and domesticating of endangered medicinal plants in a protected area, natural habitat, or a place that is only a short distance from where the plants naturally grow [4, 20, 41]. Although the populations of many wild species are under heavy pressure because of overexploitation, habitat degradation and invasive species, wild nurseries can provide an effective approach for in situ conservation of medicinal plants that are endemic, endangered, and in-demand [27, 42].

Ex situ conservation

Ex situ conservation is not always sharply separated from in situ conservation, but it is an effective complement to it, especially for those overexploited and endangered medicinal plants with slow growth, low abundance, and high susceptibility to replanting diseases [4, 43, 44]. Ex situ conservation aims to cultivate and naturalize threatened species to ensure their continued survival and sometimes to produce large quantities of planting material used in the creation of drugs, and it is often an immediate action taken to sustain medicinal plant resources [45, 46]. Many species of previously wild medicinal plants can not only retain high potency when grown in gardens far away from the habitats where they naturally occur, but can have their reproductive materials selected and stored in seed banks for future replanting [4].

Botanic gardens Botanic gardens play an important role in ex situ conservation [43], and they can maintain the ecosystems to enhance the survival of rare and endangered plant species [38]. Although living collections generally consist of only a few individuals of each species and so are of limited use in terms of genetic conservation [47], botanic gardens have multiple unique features. They involve a wide variety of plant species grown together under common conditions, and often contain taxonomically and ecologically diverse flora [48]. Botanic gardens can play a further role in medicinal plant conservation through the development of propagation and cultivation protocols, as well as undertaking programs of domestication and variety breeding [49].

Seed banks Seed banks offer a better way of storing the genetic diversity of many medicinal plants ex situ than through botanic gardens, and are recommended to help preserve the biological and genetic diversity of wild plant species [50, 51]. The most noteworthy seed bank is the Millennium Seed Bank Project at the Royal Botanic Gardens in Britain [51]. Seed banks allow relatively rapid access to plant samples for the evaluation of their properties, providing helpful information for conserving the remaining natural populations [50, 51]. The challenging tasks of seed banking are how to reintroduce the plant species back into the wild and how to actively assist in the restoration of wild populations [50].

Cultivation practice

Although wild-harvested resources of medicinal plants are widely considered more efficacious than those that are cultivated, domestic cultivation is a widely used and generally accepted practice [30, 52, 53]. Cultivation provides the opportunity to use new techniques to solve problems encountered in the production of medicinal plants, such as toxic components, pesticide contamination, low contents of active ingredients, and the misidentification of botanical origin [54]. Cultivation under controlled growth conditions can improve the yields of active compounds, which are almost invariably secondary metabolites, and ensures production stability (Table 3). Cultivation practices are designed to provide optimal levels of water, nutrients, optional additives, and environmental factors including temperature, light and humidity to obtain improved yields of target products [27, 55]. Moreover, increased cultivation contributes to decreases in the harvest volume of medicinal plants, benefits the recovery of their wild resources, and decreases their prices to a more reasonable range [4, 13, 20] (Fig. 5).

Good agricultural practices (GAP)

Good agricultural practices (GAP) for medicinal plants have been formulated to regulate production, ensure quality, and facilitate the standardization of herbal drugs [56]. A GAP approach ensures high quality, safe and pollution-free herbal drugs (or crude drugs) by applying available knowledge to address various problems [57]. GAP include comprehensive items, such as the ecological environment of production sites, germplasm, cultivation, collection, and quality aspects of pesticide detection, macroscopic or microscopic authentication, chemical identification of bioactive compounds, and inspection of metal elements [58]. Many countries actively promote the implementation of GAP. For example, Chinese authorities have promoted GAP for the growth of commonly used herbal drugs in regions where those medicinal plants are traditionally cultivated [27, 33].

Organic farming has received increasing attention for its ability to create integrated, humane, and environmentally and economically sustainable production systems

Table 3 The advantages and disadvantages of wild resource versus cultivated medicinal plant species

Characteristics	Wild resource	Cultivated species
Advantages	It is open access resource without investment	It relieves harvesting pressure on rare and threatened species
	It is natural resource and free from pesticides	It can keep genotypes being standardized or improved
	Wild resource is supposed to be more efficacious	It guarantees continuing supply of raw medicinal materials
		Production volume and price can be stable for longer periods
Disadvantages	Wild resource is becoming scarce and threatened by over-harvesting	It needs substantial investment before and during production
	There exists a risk of adulterations and resource exhaustion	It narrows genetic diversity in gene pool of wild populations
	Uncontrolled harvesting leads to the extinction of ecotype and species	Reintroduced plants can cause genetic pollution of wild resource
	There is a lack of resource inventories and related management practices	Cultivated species may have negative impacts on ecosystems
		There is a lack of successful cultivation techniques for some species

Information from Hamilton [4], Schippmann et al. [20], Liu et al. [27], and Raina et al. [54]

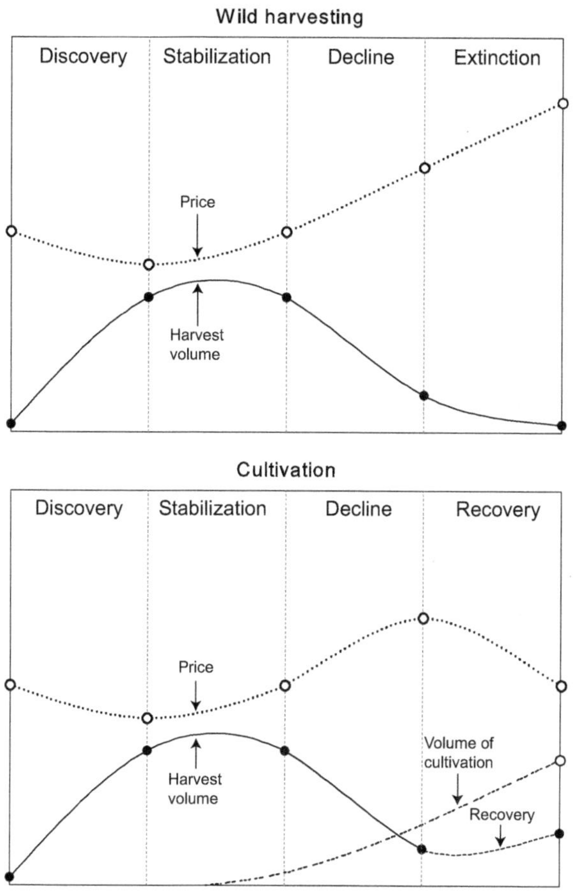

Fig. 5 Price and harvest volume variation in the transition from wild-harvesting to cultivation of medicinal plants. As wild resources decline with overharvesting, the price of raw material increases accordingly. Therefore, cultivation becomes economically feasible for price stabilization and resource recovery of medicinal plants. Data sources from Hamilton [4], Larsen and Olsen [13], Schippmann et al. [20], Chan et al. [56], and Schippmann et al. [67]

for medicinal plants, [59, 60]. The aims of organic farming of medicinal plants include producing material with better quality and high productivity, and ensuring the conservation and sustainable utilization of those plants (Table 4). The defining characteristic of organic farming is the non-use of synthetic fertilizers, pesticides and herbicides, which are not allowed according to many current organic certification standards in Europe and North America [59]. Organic farming is benign to the environment, and relies upon farm-derived renewable resources to maintain biological processes of medicinal plants and ecological balance of habitates [56, 59]. The use of organic fertilizers continuously supplies soil nutrients and improves soil stability, significantly affecting the growth of medicinal plants and the biosynthesis of essential substances. For example, when organic fertilizers were applied, the biomass yield of *Chrysanthemum balsamita* was increased and its essential oil content was high relative to those free from organic fertilizers [61]. Organic farming of medicinal plants is becoming increasingly important in the long-term development and sustainability of medicinal plants [60].

Sustainable use

For medicinal plants with limited abundance and slow growth, destructive harvesting generally results in resource exhaustion and even species extinction [13, 62]. Therefore, the sustainable use of medicinal plants should be considered, and good harvesting practices must be formulated. Root and whole-plant harvesting is more destructive to medicinal plants (e.g. herbs, shrubs and trees) than collecting their leaves and flowers or buds (Table 5). For herbal drugs made of whole plants or roots, using their leaves as a remedy can be a benign alternative. For example, Wang et al. [63] discovered that extracts from ginseng leaf-stems and roots have similar pharmacological activities, but ginseng leaf-stem has the advantage of being a more sustainable resource.

Prospects

The development of genetic engineering has led to the feasibility of large-scale biosynthesis of natural products, and advancements in tissue culture and fermentation of medicinal plants have opened new avenues for the large-scale and highly efficient production of desirable bioactive compounds. Tissue culture (including plant cell and transgenic hairy root culture) is a promising alternative for the production of rare and high-value secondary metabolites of medical importance [64]. Micropropagation via tissue encapsulation of propagules can not only facilitate storage and transportation, but also promotes higher regeneration rates [62]. When the amounts of normal seeds are insufficient for propagation, synthetic seed technology, defined as artificially encapsulated somatic embryos (or other tissues) could be used for cultivate in vitro or ex vitro, is a feasible alternative [65, 66]. Furthermore, breeding improvements can be carried out using molecular marker-based approaches applied at the genetic level, and the time required for breeding may be significantly shortened [62, 64, 65].

Table 4 The characteristics and advantages of organic farming of medicinal plants

Subjects	Characteristics and advantages of organic farming
Medicinal plants	To produce material in optimal quality and sufficient quantity
	To increase growth rate and biomass yield of medicinal plants
	To enhance the biosynthesis of efficacious substances
	To maintain the genetic diversity of medicinal plants
	To protect medicinal plants against pests and disease
Environmental effects	To prohibit the use of synthetic pesticides and fertilizers
	To promote sustainable use and proper care of production systems
	To enhance plant diversity and biotype conservation
	To protect wildlife habitats (e.g. micro-organisms, soil fora and fauna)
	To enhance soil rich in macro and microelements
	To conserve soil properties, fertility, productivity and system stability
	To use organic fertilizers and renewable resources to minimize all forms of pollution
Economic prospects	To increase market opportunity
	To maintain high market price
	To achieve optimal quality and economic returns
	To secure economic growth and social stability

Information from Rigby and Cáceres [59], Macilwain [60] and Suresh [61]

Table 5 Susceptibility of species to overharvesting regarding life forms and plant parts used

Life form	Percent (%)	Leave	Flower/bud	Fruit/seed	Bark	Root	Whole plant
Herb	52	Medium	Medium	High	None	High	High
Shrub	16	Low	Low	Low	High	High	High
Tree	22	Low	Low	Low	High	High	High

Information from Schippmann et al. [67] and Teklehaymanot and Giday [68]

Conclusion

Despite the existence of various sets of recommendations for the conservation and sustainable use of medicinal plants, only a small portion of these have achieved adequate protection of medicinal plant resources through conventional conservation in natural reserves or botanic gardens.

Abbreviations

GAP: good agricultural practices.

Authors' contributions

SC and HY conceived and designed the study. SC, HY, HL and QW carried out the article searches. HY, QW and CL performed data analysis. SC, HY, HL and QW wrote the manuscript. CL and AS revised the manuscript. All authors read and approved the final manuscript.

Author details

[1] Institute of Chinese Materia Medica, China Academy of Chinese Medical Sciences, Beijing 100700, China. [2] Institute of Medicinal Plant Development, Chinese Academy of Medical Sciences, Beijing 100193, China. [3] Shandong Center of Crop Germplasm Resources, Jinan 250100, China. [4] School of Pharmacy, Guilin Medical University, Guilin 541004, China. [5] Plant Molecular Biology Laboratory, Centre de Recherche Public-Sante´, 1526 Luxembourg, Luxembourg.

Acknowledgements

This study was supported by the National Natural Science Foundation of China (30900113) and the Natural Science Foundation of Shandong Province (ZR2013CQ038). All authors thank Dr. Xi-Wen Li, Liang Dong and Christine Leon for their helps on group discussion and manuscript polishing.

Competing interests

The authors declare that they have no competing interests.

References

1. Nalawade SM, Sagare AP, Lee CY, Kao CL, Tsay HS. Studies on tissue culture of Chinese medicinal plant resources in Taiwan and their sustainable utilization. Bot Bull Acad Sin. 2003;44:79–98.
2. Chen SL, Yao H, Han JP, Liu C, Song JY, Shi LC, Zhu YJ, Ma XY, Gao T, Pang XH, Luo K, Li Y, Li XW, Jia XC, Lin YL, Leon C. Validation of the ITS2 region as a novel DNA barcode for identifying medicinal plant species. PLoS ONE. 2010;5:e8613.
3. Chacko SM, Thambi PT, Kuttan R, Nishigaki I. Beneficial effects of green tea: a literature review. Chin Med. 2010;5:13.
4. Hamilton AC. Medicinal plants, conservation and livelihoods. Biodivers Conserv. 2004;13:1477–517.
5. Balunas MJ, Kinghorn AD. Drug discovery from medicinal plants. Life Sci. 2005;78:431–41.

6. Cole IB, Saxena PK, Murch SJ. Medicinal biotechnology in the genus *scutellaria*. In Vitro Cell Dev Plant. 2007;43:318–27.
7. Pimm S, Russell G, Gittleman J, Brooks T. The future of biodiversity. Science. 1995;269:347.
8. Bentley R, editor. Medicinal plants. London: Domville-Fife Press; 2010. p. 23–46.
9. Ross IA, editor. Medicinal plants of the world (volume 3): chemical constituents, traditional and modern medicinal uses. New Jersey: Humana Press Inc; 2005. p. 110–32.
10. Heywood VH, Iriondo JM. Plant conservation: old problems, new perspectives. Biol Conserv. 2003;113:321–35.
11. Hamilton AC. Medicinal plants in conservation and development: case studies and lessons learned. In: Kala CP, editor. Medicinal plants in conservation and development. Salisbury: Plantlife International Publisher; 2008. p. 1–43.
12. Zerabruk S, Yirga G. Traditional knowledge of medicinal plants in Gindeberet district, Western Ethiopia. S Afr J Bot. 2012;78:165–9.
13. Larsen HO, Olsen CS. Unsustainable collection and unfair trade? uncovering and assessing assumptions regarding Central Himalayan medicinal plant conservation. Biodivers Conserv. 2007;16:1679–97.
14. Uprety Y, Asselin H, Dhakal A, Julien N. Traditional use of medicinal plants in the boreal forest of Canada: review and perspectives. J Ethnobiol Ethnomed. 2012;8:1–14.
15. Huang H. Plant diversity and conservation in China: planning a strategic bioresource for a sustainable future. Bot J Linn Soc. 2011;166:282–300.
16. Rafieian-Kopaei M. Medicinal plants and the human needs. J Herb Med Pharm. 2013;1:1–2.
17. Hamilton A. Medicinal plant and conservation: issues and approaches. UK: WWF; 2003.
18. Marcy J, Balunasa A, Kinghornb D. Drug discovery from medicinal plants. Life Sci. 2005;78:431–41.
19. Srujana ST, Babu KR, Rao BSS. Phytochemical investigation and biological activity of leaves extract of plant *Boswellia serrata*. Pharm Innov. 2012;1:22–46.
20. Schippmann U, Leaman DJ, Cunningham AB, Walter S. Impact of cultivation and collection on the conservation of medicinal plants: global trends and issues. III WOCMAP congress on medicinal and aromatic plants: conservation, cultivation and sustainable use of medicinal and aromatic plants; 2005. Chiang Mai.
21. Deeb T, Knio K, Shinwari ZK, Kreydiyyeh S, Baydoun E. Survey of medicinal plants currently used by herbalists in Lebanon. Pak J Bot. 2013;45:543–55.
22. Figueiredo MSL, Grelle CEV. Predicting global abundance of a threatened species from its occurrence: implications for conservation planning. Divers Distrib. 2009;15:117–21.
23. Wagh VV, Jain AK. Status of threatened medicinal plants of Jhabua district, Madhya Pradesh, India. Ann Plant Sci. 2013;2:395–400.
24. Andel TV, Havinga R. Sustainability aspects of commercial medicinal plant harvesting in Suriname. Forest Ecol Manag. 2008;256:1540–5.
25. Soule ME, Estes JA, Miller B, Honnold DL. Strongly interacting species: conservation policy, management, and ethics. Bioscience. 2005;55:168–76.
26. Semwal DP, Saradhi PP, Nautiyal BP, Bhatt AB. Current status, distribution and conservation of rare and endangered medicinal plants of Kedarnath Wildlife Sanctuary, Central Himalayas, India. Curr Sci India. 2007;92:1733–8.
27. Liu C, Yu H, Chen SL. Framework for sustainable use of medicinal plants in China. Zhi Wu Fen Lei Yu Zi Yuan Xue Bao. 2011;33:65–8.
28. Sheikh K, Ahmad T, Khan MA. Use, exploitation and prospects for conservation: people and plant biodiversity of Naltar Valley, northwestern Karakorums, Pakistan. Biodivers Conserv. 2002;11:715–42.
29. Coley PD, Heller MV, Aizprua R, Arauz B, Flores N, Correa M, Gupta M, Solis PN, Ortega-Barría E, Romero LI, Gómez B, Ramos M, Cubilla-Rios L, Capson TL, Kursar TA. Using ecological criteria to design plant collection strategies for drug discovery. Front Ecol Environ. 2003;1:421–8.
30. Gepts P. Plant genetic resources conservation and utilization: the accomplishments and future of a societal insurance policy. Crop Sci. 2006;46:2278–92.
31. Forest F, Grenyer R, Rouget M, Davies TJ, Cowling RM, Faith DP, Balmford A, Manning JC, Proche S, Bank M, Reeves G, Terry AJ, Savolainen V. Preserving the evolutionary potential of floras in biodiversity hotspots. Nature. 2007;445:757–60.
32. Long CL, Li H, Ouyang ZQ, Yang XY, Li Q, Trangmar B. Strategies for agrobiodiversity conservation and promotion: a case from Yunnan, China. Biodivers Conserv. 2003;12:1145–56.
33. Ma J, Rong K, Cheng K. Research and practice on biodiversity in situ conservation in China: progress and prospect. Sheng Wu Duo Yang Xing. 2012;20:551–8.
34. Volis S, Blecher M. Quasi in situ: a bridge between ex situ and in situ conservation of plants. Biodivers Conserv. 2010;19:2441–54.
35. Camm J, Norman S, Polasky S, Solow A. Nature reserve site selection to maximize expected species covered. Oper Res. 2002;50:946–55.
36. Rodriguez JP, Brotons L, Bustamante J, Seoane J. The application of predictive modelling of species distribution to biodiversity conservation. Divers Distrib. 2007;13:243–51.
37. Chiarucci A, Maccherini S, De Dominicis V. Evaluation and monitoring of the flora in a nature reserve by estimation methods. Biol Conserv. 2001;101:305–14.
38. Huang H, Han X, Kang L, Raven P, Jackson PW, Chen Y. Conserving native plants in China. Science. 2002;297:935.
39. Liu J, Linderman M, Ouyang Z, An L, Yang J, Zhang H. Ecological degradation in protected areas: the case of Wolong Nature Reserve for giant pandas. Science. 2001;292:98–101.
40. Kramer AT, Havens K. Plant conservation genetics in a changing world. Trends Plant Sci. 2009;14:599–607.
41. Strandby U, Olsen CS. The importance of understanding trade when designing effective conservation policy: the case of the vulnerable *Abies guatemalensis* Rehder. Biol Conserv. 2008;141:2959–68.
42. Li XW, Chen SL. Conspectus of ecophysiological study on medicinal plant in wild nursery. Zhong Guo Zhong Yao Za Zhi. 2007;32:1388–92.
43. Havens K, Vitt P, Maunder M, Guerrant EO, Dixon K. Ex situ plant conservation and beyond. Bioscience. 2006;56:525–31.
44. Yu H, Xie CX, Song JY, Zhou YQ, Chen SL. TCMGIS-II based prediction of medicinal plant distribution for conservation planning: a case study of *Rheum tanguticum*. Chin Med. 2010;5:31.
45. Swarts ND, Dixon KW. Terrestrial orchid conservation in the age of extinction. Ann Bot. 2009;104:543–56.
46. Pulliam HR. On the relationship between niche and distribution. Ecol Lett. 2000;3:349–61.
47. Yuan QJ, Zhang ZY, Hu JA, Guo LP, Shao AJ, Huang LQ. Impacts of recent cultivation on genetic diversity pattern of a medicinal plant, *Scutellaria baicalensis* (Lamiaceae). BMC Genet. 2010;11:52–9.
48. Primack RB, Miller-Rushing AJ. The role of botanical gardens in climate change research. New Phytol. 2009;182:303–13.
49. Maunder M, Higgens S, Culham A. The effectiveness of botanic garden collections in supporting plant conservation: a European case study. Biodivers Conserv. 2001;10:383–401.
50. Li DZ, Pritchard HW. The science and economics of ex situ plant conservation. Trends Plant Sci. 2009;14:614–21.
51. Schoen DJ, Brown AHD. The conservation of wild plant species in seed banks. Bioscience. 2001;51:960–6.
52. Joshi BC, Joshi RK. The role of medicinal plants in livelihood improvement in Uttarakhand. Int J Herb Med. 2014;1:55–8.
53. Leung KW, Wong AS. Pharmacology of ginsenosides: a literature review. Chin Med. 2010;5:20.
54. Raina R, Chand R, Sharma YP. Conservation strategies of some important medicinal plants. Int J Med Aromat Plant. 2011;1:342–7.
55. Wong KL, Wong RN, Zhang L, Liu WK, Ng TB, Shaw PC, Kwok PCL, Lai YM, Zhang ZJ, Zhang YB, Tong Y, Cheung H, Lu J, Wing SC. Bioactive proteins and peptides isolated from Chinese medicines with pharmaceutical potential. Chin Med. 2014;9:19.
56. Chan K, Shaw D, Simmonds MS, Leon CJ, Xu Q, Lu A, Sutherland I, Ignatova S, Zhu YP, Verpoorte R, Williamson EM, Duezk P. Good practice in reviewing and publishing studies on herbal medicine, with special emphasis on traditional Chinese medicine and Chinese materia medica. J Ethnopharmacol. 2012;140:469–75.
57. Muchugi A, Muluvi GM, Kindt R, Kadu CAC, Simons AJ, Jamnadass RH. Genetic structuring of important medicinal species of genus *Warburgia* as revealed by AFLP analysis. Tree Genet Genome. 2008;4:787–95.

58. Makunga NP, Philander LE, Smith M. Current perspectives on an emerging formal natural products sector in South Africa. J Ethnopharmacol. 2008;119:365–75.
59. Rigby D, Cáceres D. Organic farming and the sustainability of agricultural systems. Agr Syst. 2001;68:21–40.
60. Macilwain C. Organic: is it the future of farming? Nature. 2004;428:792–3.
61. Suresh B. Organic farming: status, issues and prospects—a review. Agr Econ Res Rev. 2010;23:343–58.
62. Baker DD, Chu M, Oza U, Rajgarhia V. The value of natural products to future pharmaceutical discovery. Nat Prod Rep. 2007;24:1225–44.
63. Wang HW, Peng DC, Xie JT. Ginseng leaf-stem: bioactive constituents and pharmacological functions. Chin Med. 2009;4:20.
64. Rao SR, Ravishankar GA. Plant cell cultures: chemical factories of secondary metabolites. Biotechnol Adv. 2002;20:101–53.
65. Lata H, Chandra S, Khan IA, Elsohly MA. Propagation of *Cannabis sativa* L using synthetic seed technology. Plant Med. 2008;74:328.
66. Zych M, Furmanowa M, Krajewska-Patan A, Lowicka A, Dreger M, Mendlewska S. Micropropagation of *Rhodiola kirilowii* plants using encapsulated axillary buds and callus. Acta Biol Cracov Bot. 2005;47:83–7.
67. Schippmann U, Leaman DJ, Cunningham AB. Impact of cultivation and gathering of medicinal plants on biodiversity: global trends and issues. Inter-Department Working Group on biology diversity for food and agriculture. Rome: FAO; 2002.
68. Teklehaymanot T, Giday M. Ethnobotanical study of medicinal plants used by people in Zegie Peninsula, Northwestern Ethiopia. J Ethnobiol Ethnomed. 2007;3:12–23.

16

Anti-inflammatory activities of *Ganoderma lucidum (Lingzhi)* and *San-Miao-San* supplements in MRL/lpr mice for the treatment of systemic lupus erythematosus

Zhe Cai[1,2†], Chun Kwok Wong[1,2,3*†], Jie Dong[1,2], Delong Jiao[1,2], Man Chu[1,2], Ping Chung Leung[3], Clara Bik San Lau[3], Ching Po Lau[3], Lai Shan Tam[2,4] and Christopher Wai Kei Lam[5]

Abstract

Background: *Ganoderma lucidum* (*Lingzhi*; LZ) and *San-Miao-San* (SMS) are Chinese medicines (CMs) used to treat inflammatory ailments and numbing syndrome/arthralgia syndrome (*Bi Zheng*), respectively. Given that the main symptoms of systemic lupus erythematosus (SLE) include inflammation of the joints, joint pain, edema and palpitations of the heart because of problems associated with *Bi Zheng*, it was envisaged that LZ and SMS could be used as potential treatments for this autoimmune disease. This study aims to investigate the anti-inflammatory activity of a combination formulation containing LZ and SMS (LZ–SMS) in SLE mice.

Methods: Female adult Balb/c mice of 20–24 weeks of age were used as normal mice (n = 10), whereas female MRL/lpr mice of 12–24 weeks of age were divided into three groups (n = 10 in each group), including mild, moderate and severe SLE mice groups. The clinical characteristics of the SLE and Babl/c mice (i.e., body weight, joint thickness, lupus flare, proteinuria, leukocyturia and lymphadenopathy) were assessed. The plasma concentrations of anti-nuclear antibody (ANA) and anti-double stranded DNA antibody (anti-ds-DNA) were analyzed by an enzyme-linked immunosorbent assay, whereas the concentration of several key cytokines (IFN-γ, TNF-α, IL-6, IL-10, IL-2, IL-27, IL-12P70, IL-17A and IL-21) were analyzed by a Luminex multiplex assay. The gene expression profiles for differentiation of the T helper (Th) lymphocytes in splenic $CD4^+$ Th cells were assessed by RT-qPCR. Flow cytometry was used to measure the percentages of $CD4^+CD25^+Foxp3^+$ Treg cells and $CD19^+CD5^+CD1d^+IL\text{-}10^+$ regulatory B (Breg) cells ($IL\text{-}10^+$ Bregs).

Results: Concentrations of anti-ds-DNA in the plasma samples collected from the LZ–SMS-treated (500 mg/kg/day oral administration for 7 days followed with 50 mg/kg/day intraperitoneal administration for 7 days), moderate and severe SLE mice decreased significantly compared with the PBS treated mice ($P < 0.05$). The gene expression levels of the induced regulatory T (iTreg) and natural Treg (nTreg) cells were significantly higher than those of the Th17, Th1 and "conventional Th cells vs. Treg cells" regulated genes following the LZ–SMS treatment ($P < 0.05$). The percentages of $CD4^+CD25^+Foxp3^+$ Treg cells collected from the splenic, thymic and peripheral blood cells, as well as the percentages of $IL\text{-}10^+$ Bregs collected from the splenic and thymic cells increased significantly in the LZ–SMS-treated SLE mice ($P < 0.05$) compared with the untreated PBS group. The ratio of the percentage of $CD4^+CD25^+Foxp3^+$ Treg

*Correspondence: ck-wong@cuhk.edu.hk
†Zhe Cai and Chun Kwok Wong are co-first authors
[1] Department of Chemical Pathology, The Chinese University of Hong Kong, Prince of Wales Hospital, Shatin, N.T., Hong Kong, China
Full list of author information is available at the end of the article

cells to the percentage of $CD4^+CD25^-$ effector T cells collected from the splenic, thymic and peripheral blood cells in LZ–SMS-treated moderate and severe SLE mice increased significantly compared with the untreated PBS group ($P < 0.05$). Furthermore, a comparison with the PBS treatment group revealed significant decreases in the concentrations of several inflammatory cytokines, including IL-21, IL-10 and IL-17A ($P < 0.05$), as well as significant increases in the concentrations of IL-2 and IL-12P70 in the LZ–SMS treated SLE mice ($P < 0.05$).

Conclusion: LZ–SMS treatment led to significant increases in the percentages of $CD4^+CD25^+Foxp3^+$ Treg and $IL\text{-}10^+$ Breg cells, together with a reduction in the plasma concentrations of several inflammatory cytokines and the down-regulated expression of the corresponding cytokine related genes in SLE mice. The clinical characteristics of the LZ–SMS-treated SLE mice also improved significantly.

Background

Systemic lupus erythematosus (SLE) is a multi-systemic chronic autoimmune relapsing disease with a particularly high prevalence in middle-aged women, where it often results in damage to multiple organs, including the kidneys, skin, heart, blood vessels and central nervous system [1]. Although several drugs have been developed for this disease, which have led to considerable improvements in overall survival as well as alleviating the symptoms of severe organ damage, they are expensive and produce unwanted side effects [2–5].

Ganoderma lucidum (*Lingzhi*; LZ) has been reported to exhibit antioxidant, anti-inflammatory and analgesic effects with potential therapeutic benefits against a wide range of diseases, including hepatitis, hypertension, arthritis, bronchitis and malignancy [6–13]. LZ induced the expansion of both murine and human $CD4^+$ T cells into $Foxp3^+$ regulatory T (Treg) cells, which could be used to alleviate acute colitis [14]. LZ has also been reported to modulate the activity of peripheral mononuclear cells and suppress the production of SLE-related pathogenic cytokines, such as tumor necrosis factor-α (TNF-α), as well as interleukin (IL)-1β, IL-12 and IL-6 [5, 15–17].

San-Miao-San (SMS) is a Chinese medicine (CM) containing a 1:1:1 (w:w:w) mixture of three Chinese herbs, including *Rhizoma atractylodis* (*Cangzhu*), *Cortex phellodendri* (*Huangbai*) and *Radix achyranthis bidentatae* (*Niuxi*) [18]. This material has been used empirically for treating numbing syndrome/arthralgia syndrome (*Bi Zheng*), which is a painful obstructive syndrome caused by the invasion of exterior pathogenic factors into the muscles, tendons, bones and joints of the sufferer [5, 18]. According to CM, SLE can be generally classified into excessive and deficient syndromes and related to *Bi Zheng*, because this syndrome results in joint problems, joint pain, edema and palpitations of the heart because of its damaging effects [19]. It was therefore envisaged that the combination of SMS with *Lingzhi* could be beneficial for the treatment of SLE. The combined use of LZ and SMS (LZ–SMS) for their anti-inflammatory activities was once common practice according to CM herbalists because this combination of materials exhibits synergistic therapeutic effects [20]. Furthermore, the results of several clinical studies showed that a combined standard formulation of LZ and SMS was generally safe and well tolerated by patients suffering from rheumatoid arthritis (RA) [18, 21]. However, the in vivo anti-inflammatory mechanisms of LZ and SMS for the treatment of SLE have not yet been investigated.

We previously investigated the intracellular signal transduction mechanisms responsible for regulating the activation of human eosinophils, epithelial cells and fibroblast-like synoviocytes (FLS) during inflammation, and studied the pathological roles of cytokines in allergic and autoimmune diseases [22–25]. This study aims to investigate the anti-inflammatory activities of this combined formulation of LZ–SMS in SLE mice.

Methods

Materials

The combined LZ–SMS hot water extract formulation used in this study contained a lyophilized powder, which was prepared according to a previously reported procedure by researchers at the Institute of Chinese Medicine, The Chinese University of Hong Kong, China [18]. This extract was prepared by combining LZ 35.7 % with SMS, which consists of three Chinese herbs, including *Cangzhu* 21.4 %, *Huangbai* 21.4 % and *Niuxi* 21.4 %. The preparation was then dissolved in physiological saline, and the resulting solution was analyzed by a Limulus amoebocyte lysate assay (sensitivity limit 12 pg/mL; Biowhittaker Inc, Walkersville, MD, USA), which revealed that it did not contain any detectable lipopolysaccharide. The different herbs were authenticated in terms of their chemical composition by thin layer chromatography against a reference herb and several reference chemical markers, according to the Chinese Pharmacopoeia 2010 [26].

Mice

Female MRL/MpJ-Fas^{lpr}/2 J (MRL/lpr) mice were purchased from the Jackson Laboratory (Bar Harbor, ME,

USA) and maintained under specific pathogen-free conditions in the Laboratory Animal Services Center (LASC), The Chinese University of Hong Kong (CUHK) and Cancer Center of Prince of Wales Hospital, Hong Kong. Female adult Balb/c mice (LASC, CUHK) of 20–24 weeks of age were used as normal mice (n = 10). Adult female MRL/lpr SLE mice of 12–24 weeks of age (n = 30) were kept in a conventional animal facility. All of the experiments conducted in the present study involving live animals were carried out under strict controls according to the Animal Experimentation Ethics Committee Guide for the Care and Use of Laboratory Animals, as approved by the Animal Experimentation Ethics Committee of CUHK (Ethical approval no.: 14-012-MIS) (Additional file 1).

Monitoring of disease activity

The urine samples collected from the different groups (n = 10) of mice were analyzed for protein and leukocytes by URS-5T urine test strips (Healgen Scientific LLC, Houston, TX, USA). Female MRL/lpr mice of 12–24 weeks of age were divided into three groups (n = 10 in each group), including mild, moderate and severe SLE mice according to the following proteinuria scoring system: score 0 0–15 mg/dL, score 1 16–29 mg/dL, score 2 30–99 mg/dL, score 3 100–299 mg/dL, score 4 300–1999 mg/dL, and score 5 ≥2000 mg/dL (score 0–1: mild SLE; score 2–3: moderate SLE and score 4–5: severe SLE) [27].

Biochemical and physiological parameters

The different groups of MRL/lpr and Balb/c mice (both groups n = 5) were used to investigate the nephritic effects of the LZ–SMS formulation on the mice following the daily oral and intraperitoneal administration of this material for 14 days. The oral administration group was given 500 mg/kg/day of the LZ–SMS formulation in 400 μL of phosphate buffered saline (PBS) from day 1 to 7 (n = 5 for the lupus mice in each SLE group and Balb/c mice in the normal group). A 50 mg/kg/day dose of LZ–SMS was also prepared in 400 μL of PBS because of its limited solubility. This dose was intraperitoneally administered from day 8 to 14 into the lupus mice or normal mice (n = 5 in each case) belonging to each group. For the intraperitoneal injection of this lower dose of LZ–SMS, we only injected clear solutions of the LZ–SMS formulation (about 1.25 mg LZ–SMS/mouse daily), which were filtered prior to being injected to remove any insoluble materials. PBS was given to each mouse on a daily basis at a dose of 400 μL/mouse for 14 days according to the same protocol as that used for the PBS control (n = 5 of each group). The body weight of each mouse was measured before and after the administration of the LZ–SMS formulation to provide some indication of possible herbal toxicity [28]. Mice were also culled 1 day after the administration of the LZ–SMS formulation to investigate several immunological parameters, including the plasma concentrations of anti-nuclear antibody (ANA), anti-double stranded DNA antibody (anti-ds-DNA) and several cytokines (IL-2, IL-10, IL-27, IL-21, IL-12P70, IFN-γ, TNF-α, IL-17A and IL-6) in the whole blood. Clinical signs of lupus flare and disease severity were assessed in each group (n = 10) of MRL/lpr mice before and after the treatment process using the following four-point scale: 0–3, where 0 is normal, 1 is mild (affected areas including the snout and ears), 2 is moderate (affected area <2 cm on the snout, ears and intrascapular region) and 3 is severe (affected area >2 cm on the snout, ears and intrascapular region) [29].

Histopathological assessment

Longitudinal sections of the kidneys, which were cut through the papilla, were fixed in 4 % paraformaldehyde buffer and embedded in paraffin. The kidney sections were subsequently cut into 2-μm-thick slices and stained with periodic acid-Schiff (PAS) stain. The number of mesangial cells in the glomeruli was determined by counting their nuclei. Microscopy examination (Leica Microsystems, Wetzlar, Germany) was used to evaluate the area of the glomeruli, with 100 glomeruli being evaluated in each group. The severities of vessel infiltration, interstitial nephritis and glomerulonephritis were scored using the following macroscopic scoring system: 0, normal; 1–2, mild; 3, moderate; and 4–5, severe [30].

Quantitative real-time polymerase chain reaction (RT-qPCR)

Whole transcriptome analysis for the differentiation of the T helper (Th) cells was performed using a mouse T helper cell differentiation RT^2 profiler PCR array (Qiagen GmbH, Hilden, Germany). The RNA was extracted from splenic CD4$^+$ Th cells by an RNeasy Mini Kit (Qiagen). The splenic CD4$^+$ Th cells were purified by a mouse T helper cell isolation kit (Miltenyi Biotec, Bergisch Gladbach, Germany) with Th cell purity >95 %. The purified RNA from 1 × 10^6 splenic CD4$^+$ Th cells were analyzed according to the manufacturer's instructions for the RT^2 profiler PCR Array kit by a 384-well Applied Biosystems 7900HT Fast Real-Time PCR System (Applied Biosystems Inc., Foster City, CA, USA). The mRNA expression levels were calculated as follows:

$$\frac{\dfrac{2^{-\Delta C_T(GOI)_{expt}}}{2^{-\Delta C_T(HKG)_{expt}}}}{\dfrac{2^{-\Delta C_T(GOI)_{ctrl}}}{2^{-\Delta C_T(HKG)_{ctrl}}}} = \frac{2^{-[C_T(GOI)\,-\,\Delta C_T(HKG)]_{expt}}}{2^{-[C_T(GOI)\,-\,\Delta C_T(HKG)]_{ctrl}}} = \frac{2^{-\Delta C_{T_{expt}}}}{2^{-\Delta C_{T_{ctrl}}}} = 2^{-\Delta\Delta C_T}$$

where expt is the experiment, ctrl is the control, GOI is the gene of interest and HKG is the housekeeping gene.

Flow cytometric analyses of the $CD4^+CD25^+Foxp^+$ Treg cells, $CD4^+CD25^-$ effector T (Teff) cells and $CD19^+CD5^+CD1d^+IL\text{-}10^+$ Breg cells

Peripheral blood, splenic and thymic cells (1×10^6 cells in each case) from the MRL/lpr and Balb/c mice were stained to determine the number of $CD4^+CD25^+Foxp^+$ Treg cells [fluorescein peridinin chlorophyll protein/PerCP-conjugated $CD4^+$, allophycocyanin/APC-conjugated $CD25^+$ (BioLegend, San Diego, CA, USA) and Alexa Fluor 488-conjugated $Foxp^+$ (BD Pharmingen Corp., San Diego, CA, USA) T lymphocyte sub-populations], $CD4^+CD25^-$ Teff cells and IL-10^+ Breg cells [($CD19^+CD5^+CD1d^+$ regulatory B cell) cocktail and Phycoerythrin/Cyanine Dye 7 (PE/Cy7)-conjugated anti-IL-10 antibody (BioLegend)] by flow cytometry (Beckman Navios flow cytometer, Beckman Coulter Inc., Brea, CA, USA).

Plasma concentrations of ANA and anti-ds-DNA

The plasma ANA and anti-ds-DNA concentrations in each group were measured by an enzyme-linked immunosorbent assay (ELISA) with commercial reagent kits (Mybiosource, Inc., San Diego, CA, USA).

Plasma cytokine concentrations of MRL/lpr and Balb/c mice

Plasma was harvested and stored at −80 °C prior to being subjected to a multiplex immunoassay to measure several cytokines (i.e., IL-2, IL-10, IL-27, IL-21, IL-12P70, IFN-γ, TNF-α, IL-17A and IL-6) using a Milliplex MAP kit assay reagent (Merck Millipore, Billerica, MA, USA) with a Bio-Plex 200 suspension array system (Bio-Rad Laboratories, Hercules, CA, USA).

Statistical analysis

The results for the statistical analysis of the gene array data are described in the gene array hybridization and data analysis section. These results have been expressed as the mean ± standard deviation (SD) for normally distributed data. Non-parametric data have been expressed as the median values (interquartile range, IQR). Mann–Whitney U tests were used for the continuous variables. A comparison of the different groups was achieved by Kruskal–Wallis ANOVA, followed by Dunn's post-test for comparing the differences and calculating a P value for each pair of comparison. Two-way ANOVA was used to compare the different groups and treatments, followed by Bonferroni post-test analysis for comparing the replicate means and calculating a P value for each data pair. All hypotheses were two-tailed, and P values less than 0.05 were considered significant. All of these data were analyzed by the 6.0 for Windows version of the GraphPad Prism software (GraphPad Software, La Jolla, CA, USA).

Results

SLE disease characteristics of MRL/lpr mice

The clinical characteristics of the different mice are summarized in Table 1. The MRL/lpr mice treated with PBS were initially stratified into three subgroups (i.e., mild, moderate or severe) based on their disease activity, which provided a reflection of their proteinuria scores. The percentages of lymphadenopathy and the body weights in the different groups of MRL/lpr mice were significantly higher than those of the control mice ($P = 0.034$). Furthermore, no obvious adverse side effects were observed in the MRL/lpr mice used in the present study, as evidenced by the lack of significant loss of body weight upon LZ–SMS administration, all $P > 0.05$. All of the MRL/lpr mice in the moderate ($P < 0.001$) and severe ($P = 0.035$) groups had significantly higher proteinuria and leukocyturia scores than the control mice. However, there were no significant differences in these scores between the mild and control groups ($P = 0.056$). The joint thickness and lupus flare scores of the MRL/lpr mice in the moderate ($P = 0.036$) and severe ($P = 0.030$) groups were significantly higher than those of the control group.

Attenuation of nephritis in MRL/lpr mice treated with LZ–SMS

To confirm the immunoregulatory and therapeutic roles of LZ–SMS in vivo, we measured the nephritis clinical characteristics of the MRL/lpr mice after they had been treated with LZ–SMS or PBS. As shown in Fig. 1, the proteinuria, leukocyturia, lupus flare, glomerulonephritis, interstitial nephritis and vessel infiltrate scores for the MRL/lpr mice without LZ–SMS treatment were significantly higher than those of the Balb/c control (all $P < 0.05$). Furthermore, the results for the LZ–SMS-treated MRL/lpr mice revealed that there were obvious remissions in the extent of the nephritic disease compared with PBS treatment alone, especially in the severe SLE mice (Figs. 1, 2). Moreover, there were significant differences in the plasma concentrations of ANA and anti-ds-DNA antibodies in the moderate and severe SLE mice compared with the Balb/c control mice treated with PBS (all $P < 0.01$) (Fig. 3). Although the plasma concentrations of ANA and anti-ds-DNA antibodies in the moderate and severe SLE mice treated with LZ–SMS were significantly higher than those of the Balb/c control mice, the plasma concentrations of anti-ds-DNA in the moderate ($P < 0.001$) and severe SLE mice ($P = 0.05$) were both significantly lower than those of the PBS-treated mice.

Table 1 Clinical characteristics of MRL/lpr and Balb/c mice before treatment

	MRL/lpr (n = 30)			Balb/c
	Mild (n = 10)	Moderate (n = 10)	Severe (n = 10)	Normal (n = 10)
Clinical assessment				
Body weight, mean ± SD, g	48.0 ± 8.7$^{\&}$	49.4 ± 9.1**	48.7 ± 4.1$^{\#}$	19.2 ± 0.2
Joint thickness, mean ± SD, μm	84.3 ± 3.1	84.7 ± 2.7*	84.4 ± 2.4	79.3 ± 3.6
Lupus flare score, mean ± SD	0.7 ± 0.5	1.0 ± 0.9	1.3 ± 1.0$^{\#}$	0
Proteinuria score, mean ± SD	1.5 ± 0.5	2.8 ± 0.4***	4.0 ± 1.1$^{\#\#\#}$	0.7 ± 0.6
Leukocyturia score, mean ± SD	0.5 ± 1.2	2.0 ± 1.4*	2.5 ± 0.5$^{\#\#}$	0
Lymphadenopathy, No. (%)	10/10 (100 %)$^{\&\&\&}$	10/10 (100 %)***	10/10 (100 %)$^{\#\#\#}$	0/10 (0 %)

Joint thickness was measured in three joints of each hind paw (tarsus joint); Leukocyturia score was determined by a four-point scale (0–3, where 0 was normal and 3 was severe); No. (%), percentages of mice had lymphadenopathy among each group

SD standard deviation, *MRL/lpr* MRL/MpJ-Fas^{lpr}/2 J, *Mild* mice with mild disease activity (mild SLE, proteinuria score is 0–1), *Moderate* moderate disease activity (moderate SLE, proteinuria score is 2–3), *Severe* high disease activity (severe SLE, proteinuria score is 4–5), *Normal* age- and sex- matched healthy Balb/c mice

$^{\&}$ $P = 0.03$, $^{\&\&}$ $P = 0.008$, $^{\&\&\&}$ $P = 0.0008$, comparing between control and mild SLE mice

* $P = 0.03$, ** $P = 0.008$, *** $P = 0.0008$, comparing between control and moderate SLE mice

$^{\#}$ $P = 0.03$, $^{\#\#}$ $P = 0.008$, $^{\#\#\#}$ $P = 0.0008$, comparing between control and severe SLE mice

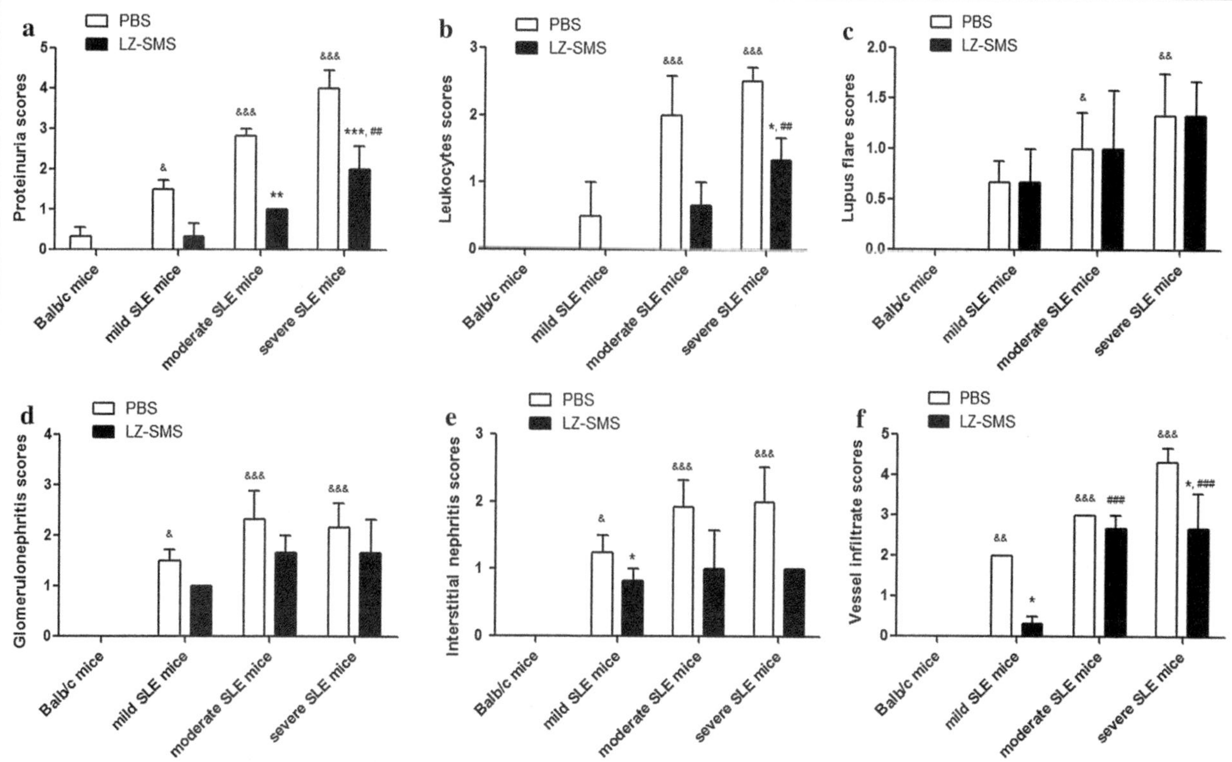

Fig. 1 Clinical characteristics of MRL/lpr mice with LZ–SMS or PBS treatment. The results of each score system of signs **a** proteinuria, **b** leukocyturia, **c** lupus flare, **d** glomerulonephritis, **e** interstitial nephritis and **f** vessels infiltration are presented as bar charts showing the arithmetic mean plus SD. * <0.05, **$P < 0.01$, ***$P < 0.001$, PBS- vs. LZ–SMS-treated MRL/lpr mice; $^{\&}P < 0.05$, $^{\&\&}P < 0.01$, $^{\&\&\&}P < 0.001$, Balb/c control mice vs. PBS-treated MRL/lpr mice; $^{\#\#}P < 0.01$, $^{\#\#\#}P < 0.001$, Balb/c control mice vs. LZ–SMS-treated MRL/lpr mice (n = 5 in each group)

Gene expression profile of Th cell differentiation

A common logarithm of gene expression revealed that the expression levels of Th1 cell-regulated genes (*Ifng, Il12rb2, Il18r1, Il18rap, Fasl* and *Tbx21*) and conventional Th cell *vs.* Treg cell-regulated genes (*Cacna1f, Chd7, Foxp3, Gata4, Hopx, Hoxa10, Hoxa3, Id2, Ikzf2, Il1r2, Il2ra, Lrrc32, Perp, Pkd2, Tnfrsf9, Trp53inp1, Uts2* and *Zeb1*) were significantly lower than those of the

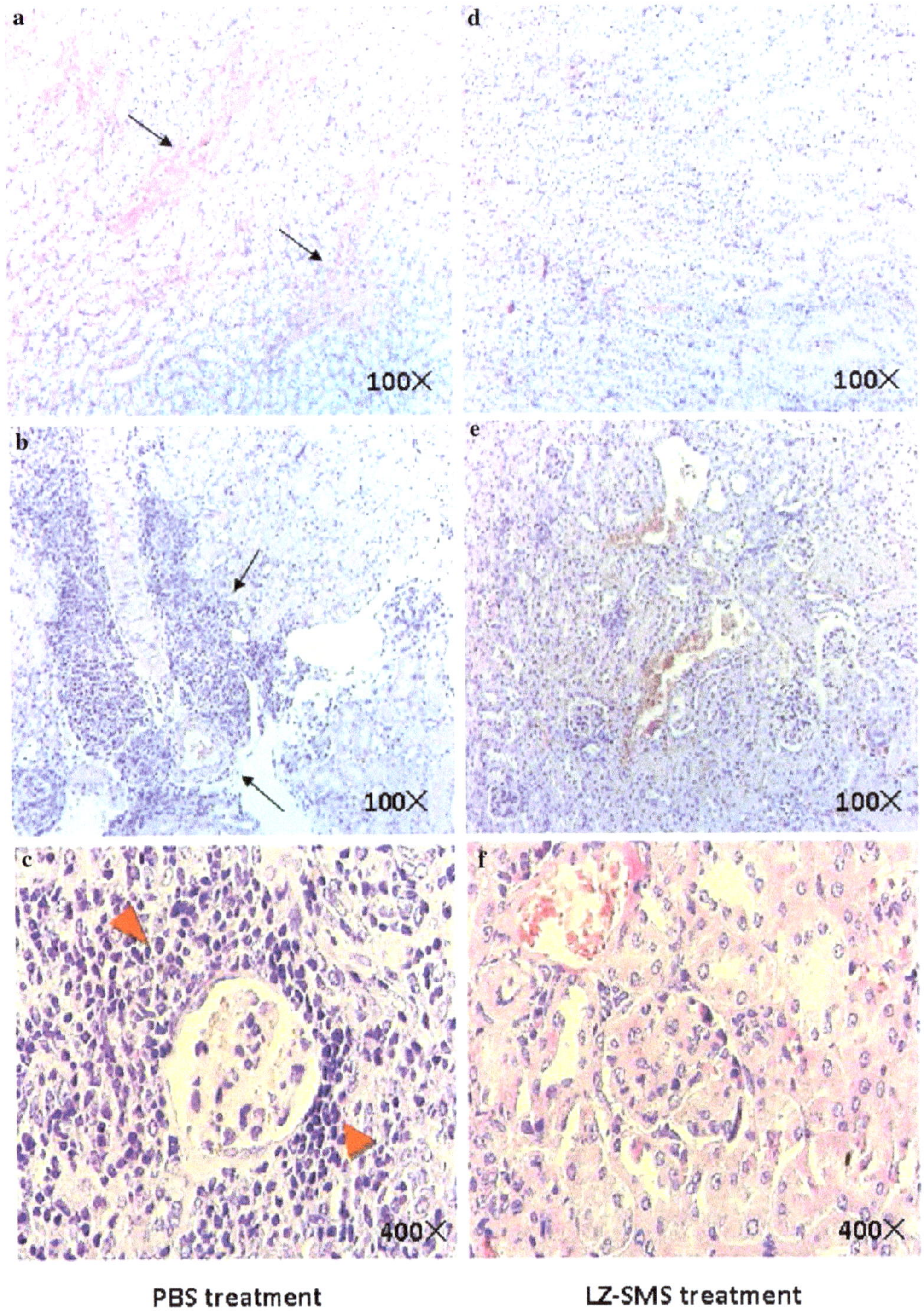

Fig. 2 Effects of LZ-SMS treatment on nephritis disease in severe MRL/lpr mice. Kidney tissues from MRL/lpr mice were collected and fixed in 4 % paraformaldehyde. The tissue sections were stained with PAS. Representative kidney histopathology in (**a**–**c**) PBS and (**d**–**f**) LZ-SMS treated SLE mice are shown. **a**, **d** PAS staining of a representative renal tubular area is shown (100×). *Black arrow* depicts the protein cast in tubular area. **b**, **e** PAS staining of a representative perivascular area is shown (100×). *Black arrow* depicts the mononuclear cells infiltration on vessel. **c**, **f** PAS staining of a representative glomerulus area is shown (400×). *Bold red arrow* depicts the mononuclear cells infiltration round glomerulus (n = 5 in each group)

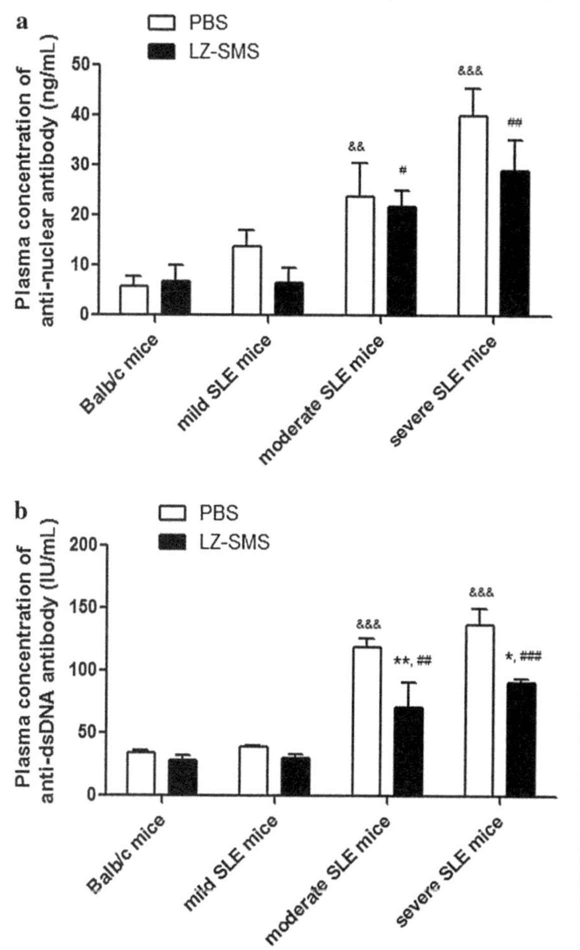

Fig. 3 Plasma concentrations of ANA and anti-ds-DNA antibody in LZ-SMS or PBS-treated MRL/lpr and Balb/c mice. Concentrations of plasma **a** ANA and **b** anti-ds-DNA are presented as *bar charts* showing the arithmetic mean plus SD. $^{*}P < 0.05$, $^{**}P < 0.01$, PBS- vs. LZ-SMS-treated MRL/lpr mice; $^{\&\&}P < 0.01$, $^{\&\&\&}P < 0.001$, Balb/c control mice vs. PBS treated MRL/lpr mice; $^{\#}P < 0.05$, $^{\#\#}P < 0.01$, $^{\#\#\#}P < 0.001$, Balb/c control mice vs. LZ-SMS treated MRL/lpr mice (n = 5 in each group)

Th2 cell-regulated genes (*Asb2, Gata3, Il13, Il1rl1, Il4, Il5* and *Pparg*) in the splenic CD4^{+} Th lymphocytes from the PBS-treated MRL/lpr mice compared with the PBS-treated Balb/c control mice (Fig. 4a). However, following LZ–SMS treatment, the mean values of the induced regulatory (iTreg) and natural Treg (nTreg) (*Ccr6, Fosl1, Foxp3, Ikzf2, Il9, Irf4, Irf8, Myb, Nr4a1, Nr4a3, Pou2f2, Rel, Tgif1* and *Tnfsf11*) regulated gene expression levels in the splenic CD4^{+} Th lymphocytes obtained from MRL/lpr mice were significantly higher than those of the Th17 cell-regulated genes (*Il17a, Il17re, Il1rl, Il21, Rora* and *Rorc*) in Th1 cells compared with the PBS treatment group (Fig. 4b). These results implied that LZ–SMS was exhibiting an immunoregulatory role towards the differentiation of splenic CD4^{+} Th cells by inducing the differentiation of CD4^{+} Th cells into iTreg cells, whilst suppressing the differentiation of Th1 and Th17 cells in vivo. Most of the Th cell differentiation-related transcription factors, as well as the cytokine and receptor genes, were found to be up-regulated (ratio > 1.0) in the MRL/lpr mice belonging to the LZ–SMS treatment group compared with those in the PBS treatment group. This was especially true for the Treg differentiation-related genes IL-2 and Foxp3, which were up-regulated by more than 1.5-fold (Table 2).

Increase in the percentages of CD4^{+}CD25^{+}Foxp3^{+} Treg cells and IL-10^{+} Breg cells in MRL/lpr mice following LZ–SMS treatment

We found that the number of CD4^{+}CD25^{+}Foxp3^{+} Treg cells in the different groups of MRL/lpr mice decreased in a linear manner compared with the Balb/c control mice both with and without LZ–SMS treatment (Fig. 5a–c). Compared with the PBS treatment group, the percentages of CD4^{+}CD25^{+}Foxp3^{+} Treg cells obtained from the splenic, thymic and peripheral blood cells in the severe SLE mice treated with LZ–SMS increased significantly (all $P < 0.05$). Furthermore, the percentage of CD4^{+}CD25^{+}Foxp3^{+} Treg cells obtained from the splenic cells in the moderate SLE mice treated with LZ–SMS was significantly higher than the value achieved with PBS treatment ($P = 0.004$). Accordingly, the percentage ratios of the CD4^{+}CD25^{+}Foxp3^{+} Treg cells to the CD4^{+}CD25^{-} effector T cells obtained from the splenic, thymic and peripheral blood cells in the severe SLE mice treated with LZ–SMS, and from thymic and peripheral blood cells in moderate SLE mice with LZ–SMS treatment were significantly increased compared with PBS treatment group (Fig. 5d, e). Finally, there was a significant increase in the percentage of IL-10^{+} Breg cells obtained from the thymic cells in mild SLE mice treated with LZ–SMS compared with the PBS-treated mice (Fig. 5g, $P < 0.001$).

Plasma concentrations of cytokines of MRL/lpr and Balb/c mice

There were decreases in the plasma concentrations of the inflammatory cytokines (IFN-γ, TNF-α and IL-6) observed in the moderate and severe SLE mice treated with LZ–SMS compared with the PBS-treated mice (Fig. 6). In particular, the plasma concentrations of the Th17 cytokines IL-21 and IL-17A in the severe SLE mice decreased significantly following their treatment with

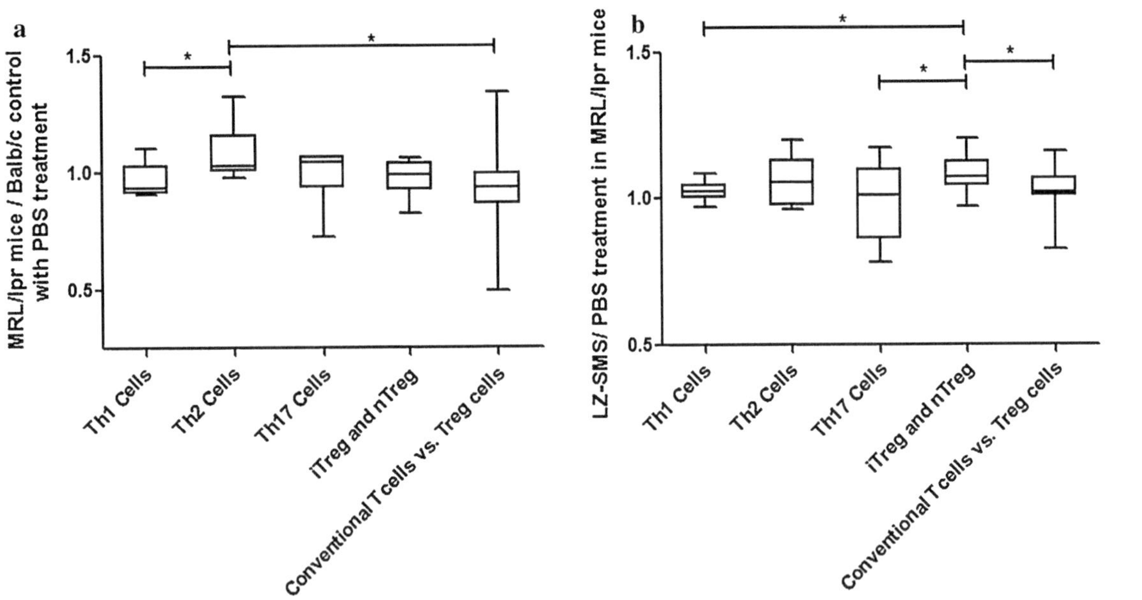

Fig. 4 RT^2 profiler PCR array of mouse Th cell differentiation. The results of gene expressions of Th1 cells, Th2 cells, iTreg and nTreg, Th17 cells and "conventional Th vs. Treg cells" in **a** PBS-treated MRL/lpr vs. Balb/c mice (in ratio) and **b** LZ-SMS-treated vs. PBS-treated MRL/lpr mice (in ratio) are presented as *box-and-whisker plots* with the median (IQR). Mann–Whitney U test was used to assess the differences of mRNA expression among different genes of Th cells. $^*P < 0.05$

the LZ–SMS material (Fig. 6c, f). In contrast, the plasma concentration of IL-2 in the severe SLE mice ($P = 0.004$), as well as the concentrations of IL-12p70 in each group of MRL/lpr mice treated with LZ–SMS increased significantly compared with those in the PBS-treated mice (Fig. 6b, d) (all $P < 0.05$). Furthermore, the plasma concentration of IL-10 in the severe SLE mice treated with LZ–SMS decreased significantly compared with that in the PBS-treated mice (Fig. 6f, $P = 0.011$). There were no significant differences in the plasma concentrations of IL-27 among the different groups of MRL/lpr mice treated with LZ–SMS compared with those in the PBS-treated mice (Fig. 6e, $P = 0.156$), even though the plasma concentrations in the moderate and severe SLE mice were significantly lower than those of the Balb/c mice (all $P < 0.01$). However, the significant differences ($P < 0.01$) observed in the IL-27 concentration in this case may not be physiologically or immunologically relevant.

Discussion

In the present study, we have evaluated the anti-inflammatory efficacy of LZ–SMS following its oral and intraperitoneal administration in MRL/lpr mice. This LZ–SMS formulation can be suspended in PBS administered at a maximum concentration of 500 mg/kg/day [5]. MRL/lpr mice were orally administered this material on a daily basis for 7 days, followed by intraperitoneal administration for a further 7 days. Notably, none of the LZ–SMS components administered in this study exceeded the toxic doses reported in humans and mice [28, 31]. MRL/lpr mice treated with LZ–SMS showed a marked decrease in the extent of the symptoms associated with their SLE disease, including improvements in proteinuria, leukocyturia, interstitial nephritis and vessel infiltration. The eldest SLE mice (20–24 weeks) showed the most severe symptoms of lupus nephritis prior to treatment. Increases were also observed in the nephritis-related clinical and biochemical indexes of the SLE mice, along with increases in age among the three different groups (mild, moderate and severe).

No data were obtained in the present study pertaining to the absorption or systemic distribution of the active ingredients of LZ–SMS. LZ contains β-glucan, which is an immunomodulating polysaccharide capable of potential interactions with pattern recognition receptors such as dectin-1. It is noteworthy that dectin-1 is a c-type lectin, which can collaborate with TLR2 to trigger innate immune responses in antigen-presenting cells [32, 33], as well as inducing a balance between pro- and anti-inflammatory responses [34–37]. Furthermore, TLR2 signaling

Table 2 Th differentiation PCR array analysis

Transcription Factors		Cytokines and receptors	
Gene	LZ-SMS PBS	Gene	LZ-SMS PBS
Fosl1	1.94	Tnf	0.98
Nr4a1	5.12	Il1r2	1.94
Nr4a3	6.46	Il17re	1.10
Hoxa10	1.06	Il21	2.01
Rel	3.22	Ccr6	1.11
Irf4	2.03	Csf2	0.79
Nfatc1	1.88	Il4	1.12
Irf8	1.57	Il18r1	1.78
Id2	1.74	Ccr3	3.61
Gata4	1.99	Ccl5	0.96
Rora	5.04	Il13ra1	0.69
Cebpb	1.72	Il1rl1	0.82
Stat1	1.58	Il18	0.84
Zbtb7b	0.83	Il2ra	0.35
Pou2f2	1.40	Ccl7	0.73
Maf	2.14	Il18rap	2.27
Stat6	0.97	Ccr4	1.34
Rorc	1.19	Il12p40	0.53
Runx1	1.29	Il1r1	3.90
Gata3	1.68	Il2	2.63
Zeb1	1.03	Ccl11	1.38
Nfatc2	2.01	Il12rb2	2.68
Foxp3	1.91	Il4ra	1.99
Nfatc2ip	1.53	Il9	6.13
Runx3	2.00	Il13	1.99
Hoxa3	1.22		
Stat4	1.41		

cDNA samples were obtained from splenic cells of 24 weeks old female MRL/lpr mice 1 day after treatment. Values represent fold increase of LZ–SMS treatment (500 mg/kg/day of LZ–SMS formulation in 400 μL PBS for day 1–7 by oral administration followed by 50 mg/kg/day of soluble LZ–SMS in 400 μL PBS for day 8–14 by intraperitoneal route) versus the PBS treatment group

could potentially enhance the proliferation of Treg cells both in vitro and in vivo, which would result in the transient suppression of Foxp3 expression and the loss of their suppressive functions. It has been shown that the expression and function of dectin-1 are defective in the peripheral blood monocytes collected from patients with SLE and RA compared with healthy controls, suggesting that dectin-1 could be involved in the pathogenesis of autoimmune inflammatory conditions [38]. Dectin-1 signaling could also make a significant contribution to the expansion of Treg cells and play a critical role in the prevention of several inflammatory conditions, such as type 1 diabetes [39]. The protocol used for the intraperitoneal administration of this combination therapy was the same as that used for its oral administration, except that the dosage used in the former of these two cases was reduced to 50 mg/kg/day because of the limited solubility of LZ–SMS.

The pronounced reduction observed in the nephritis symptoms of the mice in the present study following their treatment with LZ–SMS could be attributed to the ability of LZ–SMS to down-regulate the expression of multiple inflammatory-related genes (e.g., Th17), and Th1-cell regulated genes, as well as genes associated with the expression of inflammatory cytokines and receptors, chemokines, adhesion molecules and chronic inflammation-activated proteins [40]. These responses could also be related to the ability of LZ–SMS to up-regulate the expression of regulatory iTreg-related genes and their downstream transcription factors, such as Foxp3, Stat1 and Stat4. Although the mechanism of action for the anti-nephritic efficacy of this LZ–SMS formulation remains unclear, *Lingzhi* has been reported to regulate the production of several pro-inflammatory cytokines associated with the pathogenesis of SLE in peripheral mononuclear cells [5, 15–17].

The LZ–SMS formulation used in the present study led to an increase in the percentages of immunomodulatory $CD4^{+}CD25^{+}Foxp3^{+}$ Treg cells and IL-10^{+} Breg cells in the SLE mice compared with those in the PBS-treated SLE mice. These elevated levels of Treg cells could subsequently lead to (1) an increase in the frequency ratio of Treg to Teff cells; (2) an increase in the plasma concentration of IL-2, which could lead to an increase in the differentiation of Treg cells from naive T cells, the development of Treg cells in the thymus and the immunoregulatory roles of the Treg cells [41, 42]; or (3) considerable reductions in the amounts of several proinflammatory cytokines, including IL-21, TNF-α, IL-6 and IL-17A. Although the frequency and phenotypic characteristics of the Treg cells in the MRL/lpr mice were similar to those found in the normal mice, the inhibitory functions of the Treg cells in the MRL/lpr mice could be impaired by the LZ–SMS treatment [43]. Further functional assays are therefore required to develop a better understanding of the roles played by TLR2 and dectin-1 in Treg cells during the treatment of SLE in MRL/lpr mice with LZ–SMS. The overall results showed decreases in the plasma concentrations of ANA and anti-dsDNA antibody in the LZ–SMS-treated SLE mice (Fig. 3), indicating that the suppressive activity of LZ–SMS would be

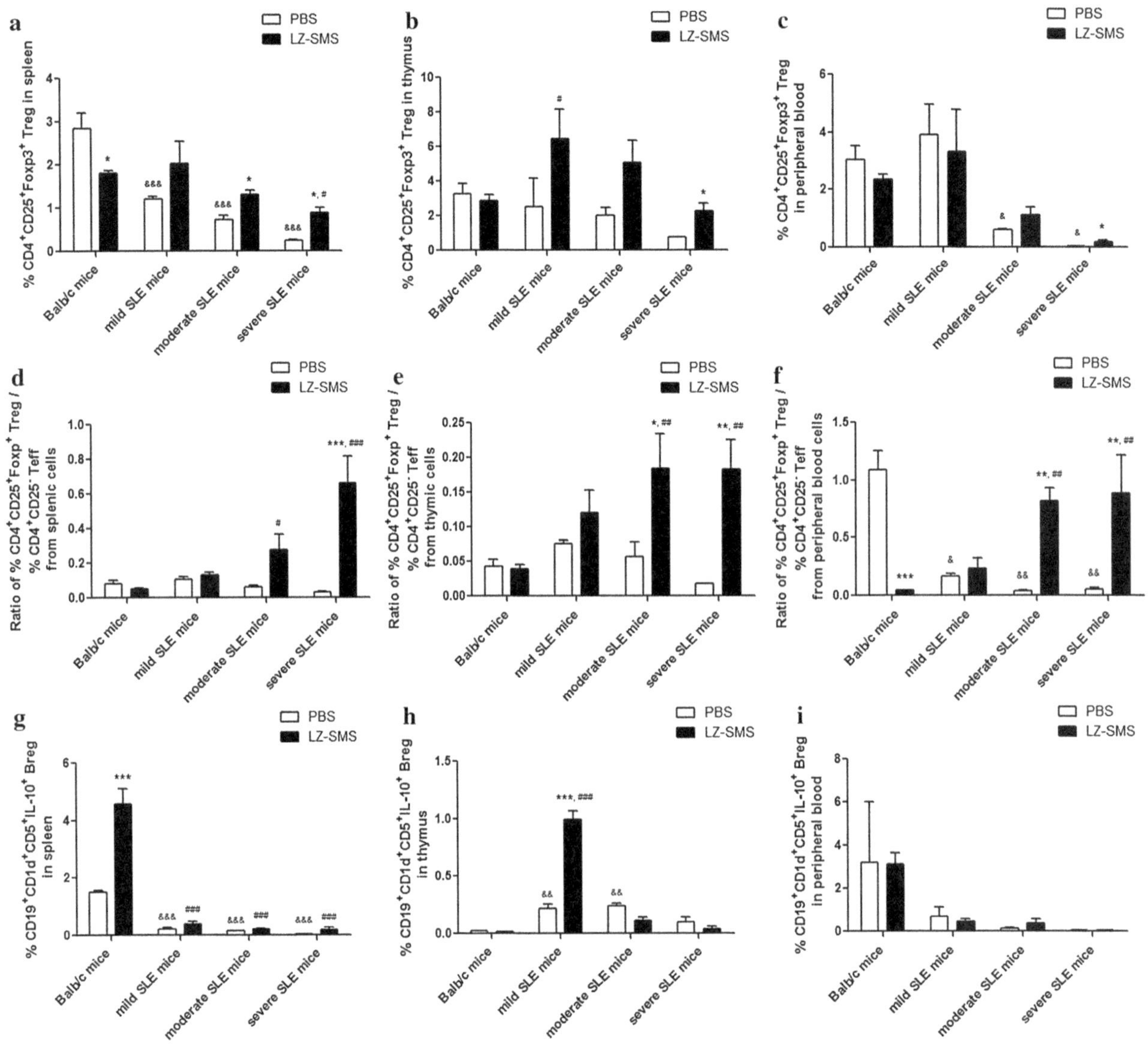

Fig. 5 Characterization of $CD4^+CD25^+Foxp3^+$ Tregs and IL-10 + Bregs in LZ–SMS or PBS-treated MRL/lpr and Balb/c mice. *Bar charts* show the arithmetic mean plus SD of the percentages of $CD4^+CD25^+Foxp3^+$ Tregs in **a** splenic, **b** thymic and **c** peripheral blood cells; and the ratios of $CD4^+CD25^+Foxp3^+$ Treg %/$CD4^+CD25^-$ effector T cell % in **d** splenic, **e** thymic and **f** peripheral blood cells; and the percentages of IL-10 + Breg cells in **g** splenic, **h** thymic and **i** peripheral blood cells. $^*P < 0.05$, $^{**}P < 0.01$, $^{***}P < 0.001$, LZ-SMS vs. PBS treatment; $^{\&}P < 0.05$, $^{\&\&}P < 0.01$, $^{\&\&\&}P < 0.001$, Balb/c control mice vs. PBS-treated MRL/lpr mice; $^{\#}P < 0.05$, $^{\#\#}P < 0.01$, $^{\#\#\#}P < 0.001$, Balb/c control mice vs. LZ-SMS-treated MRL/lpr mice (n = 5 in each group)

not only limited to $CD4^+$ Treg cells, but also related to the propagation of IL-10^+ Breg cells. However, the low frequency of IL-10^+ Breg cells in peripheral blood cells, and the reduced plasma concentration of IL-10 in the LZ–SMS-treated severe SLE mice could limit the immunoregulatory role of LZ–SMS in this context because of the exacerbation of the SLE disease.

Conclusion

Upon LZ–SMS treatment, the percentages of $CD4^+CD25^+Foxp3^+$ Treg and IL-10^+ Breg cells increased significantly in the SLE mice compared with those in the untreated mice. Furthermore, there was a decrease in the plasma concentrations of specific inflammatory cytokines, as well as a down-regulation in the expression

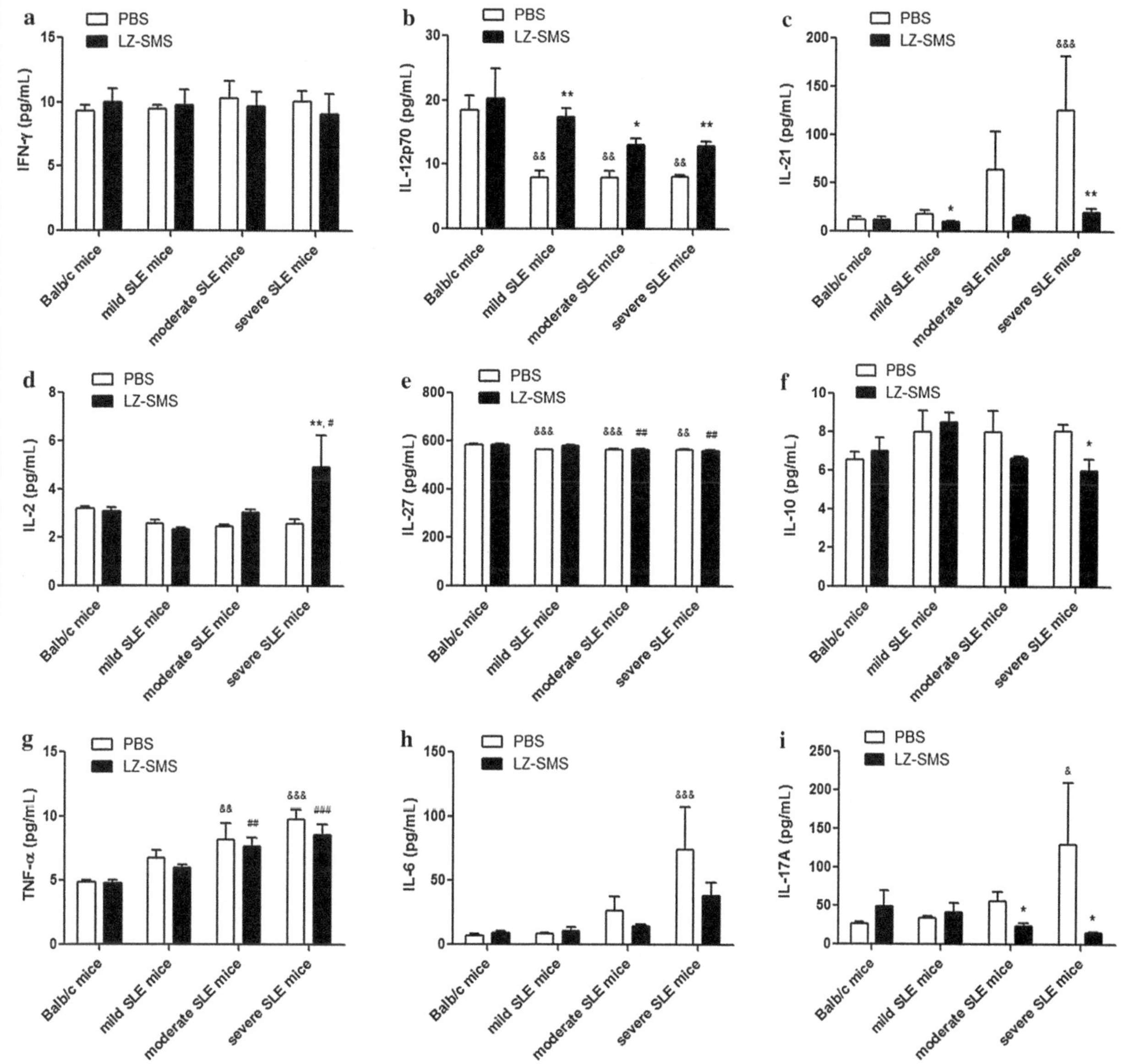

Fig. 6 Plasma concentrations of cytokines of MRL/lpr and Balb/c mice treated with LZ–SMS or PBS. *Bar charts* show the arithmetic mean values of the plasma concentrations of **a** IFN-γ, **b** IL-12P70, **c** IL-21, **d** IL-2, **e** IL-27, **f** IL-10, **g** TNF-α, **h** IL-6 and (i) IL-17A. $^{*}P < 0.05$, $^{**}P < 0.01$, LZ–SMS vs. PBS treatment; $^{\&\&}P < 0.01$, $^{\&\&\&}P < 0.001$, Balb/c control mice vs. PBS-treated MRL/lpr mice; $^{\#}P < 0.05$, $^{\#\#}P < 0.01$, $^{\#\#\#}P < 0.001$, Balb/c control mice vs. LZ–SMS-treated MRL/lpr mice (n = 5 in each group)

of the corresponding cytokine-related genes in the LZ–SMS-treated mice. The clinical characteristics of the LZ–SMS-treated SLE mice were also improved significantly.

Abbreviations

SLE: systemic lupus erythematosus; CM: Chinese medicines; LZ–SMS: *Lingzhi* and *San-Miao-San*; RA: rheumatic arthritis; FLS: fibroblast-like synoviocytes; Tregs: regulatory T cells; Bregs: regulatory B cells; ANA: anti-nuclear antibody; anti-ds-DNA: anti-double stranded DNA antibody; PAS: periodic acid-Schiff; ELISA: enzyme-linked immunosorbent assay; qPCR: quantitative real-time polymerase chain reaction; TNF-α: tumor necrosis factor-α; IFN-γ: interferon-γ; SD: standard deviation; IQR: interquartile range.

Authors' contributions

CKW, PCL and ZC conceived and designed the study. PCL, CBL and CKW obtained the funding. ZC performed the animal, molecular and biochemical assays. ZC, JD and DJ performed the animal handling experiments, MC performed the animal monitoring and molecule detection, and CPL prepared the LZ–SMS. ZC, CKW, CBL, LST and CWKL wrote the manuscript. All authors read and approved the final manuscript.

Author details

[1] Department of Chemical Pathology, The Chinese University of Hong Kong, Prince of Wales Hospital, Shatin, N.T., Hong Kong, China. [2] Shenzhen Research Institute, The Chinese University of Hong Kong, Shenzhen, China. [3] Institute of Chinese Medicine and State Key Laboratory of Phytochemistry and Plant Resources in West China, The Chinese University of Hong Kong, Hong Kong, China. [4] Department of Medicine and Therapeutics, Prince of Wales Hospital, The Chinese University of Hong Kong, Shatin, Hong Kong, China. [5] State Key Laboratory of Quality Research in Chinese Medicine, Macau Institute for Applied Research in Medicine and Health, Macau University of Science and Technology, Taipa, Macau, China.

Acknowledgements

We thank Ms. Ida Miu Ting Chu and Mr. Timmy Wai Sheng Cheng for their efforts on experimental supports. This work was supported by funding of the State Key Laboratory of Phytochemistry and Plant Resources in West China (CUHK) from HKSAR, Focused Innovations Scheme (Major Area Scheme A-Phase 2) of The Chinese University of Hong Kong.

Competing interests

The authors declare that they have no competing interests.

References

1. Mok CC, Lau CS. Pathogenesis of systemic lupus erythematosus. J Clin Pathol. 2003;56:481–90.
2. Bertsias G, Boumpas DT. Update on the management of lupus nephritis: let the treatment fit the patient. Nat Clin Pract Rheumatol. 2008;4:464–72.
3. Doria A, Iaccarino L, Ghirardello A, Zampieri S, Arienti S, Sarzi-Puttini P, Atzeni F, Piccoli A, Todesco S. Long-term prognosis and causes of death in systemic lupus erythematosus. Am J Med. 2006;119:700–6.
4. Ippolito A, Petri M. An update on mortality in systemic lupus erythematosus. Clin Exp Rheumatol. 2008;26:S72–9.
5. Lam FF, Ko IW, Ng ES, Tam LS, Leung PC, Li EK. Analgesic and anti-arthritic effects of Lingzhi and San Miao San supplementation in a rat model of arthritis induced by Freund's complete adjuvant. J Ethnopharmacol. 2008;120:44–50.
6. Lakshmi B, Ajith TA, Sheena N, Gunapalan N, Janardhanan KK. Antiperoxidative, anti-inflammatory, and antimutagenic activities of ethanol extract of the mycelium of *Ganoderma lucidum* occurring in South India. Teratog Carcinog Mutagen. 2003;Suppl 1:85–97.
7. You YH, Lin ZB. Antioxidant effect of Ganoderma polysaccharide peptide. Yao Xue Xue Bao. 2003;38:85–8.
8. Ho YW, Yeung JS, Chiu PK, Tang WM, Lin ZB, Man RY, Lau CS. *Ganoderma lucidum* polysaccharide peptide reduced the production of proinflammatory cytokines in activated rheumatoid synovial fibroblast. Mol Cell Biochem. 2007;301:173–9.
9. Kabir Y, Kimura S, Tamura T. Dietary effect of *Ganoderma lucidum* mushroom on blood pressure and lipid levels in spontaneously hypertensive rats (SHR). J Nutr Sci Vitaminol. 1988;34:433–8.
10. Kanmatsuse K, Kajiwara N, Hayashi K, Shimogaichi S, Fukinbara I, Ishikawa H, Tamura T. Studies on *Ganoderma lucidum*. I. efficacy against hypertension and side effects. Yakugaku Zasshi. 1985;105:942–7.
11. Li YQ, Wang SF. Anti-hepatitis B activities of ganoderic acid from *Ganoderma lucidum*. Biotechnol Lett. 2006;28:837–41.
12. Wasser SP, Weis AL. Therapeutic effects of substances occurring in higher Basidiomycetes mushrooms: a modern perspective. Crit Rev Immunol. 1999;19:65–96.
13. Yuen JW, Gohel MD. Anticancer effects of Ganoderma lucidum: a review of scientific evidence. Nutr Cancer. 2005;53:11–7.
14. Hsu HY, Kuan YC, Lin TY, Tsao SM, Hsu J, Ma LJ, Sheu F. Reishi protein LZ-8 induces FOXP3(+) treg expansion via a CD45-dependent signaling pathway and alleviates acute intestinal inflammation in mice. Evid Based Complement Alternat Med. 2013: 513542.
15. Maczynska I, Millo B, Ratajczak-Stefanska V, Maleszka R, Szych Z, Kurpisz M, Giedrys-Kalemba S. Proinflammatory cytokine (IL-1beta, IL-6, IL-12, IL-18 and TNF-alpha) levels in sera of patients with subacute cutaneous lupus erythematosus (SCLE). Immunol Lett. 2006;102:79–82.
16. Sun KH, Yu CL, Tang SJ, Sun GH. Monoclonal anti-double-stranded DNA autoantibody stimulates the expression and release of IL-1beta, IL-6, IL-8, IL-10 and TNF-alpha from normal human mononuclear cells involving in the lupus pathogenesis. Immunol. 2000;99:352–60.
17. Umare V, Pradhan V, Nadkar M, Rajadhyaksha A, Patwardhan M, Ghosh KK, Nadkarni AH. Effect of proinflammatory cytokines (IL-6, TNF- alpha, and IL-1 beta) on clinical manifestations in Indian SLE patients. Mediators Inflamm. 2014: 385297.
18. Li EK, Tam LS, Wong CK, Li WC, Lam CW, Wachtel-Galor S, Benzie IF, Bao YX, Leung PC, Tomlinson B. Safety and efficacy of *Ganoderma lucidum* (lingzhi) and San Miao San supplementation in patients with rheumatoid arthritis: a double-blind, randomized, placebo-controlled pilot trial. Arthr Rheum. 2007;57:1143–50.
19. Chen DP, Wong CK, Leung PC, Fung KP, Lau CB, Lau CP, Li EK, Tam LS, Lam CW. Anti-inflammatory activities of Chinese herbal medicine sinomenine and Liang Miao San on tumor necrosis factor-alpha-activated human fibroblast-like synoviocytes in rheumatoid arthritis. J Ethnopharmacol. 2011;137:457–68.
20. Lau KM, Lai KK, Liu CL, Tam JC, To MH, Kwok HF, Lau CP, Ko CH, Leung PC, Fung KP, Poon SK, Lau CB. Synergistic interaction between Astragali Radix and Rehmanniae Radix in a Chinese herbal formula to promote diabetic wound healing. J Ethnopharmacol. 2012;141:250–6.
21. Bao YX, Wong CK, Li EK, Tam LS, Leung PC, Yin YB, Lam CW. Immunomodulatory effects of lingzhi and san-miao-san supplementation on patients with rheumatoid arthritis. Immunopharmacol Immunotoxicol. 2006;28:197–200.
22. Cheung PFY, Wong CK, Lam CWK. Molecular mechanisms of cytokine and chemokine release from eosinophils activated by IL-17F and IL-23: implications for Th17 lymphocyte-mediated allergic inflammation. J Immunol. 2008;180:5625–35.
23. Lit LC, Wong CK, Tam LS, Li EK, Lam CW. Raised plasma concentration and ex vivo production of inflammatory chemokines in patients with systemic lupus erythematosus. Ann Rheum Dis. 2006;65:209–15.
24. Wong CK, da Chen P, Tam LS, Li EK, Yin YB, Lam CW. Effects of inflammatory cytokine IL-27 on the activation of fibroblast-like synoviocytes in rheumatoid arthritis. Arthr Res Ther. 2010;12:R129.
25. Wong CK, Li ML, Wang CB, Ip WK, Tian YP, Lam CW. House dust mite allergen Der p 1 elevates the release of inflammatory cytokines and expression of adhesion molecules in co-culture of human eosinophils and bronchial epithelial cells. Int Immunol. 2006;18:1327–35.
26. Ip SP, Zhao M, Xian Y, Chen M, Zong Y, Tjong YW, Tsai SH, Sung JJ, Bensoussan A, Berman B, Fong HH, Che CT. Quality assurance for Chinese herbal formulae: standardization of IBS-20, a 20-herb preparation. Chin Med. 2010;5:8.
27. Mills JA. Systemic lupus erythematosus. N Engl J Med. 1994;330:1871–9.
28. Chiu SW, Wang ZM, Leung TM, Moore D. Nutritional value of *Ganoderma* extract and assessment of its genotoxicity and anti-genotoxicity using comet assays of mouse lymphocytes. Food Chem Toxicol. 2000;38:173–8.
29. Lipsky PE. Systemic lupus erythematosus: an autoimmune disease of B cell hyperactivity. Nat Immunol. 2001;2:764–6.
30. Watson ML, Rao JK, Gilkeson GS, Ruiz P, Eicher EM, Pisetsky DS, Matsuzawa A, Rochelle JM, Seldin MF. Genetic-analysis of Mrl-Lpr Mice—relationship of the fas apoptosis gene to disease manifestations and renal disease-modifying loci. J Exp Med. 1992;176:1645–56.
31. Chang R. Effective dose of *Ganoderma* in humans. In: Buchanan PK, Hseu RS, Moncalvo JM, editors. Proceedings of the Contributed Symposium 59A, B of the 5th International Mycological Congress; 1994. p. 101–113.
32. Goodridge HS, Underhill DM. Fungal Recognition by TLR2 and Dectin-1. Handb Exp Pharmacol. 2008;183:87–109.
33. Underhill DM. Collaboration between the innate immune receptors dectin-1, TLRs, and nods. Immunol Rev. 2007;219:75–87.
34. Sing A, Reithmeier-Rost D, Granfors K, Hill J, Roggenkamp A, Heesemann J. A hypervariable N-terminal region of Yersinia LcrV determines Toll-like receptor 2-mediated IL-10 induction and mouse virulence. Proc Natl Acad Sci. 2005;102:16049–54.
35. Kiura K, Kataoka H, Yasuda M, Inoue N, Shibata K. The diacylated lipopeptide FSL-1 induces TLR2-mediated Th2 responses. FEMS Immunol Med Microbiol. 2006;48:44–55.

36. Martin M, Schifferle RE, Cuesta N, Vogel SN, Katz J, Michalek SM. Role of the phosphatidylinositol 3 kinase-Akt pathway in the regulation of IL-10 and IL-12 by *Porphyromonas gingivalis* lipopolysaccharide. J Immunol. 2003;171:717–25.
37. Polumuri SK, Toshchakov VY, Vogel SN. Role of phosphatidylinositol-3 kinase in transcriptional regulation of TLR-induced IL-12 and IL-10 by Fc gamma receptor ligation in murine macrophages. J Immunol. 2007;179:236–46.
38. Salazar-Aldrete C, Galan-Diez M, Fernandez-Ruiz E, Nino-Moreno P, Estrada-Capetillo L, Abud-Mendoza C, Layseca-Espinosa E, Baranda L, Gonzalez-Amaro R. Expression and function of dectin-1 is defective in monocytes from patients with systemic lupus erythematosus and rheumatoid arthritis. J Clin Immunol. 2013;33:368–77.
39. Karumuthil-Melethil S, Perez N, Li R, Vasu C. Induction of innate immune response through TLR2 and dectin 1 prevents type 1 diabetes. J Immunol. 2008;181:8323–34.
40. Barnes PJ. How corticosteroids control inflammation: quintiles prize lecture 2005. Br J Pharmacol. 2006;148:245–54.
41. Setoguchi R, Hori S, Takahashi T, Sakaguchi S. Homeostatic maintenance of natural Foxp3(+) CD25(+) CD4(+) regulatory T cells by interleukin (IL)-2 and induction of autoimmune disease by IL-2 neutralization. J Exp Med. 2005;201:723–35.
42. Brandenburg S, Takahashi T, de la Rosa M, Janke M, Karsten G, Muzzulini T, Orinska Z, Bulfone-Paus S, Scheffold A. IL-2 induces in vivo suppression by CD4(+)CD25(+)Foxp3(+) regulatory T cells. Eur J Immunol. 2008;38:1643–53.
43. Parietti V, Monneaux F, Decossas M, Muller S. Function of $CD4^{+}CD25^{+}$ Treg cells in MRL/lpr mice is compromised by intrinsic defects in antigen-presenting cells and effector T cells. Arthr Rheum. 2008;58:1751–61.

17

Rapid differentiation of *Xihuangcao* from the three *Isodon* species by UPLC-ESI-QTOF-MS/MS and chemometrics analysis

Lai Lai Wong[1], Zhitao Liang[1,2], Hubiao Chen[1,2] and Zhongzhen Zhao[1,2*]

Abstract

Background: *Isodon lophanthoides*, *I. lophanthoides* var. *graciliflorus* and *I. serra* are the three botanical sources of *Xihuangcao*, which are often used indiscriminately in herbal products. The aim of this study was to develop a rapid and accurate analytical method to identify the three different botanical sources of *Xihuangcao* by combining UPLC-ESI-QTOF-MS with chemometrics analysis.

Methods: Fifteen batches of plants were collected as reference materials and their chemical profiles were analyzed by UPLC-ESI-QTOF-MS. These data were subsequently processed by statistical methods, including principal component analysis (PCA), hierarchical cluster analysis (HCA) and orthogonal partial least squared discriminant analysis (OPLS-DA). An automated sample class prediction model was also built using Naive Bayes as a class prediction algorithm to rapidly determine the source species of twenty-seven batches of commercial *Xihuangcao* samples.

Results: The base peak chromatograms of the three authenticated species showed different patterns and twenty-seven peaks were chosen, including six diterpenoids, one phenolic acid and two glycosides to distinguish among these three species. The results showed good differentiation among the three species by PCA, HCA and OPLS-DA. *Isodon lophanthoides* var. *graciliflorus* was found to be the major botanical source of the commercial samples.

Conclusion: UPLC-ESI-QTOF-MS and subsequent chemometrics analysis were demonstrated effective to differentiate among the three different species of plants used as *Xihuangcao*.

Background

Xihuangcao is a folk medicine that is commonly used in southern China as a *dampness*-draining, antiicteric and liver protection herb [1]. Furthermore, clinical research has highlighted the beneficial effects of *Xihuangcao* for the treatment of hepatitis with jaundice, leading to the development and commercialization of numerous proprietary medicines and functional food products based on *Xihuangcao* [1]. Four different plants have been recorded as sources of *Xihuangcao*, including *Isodon lophanthoides* (Buch.-Ham. ex D. Don) Hara (IL), *I. lophanthoides* var. *graciliflorus* (Benth.) H. Hara (ILG), *I. lophanthoides* var. *gerardianus* (Benth.) H. Hara and *I. serra* (Maxim.) Kudo (IS) [2]. According to a taxonomic revision, the plants in this genus have been much confused, especially for the varieties of *I. lophanthoides*. A new classification of *I. lophanthoides* and its varieties was suggested in 2004, in which *I. lophanthoides* var. *gerardianus* and *I. lophanthoides* var. *graciliflorus* were merged as *I. lophanthoides* var. *graciliflorus* (ILG) [3]. However, some experts believe that IS should not be used as *Xihuangcao* because its leaves do not have yellow juice when they are rubbed, which is recorded as a major characteristic of *Xihuangcao* in several ancient herbal medicine books [4]. Recent studies have also demonstrated the chemical compositions of IL, ILG and IS are different, which diterpenoids in IL and ILG are mainly abietane and tricyclic types and that of IS are *ent*-kaurane type; thus, they should not be used as one herb [1, 4].

Although *Xihuangcao* has multiple botanical sources, most of the *Xihuangcao*-based products do not

*Correspondence: zzzhao@hkbu.edu.hk
[1] School of Chinese Medicine, Hong Kong Baptist University, Kowloon, Hong Kong Special Administrative Region, People's Republic of China
Full list of author information is available at the end of the article

specify the species used. The development of an analytical method to identify the three different source species of *Xihuangcao* is therefore strongly desired to ensure the safe and effective use of these herbal products. IL and its variety ILG are difficult to distinguish based on their morphological or microscopic features [5, 6]. In contrast, IS can be readily distinguished from IL and ILG based on its microscopic features, but this method cannot be applied to differentiate between samples of different sources in their extracted forms. It is noteworthy that *Xihuangcao* has not yet been recorded in *The Pharmacopoeia of the People's Republic of China*. The only official method available for the analysis of *Xihuangcao* is recorded in the *Guangdong Chinese Materia Medica Standards*. According to this method, samples for analysis are compared with a reference material (*I. lophanthoides* var. *graciliflorus*) by thin-layer chromatography with no provision for differentiating between the three species [2]. Although numerous studies have been conducted in recent years concerning *Xihuangcao*, most of these studies have limited to the chemical separation or pharmacological evaluation [7–10]. A few chemical analytical studies have been published, but each study analyzed a single species only [11, 12].

Chromatographic fingerprinting is an effective analytical method for identifying samples based on a comparison of their chemical profiles. Ultra-performance liquid chromatography (UPLC) can be used to separate a wide variety of compounds with superior resolution over a short period of time, and can also be coupled with mass spectrometry (MS). The major drawback of this method is that it can be time consuming to analyze all the MS data generated from a large number of samples. Chemometrics solves this problem by statistical analysis to distinguish between different species, thereby avoiding the manual comparison of huge amounts of raw MS data. Furthermore, class prediction models, which can be built based on the statistical interpretation of known reference samples can be used for automated classification of unknown samples.

The aim of this study was to identify the three botanical sources of *Xihuangcao* by ultra-performance liquid chromatography coupled with electrospray ionization quadrupole time-of-flight mass spectrometry (UPLC-ESI-QTOF-MS) in combination with chemometrics analysis.

Methods

Chemicals and reference standards

All chemicals and reference standards used in this study were purchased as the HPLC grade. Oridonin (purity ≥98%) and rosmarinic acid (purity ≥98%) were purchased from Chengdu Must Bio-Technology Co., Ltd (Chengdu, China). Schaftoside (purity ≥98%) was purchased from Chengdu Biopurify Phytochemicals Ltd (Chengdu, China). Methanol and acetonitrile were purchased from E. Merck (Darmstadt, Germany). Formic acid (purity 96.0%) was purchased from Tedia Company Inc. (Fairfield, OH, USA). Water was obtained from a Milli-Q water purification system (Millipore, Bedford, MA, USA).

Plant materials and sample preparation

Fifteen batches of plant samples were collected in southern China as reference materials, including four batches of *I. lophanthoides* var. *lophanthoides,* seven batches of *I. lophanthoides* var. *graciliflorus* and four batches of *I. serra* (Table 1; Fig. 1). These samples were authenticated

Table 1 Plant samples of *Xihuangcao* collected

Sample no.	Species	Source	Date of collection
IL-01	*Isodon lophanthoides*	Baiyun, Guangdong Province (transplant from Fujian)	July 2012
IL-02	*Isodon lophanthoides*	Baiyun, Guangdong Province	July 2012
IL-03	*Isodon lophanthoides*	Yingde, Guangdong Province	July 2012
IL-04	*Isodon lophanthoides*	Yingde, Guangdong Province	July 2012
ILG-01	*Isodon lophanthoides* var. *graciliflora*	Pingyuan, Guangdong Province	July 2012
ILG-02	*Isodon lophanthoides* var. *graciliflora*	Pingyuan, Guangdong Province	July 2012
ILG-03	*Isodon lophanthoides* var. *graciliflora*	Heping, Guangdong Province	July 2012
ILG-04	*Isodon lophanthoides* var. *graciliflora*	Baiyun, Guangdong Province	July 2012
ILG-04	*Isodon lophanthoides* var. *graciliflora*	Shatin, Hong Kong	August 2013
ILG-05	*Isodon lophanthoides* var. *graciliflora*	Meizhou, Guangdong Province	September 2013
ILG-06	*Isodon lophanthoides* var. *graciliflora*	Panyu, Guangdong Province	February 2014
IS-01	*Isodon serra*	Yingde, Guangdong Province	July 2012
IS-02	*Isodon serra*	Baiyun, Guangdong Province	July 2012
IS-03	*Isodon serra*	Zhaoqing, Guangdong Province	July 2012
IS-04	*Isodon serra*	Panyu, Guangdong Province	February 2014

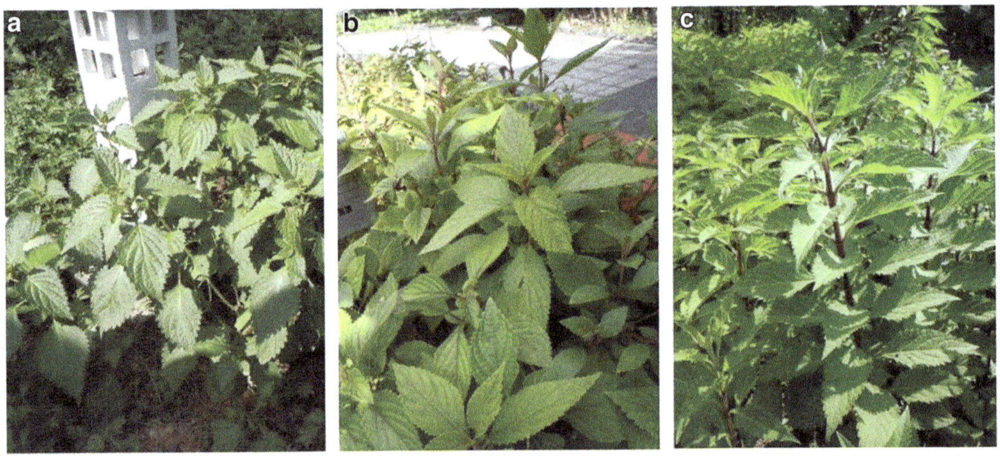

Fig. 1 The botanical sources of *Xihuangcao*: **a** *I. lophanthoides*, **b** *I. lophanthoides* var. *graciliflorus* and **c** *I. serra*

by Prof. Zhongzhen Zhao (School of Chinese Medicine, Hong Kong Baptist University, Hong Kong) based on their morphological characteristics [3, 13]. Twenty-seven samples of commercial batches of *Xihuangcao* were collected from retail markets in Guangdong and Guangxi (Table 2; Fig. 2).

Table 2 Commercial *Xihuangcao* samples collected and the identification result

Sample no.	Producing area	Usage	Species identified
Sample 01	Shangsha, Guangdong	Ingredient of soup	*Isodon lophanthoides* var. *graciliflorus*
Sample 02	Meizhou, Guangdong	Ingredient of soup	*Isodon lophanthoides* var. *graciliflorus*
Sample 03	Guangxi	Herb tea	*Ampelopsis grossedentata*
Sample 04	Huizhou, Guangdong	Herb tea	*Ampelopsis grossedentata*
Sample 05	Yulin, Guangxi	Decoction pieces	*Isodon serra*
Sample 06	Yulin, Guangxi	Herb tea	*Ampelopsis grossedentata*
Sample 07	Shaoguan, Guangdong	Herb tea	*Isodon serra*
Sample 08	Meizhou, Guangdong	Ingredient of soup	*Isodon lophanthoides* var. *graciliflorus*
Sample 09	Taiping, Guangxi	Herb tea	*Ampelopsis grossedentata*
Sample 10	Wengyuan, Guangdong	Herb tea	*Isodon serra*
Sample 11	Wengyuan, Guangdong	Herb tea	*Ampelopsis grossedentata*
Sample 12	Guangdong	Herb tea	*Isodon serra*
Sample 13	Meizhou, Guangdong	Ingredient of soup	*Isodon lophanthoides* var. *graciliflorus*
Sample 14	Heyuan, Guangdong	Herb tea	*Ampelopsis grossedentata*
Sample 15	Guangdong	Herb tea	*Ampelopsis grossedentata*
Sample 16	Meizhou, Guangdong	Ingredient of soup	*Isodon lophanthoides* var. *graciliflorus*
Sample 17	Meizhou, Guangdong	Ingredient of soup	Unknown
Sample 18	Jiangxi	Decoction pieces	*Isodon serra*
Sample 19	Meizhou, Guangdong	Ingredient of soup	*Isodon lophanthoides* var. *graciliflorus*
Sample 20	Huizhou, Guangdong	Herb tea	*Ampelopsis grossedentata*
Sample 21	Meizhou, Guangdong	Ingredient of soup	*Isodon lophanthoides* var. *graciliflorus*
Sample 22	Meizhou, Guangdong	Ingredient of soup	*Isodon lophanthoides* var. *graciliflorus*
Sample 23	Longyan, Fujian	Herb tea	*Isodon lophanthoides* var. *graciliflorus*
Sample 24	Meizhou, Guangdong	Ingredient of soup	*Isodon lophanthoides* var. *graciliflorus*
Sample 25	Meizhou, Guangdong	Ingredient of soup	*Isodon lophanthoides* var. *graciliflorus*
Sample 26	Meizhou, Guangdong	Decoction pieces	*Isodon serra*
Sample 27	Meizhou, Guangdong	Decoction pieces	*Isodon lophanthoides* var. *graciliflorus*

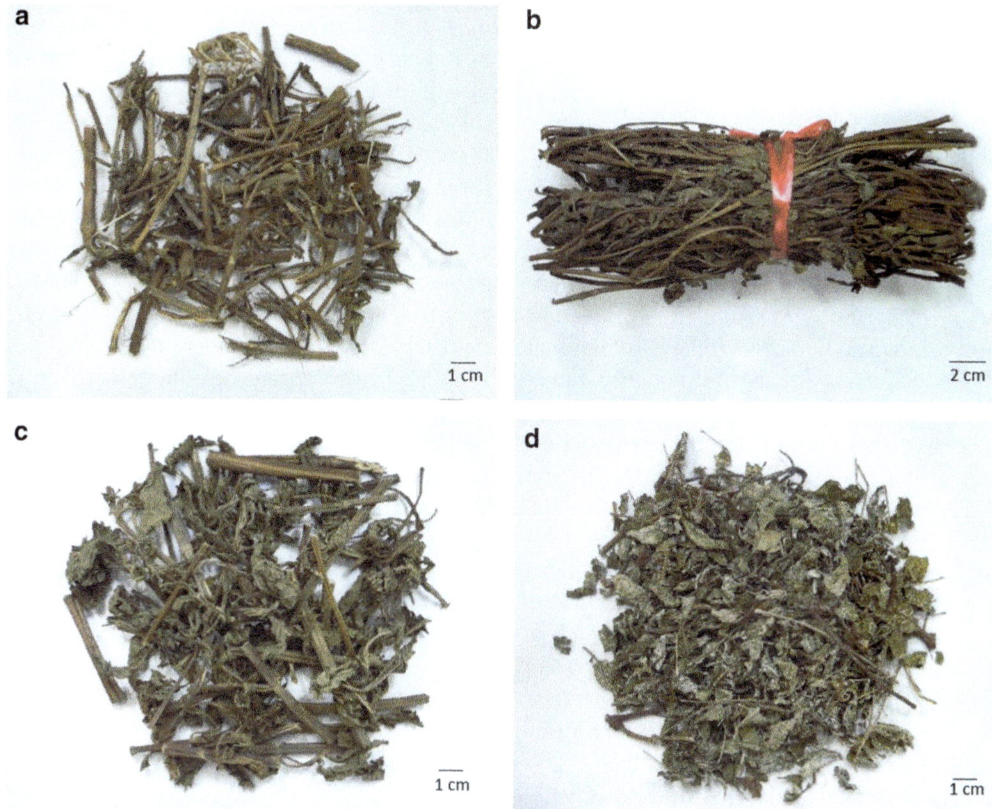

Fig. 2 Photos of some of the commercial *Xihuangcao* samples collected in this study: **a**, **b** *I. lophanthoides* var. *graciliflorus*, **c** *I. serra* and **d** *Ampelopsis grossedentata*

For the preparation of the reference materials, the roots were removed from the plants together with any foreign matter, and the remaining materials were dried under the sun. All of the dried samples were then powdered in a blender. A sample (0.5 g) of the powdered material was then accurately weighed into a centrifuge tube followed by 10 mL of methanol, and the resulting mixture was sonicated for 30 min at room temperature. The supernatant was then centrifuged at 25,920×*g* for 10 min on an Eppendorf 5810 centrifuge (Eppendorf, Hamburg, Germany). The extract (0.2 mL) was then diluted with 0.8 mL of methanol and transferred into a brown HPLC vial for injection.

UPLC-ESI-QTOF-MS analysis

UPLC-ESI-QTOF-MS analysis was performed on an Agilent 6540 accurate mass Q-TOF LC/MS system (Agilent Technologies, Santa Clara, CA, USA). Chromatography was performed on a UPLC C_{18} analytical column (2.1 × 5 mm, I.D. 1.7 μm, ACQUITY UPLC® BEH, Waters, Milford, MA, USA). The mobile phase used for the elution of the column consisted of 0.1% (v/v) formic acid in water (solvent A) and 0.1% (v/v) formic acid in acetonitrile (solvent B). A gradient elution was performed as follows: 0–15 min, 10–45% B; 15–23 min, 45–70% B; 23–25 min, 70–100% B. The flow rate was set at 0.4 mL/min with an injection volume of 2 μL, whilst the column temperature was maintained at 40 °C.

Detection by ESI-QTOF-MS/MS was performed in positive ion mode. The source parameters were set as follows: gas temperature, 300 °C; gas flow, 8.0 L/min; nebulizer pressure, 45 psi; sheath gas temperature, 350 °C; sheath gas flow, 8.0 L/min. The scan source parameters were set as follows: VCap, 3500; nozzle voltage, 500 V; fragmentation voltage, 120 V. Reference masses were used at *m/z* 121.0508 (purine) and 922.0097 (hexakisphosphazine). Automatic MS/MS was performed using a fixed collision energy of 15 eV.

Qualitative analysis

Data were analyzed using the Agilent MassHunter Workstation Software-Qualitative Analysis software (version B.06.00, build 6.0.633.0, Agilent Technologies Inc., 2012) with the following settings: extraction restrict retention time, 2–25 min; peak height, ≥100 counts; charge state, 1; peck spacing tolerance, 0.0025 *m/z* plus

7.0 ppm; compound relative height, ≥2.5%; absolute height, ≥2000 counts; elements of C, H, O from 3 to 60, 0 to 120 and 0 to 30, respectively, for generating the formulae.

Statistical analysis

Statistical analyses and class prediction of the UPLC-MS/MS results were carried out using the Agilent MassHunter Mass Profiler Professional Software (version B.02.02, Agilent Technologies Inc., 2011). Data were initially exported from the Mass Hunter Workstation before being imported into the Mass Profiler Professional Software with the following settings: abundance filtering with minimum absolute abundance, 5000 counts; all charge states permitted; retention time (RT) correction with a maximum of 0.5% plus 0.5 min; mass window 5.0 ppm plus 2.0 mDa; compound alignment with RT window 0.1% plus 0.15 min. One-way analysis of variance (ANOVA) was used with a *P* value of 0.05 to further filter these data. A 3D principal component analysis (PCA) was conducted on all of the samples. A hierarchical cluster analysis (HCA) was also conducted with the following settings: cluster on conditions, Euclidean as the distance metric, centroid as the linkage rule. An automated sample class prediction model was built based on the UPLC-MS/MS results of the reference plants with the following settings: Naive Bayes as the class prediction algorithm; validation type, N-fold; number of folds, 3; number of repeats, 10.

SIMCA (version 13.0.3.0, Umetrics AB 2013) was used to analyze selected peaks. The peak volumes were manually imported as X-variables, with the sample number as a primary ID, peak number as a secondary ID and sample speciation as a class ID. The model type was set using orthogonal partial least squared discriminant analysis (OPLS-DA), where the significant components were calculated using an "Autofit" function.

Results and discussion

Chromatographic profiling of the reference plants

The UPLC-ESI-QTOF-MS/MS chromatograms revealed the chemical profiles of the three different *Isodon* species, and typical base peak chromatograms (BPC) of these three species are shown in Fig. 3. The chemical profiles of IL and ILG were similar, whereas the chemical profile of IS was considerably different. By comparing the samples of the different batches of IS, IL and IL, we were able to select 11, 17 and 13 common peaks for each species, respectively. One common peak (peak 5) was found in all three species. Thirteen common peaks were found in the chromatograms of IL and ILC, namely peaks 1, 2, 5, 13, 14, 19, 21, 22, 23, 24, 25, 26 and 27. The main difference between IL and ILG was that peaks 4, 16, 17 and 20 only appeared in IL. Moreover, peak 13 was absent or only detected in small quantities in ILG, but was distinct in IL; peak 14 was absent or only detected in small quantities in IL, but was distinct in ILG; peak 22 was present in much higher quantities in IL than ILG; and peak 27 was detected in higher quantities than peak 26 in IL, and vice versa in ILG. However, 10 specific peaks (peaks 3, 6, 7, 8, 9, 10, 11, 12, 15 and 18) were only detected in the chromatogram of IS.

All of the raw UPLC-MS data for the reference plants were examined using the Agilent MassHunter Mass Profiler Professional Software to further validate the differences between the three *Isodon* species. PCA was conducted, which exposed the variance between the samples by converting the numerous variables into principal components. The UPLC-MS data for the plants were imported for the calculation. Following the reduction of these data by statistical means, including ANOVA and the use of a frequency filter, three principal components were calculated. The PCA plot with principal components 1 (41.20%), 2 (22.26%) and 3 (7.42%) is shown in Fig. 4. The samples were distinctively clustered in three groups, which were correlated with the three species. The UPLC-MS features of the three species were different and these data could be used to distinguish between the three species. HCA was also used to interpret the relationships between the three different species. By comparing the detected *m/z* signals and signal intensities of the UPLC-MS data, samples were organized into clusters based on the similarity in their MS profiles. Figure 5 shows the dendrogram of hierarchical clustering, where the samples have been grouped into three branches correlating to the three species. These data highlighted the closer

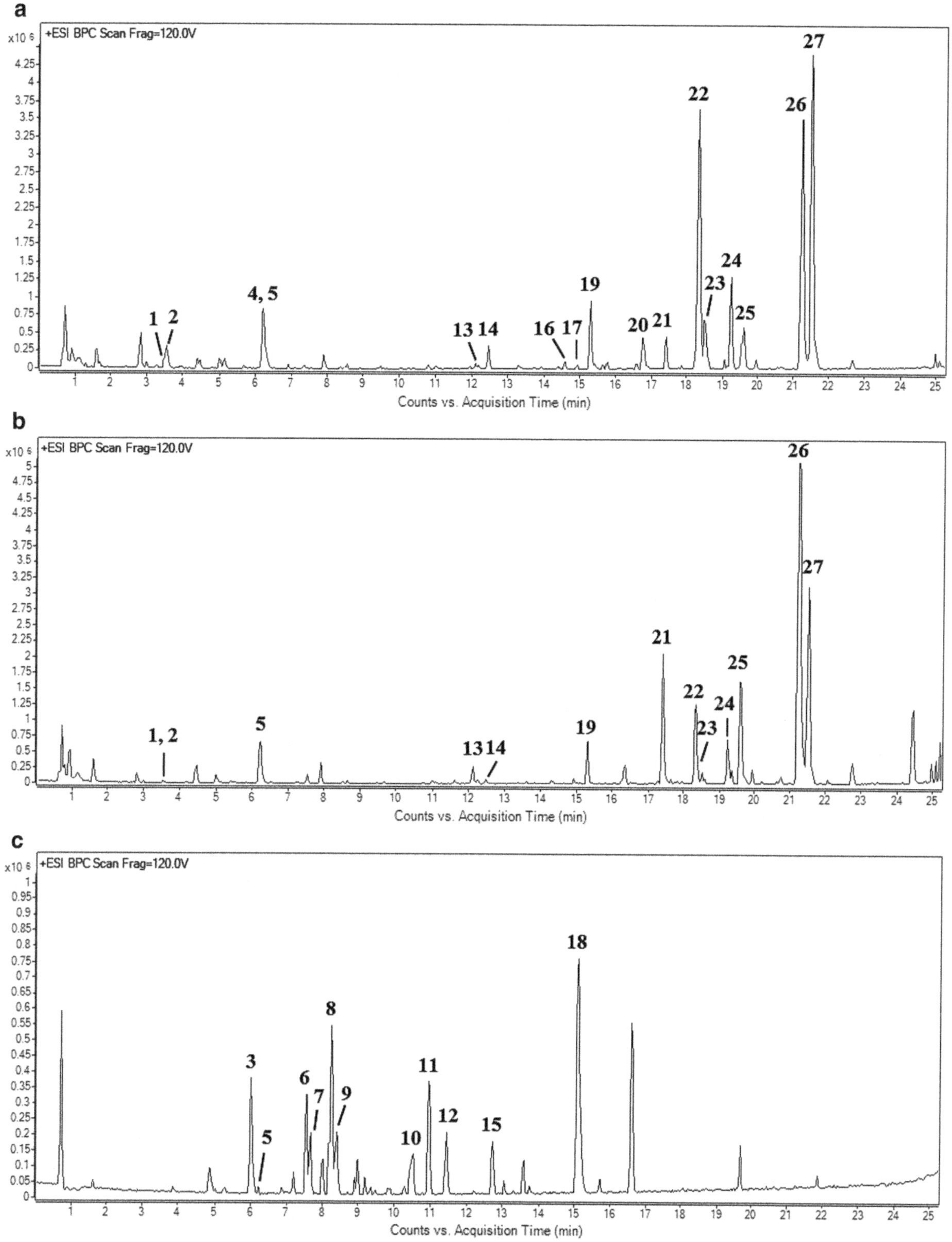

Fig. 3 Typical BPC chromatograms of **a** *I. lophanthoides*, **b** *I. lophanthoides* var. *graciliflorus* and **c** *I. serra*

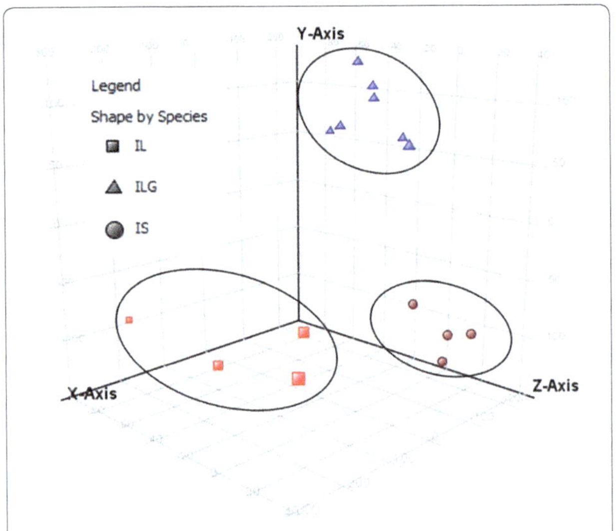

Fig. 4 3D PCA plot of the samples

relationship between IL and ILG compared with IS. The HCA results therefore supported those of the PCA, and revealed the phylogenetic relationships between the three *Isodon* species.

Twenty-seven different peaks were selected from the chromatograms of the three different species to allow for their differentiation. Furthermore, the ability of these peaks to distinguish between the different species was verified by OPLS-DA. A 3D OPLS-DA is shown in Fig. 6, where the samples were separated into three groups by species. The consistency observed between these results and those obtained using the MS data highlighted the representative nature of the selected peaks.

Peak assignments and the interpretation of MS/MS spectra

Peak assignments for the three species were conducted according to the references, standard compounds and possible fragmentation pathways. The details of the peaks identified from the three *Isodon* species are summarized in Table 3, and the structures of the identified compounds are shown in Fig. 7.

Peak 5 was common to all three species. The dominant mass ion for peak 5 had an *m/z* value of 163.0392, which was consistent with the MS data of rosmarinic acid resulted from the cleavage of its ester bond, weak *m/z* 383.0724 $[M+Na]^+$ and *m/z* 343.0814 $[M+H-H_2O]^+$ ions also found, which provided evidence that this peak could be attributed to rosmarinic acid [12, 14].

Diterpenoids are the major active compounds in *Isodon* species [15]. More than 500 diterpenoids have been isolated from plants belonging to this genus and a number of them have been reported to exhibit strong antibacterial, anti-inflammatory and anticancer activities [15]. Six *ent*-kaurane type diterpenoids were identified from IS in this study, including lasiodonin (peak 3), oridonin (peak 7), ponicidin (peak 8), lasiokaurin (peak 10), shikokianin (peak 13) and shikokianidin (peak 18) [11, 16]. Their chemical structures are shown in Fig. 7. The loss of H_2O (−18 Da) from a hydroxyl group, AcOH (−60 Da) or $CH_2{=}CO$ (−42 Da) from an acetate group, CO (−28 Da) from the D ring and CH_2O (−30 Da) from the C-20 oxygenated B ring were identified as the dominant fragmentation processes in the tandem MS/MS spectra of these compounds.

Abietane and tricyclic diterpenoids have been reported to be the major diterpenoids found in IL and ILG. Diterpenoids of this type have only ever been found in a few *Isodon* species, including *I. grandifolia* and *I. forrestii* [17]. Information pertaining to diterpenoids of this type is therefore limited. Based on the fragmentation pattern of salvialeriafone, which is a diterpenoid found in the genus *Salvia* with a similar skeletal structure to those found in IL and ILG, the proposed fragmentation of the diterpenoids was the loss of CO (−28 Da) and H_2O (−18 Da) from their C ring after the removal of their side chains or other functional groups [18]. Although more than thirty diterpenoids were isolated from IL, ILG, *I. lophanthoides* var. *gerardianus* and *I. lophanthoides* var. *micranthus* [6, 8–10, 19], none of them showed identical molecular weight and possible fragmentation pathways to the peaks in this study. However, the calculated formulae and MS/MS fragments $-C_3H_4$ (−40 Da), $-C_3H_6$ (−42 Da) and $-C_5H_8$ (−68 Da) (removal of side chain from C ring) indicated that most of the peaks could be attributed to abietane-type diterpenoids. Furthermore, two of the peaks in the chromatograms for IL and ILG were identified as glycosides schaftoside (peak 1) and isoschaftoside

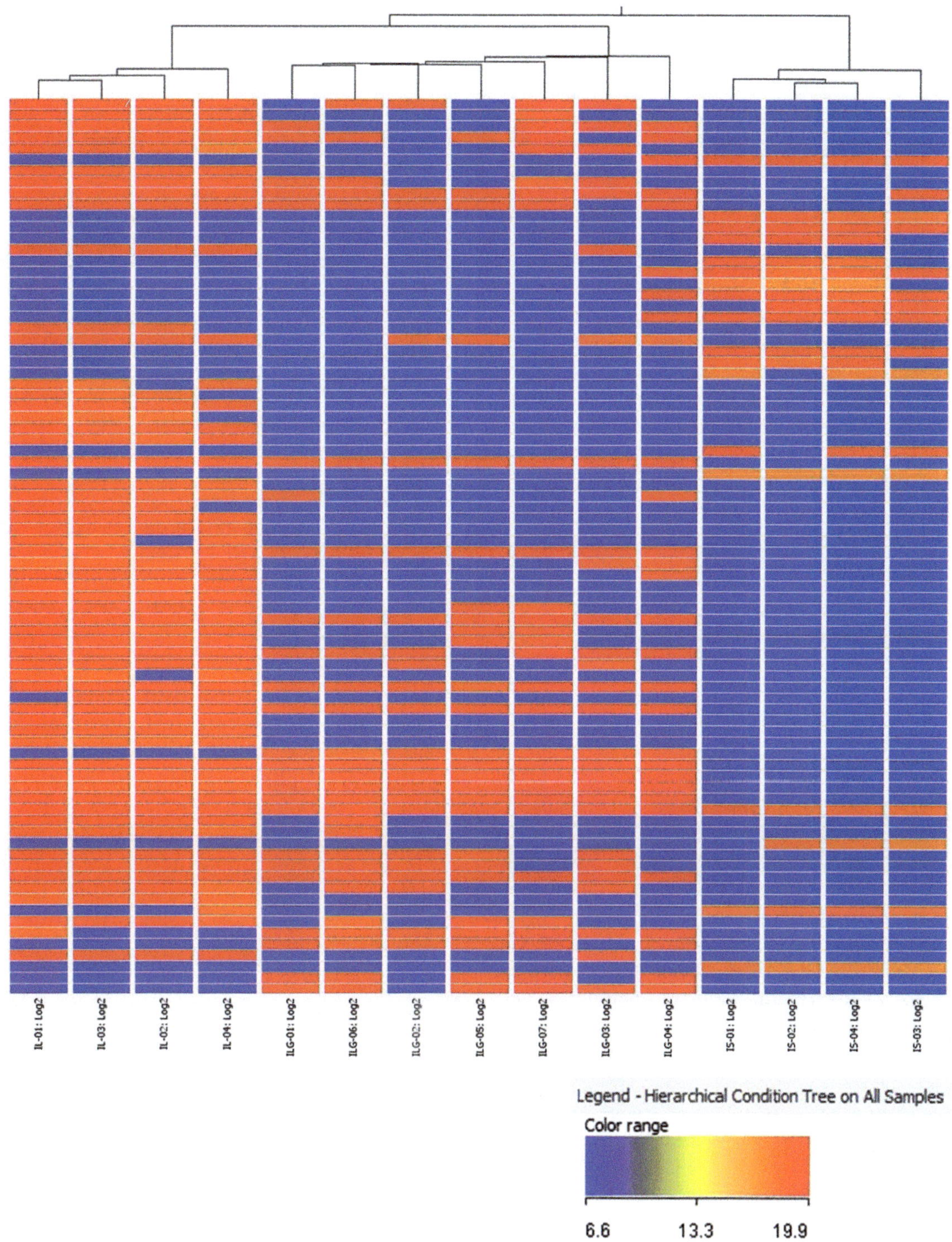

Fig. 5 Hierarchical cluster analysis heat map for the association of compounds detected in samples. Each *line* represents an *m/z* signal detected in MS, whereas the *color* indicates the log_2-transformed *m/z* signal intensities

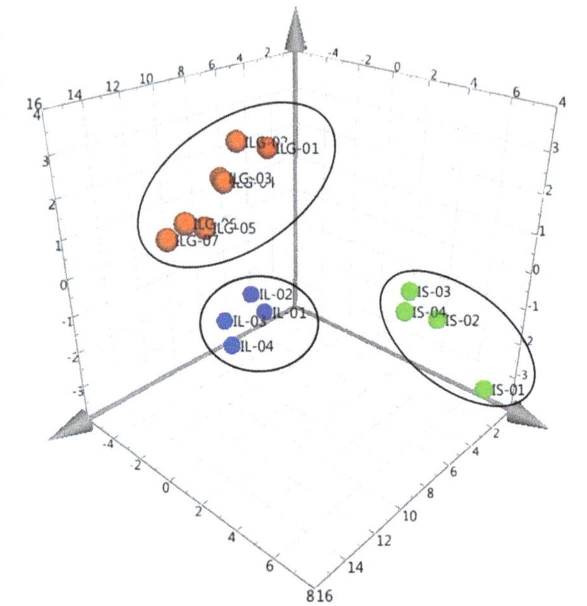

Fig. 6 The OPLS-DA plot of samples using the selected peaks

(peak 2) based on comparisons with standards and references [13, 20].

Identification of commercial samples

Based on the UPLC-MS data generated using the reference plants, we proceeded to investigate the identification of the 27 batches of commercial *Xihuangcao*. Fundamental morphologic and microscopic identification of *Xihuangcao* and several related species were done in our previous study. In terms of the morphological features of the 27 samples evaluated in this study, eight of the samples (samples 03, 04, 06, 09, 11, 14, 15, and 20) obviously did not contain plants belonging to the genus *Isodon*, which have white powders on their surface and leaves 1- or 2-pinnate (Fig. 2d). The microscopic features of these samples were also different from those of the *Isodon* species according to our preliminary studies. These samples were therefore identified as *Ampelopsis grossedentata* (Hand.-Mazz.), which is a common adulterant of *Xihuangcao* [21]. Preliminary analysis of *A. grossedentata* by UPLC-MS showed its chemical composition differed considerably from those of the *Isodon* species (Additional file 1: Figure S1), hence the UPLC-MS data for these eight batches were excluded from the automated sample class prediction.

A prediction model was initially built using the UPLC-MS data generated form the 15 reference plants. Significant signals were identified via a series of statistical calculations and filtration processes, followed by a statistical validation step, which showed the accuracy of the prediction for each class. The model was finally visualized by PCA. In this model, naive Bayesian classifier, which is a multi-class parameter-based statistical classifier, was used. The UPLC-MS data of the remaining 19 commercial samples were imported and classified using the prediction model. Twelve samples were predicted as ILG (samples 01, 02, 08, 13, 16, 19, 21, 22, 23, 24, 25 and 27), whereas six samples were predicted as IS (samples 05, 07, 10, 12, 18 and 26) with a high confidence measure of 1.000 in both cases. The only major exception was sample 17, which was predicted to be IS with a low confidence measure of 0.692. A representative prediction report is shown in Fig. 8. The UPLC-MS data for this sample was converted into three principal components and compared with those of the model. Manual identification of the samples using the 27 characteristic peaks was also conducted to further confirm the result. All of these results were consistent with those of the automated prediction, except for sample 17, which showed a low confidence measure. This sample could not be identified as one of the three *Isodon* species.

According to the species identification results, ILG was the major source of *Xihuangcao*, whereas IS was found in approximately one-quarter of the samples (22%) and IL was not used at all. *Xihuangcao* is mainly sold as a special local product in the markets for the preparation of soup or herbal tea. IS has a very bitter taste, whereas IL and ILG are only slightly bitter, which could explain why IS

Table 3 Identification information of the selected peaks

Peak no.	Retention time (min)	MS^1 m/z (relative abundance)	MS^2 m/z of the molecular ion (relative abundance)	Identity/classification	Calculated formula	Calculated mass	Mass accuracy (ppm)
1	3.47	587.1347 $[M+Na]^+$ (30), 565.1537 $[M+H]^+$ (100)	565.1522 $[M+H]^+$(59), 547.1419 $[M+H-H_2O]^+$(100), 529.1325 $[M+H-2H_2O]^+$(47), 511.1227 $[M+H-3H_2O]^+$(28), 499.1208 $[M+H-2H_2O-CH_2O]^+$(42), 493.1086 $[M+H-4H_2O]^+$(13), 481.1106 $[M+H-3H_2O-CH_2O]^+$(17), 469.1112 $[M+H-2H_2O-C_2H_4O_2]^+$(31), 457.1105 $[M+H-H_2O-C_3H_6O_3]^+$(33), 445.1118 $[M+H-5H_2O-CH_2O]^+$(40)	Schaftoside	$C_{26}H_{28}O_{14}$	564.1479	−2.66
2	3.54	587.1347 $[M+Na]^+$ (24), 565.1538 $[M+H]^+$ (100)	565.1538 $[M+H]^+$(100), 547.1428 $[M+H-H_2O]^+$(71). 529.1332 $[M+H-2H_2O]^+$(64), 511.1213$[M+H-3H_2O]^+$ (56), 499.1217 $[M+H-2H_2O-CH_2O]^+$(28), 481.1108 $[M+H-3H_2O-CH_2O]^+$(17), 445.1111 $[M+H-5H_2O-CH_2O]^+$(14), 427.1012 $[M+H-H_2O-C_4H_8O_4]^+$(86), 409.0906 $[M+H-2H_2O-C_4H_8O_4]^+$(38)	Isoschaftoside	$C_{26}H_{28}O_{14}$	564.1479	−2.48
3	5.98	387.1765 $[M+Na]^+$ (100), 365.1949 $[M+H]^+$ (70), 347.1843 $[M+H-H_2O]^+$ (35)	347.1843 $[M+H-H_2O]^+$ (100), 329.1744 $[M+H-2H_2O]^+$(46), 311.1631 $[M+H-3H_2O]^+$ (84), 299.1637 $[M+H-2H_2O-CH_2O]^+$(64), 283.1685 $[M+H-3H_2O-CO]^+$(37), 281.1524 $[M+H-3H_2O-CH_2O]^+$(61), 265.1568 $[M+H-4H_2O-CO]^+$(21), 253.1568 $[M+H-3H_2O-CH_2O-CO]^+$(14)	Lasiodonin	$C_{20}H_{28}O_6$	364.1886	−2.75
4	6.21	629.1450 $[M+Na]^+$ (2), 607.1645 $[M+H]^+$ (100)	607.1634$[M+H]^+$ (100), 589.1527 $[M+H-H_2O]^+$(54), 571.1417 $[M+H-2H_2O]^+$(35), 553.1315 $[M+H-3H_2O]^+$(29), 541.1323 $[M+H-2H_2O-CH_2O]^+$(14), 523.1222$[M+H-3H_2O-CH_2O]^+$(13), 469.1110 $[M+H-H_2O-C_4H_8O_4]^+$ (12), 427.1011 $[M+H-2H_2O-C_2H_4O_2]^+$(45), 409.0902 $[M+H-3H_2O-C_2H_4O_2]^+$ (22)	Glycoside	$C_{28}H_{30}O_{15}$	606.1584	−1.48
5	6.22	383.0724 $[M+Na]^+$ (20), 343.0805 $[M+H-H_2O]^+$ (11), 163.0385 $[M+H-C_9H_{10}O_5]^+$ (100)	163.0385 $[M+H-C_9H_{10}O_5]^+$(100), 145.0287 $[M+H-C_9H_{12}O_6]^+$(6)[a]	Rosmarinic acid	$C_{18}H_{16}O_8$	360.0845	−1.94
6	7.55	387.1765 $[M+Na]^+$ (100), 365.1950 $[M+H]^+$ (49), 347.1841 $[M+H-H_2O]^+$ (22)	347.1838 $[M+H-H_2O]^+$(16), 329.1739 $[M+H-2H_2O]^+$(30), 311.1631 $[M+H-3H_2O]^+$(100), 299.1637 $[M+H-2H_2O-CH_2O]^+$(23), 283.1680 $[M+H-3H_2O-CO]^+$(23), 281.1528 $[M+H-3H_2O-CH_2O]^+$(30)	C-20 oxygenated *ent*-kaurane diterpenoids	$C_{20}H_{28}O_6$	364.1886	−2.47
7	7.67	387.1771 $[M+Na]^+$ (100), 365.1942 $[M+H]^+$ (7), 347.1847 $[M+H-H_2O]^+$ (73)	347.1834 $[M+H-H_2O]^+$(14), 329.1740 $[M+H-2H_2O]^+$(22), 311.1630 $[M+H-3H_2O]^+$ (20), 301.1789 $[M+H-2H_2O-CO]^+$(100), 299.1630 $[M+H-2H_2O-CH_2O]^+$(23), 283.1685 $[M+H-3H_2O-CO]^+$(68), 281.1528 $[M+H-3H_2O-CH_2O]^+$(59)[a]	Oridonin	$C_{20}H_{28}O_6$	364.1886	−1.92
8	8.27	747.3332 $[2M+Na]^+$ (100), 385.1610 $[M+Na]^+$ (85), 363.1794 $[M+H]^+$ (44)	363.1788 $[M+H]^+$(18), 345.1686 $[M+H-H_2O]^+$(32), 327.1577 $[M+H-2H_2O]^+$(53), 309.1490 $[M+H-3H_2O]^+$(25), 299.1627 $[M+H-2H_2O-CO]^+$(73), 281.1529 $[M+H-2H_2O-COOH]^+$(100), 253.1569 $[M+H-2H_2O-COOH-CO]^+$(20)[a]	Ponicidin	$C_{20}H_{26}O_6$	362.1729	−1.10

Table 3 continued

Peak no.	Retention time (min)	MS^1 m/z (relative abundance)	MS^2 m/z of the molecular ion (relative abundance)	Identity/ classification	Calculated formula	Calculated mass	Mass accuracy (ppm)
9	8.39	385.1613 $[M+Na]^+$ (100), 367.1510 $[M-H_2O+Na]^+$ (11), 345.1688 $[M+H-H_2O]^+$ (52)	345.1681 $[M+H-H_2O]^+$(100), 327.1576 $[M+H-2H_2O]^+$(13), 309.1474 $[M+H-3H_2O]^+$(35), 299.1620 $[M+H-2H_2O-CO]^+$(23), 281.1530 $[M+H-2H_2O-COOH]^+$(67), 271.1678 $[M+H-2H_2O-2CO]^+$(15), 253.1559 $[M+H-2H_2O-COOH-CO]^+$(12)	*ent*-kaurane diterpenoids	$C_{20}H_{26}O_6$	362.1729	−2.21
10	10.41	429.1878 $[M+Na]^+$ (100), 407.2065 $[M+H]^+$ (23), 389.1957 $[M+H-H_2O]^+$ (3)	389.1956 $[M+H-H_2O]^+$(18), 329.1725 $[M+H-H_2O-AcOH]^+$(36), 311.1162 $[M+H-2H_2O-AcOH]^+$(13), 299.1629 $[M+H-H_2O-AcOH-CH_2O]^+$(100), 281.1529 $[M+H-2H_2O-AcOH-CH_2O]^+$(30),253.1572 $[M+H-2H_2O-AcOH-CH_2O-CO]^+$(45)	Lasiokaurin	$C_{22}H_{30}O_7$	406.1991	0.25
11	10.96	429.1875 $[M+Na]^+$ (100), 407.2058 $[M+H]^+$ (3), 389.1956 $[M+H-H_2O]^+$ (42)	371.8261 $[M+H-2H_2O]^+$(14), 343.1874 $[M+H-2H_2O-CO]^+$ (11), 329.1751 $[M+H-H_2O-AcOH]^+$(85), 311.1630 $[M+H-2H_2O-AcOH]^+$(64), 299.1615 $M+H-H_2O-AcOH-CH_2O]^+$(72), 283.1686 $[M+H-2H_2O-AcOH-CO]^+$(89), 281.1526 $[M+H-2H_2O-AcOH-CH_2O]^+$(100), 265.1580 $[M+H-3H_2O-AcOH-CO]^+$(46), 253.1576 $[M+H-2H_2O-AcOH-CH_2O-CO]^+$ (61)	C-20 oxygenated *ent*-kaurane diterpenoids	$C_{22}H_{30}O_7$	406.1991	−1.97
12	11.47	471.1983 $[M+Na]^+$ (100), 449.2159 $[M+H]^+$ (47)	389.1948 $[M+H-AcOH]^+$(12), 371.1841 $[M+H-H_2O-AcOH]^+$(21), 329.1743 $[M+H-2AcOH]^+$(22), 311.1633 $[M+H-H_2O-2AcOH]^+$(100), 293.1531 $[M+H-2H_2O-2AcOH]^+$(15), 283.1688 $[M+H-H_2O-2AcOH-CO]^+$(24), 281.1527 $[M+H-H_2O-2AcOH-CH_2O]^+$(66)	Shikokianin	$C_{24}H_{32}O_8$	448.2097	−2.45
13	12.07	353.1714 $[M+Na]^+$ (100), 313.1794 $[M+H-H_2O^{\cdot+}$ (14)	295.1669 $[M+H-2H_2O]^+$ (4), 277.1590 $[M+H-3H_2O]^+$(23), 237.1273 $[M+H-3H_2O-C_3H_4]^+$(100), 209.0948 $[M+H-3H_2O-C_5H_8]$ (17)	Abietane diterpenoids	$C_{20}H_{26}O_4$	330.1831	−2.73
14	12.45	353.1714 $[M+Na]^+$ (38). 331.1889 $[M+H]^+$ (4), 313.1798 $[M+H-H_2O^{\cdot+}$ (100)	253.1219 $[M+H-2H_2O-C_3H_6]^+$(9), 227.1056 $[M+H-2H_2O-C_5H_8]^+$(100), 212.0822$[M+H-2H_2O-C_5H_8-CH_3]^+$(14), 209.0955 $[M+H-3H_2O-C_5H_8]^+$(16), 199.1114 $M+H-2H_2O-C_5H_8-CO]^+$(21)	Abietane diterpenoids	$C_{20}H_{26}O_4$	330.1831	−2.73
15	12.73	413.1925 $[M+Na]^+$ (100), 391.2103 $[M+H]^+$ (16), 373.1998 $[M+H-H_2O^{\cdot+}$ (10)	391.2000 $[M+H]^+$(6), 373.2000 $[M+H-H_2O]^+$(50), 313.1781 $[M+H-H_2O-AcOH]^+$(66), 295.1673 $[M+H-2H_2O-AcOH]^+$(50), 283.1678 $[M+H-H_2O-AcOH-CH_2O]^+$(100), 267.1730 $[M+H-2H_2O-AcOH-CO]^+$(57), 265.1576 $[M+H-2H_2O-AcOH-CH_2O]^+$(22)	C-20 oxygenated *ent*-kaurane diterpenoids	$C_{22}H_{30}O_6$	390.2042	-2.31
16	14.53	417.2266 $[M+H]^+$ (100) 357.2056 $[M+H-AcOH]^+$ (91)	315.1940 $[M+H-AcOH-CH_2{=}CO]^+$(100), 297.1841 $[M+H-2AcOH]^+$(75), 279.1726 $[M+H-H_2O-2AcOH]^+$(26), 255.1369 $[M+H-2AcOH-C_3H_6]^+$(48), 229.1214 $[M+H-2AcOH-C_5H_8]^+$(26)	Abietane diterpenoids	$C_{24}H_{32}O_6$	416.2199	−1.44

Table 3 continued

Peak no.	Retention time (min)	MS^1 m/z (relative abundance)	MS^2 m/z of the molecular ion (relative abundance)	Identity/classification	Calculated formula	Calculated mass	Mass accuracy (ppm)
17	14.89	375.2161 $[M+H]^+$ (100), 315.1947 $[M+H-AcOH]^+$ (27)	315.1946 $[M+H-AcOH]^+$(87), 297.1846 $[M+H-H_2O-AcOH]^+$(68), 287.1998 $[M+H-AcOH-CO]^+$(22), 279.1723 $[M+H-2H_2O-AcOH]^+$(13), 273.1468 $[M+H-AcOH-C_3H_6]$(16), 255.1369 $[M+H-3H_2O-AcOH]^+$(19), 229.1220 $[M+H-H_2O-AcOH-C_5H_8]^+$(100), 205.1215 $[M+H-AcOH-C_7H_{10}O]^+$(48)	Abietane diterpenoids	$C_{22}H_{30}O_5$	374.2093	−1.34
18	15.07	513.2076 $[M+Na]^+$ (100), 508.2521 $[M+NH4]^+$ (4), 491.2253 $[M+H]^+$ (3)	431.2025 $[M+H-AcOH]^+$(8), 389.1976 $[M+H-AcOH-CH_2{=}CO]^+$(22), 371.1830 $[M+H-2AcOH]^+$(49), 329.1740 $[M+H-2AcOH-CH_2{=}CO]^+$(100), 311.1634 $[M+H-H_2O-2AcOH-CH_2{=}CO]^+$(38), 283.1708 $[M+H-H_2O-2AcOH-CH_2{=}CO-CO]^+$(29)[b]	Shikokianidin	$C_{26}H_{34}O_9$	490.2203	−3.88
19	15.28	411.1765 $[M+Na]^+$ (17), 389.1946 $[M+H]^+$ (100)	371.1847 $[M+H-H_2O]^+$(15) 311.1633$[M+H-H_2O-AcOH]^+$ (38), 269.1164 $[M+H-H_2O-AcOH-C_3H_6]^+$ (34), 243.1015 $[M+H-H_2O-AcOH-C_5H_8]^+$(100), 225.0903$[M+H-2H_2O-AcOH-C_5H_8]^+$ (11)	Abietane diterpenoids	$C_{22}H_{28}O_6$	388.1886	−3.35
20	16.78	455.2022 $[M+Na]^+$ (13), 433.2203 $[M+H]^+$ (100)	331.1889 $[M+H-AcOH-CH_2{=}CO]^+$(19), 313.1785 $[M+H-2AcOH]^+$(100), 271.1332 $[M+H-2AcOH-C_3H_6]^+$(13), 245.1164 $[M+H-2AcOH-C_5H_8]^+$(19), 219.1012$[M+H-2AcOH-C_7H_{10}]^+$(37), 205.0855$[M+H-2AcOH-C_8H_{12}]^+$ (37)	Abietane diterpenoids	$C_{24}H_{32}O_7$	432.2148	−4.16
21	17.42	353.1716 $[M+Na]^+$ (22), 331.1894 $[M+H]^+$ (100)	313.1793 $[M+H-H_2O]^+$(100), 257.1168 $[M+H-H_2O-C_4H_8]^+$(11), 243.1014 $[M+H-H_2O-C_5H_{10}]^+$(74)	Abietane diterpenoids	$C_{20}H_{26}O_4$	330.1831	−2.12
22	18.32	395.1816 $[M+Na]^+$ (26), 373.2015 $[M+H]^+$ (100), 355.1896 $[M+H-H_2O]^+$ (10)	355.1892 $[M+H-H_2O]^+$ (9), 337.1791 $[M+H-2H_2O]^+$(14), 295.1684 $[M+H-2H_2O-CH_2{=}CO]^+$(42), 277.1578 $[M+H-2H_2O-AcOH]^+$(26), 253.1219 $[M+H-2H_2O-CH_2{=}CO-C_3H_6]^+$(87), 239.1059 $[M+H-2H_2O-CH_2{=}CO-C_4H_8]^+$(34), 227.1066 $[M+H-2H_2O-CH_2{=}CO-C_5H_8]^+$(100), 211.1112 $[M+H-2H_2O-CH_2{=}CO-C_4H_8-CO]^+$(24), 209.0956 $[M+H-2H_2O-AcOH-C_5H_8]^+$(50)	Abietane diterpenoids	$C_{22}H_{28}O_5$	372.1937	1.34
23	18.52	381.2025 $[M+Na]^+$ (100), 359.2210 $[M+H]^+$ (20)	299.1999 $[M+H-AcOH]^+$(100), 271.1680 $[M+H-AcOH-C_2H_4]^+$(25)	Diterpenoids	$C_{22}H_{30}O_4$	358.2144	−1.95
24	19.23	435.1745 $[M+2Na]^+$ (7), 413.1926 $[M+Na]^+$ (100), 373.2005 $[M+H-H_2O]^+$ (8), 313.1793 $[M+H-H_2O-AcOH]^+$ (10)	355.1857 $[M+H-2H_2O]^+$(7), 313.1798 $[M+H-H_2O-AcOH]^+$(93), 295.1678 $[M+H-2H_2O-AcOH]^+$(25), 285.1827 $[M+H-H_2O-CO]^+$(9), 280.1427 $[M+H-2H_2O-AcOH-CH_3]^-$(13), 271.1673 $[M+H-H_2O-AcOH-CH_2{=}CO]^+$(61), 253.1232 $[M+H-2H_2O-AcOH-C_3H_6]^+$(44), 243.1749 (13), 227.1038 $[M+H-2H_2O-AcOH-C_5H_8]^+$(17)[a]	Abietane diterpenoids	$C_{22}H_{30}O_6$	390.2042	−2.05
25	19.61	647.3333 $[2M+Na]^+$ (100), 335.1610 $[M+Na]^+$ (94), 313.1794 $[M+H]^+$ (17)	295.1685 $[M+H-H_2O]^+$(13), 277.1583 $[M+H-2H_2O]^+$(43), 237.1271 $[M+H-2H_2O-C_3H_4]^+$(100), 227.1062$[M+H-H_2O-C_5H_8]^+$ (25), 209.0953 $[M+H-2H_2O-C_5H_8]^+$(15)	Abietane diterpenoids	$C_{20}H_{24}O_3$	312.1725	−1.28

Table 3 continued

Peak no.	Retention time (min)	MS¹ m/z (relative abundance)	MS² m/z of the molecular ion (relative abundance)	Identity/classification	Calculated formula	Calculated mass	Mass accuracy (ppm)
26	21.22	337.1765 $[M+Na]^+$ (40), 315.1950 $[M+H]^+$ (2), 297.1856 $[M+H-H_2O]^+$ (100)	297.1843 $[M+H-H_2O]^+$(17), 279.1736 $[M+H-2H_2O]^+$ (10), 227.1061 $[M+H-H_2O-C_5H_{10}]^+$(100), 212.0830 $[M+H-H_2O-C_5H_{10}-CH_3]^+$(18), 199.1117 $[M+H-H_2O-C_5H_{10}-CO]^+$(19)	Diterpenoids	$C_{20}H_{26}O_3$	314.1882	−1.59
27	21.5	455.2033 $[M+Na]^+$ (100), 450.2478 $[M+NH4]^+$ (8)	373.1997 $[M+H-AcOH]^+$ (8), 313.1788 $[M+H-2AcOH]^+$(100), 295.1682 $[M+H-H_2O-2AcOH]^+$(31), 253.1201 $[M+H-H_2O-2AcOH-C_3H_6]^+$ (4)[b]	Abietane diterpenoids	$C_{24}H_{32}O_7$	432.2148	−1.62

[a] Tandem MS/MS spectra of the $[M+H-H_2O]^+$ was listed as the amount of $[M+H]^+$ ion is too low

[b] Tandem MS/MS spectra of the $[M+NH4]^+$ was listed as the amount of $[M+H]^+$ ion is too low

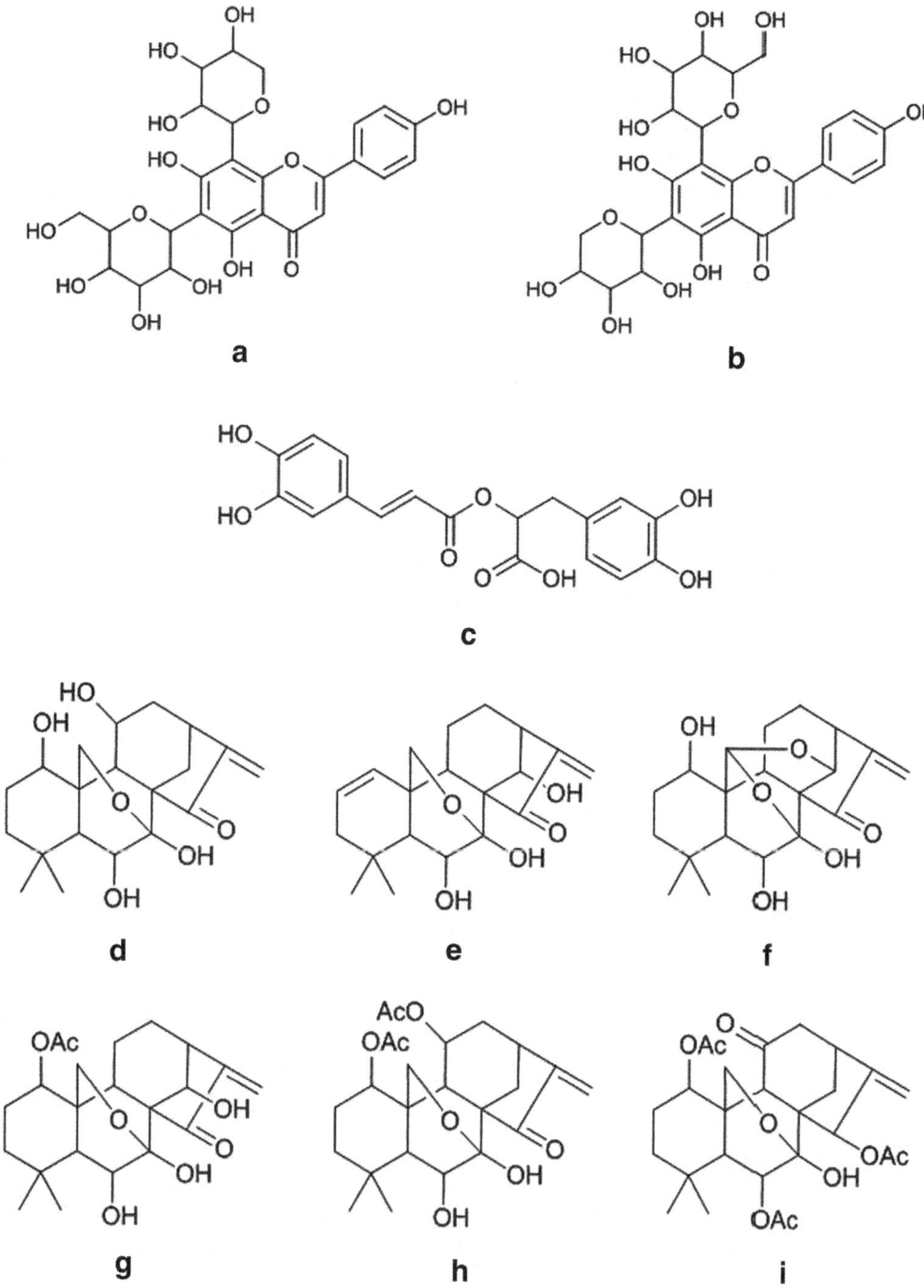

Fig. 7 Chemical structures of the identified compounds. **a** Schaftoside; **b** Isoschaftoside; **c** Rosmarinic acid; **d** Lasiodonin; **e** Oridonin; **f** Ponicidin; **g** Lasiokaurin; **h** Shikokianin; **i** Shikokianidin

was found in small quantities in the *Xihuangcao* samples in this market investigation. IL is an annual or short-lived perennial herb, whereas its variety ILG is an undershrub capable of reaching more than 1 m in height [3]. ILG is therefore more desirable for cultivation in terms of its production yield. The large proportion of adulterant (44%) found in this study also raises concerns about the quality of the *Xihuangcao* being sold in retail markets.

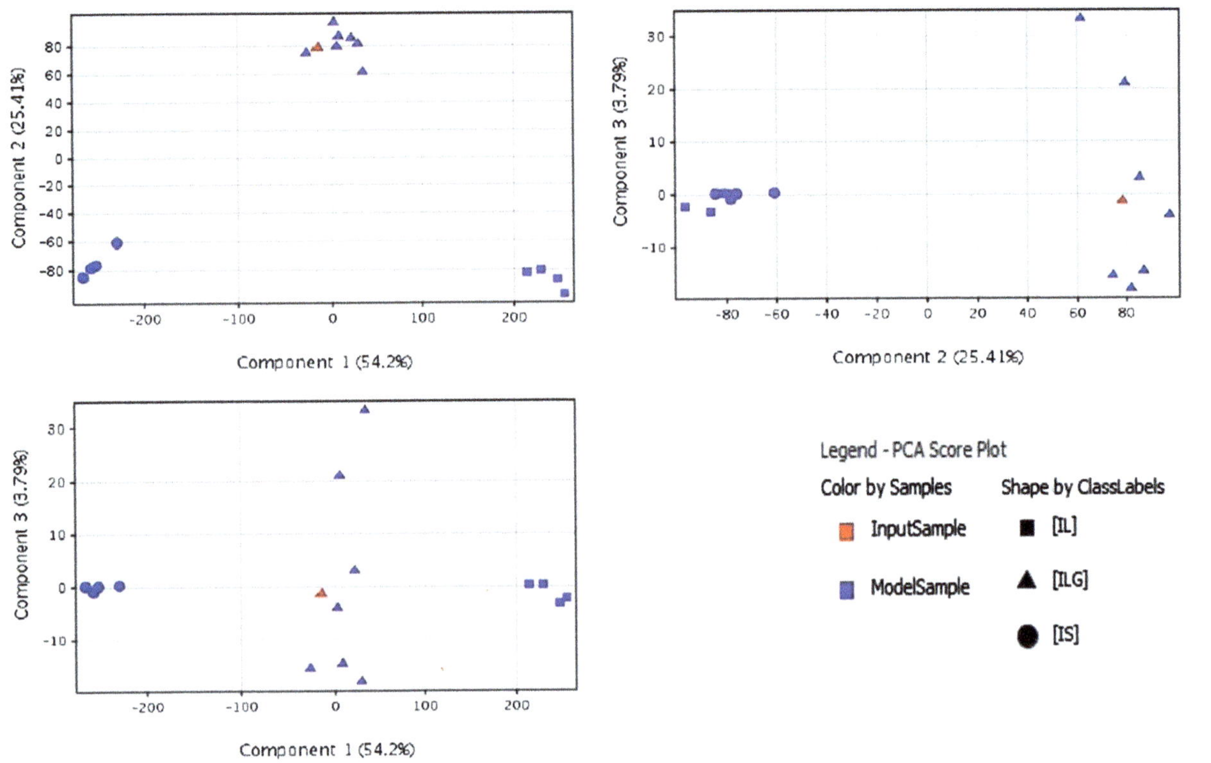

Fig. 8 Prediction report of sample 02

Conclusion

UPLC-ESI-QTOF-MS and subsequent chemometrics analysis were demonstrated effective to differentiate among the three different species of plants used as *Xihuangcao*.

Abbreviations

BPC: base peak chromatogram; HCA: hierarchical cluster analysis; IL: *Isodon lophanthoides*; ILG: *Isodon lophanthoides* var. *graciliflorus*; IS: *Isodon serra*; MS: mass spectrometry; ANOVA: one-way analysis of variance; OPLS-DA: orthogonal partial least squared discriminant analysis; PCA: principal component analysis; UPLC: ultra-performance liquid chromatography; UPLC-ESI-QTOF-MS: ultra-performance liquid chromatography coupled with electrospray ionization quadrupole time-of-flight mass spectrometry.

Authors' contributions

HBC and ZZZ conceived the study. LLW and ZTL designed the study. LLW, ZTL collected the plant materials and samples. LLW conducted the sample preparation, UPLC analysis, and analyzed the data. LLW, ZTL wrote the manuscript. ZTL revised the manuscript. All authors read and approved the final manuscript.

Author details

[1] School of Chinese Medicine, Hong Kong Baptist University, Kowloon, Hong Kong Special Administrative Region, People's Republic of China. [2] Research Center for Pharmacognosy, Institute of Chinese Materia Medica, Academy of Chinese Medical Sciences, Beijing, People's Republic of China.

Acknowledgements

We would like to thank Ms. Qiaohua Deng and Mr. Weiliang Zhang form Hutchison Whampoa Guangzhou Baiyunshan Chinese Medicine Company Limited for the help in the collection of reference plants, also Mr. Alan Ho from the School of Chinese Medicine, Hong Kong Baptist University for his kind technical support.

Competing interests

The authors declare that they have no competing interests.

References

1. Wu JF. Literature review of *Xihuangcao*. Shi Zhen Guo Yi Guo Yao. 2003;14(8):498–500.
2. Guangdong Food and Drug Administration. Guangdong Chinese Materia Medica Standards, vol. 2. Guangdong: Guangdong Science & Technology Press; 2011. p. 347–53.
3. Suddee S, Paton AJ, Parnell JAN. A taxonomic revision of tribe *Ocimeae* Dumorts. (Lamiaceae) in continental South East Asia. Kew Bull. 2004;59(3):379–414.

4. Fu L, Deng QH, Ceng FY, Yr YS. Research of the name of Chinese medicine Xihuangcao. Zhong Yao Cai. 2012;35(3):493–5.
5. Chen JN, Jiang DX, Zhao AG, Lai XP. Microscopic identification of medicinal material of Herba Rabdosiae Serrae. Guang Zhou Zhong Yi Yao Da Xue Xue Bao. 2006;23:52–5.
6. Zhang Q, Pan CM. The comparative studies on the morphology of *I. serra*, *I. lophanthoides*, *I. lophanthoides* var. *geradiana* and *I. lophanthoides* var. *graciliflorus*. Pharm Today. 2012;22(1):21–4.
7. Liang YG, Xie HH, Wu P, Jiang YM, Wei XY. Podocarpane, isopimarane, and abietane diterpenoids from *Isodon lophanthoides* var. *graciliflorus*. Food Chem. 2013;136:1177–82.
8. Yang LB, Li L, Huang SX, Pu JX, Zhao Y, Ma YB, Chen JJ, Leung CH, Tao ZM, Sun HD. Anti-hepatitis B virus and cytotoxic diterpenoids from *Isodonlophanthoides* var. *gerardianus*. Chem Pharm Bull (Tokyo). 2011;59(9):1102–5.
9. Zhao AH, Li SH, Li YW, Huan QB, Zhao QS, Lin ZW, Sun HD. Two New Abietane Quinones from *Isodon lophanthoides* var *micranthus*. Chin Chem Lett. 2003;14(6):591–3.
10. Zhou W, Xie H, Wu P, Wei X. Abietane diterpenoids from *Isodon lophanthoides* var. *graciliflorus* and their cytotoxicity. Food Chem. 2013;136:1110–6.
11. Liu PW, Du TF, Zhang XW, Sheng XN, Shi XW, Zhai CC, Zhu H, Wang N, Zhang LT. Rapid analysis of 27 components of *Isodon Serra* by LC-ESI-MS-MS. Chromatographia. 2010;72:265–73.
12. Flora of China: TaxonId 210000832—*Isodon serra*. Beijing: Flora of China Editorial Board. 2013. http://foc.eflora.cn/content.aspx?TaxonId=210000832. Accessed 12 Jun 2014.
13. Kuang YH, Liang S, Yao XH, Huang L, Lin Q. Determination of isoschaftoside, schaftoside and romarinic acid in *Isodon lophanthoides* var. *gracili-flora* by HPLC. Zhong Cheng Yao. 2013;35(3):570–3.
14. MassBank Record: PR040220—Rosmarinic acid. Tokyo: MassBank Project. 2014. http://www.massbank.jp/jsp/Dispatcher.jsp?type=disp&id=PR040220&site=1. Accessed 12 Jun 2014.
15. Sun HD, Huang SX, Han QB. Diterpenoids from *Isodon* species and their biological activities. Nat Prod Rep. 2006;23:673–98.
16. Sun HD, Xu YL, Jiang B. Diterpenoids from *Isodon* species. Beijing: Science Publishing House; 2001. p. 245.
17. Zhang L, Zhou GX, Li Q, Dai Y, Ye WC, Yao XS. Chemical constituents of *Isodon lophanthoides* (Buch. –Ham. ex D. Don) Hara var. *gerandianus* (Benth.) Hara. Shen Yang Yao Ke Da Xue Xue Bao. 2006;23(12):768–70.
18. Musharraf SG, Goher M, Hussain A, Choudhary ML. Electrospray tandem mass spectrometric analysis of a dimeric conjugate, salvialeriafone and related compounds. Chem Cent J. 2012;6:120.
19. Sun HD, Xu YL, Jiang B. Diterpenoids from *Isodon* species. Beijing: Science Publishing House; 2001. p. 119.
20. Colombo R, Yariwake JH, McCullaghb M. Study of C- and O-glycosylflavones in sugarcane extracts using liquid chromatography—exact mass measurement mass spectrometry. J Braz Chem Soc. 2008;19(3):483–90.
21. Deng QH. Study on distribution and development of Herba Isodonis Lophanthoidis. Jin Ri Yao Xue. 2009;19(9):21–5.

18

An investigation of fungal contamination on the surface of medicinal herbs in China

Run-sheng Zheng[1,2†], Wen-li Wang[1,2†], Jing Tan[1,2], Hui Xu[1,2*], Ruo-ting Zhan[1,2] and Wei-wen Chen[1,2]

Abstract

Background: The dried parts of medicinal herbs are susceptible to the infection of fungi during pre- or post-harvest procedure. This study aimed to investigate the presence of fungi and their metabolites mycotoxins on the surface of medicinal herbs collected from China.

Methods: Forty-five retail samples of 15 different medicinal herbs were collected from 3 different regions in China. Then the potential fungi were immediately washed off from the surface of each sample with 0.1% Tween-20 followed by incubation of the rinse on petri-dish with potato dextrose agar containing chloramphenicol at 28 °C. The obtained fungi were isolated as single colonies and then characterized by morphology and molecular identification using internal transcribed spacer (ITS) sequencing with extracted DNA. Meanwhile, the mycotoxin-producing potential of the isolates was studied by liquid chromatography-tandem mass spectrometry (LC-MS/MS).

Results: A total of 126 fungi were identified from the surface of samples by morphology and ITS sequencing, with *Aspergillus* and *Penicillium* genera as the predominant contaminants. The mycotoxin-producing potential analysis showed that 6 of 8 *A. versicolor* isolates could produce sterigmatocystin. All 3 *A. aculeatus* isolates produced ochratoxin A, but only 1 of 3 *A. flavus* strains produced aflatoxins B_1 and B_2 without G_1 and G_2. Although the sample contamination ratios were high (≥95.6%), there was no significant difference ($\chi^2 = 1.05$, $P = 1.0$) among the samples from 3 regions, which demonstrates the prevalent fungal contamination in the herbal medicines.

Conclusion: The prevalent contamination phenomenon of fungi and high potential risk of sterigmatocystin and ochratoxin A were observed in 45 medicinal herbs collected from China.

Background

With the popular and extensive use of medicinal herbs all over the world, safety issues related to the contamination with microbial organisms has become a major concern [1–4]. Most of fungi are toxigenic in nature, and some other non-toxigenic species may impart a mouldy odour and taste [5]. In the pre-harvest stage, medicinal herbs are susceptible to indigenous fungi in the soil where they were grown. The dried part of medicinal herbs may be exposed to fungal contamination during post-harvest. Different taxonomic groups of fungi were detected in medicinal plant samples collected from different regions, suggesting *Aspergillus* and *Penicillium* groups as the most predominant genera [6–8]. Many species of *Aspergillus* and *Penicillium* genera are known mycotoxin-producers, which may pose a great threat to public health [5].

Mycotoxigenic fungi could produce a wide variety of mycotoxins. Aflatoxins (B_1, B_2, G_1, and G_2) are a family of structurally related toxic secondary metabolites which mainly produced by certain strains of *Aspergillus flavus* (*A. flavus*) and *Aspergillus Parasiticus* (*A. parasiticus*) [9, 10]. Aflatoxin B_1 (AFB_1) was classified as a Group I carcinogen by the World Health Organization for Research on Cancer in 1993 [11]. Sterigmatocystin (ST), the stable intermediate in the final steps of aflatoxin biosynthesis

*Correspondence: zyfxsherry@gzucm.edu.cn
†Run-sheng Zheng and Wen-li Wang contributed equally to this work
[1] Research Centre of Chinese Herbal Resource Science and Engineering, Guangzhou University of Chinese Medicine, Guangzhou, China
Full list of author information is available at the end of the article

in the aflatoxin-producing fungi *A. flavus* and *A. parasiticus*, was proven to be another carcinogenic mycotoxin [12]. Some certain stains, e.g., *A. versicolor, A. sydowi, A. nidulans, Bipolaris, Chaetomium* and *Emericella* spp. could also produce ST [13–16]. Produced by *P. verrucosum, P. nordicum* and *A. carbonarius* [17–19], another mycotoxin ochratoxin A (OTA) could cause a series of adverse effects in animals and humans, including teratogenicity, immunotoxicity, genotoxicity and mutagenicity [20–22].

This study aimed to investigate the presence of fungi on the surface of 45 medicinal herbs samples of fifteen herbs collected from Hunan, Hubei and Guangxi Province, China, by the characterization of morphology and ITS sequencing, followed by analysis of mycotoxigenic potential of isolated fungi using LC-MS/MS for the measurement of AFB_1, AFB_2, AFG_1, AFG_2, ST and OTA.

Methods

Chemicals and reagents

Standard solutions of AFB_1, AFB_2, AFG_1 and AFG_2, and OTA and ST powder standards were purchased from Supelco Sigma-Aldrich (St Louis, MO, USA). Potato dextrose agar (PDA) with chloramphenicol (0.1 g/L) was obtained from Huan-Kai (Guangzhou, China). LC-grade acetonitrile and methanol were bought from Merck (Darmstadt, Germany). Ultra-pure water was obtained from a Millipore Q system (Millipore, France). The other reagents were of analytical grade and bought from local producers.

Samples collection

Fifteen kinds of most commonly-used medicinal herbs (Table 1) were chosen for analysis. During July and August of 2010, about 30 g of each kind of medicinal herb were purchased from a random herbal medicine store in Hunan, Hubei and Guangxi province (China), respectively. The herbs were authenticated by an experienced pharmacist for traditional Chinese medicine according to Chinese Pharmacopeia [23]. Each sample was instantly put into a sterile polythene bag, sealed properly, shipped to the laboratory and stored at 4 °C prior to use. The detail information of each sample was given as Additional file 1: Table S1. The samples were processed as soon as possible to avoid second contamination.

Isolation of the fungi

Five grams of each sample (2.5 g was used for flower samples) was mixed with 30 mL 0.1% Tween-20 and vortexed (Vortex-5, Qilinbeier, China) for 3 min. Then the mixture was filtrated through a disposable syringe with sterile cotton and the filtrate was centrifuged (3-18 K, Satorius, Germany) at 2600×*g* for 10 min. After dissolving the pellet in 300 μL sterile 40% glycerol, serial decimal dilutions were performed. For incubation, 100 μL aliquots of each dilution were plated in duplicate onto PDA containing chloramphenicol (0.1 g/L), which were cultured at 28 °C for 7–10 days. Meanwhile, a sample without medicinal herbs was prepared in parallel and used as the negative control. The fungal colonies were then transferred to fresh PDA plates to obtain pure cultures, with 0.1% Tween-20 as negative control.

Morphological observation

The purified isolates were cultured with 1 or 3 point inoculations for 7 days on PDA at 28 °C. When the colony characteristics and pigment production were noted, the conidia and conidial head were observed microscopically (Smart, Optec, China) for morphological identification by lactophenol cotton blue stain. Taxonomic identification results were classified based on Manual of fungal Identification into Aspergillus, Penicillium and Fusicladium *etc* [24–27].

Molecular identification by ITS primers

After the pure isolates were grown on PDA at 28 °C for 7 days, the mycelia were harvested. DNA extraction was performed using the Lysis Buffer for Microorganism to Direct PCR kit (Takara, Dalian, China) according to the manufacturer's instructions. Fungal mycelium was added to 50 μL lysis buffer and incubated at 80 °C for 15 min. After centrifugation, the supernatant was collected and used as the polymerase chain reaction (PCR) template. Positive control was performed with the standard strain *Aspergillus flavus* NRRL3357.

PCR amplification was performed in a 50 μL reaction prepared by mixing 25 μL 2× Power *Pfu* PCR Mixture (Bioteke, Beijing, China), 2.5 μL oligonucleotide primers (10 μmol/L) and 5 μL DNA template. Two pairs of primers (Table 2) were used to amplify ITS1, 5.8S and ITS2 in rDNA regions. The novel primers of Wen1-F and Wen1-R were designed according to the ITS sequences of *Penicillium expansu* (AJ005676.1) and *P. janthinellum* (GU565108.1). The amplification program was as follows: pre-denaturation at 95 °C for 5 min; 35 cycles of 30 s at 95 °C, 30 s at 55 °C and 1 min at 72 °C; and final extension at 72 °C for 10 min. The sequence analysis was performed at Huada Co. Ltd. (Guangzhou, China) and the sequencing results were analysed with the BLAST program of the National Centre for Biotechnology Information (NCBI) by searching NCBI nucleotide database (RRID:SCR_004860) for identification of the genus and species of the isolates.

Table 1 Number of different fungal species isolated from different medicinal herbs

Name of Samples	No. of samples	Fungal species[a]									
		A. flavus	*A. versicolor*	*A. aculeatus*	Other *Asper-gillus* spp.	*Euro-tium* spp.	*Penic-illium* spp.	*Clados-porium* spp	*Fusa-rium* spp.	Others	Total
Bulbus *Fritillariae cir-rhosae*	3	–[b]	–	–	–	1	2	–	–	1	4
Cortex *Eucommiae*	3	–	–	–	–	–	2	–	–	1	3
Cortex *Magnoliae officinalis*	3	–	–	–	0	1	–	–	–	1	2
Flos *Carthami*	3	2	–	–	2	1	2	–	–	6	13
Flos *Lonicerae japoni-cae*	3	–	–	–	–	1	2	–	–	0	3
Fructus *Lycii*	3	1	1	–	1	–	–	–	–	4	7
Herba *Andrographis*	3	–	1	–	3	4	5	2	–	3	18
Radix *Angelicae sinensis*	3	–	–	1	1	1	3	–	1	–	7
Radix *Astragali*	3	–	–	–	3	–	2	3	–	4	12
Radix *Codcnopsitis Pilosulas*	3	–	–	1	–	–	5	–	1	1	8
Radix *et* Rhizoma *Glycyrrhizae*	3	–	2	1	2	–	2	1	1	6	15
Radix *Notoginseng*	3	–	1	–	1	–	2	–	–	2	6
Radix *Panacis quinque-folii*	3	–	–	–	–	–	3	2	–	6	11
Radix *Pseudostellariae*	3	–	1	–	–	–	3	1	–	–	5
Semen *Armeniacae amarae*	3	–	2	–	2	5	2	1	–	–	12
Total	45	3	8	3	14	14	35	10	3	36	126

[a] The strains were deposited in Research Centre of Chinese Herbal Resource Science and Engineering, Guangzhou University of Chinese Medicine, Guangzhou, China

[b] Not found

Table 2 Oligonucleotide primers used for molecular identification

Primer name	Primer sequence	Amplification product (bp)	Annotation	Gene targeted
Wen1-F	5′-TCCAACCTCCCACCCGTGTTTA-3′	400	This study	ITS1-5.8S-ITS2
Wen1-R	5′-AAGCCCCTACGCTCGAGGA-3′			
ITS1	5′-TCCGTAGGTGAACCTGCG-3′	500 ~ 700	[32]	
ITS4	5′-TCCTCCGCTTATTGATATGC-3′			

Mycotoxin-producing potential analysis

The assay was to aim to determine AFB_1, AFB_2, AFG_1, AFG_2, OTA and ST. Therefore, only the potential producer,according to literatures, were screened and the other 16 strains were excluded. Among the total isolates obtained from the samples, 110 strains potentially producing 6 mycotoxins were grown in Sabouraud dextrose medium (SD) at 28 °C for 10 days. Then 5 mL the culture broth was extracted with ethyl acetate followed by dichloromethane [28] and the organic layers were combined and then evaporated to dryness. After that, the residues were dissolved in 1.5 mL ethanol and injected into liquid chromatography-tandem mass spectrometry (LC–MS/MS) for determination of AFB_1, AFB_2, AFG_1, AFG_2, OTA and ST. Meanwhile, the standard strain *Aspergillus flavus* NRRL3357 were used as positive control.

Liquid chromatography separation of 10 μL sample was performed on a Hypersil GOLD C_{18} (100 × 2.1 mm, 3 μm) column. The mobile phase consisted of (A) water containing 4 m mol/L NH_4Ac–0.1% HCOOH and (B) methanol and the flow rate was 300 μL/min. A gradient elution program was applied: 0–10 min, 20–85% B; 10–15 min, 85–100% B; 15–20 min, 100% B. The mass spectrometer was operated in the ESI^+ mode using selective reaction monitoring (SRM). High-purity nitrogen was used as the drying and ionisation gas. Argon was used as the collision gas for collision-induced dissociation. The capillary voltage was set at 3.50 kV and the capillary temperature was 350 °C. The SRM transitions used to detect mycotoxins were listed in Table 3 and chromatograms of 6 mycotoxins in standard solution and representative samples were showed in the Fig. 1.

Statistical analysis

Software RStudio (R version 3.2.2) [29] was used for the data analysis, where the comparison of fungal contamination ratios was performed by Pearson's Chi squared test with simulated *P* value (based on 2000 replicates).

Results and discussion

Fungal contamination

The association between fungal species and herbal medicines is not fully understood due to the complicated contamination causes including extrinsic (environmental and geographical) and intrinsic (constituents of each herbal species) factors [30, 31]. Forty-five samples of 15 common medicinal herbs were investigated in this study to reveal the main contaminating fungi and provide some relevant references for quality control on medicinal herbs in China.

In this study, morphological analysis as well as molecular identification using ITS sequencing were applied to analyse fungal diversity. As not all the strains could be amplified by the primer pair ITS1/ITS4 [32], a novel primer pairs Wen1F/Wen1R were designed for the ITS regions of the fungi by Primer-BLAST of NCBI (Table 2). A total of 126 isolated strains were successfully amplified. It is notable that the primers of Wen1F/Wen1R tended to be biased towards the amplification of *Aspergillus* and *Penicillium*, which agreed with the view on the potential primers bias during PCR in fungal diversity exploring [33].

As a result, 126 strains were isolated (Table 1) illustrating the two main genera identified were *Aspergillus* (28 isolates) and *Penicillium* (35 isolates). Among

Table 3 The ESI-MS/MS parameters, retention time, SRM transitions and LOD for 6 mycotoxins

Mycotoxin	RT (min)	Precursor ion (m/z)	Product ions (m/z)	Collision energy (eV)	LOD (ng/L)
Aflatoxin B_1	10.20	313 $[M+H]^+$	285/241	23/37	5.20
Aflatoxin B_2	9.82	315 $[M+H]^+$	287/259	27/31	6.30
Aflatoxin G_1	9.41	329 $[M+H]^+$	243/200	27/45	10.60
Aflatoxin G_2	8.96	331 $[M+H]^+$	313/245	26/30	5.80
Ochratoxin A	13.22	404 $[M+H]^+$	239/358	25/15	25.00
Sterigmatocystin	13.44	325 $[M+H]^+$	281/310	36/25	1.56

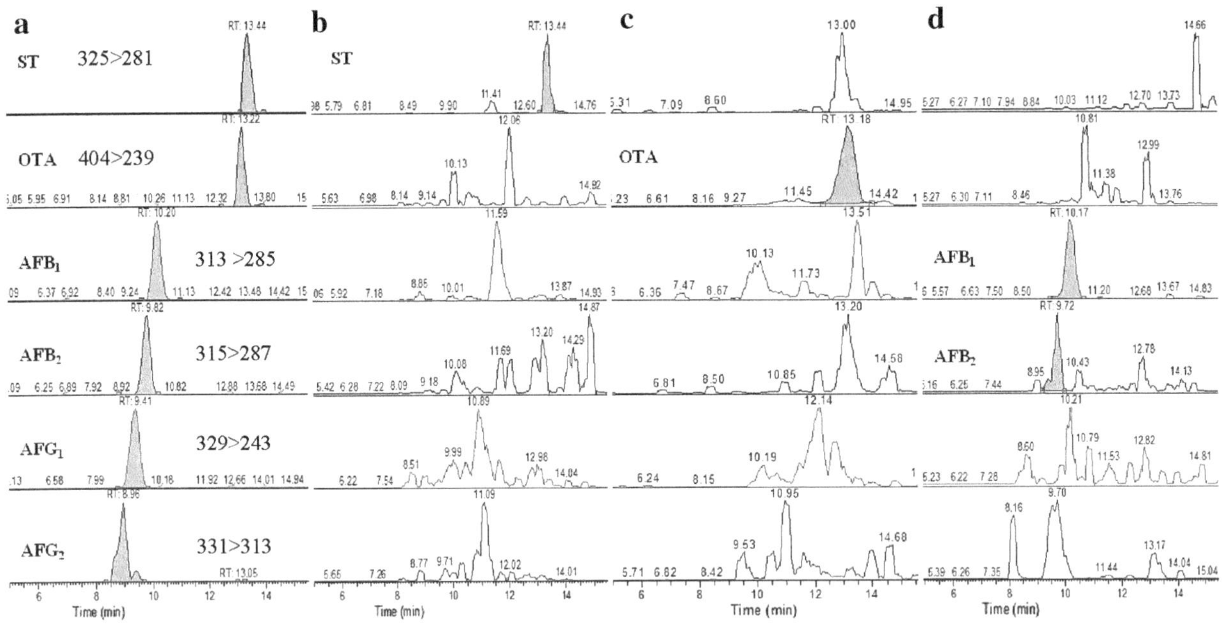

Fig. 1 SRM Chromatograms of 6 mycotoxins in standard solution (**a**), *A. versicolor* isolated from Herba *Andrographis* (**b**), *A. aculeatus* isolated from Radix *Angelicae sinensis* (**c**) and *A. flavus* isolated from *Fructus lycii* (**d**)

of 28 *Aspergillus* recovered, *A. versicolor* (8 strains) was the dominant species, followed by the *A. fumigatus* (4 strains), *A. aculeatus* (3 strains) and *A. flavus* (3 strains). Other members of the *Aspergillus* group were detected at lower level. The colonies and microscopic morphologies of *A. flavus, A. aculeatus* and *A. versicolor* isolated from Fructus *Lycii*, Radix *Angelicae Sinensis* and Radix *et* Rhizoma *Glycyrrhizae*, respectively, were shown in Fig. 2.

Although the average of fungal contamination ratio (95.6%) are extremely high in 45 samples collected from 3 places (93.3, 93.3, 100% for samples from Hubei, Hunan and Guangxi, respectively), Pearson's Chi squared test indicated there is no significant difference among 3 groups by $P = 1.0$. This further proved the prevalent fungal contamination phenomenon across the collected herbal medicine and should rise our attention.

Overall, the observation of *Aspergillus* and *Penicillium* spp. as the most frequently contaminant was consistent with previous reports. Efuntoye [30] found that *A. niger, A. flavus, F. moniliforme, Trichoderma viride, P. expansum* and *Mucor fragilis* were the dominant species in sundried herbs. Roy et al. [34] reported that 52% of 152 samples were contaminated with species from the *Aspergillus* genus, while Halt [35] found that the most predominant fungi detected in 62 samples of medicinal plant material and 11 herbal tea samples were *Aspergillus* and *Penicillium*.

In comparison, fungi from other genera including *Eurotium, Cladosporium* was detected at a low incidence in this study, which was also consistent with the study from Song et al. [3]. *Cladosporium* spp. is the common and widespread fungi on land and in air [36, 37]. Although there are no publications regarding its ability of producing toxin, they do produce odours likely relating to some volatile organic compounds.

Mycotoxigenic potentials of the fungal isolates

As documented in Table 3, the LC-MS/MS method showed an outstanding sensitive, with the limit of detection (LOD) from 1.56 to 25.00 ng/L determined in 3 times of the ratio of signal to noise (S/N). The data on the mycotoxin-producing potentials of the fungal isolates were presented in Table 4. Of the 3 *A. flavus* isolates, only 1 strain from Fructus *Lycii* produced AFB_1 and AFB_2 but not AFG_1 and AFG_2. The inability of the other 2 strains to produce aflatoxins might be a result of some mutation in the biosynthetic gene cluster of aflatoxins [38].

Another mycotoxin ST, which was overlooked in many reports except a study of mycotoxins screening in medicinal herbs [39], presented in 6 of the 8 *A. versicolor* isolates by the analysis of LC-MS/MS. To evaluate human exposure to this mycotoxin and more importantly, monitor medicinal herbs for existing or future legal compliance, suitable and simple analytical procedures are necessary

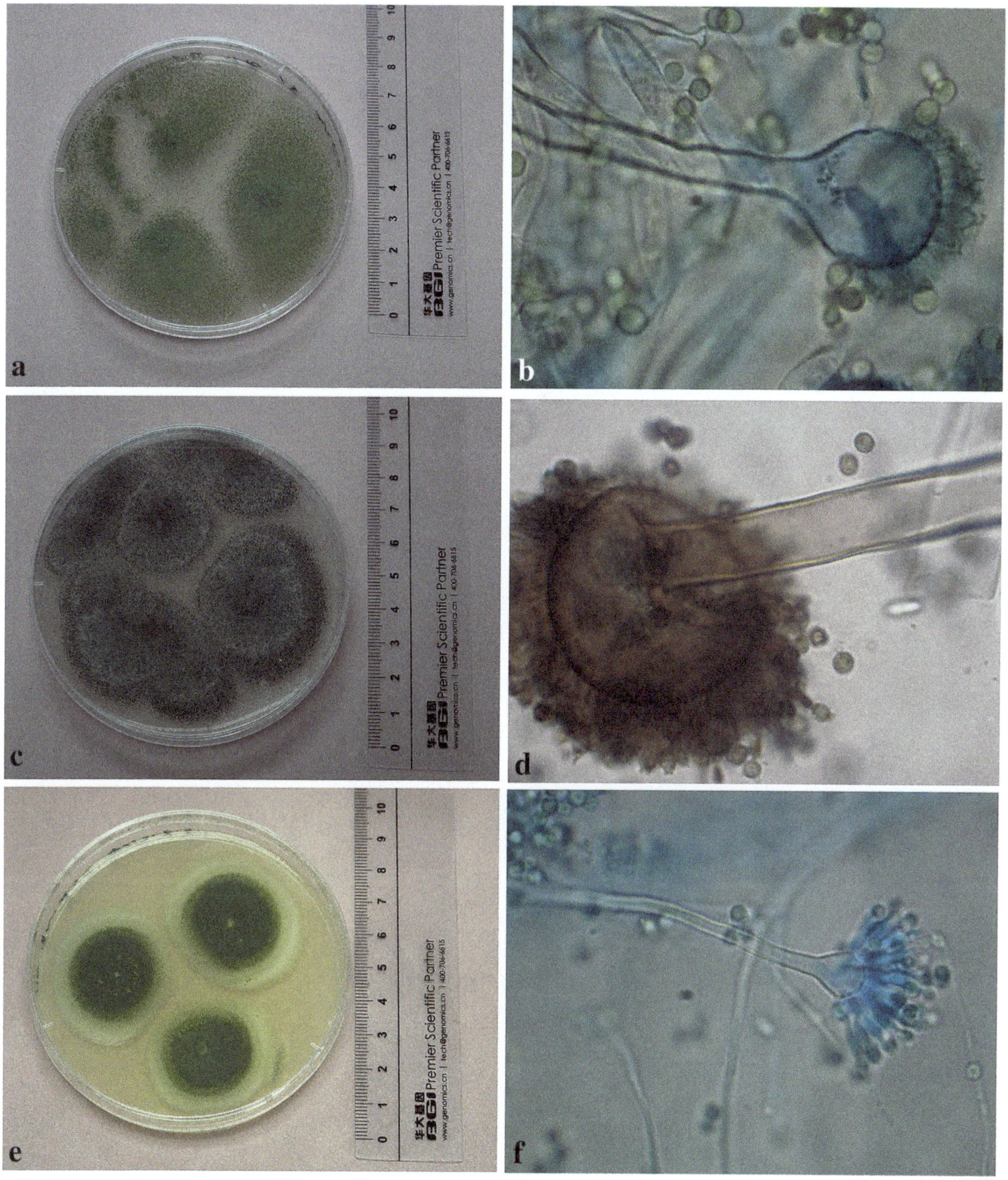

Fig. 2 Colony morphologies and microscopic characteristic of some fungal isolates. **a**, **b** *A. flavus*; **c**, **d** *A. aculeatus*; **e**, **f** *A. versicolor*. **a**, **c** and **e** Colonies after incubation for 7 days at 25 °C on PDA. **b**, **d** and **f** conidial heads and conidiophores. Magnification 10 × 100

to precisely analyse it and its contamination phenomenon in these samples even all the medicinal herbs.

Consistent to Blank et al. [40], all the *A. aculeatus* strains isolated in this study produced OTA. Although it has been reported that a number of *Penicillium* strains are OTA producers [17, 19, 41], none of 35 *Penicillium* strains in this study produced OTA, which has to be further confirmed. Moreover, the contaminant *A. fumigatus* still should not be neglected, even though neither the *A. fumigatus*, *Cladosporium* spp. strains nor the *Penicillium* spp. produced detectable mycotoxins. Because *A. fumigatus* is thermos-tolerant and has the ability to excrete

Table 4 Toxigenic potentials of the isolates from 45 samples of medicinal herbs

Fungi	Source	No. of strains isolated	No. of positive strains	Toxin production[a]
A. flavus	Flos *Carthami*	2	0	–[b]
A. flavus	Fructus *Lycii*	1	1	AFB_1, AFB_2
A. versicolor	Radix *et* Rhizoma *Glycyrrhizae*	2	2	ST
A. versicolor	Semen *Armeniacae amarae*	2	1	ST
A. versicolor	Herba *Andrographis*	1	1	ST
A. versicolor	Radix *Pseudostellariae*	1	1	ST
A. versicolor	Fructus *Lycii*	1	1	ST
A. versicolor	Radix *Notoginseng*	1	0	–
A. aculeatus	Radix *et* Rhizoma *Glycyrrhizae*	1	1	OTA
A. aculeatus	Radix *Codcnopsitis pilosulas*	1	1	OTA
A. aculeatus	Radix *Angelicae sinensis*	1	1	OTA

[a] Mycotoxins determined including AFB_1, AFB_2, AFG_1, AFG_2, OTA and ST

[b] Below the detection limits

hydrolytic extracellular enzymes that consequently allow opportunistic colonisation in lung tissue [42].

Conclusion

The prevalent contamination phenomenon of fungi observed in 45 medicinal herbs collected from China and the mycotoxigenic potential of some fungal isolates suggested appropriate procedures should be engaged to protect medicinal herbs from being contaminated.

Abbreviations

AFB_1: aflatoxin B_1; AFB_2: aflatoxin B_2; AFG_1: aflatoxin G_1; AFG_2: aflatoxin G_2; ITS: internal transcribed spacer; LC-MS/MS: liquid chromatography-tandem mass spectrometry; LOD: limit of detection; NCBI: National Centre for Biotechnology Information; OTA: ochratoxin A; PCR: polymerase chain reaction; PDA: potato dextrose agar; SD: sabouraud dextrose medium; SRM: selective reaction monitoring; ST: sterigmatocystin.

Authors' contributions

HX conceived and designed the study and performed the data analysis. RSZ, WLW and JT performed the experiments, analyzed data and wrote the manuscript. RTZ and WWC collected, authenticated medicinal herb samples and revised the manuscript. All authors have read and approved the final manuscript.

Author details

[1] Research Centre of Chinese Herbal Resource Science and Engineering, Guangzhou University of Chinese Medicine, Guangzhou, China. [2] Key Laboratory of Chinese Medicinal Resource from Lingnan, Ministry of Education, Guangzhou University of Chinese Medicine, Guangzhou, China.

Acknowledgements

This work was financially supported by the Project Based Personnel Exchange Program between the China Scholarship Council and the German Academic Exchange Service, and the Science and Technology Project of Guangdong Province (Grant No. 2015A030401083). The authors thank Mr. Li Dingmiao and Mr. Chen Jiamin for their technical assistance and Miss Chen Huizhi for her comments on the manuscript.

Competing interests

The authors declare that they have no competing interests.

References

1. Limyati DA, Juniar BL. Jamu Gendong, a kind of traditional medicine in Indonesia: the microbial contamination of its raw material and endproduct. J Ethnopharmacol. 1998;63:201–8.
2. Rizzo I, Vedoya G, Maurutto S, Haidukowski M, Varsavsky E. Assessment of toxigenic fungi on Argentinean medicinal herbs. Microbiol Res. 2004;159:113–20.
3. Song MF, Chen J, Li XL, Tang DY, Sun BD, Gao WW. Primary investigation of contaminating fungi on *Panax notoginseng* and *Amomum tsaoko* in Yunnan. Zhong Guo Zhong Yao Za Zhi. 2012;37:1734–6.
4. Song MF, Chen J, Li XL, Tang DY, Sun BD, Gao WW. Primary investigation of contaminating fungi on *Gynostemma pentaphyllum* in Yunnan. Shi Zhen Guo Yi Guo Yao. 2012;23:2016–7.
5. Sekar P, Yamnam N, Ponmurugan K. Screening and characterization of mycotoxin producing fungi from dried fruits and grains. Adv Biotech. 2008;7:12 5.
6. Aziz NH, Youssef YA, El-Fouly MZ, Moussa LA. Contamination of some common medicinal plant samples and spices by fungi and their mycotoxins. Bot Bull Acad Sinica. 1998;39:279–85.
7. Bugno A, Almodovar AAB, Pereira TC, Pinto TJA, Sabino M. Occurrence of toxigenic fungi in herbal drugs. Braz J Microbiol. 2006;37:47–51.
8. Moorthy K, Prasanna I, Thajuddin N, Arjunan S, Gnanendra TS, Zahir Hussain MI. Occurrence of mycopopulation in spices and herbal drugs. Int J Biol Technol. 2010;1:6–14 **(special issue)**.
9. Kim DM, Chung SH, Chun HS. Multiplex PCR assay for the detection of aflatoxigenic and non-aflatoxigenic fungi in meju, a Korean fermented soybean food starter. Food Microbiol. 2011;28:1402–8.
10. Mateo EM, Gil-Serna J, Patino B, Jiménez M. Aflatoxins and ochratoxin A in stored barley grain in Spain and impact of PCR-based strategies to assess the occurrence of aflatoxigenic and ochratoxigenic *Aspergillus* spp. Int J Food Microbiol. 2011;149:118–26.
11. International Agency for Research on Cancer (IARC). IARC monographs on the evaluation of carcinogenic risks to humans. Some naturally occurring substances: food items and constituents, heterocyclic aromatic amines and mycotoxins. lyon: IARC Press; 1993. p. 362.

12. Yu J, Chang PK, Cary JW, Wright M, Bhatnagar D, Cleveland TE, Payne GA, Linz JE. Comparative mapping of aflatoxin pathway gene clusters in *Aspergillus parasiticus* and *Aspergillus flavus*. Appl Environ Microbiol. 1995;61:2365–71.
13. Lepom P, Kloss H. Production of sterigmatocystin by *Aspergillus versicolor* isolated from roughage. Mycopathologia. 1988;101:25–9.
14. Rabie CJ, Lübben A, Marais GJ, van Vuuren HJ. Enumeration of fungi in barley. Int J Food Microbiol. 1997;35:117–27.
15. Atalla MM, Hassanein NM, El-Beih AA, Youssef YA. Mycotoxin production in wheat grains by different Aspergilli in relation to different relative humidities and storage periods. Nahrung. 2003;47:6–10.
16. Versilovskis A, De Saeger S. Sterigmatocystin: occurrence in foodstuffs and analytical methods—an overview. Mol Nutr Food Res. 2010;54:136–47.
17. Pitt JI. Penicillium viridicatum, Penicillium verrucosum, and production of ochratoxin A. Appl Environ Microbiol. 1987;53:266–9.
18. Horie Y. Productivity of ochratoxin A of Aspergillus carbonarius in Aspergillus section Nigri. Nippon Kingakukai Kaiho. 1995;36:73–6.
19. Lund F, Frisvad JC. *Penicillium verrucosum* in wheat and barley indicates presence of ochratoxin A. J Appl Microbial. 2003;95:1117–23.
20. Kuiper-Goodman T, Scott PM. Risk assessment of the mycotoxin ochratoxin A. Biomed Environ Sci. 1989;2:179–248.
21. O'Brien E, Dietrich DR. Ochratoxin A: the continuing enigma. Crit Rev Toxicol. 2005;35:33–60.
22. Pfohl-Leszkowicz A, Manderville RA. Ochratoxin A: an overview on toxicity and carcinogenicity in animals and humans. Mol Nutr Food Res. 2007;51:61–99.
23. Chinese Pharmacopeia Commission. The 2015 Edition of Pharmacopoeia of the People's Republic of China, vol. 1. Beijing: China Medical Science and Technology Press; 2015.
24. Wei J. Manual of fungal identification. Shanghai: Shanghai Scientific & Technical Publisher; 1979.
25. Qi Z. Fungi of China: Aspergillus and Related Teleomorphs, vol. 5. Beijing: Science Publisher; 1997.
26. Kong H. Fungi of China (Vol. 35): Penicillium and Related Teleomorphs. Beijing: Science Publisher; 2007.
27. Zhang Z. Fungi of China (Vol. 14): Gladaxporism, Fusicladium, Pyricularia. Beijing: Science Publisher; 2003.
28. Delmulle B, De Saeger S, Adams A, De Kimpe N, Van Peteghem C. Development of a liquid chromatography/tandem mass spectrometry method for the simultaneous determination of 16 mycotoxins on cellulose filters and in fungal cultures. Rapid Commun Mass Spectrom. 2006;20:771–6.
29. R Core Team. R: a language and environment for statistical computing. Vienna: R Foundation for Statistical Computing; 2015.
30. Efuntoye MO. Fungi associated with herbal drug plants during storage. Mycopathologia. 1996;136:115–8.
31. Mandeel QA. Fungal contamination of some imported spices. Mycopathologia. 2005;159:291–8.
32. Sampietro DA, Marín P, Iglesias J, Presello DA, Vattuone MA, Catalan CAN, Gonzalez Jaen MT. A molecular based strategy for rapid diagnosis of toxigenic Fusarium species associated to cereal grains from Argentina. Fungal Biol. 2010;114:74–81.
33. Bellemain E, Carlsen T, Brochmann C, Coissac E, Taberlet P, Kauserud H. ITS as an environmental DNA barcode for fungi: an in silico approach reveals potential PCR biases. BMC Microbiol. 2010;10:189.
34. Roy AK, Sinha KK, Chourasia HK. Aflatoxin contamination of some common drug plants. Appl Environ Microbiol. 1988;54:842–3.
35. Halt M. Moulds and mycotoxins in herb tea and medicinal plants. Eur J Epidemio. 1998;14:269–74.
36. Crous PW, Braun U, Schubert K, Groenewald JZ. Delimiting Cladosporium from morphologically similar genera. Stud Mycol. 2007;58:33–56.
37. Chiba S, Okada S, Suzuki Y, Watanuki Z, Mitsuishi Y, Igusa R, Sekii T, Uchiyama B. Cladosporium species related Hypersensitivity Pneumonitis in household environments. Intern Med. 2009;48:363–7.
38. Wilkinson JR, Kale SP, Bhatnagar D, Yu J, Ehrlich KC. Expression profiling of non-aflatoxigenic *Aspergillus parasiticus* mutants obtained by 5-azacytosine treatment or serial mycelial transfer. Toxins. 2011;3:932–48.
39. Zheng RS, Wang WL, Xu H, Zhan RT, Chen WW. Simultaneous determination of aflatoxin B_1, B_2, G_1, G_2, ochratoxin A and sterigmatocystin in traditional Chinese medicines by LC-MS-MS. Anal Bioanal Chem. 2014;406:3031–9.
40. Blank G, Nwoko U, Frohlich A, Marquardt R. Ochratoxin A production in relation to the growth morphology of Aspergillus alutaceus. Food Sci Technol. 1998;31:210–4.
41. Geisen R, Mayer Z, Karolewiez A, Färber P. Development of a real time PCR system for detection of *Penicillium nordicum* and for monitoring ochratoxin A production in foods by targeting the ochratoxin polyketide synthase gene. Syst Appl Microbiol. 2004;27:501–7.
42. St Leger RJ, Screen SE. In vitro utilization of mucin, lung polymers, plant cell walls and insect cuticle by *Aspergillus fumigatus*, *Metarhizium anisopliae* and *Haematonectria haematococca*. Mycol Res. 2000;104:463–71.

19

Quality control of *Lycium chinense* and *Lycium barbarum cortex* (*Digupi*) by HPLC using kukoamines as markers

Yuan-Yuan Li[1,3†], Rui Di[1†], Wing-Leung Hsu[1], Ye-Qing Huang[1] and Hon-Yeung Cheung[1,2*]

Abstract

Background: Lycii Cortex (LyC), composed of *Lycium chinense* and *Lycium barbarum cortex* and having the Chinese name Digupi, is used to treat chronic diseases like cough, hypertension, and diabetes in Eastern Asia. However, chromatographic methods, such as TLC and HPLC, to determine the phytochemical composition of LyC have not been included in any official compendiums. This study aims to establish a validated HPLC method for quality control of LyC.

Methods: Kukoamines A and B (KA and KB, respectively) were selected as markers for the HPLC method. An acetic acid solution was adopted for sample extraction because it facilitated the release of kukoamines and effectively prevented their degradation. Optimal separation of the kukoamine isomers was achieved on hydrophilic ligand-coated C18 columns with a gradient elution of acetonitrile and 0.1% (v/v) trifluoroacetic acid. The average contents and proposed contents for LyC were calculated with a *t* test and an uncertainty test based on 16 batches of authentic samples.

Results: The method was validated with linearity ($r^2 = 0.9999$ for both KA and KB), precision (RSD = 1.29% for KA and 0.57% for KB), repeatability (RSD = 1.81% for KA and 0.92% for KB), and accuracy (recovery of 90.03–102.30% for KA, and 98.49–101.67% for KB), indicating that the method could offer reliable results for quality control analysis of LyC. At the 95% confidence level, the calculated content limits were 1.45 mg/g for KA and 4.72 mg/g for KB.

Conclusion: Compared with conventional morphological identification, the HPLC method involving KA and KB contents offers precise, objective, and quantitative results for quality control of LyC.

Background

Lycii Cortex (LyC) is used to treat chronic diseases like cough, hypertension, and diabetes in Eastern Asia [1–3]. Although pharmacopeias from China, Japan, and Korea have officially stipulated the source of LyC as the root bark of *Lycium chinense* and *Lycium barbarum* [4–6], the herb is often misused or adulterated with other cortexes having similar appearances. Contemporary authentication of LyC relies on morphological identification [4–6]. In contrast, inspections based on characteristic constituents are practical and objective, because monitoring of phytochemical markers is normally not only genus-specific, but also herbal function-related [7–9].

Chromatographic techniques are commonly used for both qualitative and quantitative purposes with reliable results [10]. However, a genuine chromatographic method for LyC involving unique markers is still missing in official compendiums. Although some phytochemicals such as phenolic acids and flavonoids have been recommended as markers for quality assessment for LyC [11–13], they are neither unique nor abundant in this herb. Hence, they should not be adopted.

Recently, kukoamines A and B (KA and KB, respectively) were recommended by us as unique markers for LyC [14], because they are truly bioactivity-related, genus-specific, and content-abundant in this herb. Although the LC–MS/

*Correspondence: cheung.honyeung@cityu.edu.hk
†Yuan-Yuan Li and Rui Di contributed equally to this work
[1] Research Group for Bioactive Products, Department of Biomedical Sciences, City University of Hong Kong, Hong Kong SAR, China
Full list of author information is available at the end of the article

MS method is considered to provide simultaneous and precise determination of numerous phytochemical constituents [14, 15], the high cost of the equipment and its operation has made this method less practical for daily quality control inspections.

This study aims to provide a validated method for quality control of LyC with reference to KA and KB. Based on the developed method, multiple batches of LyC were investigated and the content limits were statistically calculated.

Methods

Reagents

Methanol and acetonitrile (HPLC grade) were purchased from Labscan Asia (Thailand). Trifluoroacetic acid (TFA) and acetic acid (both HPLC grade) were purchased from Fluka (Switzerland). All other chemicals were of analytical grade. Water was prepared using a Millipore MilliQ-Plus system (Millipore, USA). KA and KB (Fig. 1) were extracted and purified by our group (purity: higher than 98%) [16].

Plant materials

Dried root bark samples of *L. chinense* and *L. barbarum* were collected from different regions in China and a local market in Hong Kong (Table 1). At least 2 kg of each bark was collected. The species of the plants were identified by Dr. Zhi-Feng Zhang (Ethnic Pharmaceutical Institute, Southwest University for Nationalities). The voucher specimens (DGP-JXXS-001, DGP-HBQL-001, and DGP-JXJJ-001) were stored in the Department of Health, Hong Kong Government SAR.

LyC sliced samples, with the commercial names Hong Digupi (RLyC) and Bai Digupi (WLyC), were provided by herb stores from the Hehuachi herbal market in Chengdu (Sichuan Province, China). These samples had unclear sources, and were classified based on traditional experience. LyC extracts (Nos. 01–03) were bought from herbal extract companies in Sichuan, Shanxi, and Hubei. These extracts were claimed to be extracted from LyC.

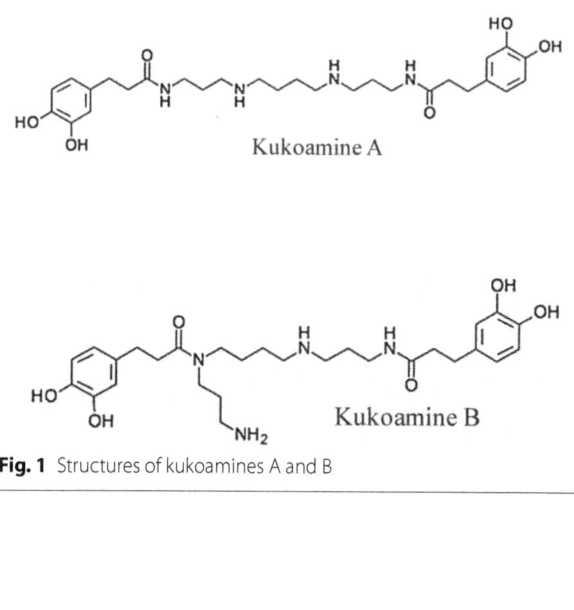

Fig. 1 Structures of kukoamines A and B

Chromatographic conditions

The HPLC analysis was performed on an Agilent 1260 system (Agilent, USA) equipped with an on-line degasser (G1322A; Agilent, USA), a binary bump (G1312C; Agilent, USA), an autosampler (G1329B; Agilent, USA), a column oven (G1316A; Agilent, USA), and a diode array detector (G1315D; Agilent, USA). A Zorbax C18 SB-AQ column (250 mm × 4.6 mm i.d., 5 μm; Agilent, USA) was used for the separation. A mobile phase consisting of 0.1% TFA (A) and acetonitrile (B) was applied for the separation with the following gradient program: 0–15 min, 12–16% B; 15–35 min, 16–22% B. The flow rate was 1.0 mL/min and the column oven was set at 40 °C. The detection wavelength was 280 nm.

Sample preparation

Each LyC sample was cut into small pieces and pulverized into a powder (passed through a 200-mesh sieve). The herbal powder (0.5 g) was accurately weighed. The extraction solvent was a 50% methanol aqueous solution containing 0.5% acetic acid (v/v). After addition of 20 mL of the extraction solvent, the mixture was sonicated in an ultrasonic bath (100 W, AC-120H; MRC, Germany) for 30 min and then centrifuged at 2880×*g* for 10 min (Allegra X-15R; Beckman Coulter, USA). The supernatant was transferred into a 50-mL volumetric flask and the pellet was re-extracted with another 20 mL of extraction solvent for 30 min. After centrifugation, the extracted solution was transferred to the same volumetric flask. Next, 10 mL of extraction solvent was used to wash the tube, and the washing solution was also added to the volumetric flask and filled to the mark. The prepared sample solution was filtered through a 0.22-μm pore-size filter before injection.

Method validation

Calibration curves for KA and KB were constructed by plotting the peak area versus the standard concentration. The calibration curves ranged from 3.91–250.00 mg/L for KA and 4.12–263.50 mg/L for KB. The method precision was measured by the relative standard deviation (RSD; %) of the peak areas determined for six successive injections of the standard solution. The repeatability test was measured by injection of five replicate samples for the proposed sample preparation and determination methods. The repeatability was calculated by the RSD

Table 1 Production areas and species of Lycii Cortex samples and the contents of kukoamines A and B

Batch no.	Species	Origin	Collection year	Content of KA[a] (mg/g)	Content of KB[a] (mg/g)
LC 1	*L. chinense*	Jiangxi	2011	9.65 ± 0.26	5.03 ± 0.13
LC 2	*L. chinense*	Jiangxi	2011	4.38 ± 0.27	13.27 ± 0.04
LC 3	*L. chinense*	Jiangxi	2011	3.33 ± 0.18	13.50 ± 0.18
LC 4	*L. chinense*	Jiangxi	2011	1.82 ± 0.13	3.39 ± 0.22
LC 5	*L. chinense*	Gansu	2011	3.83 ± 0.03	13.29 ± 0.14
LC 6	*L. chinense*	Shangxi	2011	6.34 ± 0.11	22.08 ± 0.11
LC 7	*L. chinense*	Neimenggu	2011	1.13 ± 0.02	3.49 ± 0.02
LC 8	*L. chinense*	Neimenggu	2011	4.87 ± 0.04	14.27 ± 0.27
LC 9	*L. barbarum*	Ningxia	2011	1.86 ± 0.09	6.80 ± 0.18
LC 10	*L. barbarum*	Ningxia	2011	1.93 ± 0.02	6.65 ± 0.01
LC 11	*L. barbarum*	Ningxia	2011	4.06 ± 0.23	16.88 ± 0.38
LC 12	*L. barbarum*	Ningxia	2011	1.47 ± 0.01	4.76 ± 0.23
LC 13	*L. barbarum*	Ningxia	2011	3.96 ± 0.29	19.02 ± 0.11
LC 14	*L. chinense*	Hong Kong	2011	1.29 ± 0.03	3.47 ± 0.15
LC 15	*L. chinense*	Hong Kong	2012	4.25 ± 0.04	18.45 ± 0.60
LC 16	*L. chinense*	Hong Kong	2012	1.75 ± 0.02	7.60 ± 0.02

[a] The content was converted to the dry basis. The experiments for each sample were performed in triplicate (n = 3), and the results are presented as the mean ± standard deviation

of the contents obtained from the five replicate samples [17]. The sample recovery was assessed by adding known amounts of individual standards into an accurately weighted sample. Three concentrations were investigated and triplicate measurements were performed for each concentration. Recovery was calculated with the following equation [16]:

$$\text{Recovery (\%)} = 100 \times (\text{amount found} - \text{original amount})/\text{amount spiked}$$

The method detection limit (MDL) and limit of quantitation (LOQ) were determined according to the guidelines in Validation of Analytical Procedures: Methodology (Q2B) [18].

Statistical analysis

The contents of samples were presented as the mean ± standard deviation. The proposed content limit for each analyte was calculated according to the contents from multiple batches with consideration of the standard uncertainty of the precision, bias, purity of reference substance, and water content (the calculation equation is shown in Additional file 1). The calculation was based on the ISO "Guide to the Expression of Uncertainty in Measurement" [19], EURACHEM/CITAC document "Quantifying Uncertainty in Analytical Measurement" [20], and LGC document "Development and Harmonization of Measurement Uncertainty Principles" [21]. The mean differences for KA and KB in the two species of *L. chinense* and *L. barbarum* were evaluated by analysis of variance (ANOVA). If the *P* value was less than 0.05, a follow-up post hoc test was conducted.

Results and discussion

Establishment of HPLC conditions for determination of kukoamines

Selection of column, mobile phase, and detection wavelength

KA and KB are water-soluble spermine alkaloids with multiple amino and amide groups [22, 23] that cause peak tailing on the C_{18} packing material. Three kinds of C_{18} columns with special coatings on the packing surface, i.e., Zorbax C_{18} BDS, Zorbax C_{18} Extended, and Zorbax C_{18} SB-AQ (all from Agilent, USA), were compared for the analyte retention behaviors. The kukoamines showed better retention on the Zorbax C_{18} SB-AQ column, owing to the better affinity of the extremely water-soluble analytes for the hydrophilic packing surface.

The influence of acids on the separation was investigated (Table 2). Within the pH range of 2.0–2.5, TFA was superior to phosphoric acid and formic acid in obtaining satisfactory peak resolution and symmetry. Furthermore, the peak sequence of KA and KB observed with TFA was the opposite to that observed with the other two acids. This difference was caused by the formation of ion pairs [24], which greatly altered the interaction between the analytes and the packing surface. Owing to the better separation performance, TFA was chosen as the acid for the mobile phase. The detection wavelength chosen for the kukoamines was 280 nm, based on the characteristic UV absorption of the *o*-dihydrocaffeoyl groups in the analytes.

Table 2 Influence of acids on chromatographic behaviors of kukoamines

Aqueous phase[a] (v/v)	Analytes	Retention time (min)	Plates[b]	R[c]	T[d]
Water	KA	15.3	126	0.8	2.30
	KB	20.9	52		4.40
0.2% Formic acid (v:v) pH 2.5	KA	34.6	4557	1.0	3.02
	KB	37.8	4632		3.06
0.1% Phosphate acid (v:v) pH 2.0	KA	35.1	3954	0.7	2.01
	KB	37.9	3249		2.52
0.1% Trifluoroacetic acid (v:v) pH 2.0	KA	47.3	10,091	2.6	1.10
	KB	37.1	10,887		1.12

[a] The exp eriment was conducted on an Agilent Zorbax C_{18} SB-AQ column (250 mm × 4.6 mm i.d., 5 μm) with fixed proportions of acetonitrile and aqueous phase (16:84). The aqueous phase was investigated with different acids

[b] The number of theoretical plates was calculated as $N = 5.54\ (t_R/W_{h/2})^2$, where t_R is the retention time and $W_{h/2}$ is the peak width at half height

[c] The resolution R refers to the resolution between KA and KB. It was calculated as $R = 2\ (t_A - t_B)/(W_A + W_B)$, where t_A and t_B are the retention times and W_A and W_B are the peak widths

[d] The tailing factor T was calculated as $T = W_{0.05h}/2f$, where $W_{0.05h}$ is the peak width at 5% peak height and f is the width start point at 5% peak height to the time of the maximum point

Influence of pH on the stability of the kukoamines

A stability test for the analytes was performed, and the results are shown in Fig. 2. KA and KB were not stable in neutral solution (pH = 7), as they were found to decrease by about 30% after exposure in air for 21 h. This change might arise through oxidation of the *o*-dihydrocaffeoyl moieties into quinones [25]. In contrast, it was found that when the pH was adjusted to 2.5–3 by acetic acid, KA and KB remained constant within the investigated period. This protective effect can be explained by the formation of hydrogen bonds between the phenolic hydroxyl groups and the solvent molecules in the acidic solution, which greatly protected the phenolic hydroxyl groups from oxidization [26]. Therefore, an acidic solution (0.5% acetic acid aqueous solution, v/v) was preferred for both the standard and sample solutions.

Optimization of kukoamine extraction procedures

Key factors influencing the extraction efficiency, specifically the extraction solvent and number of extraction rounds, were optimized to completely extract the analytes for analysis. The 50 and 80% methanol solutions (v/v) showed similar performances, which were much higher than those for the other concentrations (Fig. 3a). The optimal concentration of methanol for extraction was found to be 50% (v/v) from the aspect of eco-friendliness. Figure 3b shows the effects of acids on the extraction efficiency. The acidic solution was about one-fold more potent than the neutral solution for kukoamine extraction. Therefore, 0.5% acetic acid (v/v) was adopted, because it facilitated the release of alkaloids from the powder to the solvent. The influence of the number of extraction rounds was also examined (Fig. 3c). When samples were sonicated twice, almost all of the kukoamines were completely extracted. Therefore, two extractions were chosen for our extraction procedure.

Method validation

The established method was validated for its detection limit (MDL), quantification limit (LOQ), linearity, precision, reproducibility, and recovery. As shown in Table 3, the high correlation coefficient ($r^2 = 0.9999$; $P < 0.05$) indicated good linearity between the concentrations of kukoamines and their peak areas. The MDL and LOQ were derived from the responses of the analytes to UV, and were found to be 1.76 and 8.78 μg/mL for kukoamine A, and 1.86 and 9.29 μg/mL for kukoamine B, respectively. The RSD (%) in the recovery, precision, and reproducibility tests were all less than 2%. The good recovery obtained further suggested that the method was accurate and reliable.

Quantification results and proposed contents

The validated method was applied to investigation of the LyC samples from different locations, which covered most of the production regions in China. The post-harvest treatment of the herb strictly followed the procedures described in the professional compendiums to ensure quality consistency [4, 27]. A typical chromatogram of LyC and the overlay chromatograms for multiple batches are shown in Fig. 4a, b. The chromatographic patterns of all samples, regardless of whether they were *L. barbarum* or *L. chinense*, were highly consistent, although the abundance of some peaks varied remarkably. With the proposed chromatographic methods, the common peaks (1–6) in Fig. 4b could be used as the fingerprinting features for LyC authentication. The contents of KA and KB in the investigated LyC samples were in the ranges of 1.13–9.65 and 3.39–22.08 mg/g, respectively

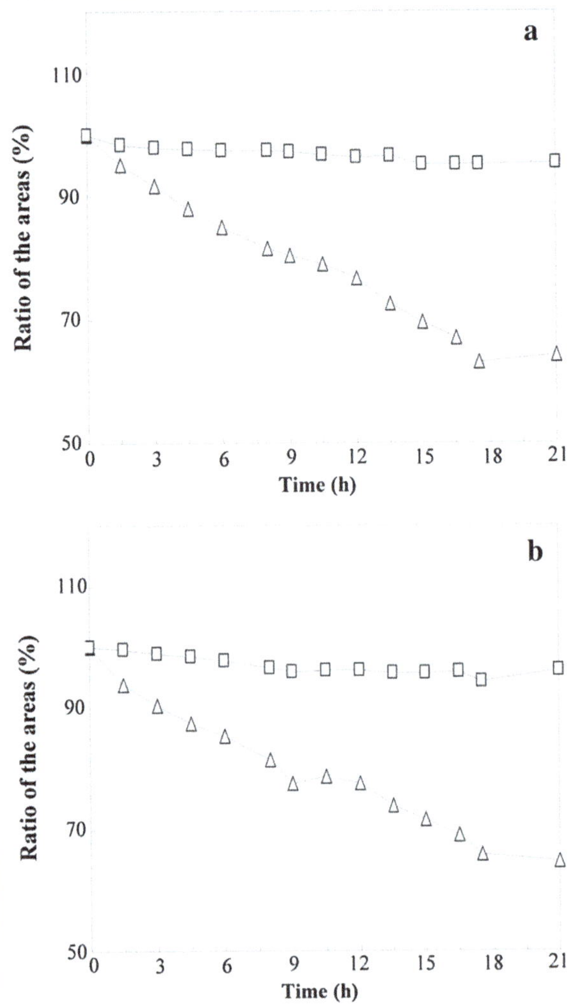

Fig. 2 Kukoamines A (**a**) and B (**b**) are stable in sample solution at pH 2.5 (*open square*), but not at pH 7.0 (*triangle*)

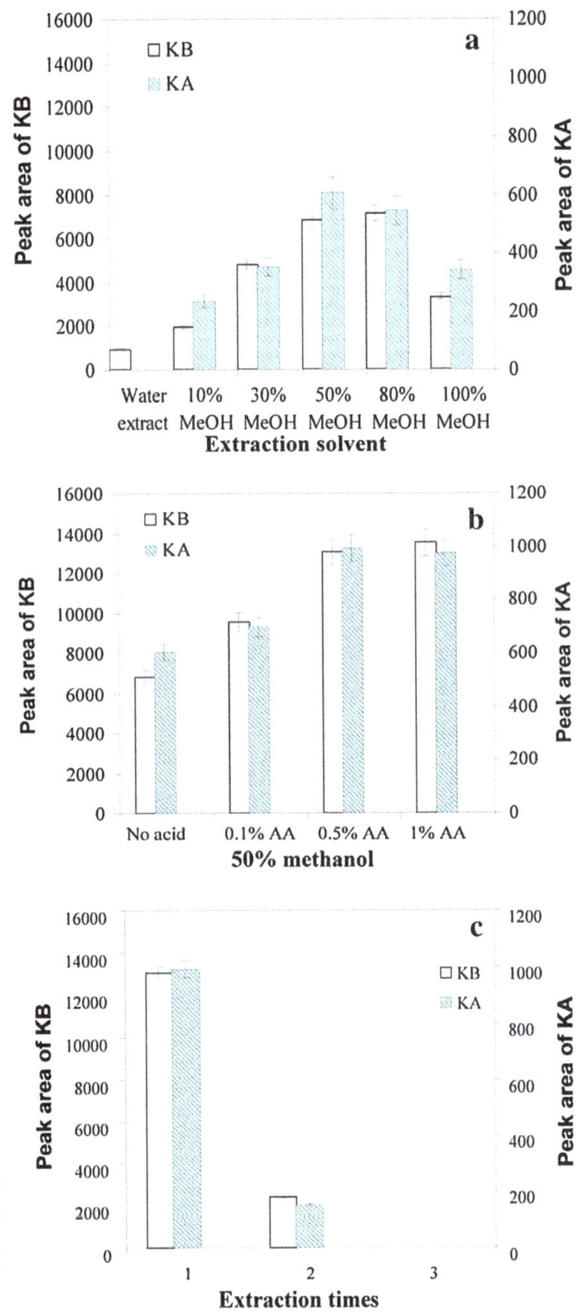

Fig. 3 Influence of methanol concentration (**a**), acetic acid concentration (**b**), and number of extraction rounds (**c**) on the extraction efficiency of kukoamines in LyC. The experiments for each condition were performed in triplicate (n = 3) and the results are presented as the mean ± standard deviation

(Table 1). In general, KB was more abundant than KA in the LyC samples.

The LyC samples from *L. chinense* and *L. barbarum* did not differ significantly from each other in their kukoamine contents when compared by one-way ANOVA (Additional file 1). These findings demonstrated that both plants can produce LyC with equivalent quality.

Geography, soil, and climate can cause fluctuations in herbal constituents [28–30]. Nevertheless, the secondary metabolites in LyC, KA and KB, typically fitted a normal distribution model [19–21]. Therefore, we estimated the content ranges of KA and KB for the LyC population using data from the collected representative samples by statistical inference [19–21] (Additional file 2). At the 95% confidence level, the calculated content limits were 1.45 mg/g for KA and 4.72 mg/g for KB (Table 4). These content limits could be used as reference values to judge the quality of LyC samples (Table 4).

Application of the HPLC method for quality control of LyC

Five batches of unauthenticated samples, which were claimed to be LyC sliced pieces and extracts, were tested by the established method and then judged by the calculated quality criteria. As shown in Fig. 5, only the crude material called "Hong Digupi" and the extract powder

Table 3 Linearity, precision, repeatability, recovery, MDL, and LOQ of the established method

Parameter	Kukoamine A	Kukoamine B
Linearity (12 points)	3.91–250.00 mg/L; $r^2 = 0.9999$[a]	4.12–263.50 mg/L; $r^2 = 0.9999$[a]
Precision (RSD)[b], %	1.29	0.57
Repeatability (RSD)[c], %	1.81	0.92
Mean recovery (n = 5)[d]	95.89% 90.03–102.30%	100.32% 98.49–101.67%
MDL (μg/mL)	1.76	1.86
LOQ (μg/mL)	8.78	9.29

MDL method detection limit, *LOQ* limit of quantification

[a] r^2, square of correlation coefficient for the linear regression ($P < 0.05$)

[b] Precision was tested based on six injections of a standard solution with 62.50 μg/mL kukoamine A and 131.75 μg/mL kukoamine B. RSD (%) = 100 × SD/mean

[c] Repeatability was tested on five replicate samples

[d] Recovery (%) = 100 × (amount found − original amount)/amount spiked. The results were presented as the mean recovery and recovery range. The amounts of spiked components for the recovery test were 10.4, 20.8, and 41.6 mg for KB, and 1.5, 3.0, and 4.5 mg for KA

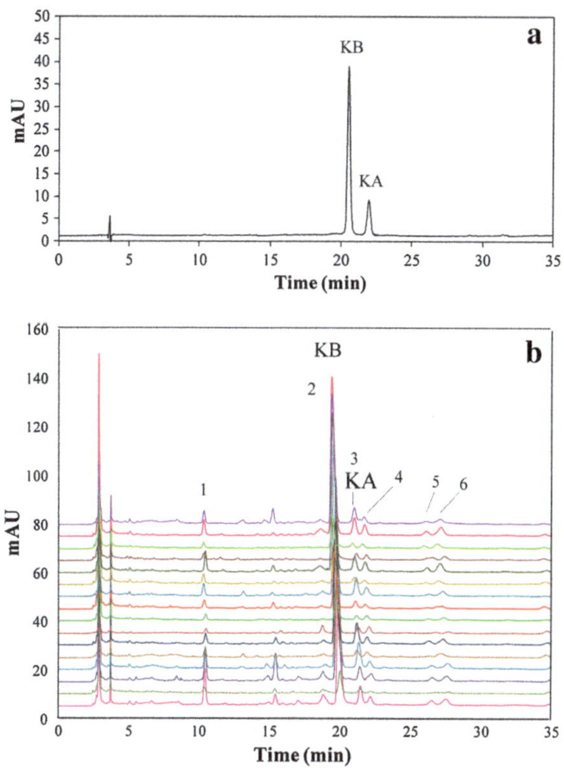

Fig. 4 HPLC chromatogram of mixed standards (**a**) and fingerprint profiles of LyC (**b**) from multiple batches. The numbers 1–6 in **b** indicate the common fingerprinting peaks for identification

from Sichuan presented the proper amounts of kukoamines, while other samples did not contain any kukoamines. The "Bai Digupi" on the market was actually not from the root bark of either *L. chinense* or *L. barbarum*. The lack of kukoamines in the investigated LyC extract powder might be caused by an inappropriate extraction method that damaged the major bioactive compounds, or extraction from the wrong source plants.

Compared with the conventional morphological identification, the proposed HPLC method for monitoring the characteristic constituents KA and KB provides a simple and universal way to measure the quality of LyC samples. The method and calculated content limits presented in this article could support amendments to the quality standards for LyC in official compendiums.

Table 4 Mean contents and proposed content limits for kukoamines A and B in Lycii Cortex

Parameters	KA	KB
Ca[a]	3.49	10.75
SD[b]	2.51	6.31
RSD[c]	71.91	58.73
n[d]	16	
$t^{e}_{critical}$	2.131	
uc (C)[f]	0.46	2.67
Calculated limit[g]	1.45	4.72
Outlier[h]	0	0
Failing rate (%)[i]	12.50	18.75

[a] Ca, average content of klkukoamines in samples (mg/g)

[b] SD, standard deviation of the contents in all samples

[c] RSD (%) = 100 × SD/mean

[d] n, sample size

[e] $t_{critical}$, critical value for a 95% confidence interval when the sample size was 16

[f] *uc* (C), combined standard uncertainty of the kukoamine B content in the sample (mg/g). The calculation is shown in the supplementary data section

[g] Calculated limit for kukoamines in the sample. The calculation is shown in the supplementary data section

[h] Number of outlier samples. The data are referenced to Table 1

[i] Percentage of samples with kukoamine contents outside the calculated limits

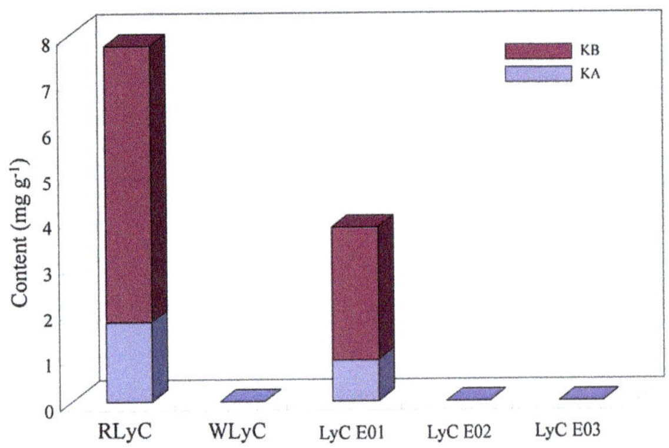

Fig. 5 Quality assessment of LyC sliced samples and extracts from markets. *RLyC* Hong Digupi, *WLyC* Bai Digupi, *LyC E 01–03* LyC extracts from manufacturers 01–03

Conclusion

The developed method could be applied for quality inspection of LyC in the food and pharmaceutical manufacturing industries.

Abbreviations

LyC: Lycii Cortex; KA: kukoamine A; KB: kukoamine B; HPLC: high performance liquid chromatography; LOQ: limit of quantification; MDL: method detection limit; RSD: relative standard deviation; TFA: trifluoroacetic acid.

Authors' contributions

LYY and DR conceived and designed the study. CHY secured financial support and oversaw the whole study. DR, LYY, and HWL performed the experiments. HYQ performed the statistical analysis. LYY and DR drafted the manuscript and CHY revised it. All authors read and approved the final manuscript.

Author details

[1] Research Group for Bioactive Products, Department of Biomedical Sciences, City University of Hong Kong, Hong Kong SAR, China. [2] Key Laboratory of Biochip Technology, Shenzhen Biotech and Health Centre, City University of Hong Kong, Shenzhen 518057, China. [3] Present Address: System and Translational Science Center, RTI International, Research Triangle Park, NC 27709, USA.

Acknowledgements

The authors also extend their gratitude to Mr. William T. Mahan for language editing.

Competing interests

The authors declare that they have no competing interests.

Funding

Hong Kong Chinese Materia Medica Standards, Department of Health, Hong Kong Government, SAR, China, for the CityU project (No. 9210029).

References

1. Ministry of Health of RP China. Document for further management of materials for manufacture functional food. 2002. http://www.moh.gov.cn/zhuzhan/wsbmgz/201304/e33435ce0d894051b15490aa3219cdc4.shtml.
2. Yao X, Peng Y, Xu LJ. Phytochemical and biological studies of Lycium medicinal plants. Chem Biodivers. 2011;8:976–1010.
3. Potterat O. Goji (*Lycium barbarum* and *L. chinese*): phytochemistry, pharmacology and safety in the perspective of traditional uses and recent popularity. Planta Med. 2010;76:7–19.
4. Committee of National Pharmacopoeia. Pharmacopoeia of the People's Republic of China. Beijing: Chemical Industry Press; 2010. p. 115.
5. Ministry of Health. Labor and welfare: The Japanese pharmacopoeia. Tokyo: Pharmaceuticals and Medical Devices Agency; 2012. p. 1686.
6. Korea Food and Drug Administration. The Korean herbal pharmacopoeia. Seoul: Ministry of health family welfare of South Korea; 2007. p. 1058–9.
7. Liang XM, Jin Y, Wang YP. Qualitative and quantitative analysis in quality control of traditional Chinese medicines. J Chromatogr A. 2009;1216:2033–44.
8. Lau AJ, Woo SO, Koh HL. Analysis of saponins in raw and steamed *Panax notoginseng* using high-performance liquid chromatography with diode array detection. J Chromatogr A. 2003;1011:77–87.
9. Shi Z, He J, Yao T. Simultaneous determination of cryptotanshinnone, tanshinone I and tanshinone IIA in traditional Chinese medicinal preparations containing Radix salvia miltiorrhiza by HPLC. J Pharm Biomed Anal. 2005;37:481–6.
10. Wu HF, Guo J, Chen SL. Recent developments in qualitative and quantitative analysis of photochemical constituents and their metabolites using liquid chromatography-mass spectrometry. J Pharm Biomed Anal. 2012;72:267–91.
11. Chu QC, Fu L, Lin M. Study on bioactive ingredients in Cortex Lycii by capillary zone electrophoresis with amperometric detection. Chin J Anal Chem. 2005;33:1611–4.
12. Li K, Chen XH, Bi KS. Determination of vanillic acid in Cortex Lycii by RP-HPLC. Chin Tradit Herbal Drugs. 2005;36:446–7.
13. Li K, Li Q, Yuan JS. Determination of scopoletin in Cortex Lycii by RP-HPLC. Chin Pharm J. 2005;40:1741–2.
14. Li YY, Di R, Baibado JT. Identification of kukoamines as the novel markers for quality assessment of Lycii Cortex. Food Res Int. 2014;35:373–80.
15. Zhang JX, Guan SH, Yang M. Simultaneous determination of 24 constituents in Cortex Lycii using high-performance liquid chromatography-triple quadrupole mass spectrometry. J Pharm Biomed Anal. 2013;77:63–70.
16. Cheung HY, Li YY, Di R, Process for isolating kukoamine. USP 9012687B2.
17. US Environmental Protection Agency. Technique support document for the assessment of detection and quantitation approaches. EPA-821-R-03-005, Washington D.C. 2003.
18. ICH, H. T. G. Validation of Analytical Procedure: Methodology (Q2B). International conference on harmonization. USA; 1997.
19. International Organization for the Standardization: ISO/IEC Guide 98-3 uncertainty of measurement—part 3: guide to the expression of uncertainty in measurement (GUM: 1995). Geneva; 2008.
20. Ellison SLR, Roesslein M, Williams A. EURACHEM/CITAC Guide: quantifying uncertainty in analytical measurement, 2nd ed. 2000. http://www.vtt.fi/ket/eurachem/quam2.pdf.
21. Barwick VJ, Ellison SLR. VAM Project 3.2.1 Development and Harmonisation of Measurement Uncertainty Principles Part (d): Protocol for Uncertainty Evaluation from Validation Data, Version 5.1, LGC (Teddington) Limited. 2000. http://blpd.dss.go.th/knowledge_el/VAM_uncertainty-0452.pdf.
22. Parr A, Mellon FA, Colquhoun IJ. Dihydrocaffeoyl polyamines (kukoamine and allies) in potato (*Solanum tuberosum*) tuber detected during metabolite profiling. J Agr Food Chem. 2005;53:5461–6.
23. Rogoza LN, Salakhutdinov NF, Tolstikov GA. Plant alkaloids of the polymethyleneamine series. Russ Chem Rev. 2005;74:381–96.

24. Cai B, Li J. Evaluation of trifluoroacetic acid as an ion-pair reagent in the separation of small ionizable molecules by reversed-phase liquid chromatography. Anal Chim Acta. 1999;399:249–58.
25. Li YY, Wang H, Zhao C, Huang Y, Tang X, Cheung HY. Inentification and characterization of kukoamine metabolites by multiple ion monitoring triggered enhanced product ion scan method with a triple-quadruple linear ion trap mass spectrometer. J Agric Food Chem. 2015;63:10785–90.
26. Sjödin M, Irebo T, Utas JE, Lind J, Merényi G, Akermark B, Hammarström L. Kinetic effects of hydrogen bonds on proton-coupled electron transfer from phenols. J Am Chem Soc. 2006;128:13076–83.
27. Wagner H, Bauer R, Melchart D. Chromatographic fingerprint analysis of herbal medicines: thin-layer and high performance liquid chromatography of Chinese drugs (vol 1). New York: Springer; 2011. p. 509–19.
28. Yi LZ, Yuan DL, Liang YZ. Quality control and discrimination of Percarpium Citri Reticulatae and Pericarpium Citri Reticulatae Viride based on high-performance liquid chromatographic fingerprints and multivariate statistical analysis. Anal Chim Acta. 2007;588:207–15.
29. Liang YZ, Xie PS, Chan K. Quality control of herbal medicines. J Chromatogr A. 2004;812:53–70.
30. Zhao ZZ, Yuen JPS, Wu J. A system study on confused species of Chinese Materia Medica in the Hong Kong market. Ann Acad Med Singapore. 2006;35:764–9.

The neuroprotective effects of *Tao-Ren-Cheng-Qi Tang* against embolic stroke in rats

Ling-Wei Hsu[1†], Wei-Cheng Shiao[1,2†], Nen-Chung Chang[3], Meng-Che Yu[1], Ting-Lin Yen[1], Philip Aloysius Thomas[4], Thanasekaran Jayakumar[1*] and Joen-Rong Sheu[1,5*]

Abstract

Background: Combinations of the traditional Chinese and Western medicines have been used to treat numerous diseases throughout the world, and there is a growing body of evidence showing that some of the herbs used in traditional Chinese medicine elicit significant pharmacological effects. The aim of this study was to demonstrate the neuroprotective effects of *Tao-Ren-Cheng-Qi Tang* (TRCQT) in combination with aspirin following middle cerebral artery occlusion (MCAO)—induced embolic stroke in rats.

Methods: A blood clot was embolized into the middle cerebral artery of rats to induce focal ischemic brain injury. After 24 h of MCAO occlusion, the rats were arbitrarily separated into five groups and subjected to different oral treatment processes with TRCQT and aspirin for 30 days before being evaluated in terms of their neurological behavior using a four-point system. The rats were sacrificed at 30 days after drug treatment and the infarct volumes were measured using a 2,3,5-triphenyltetrazolium chloride staining method. Tumor necrosis factor-α (TNF-α), c-Jun N-terminal kinases (JNK), activated caspase-3 and Bax were detected by western blot analysis. The apoptotic cells were identified by Terminal deoxynucleotidyl transferase dUTP nick end labeling (TUNEL) staining. ROS generation was also measured by electron spin resonance spectrometry.

Results: Rats treated with TRCQT alone or in combination with aspirin showed a significantly reduced infarct volume ($P < 0.001$) and improved neurological outcome compared with those treated with distilled water. Rats treated with TRCQT alone ($P = 0.021$) or in combination with aspirin ($P = 0.02$) also showed significantly reduced MCAO-induced expression levels of TNF-α and pJNK ($P < 0.001$) in their ischemic regions. Rats treated with TRCQT alone or in combination with aspirin showed decreased apoptosis by a reduction in the number of TUNEL positive cells, which inhibited the expression of activated caspase-3 ($P = 0.038$) and Bax ($P = 0.004$; $P = 0.003$). TRCQT also led to a significant concentration-dependent reduction in the formation of hydroxyl radicals ($P < 0.001$).

Conclusions: TRCQT reduced brain infarct volume and improved neurological outcomes by reducing apoptosis, attenuating the expression of TNF-α and p-JNK, and reducing the formation of hydroxyl radicals in MCAO-induced embolic stroke of rats.

Background

The incidence of stroke has markedly increased in developing countries over the past four decades [1]. Most strokes are caused by a thromboembolism, which disrupts cerebral blood flow, leading to oxygen and glucose deprivation in cells [2]. Secondary strokes who the individuals have a stroke history often have a higher rate of death and disability because of existing damage to the parts of the brain injured by the original stroke. Aspirin has been used to prevent secondary stroke. The incidence of cerebral hemorrhage and other bleeding events

*Correspondence: tjaya_2002@yahoo.co.in; sheujr@tmu.edu.tw
†Ling-Wei Hsu and Wei-Cheng Shiao contributed equally to this work
[1] Graduate Institute of Medical Sciences, College of Medicine, Taipei Medical University, Taipei, Taiwan
Full list of author information is available at the end of the article

is higher in China than it is in people from other high-income countries [3]. Ischemic brain tissue can be partially prevented from sprouting into infarction by several neuroprotective drugs [4]. It is noteworthy however, that numerous experimentally effective neuroprotective drugs have failed in clinical trials in human because of serious side effects [5].

Chinese medicines (CMs) usually contain a large number of compounds, which can affect multiple targets [6, 7], and several CMs have been used to treat stroke [8]. Previous studies have reported that the well-known Chinese formula *Tao-Hong-Si-Wu Tang* can be used to treat type 2 diabetes [9], as well as several mental disorders, including periodic psychosis, mania, neurosis, menopausal syndrome and involutional depression [10]. However, *Tao-Ren-Cheng-Qi Tang* (TRCQT) has not been clinically or experimentally used to treat stroke. In this study, we have used TRCQT, which consists of *Tao Ren* (*Prunus persica* (L.) Batsch., 5.0 g), *Gui Zhi* (*Cinnamon Twig.*, 5.0 g), *Mang Xiao* (*Natrii Sulfas*, 5.0 g), *Zhi Gan Cao* (*Radix Glycyrrhizae Preparata.*, 5.0 g) and *Da Huang* (*Radix et Rhizoma Rhei.*,10 g), to treat ischemic stroke in a rat animal model. The aim of this study was to demonstrate the neuroprotective effects of TRCQT in combination with aspirin following a middle cerebral artery occlusion (MCAO)-induced embolic stroke in rats.

Methods

Tao-Ren-Cheng-Qi Tang

A dried powder sample of TRCQT (Batch Number, 161342) was purchased from the Sun Ten Pharma. Co. (Taichung, Taiwan). The composition of a 30-g portion of this material was as follows: *Tao Ren* 5.0 g, *Gui Zhi* 5.0 g, *Mang Xiao* 5.0 g, *Da Huang* 10 g, *Zhi Gan Cao* 5.0 g. Thirty grams of this herbal mixture was extracted with water, yielding 7.0 g of dry extract (30.0:7.0 = 4.3:1). This material was mixed with 5 g of corn starch to give 12 g of final product. For sample preparation, the dried extract of TRCQT was dissolved in sterilized saline water (0.9% NaCl) at a concentration of 0.5 g/kg.

Reagents

3-(4,5-Dimethylthiazol-2-yl)-2,5-diphenyltetrazolium bromide (MTT) and propidium iodide (PI) were purchased from Sigma-Aldrich (St. Louis, MO, USA). TNF-α, JNK, Bax and activated caspase-3 antibodies were purchased from Cell Signaling Technology (Beverly, MA, USA). The anti-α-tubulin mAb was purchased from Neo Markers (Fremont, CA, USA). The Hybond-P polyvinylidene difluoride membrane, enhanced chemiluminescence (ECL) western blotting detection reagent and analysis system, horseradish peroxidase (HRP)-conjugated donkey anti-rabbit immunoglobulin G (IgG) and sheep anti-mouse IgG were purchased from Amersham (Buckinghamshire, UK).

MCAO-induced ischemia rat model

Healthy male Wistar rats (250–300 g) were used in this study. All of the animal studies were conducted in accordance with the standards established in the Guide for the Care and Use of Laboratory Animals, which was published by the Institutional Animal Care and Use Committee (IACUC) of Taipei Medical University (Additional file 1). The animal studies were also performed in accordance with the ARRIVE guideline (Additional file 2). Thirty rats were acclimated for 20 days before dosing, but only 25 of these animals were used the following experiments. All of the rats were kept at 37 °C in groups of five under a 12-h dark/light cycle with ad libitum access to food and water before the surgery. The rats were subjected to MCAO-induced ischemia by the administration of an autologous blood clot, as described in our previous studies [11, 12]. After surgery, the rats were housed individually under similar environmental conditions and were found to be free of apparent infection or inflammation, as well as showing no neurological deficits. In this study, at 24 h after MCA occlusion, the rats were arbitrarily separated into five groups of five rats each, including (group 1) sham-operated; (group 2) orally treated with distilled water for 30 days, followed by thromboembolic occlusion; (groups 3 and 4) treated with aspirin (5 mg/kg) and TRCQT (0.5 g/kg) alone for 30 days, followed by thromboembolic occlusion; and (group 5) treated with TRCQT (0.5 g/kg) combined with aspirin (5 mg/kg), followed by thromboembolic occlusion.

Neurological functional tests

To assess the neurobehavioral scoring of the animals, a sensorimotor integrity was measured for 30 days after MCAO by an investigator with no prior knowledge of the group allocation (Additional file 3) [13]. The neurologic scores were measured by using a 4-point sliding scale. Each rat was examined for resistance to lateral push (score = 4), open field circling (score = 3) and shoulder adduction (score = 2) or contralateral forelimb flexion (score = 1) when held by the tail. Rats extending both forelimbs towards the floor and not showing any other signs of neurologic impairment were scored 0. In this study, all of the rats subjected to MCAO either exhibited a neurologic score of 4 when they were examined 24 h after ischemia or immediately before reperfusion, or were excluded from the study.

Quantification of brain infarct volume

At 24 h after reperfusion, the rats were anesthetized and their brains were removed and cut into 2-mm-thick slices. The slices were then immersed in a 2% solution of 2,3,5-triphenyltetrazolium chloride (TTC) in phosphate-buffered saline at 37 °C for 30 min and fixed in 4% phosphate buffered formalin. The infarct areas of each slice were determined using a computerized image analyzer (Image-Pro plus). These areas were then summed and multiplied by the slice thickness to give the infarct volumes of each slice, which were calculated according to the method reported by Hsiao's group [11]. None of the animals died during these experiments.

Western blot analysis

After 30 days of TRCQT treatment followed by thromboembolic occlusion, the rat brain tissues were collected and homogenized, followed by sonication in a lysis buffer containing 20 mM Tris–HCl (pH 7.5), 1 mM $MgCl_2$, 125 mM NaCl, 1% Triton X-100, 1 mM phenylmethylsulfonyl fluoride, 10 μg/mL leupeptin, 10 μg/mL aprotinin, 25 mM β-glycerophosphate, 50 mM sodium fluoride and 100 μM sodium orthovanadate. The expression levels of TNF-α, phospho-JNK, activated caspase-3 and Bax-2 were analyzed by immunoblotting, as described previously by Rodrigo et al. [14] with minor modifications. A mixture of tris-buffered saline and Tween 20 (TBST) buffer containing 0.1% Tween 20 was used to wash the membranes.

Detection of DNA fragmentation by TUNEL assay

The in situ detection of DNA fragmentation in the brain tissues of the rats was performed 30 days after TRCQT treatment followed by thromboembolic occlusion using a TUNEL detection kit (Millipore, Billerica, Massachusetts, USA). Briefly, brain tissues were fixed in 4% formaldehyde and embedded in paraffin wax. Five micrometer sections of the embedded material were then cut and washed for 30 min in PBS. The sections were then equilibrated in water for 30 min at 37 °C, before being incubated in a mixture of Proteinase K (250 μL) enzyme at 37 °C for 30 min. The proteinase K digestion process was stopped by washing the sections with PBS (four 2-min wash cycles). The sections were then incubated in terminal deoxynucleotidyl transferase (TdT) buffer [2.5 mM Tris–HCl (pH 6.6), 0.2 M potassium cacodylate, 2.5 mM $CoCl_2$, 0.25 mg/mL bovine serum albumin (BSA)] for 10 min, followed by 60 min at 37 °C in a TdT end-labeling cocktail. The TdT end-labeling cocktail was removed and the reaction was stopped, and the resulting sections were washed in PBS. The sections were incubated in Avidin-FITC in the dark for 30 min at 37 °C and then washed in PBS to end the reaction. The sections were then counterstained with PI for 10 min at 37 °C and mounted on a cover slip. Only the green-stained cells were counted as belonging to the apoptotic phenotype and the density of apoptotic cells was detected by immuno-fluorescent microscopy (TCS SP5, Leica, Mannheim, Germany) by counting the green-stained cells.

Measurements of hydroxyl radical ($OH^{\cdot-}$) formation by electron spin resonance (ESR) spectrometry

ESR experiments were conducted according to the method reported by Chou et al. [15] using a Bruker EMX ESR spectrometer (Billerica, MA, USA). Briefly, a Fenton reaction solution (50 μm $FeSO_4$ + 2 mM H_2O_2) was pretreated with a solvent control (0.1% DMSO) or TRCQT (0.3, 0.7 and 1.3 mg/mL) for 10 min. The rate of hydroxyl radical-scavenging activity was defined by the following equation:

$$\text{Inhibition rate} = 1 - [\text{signal height (TRCQT)}/\text{signal height (control)}]$$

Statistical analysis

The results were expressed as the mean ± SD and were accompanied by the number of observations. The experiments were assessed by analysis of variance (ANOVA), version 9.2 (SAS Inc., Cary, NC, USA), using the Newman–Keuls method. A P value of less than 0.05 was considered statistically significant. Concentration-dependent effects were determined by visual inspection of the results.

Results

Effect of TRCQT, aspirin alone, or in combination on infarct volume

The effects of TRCQT and aspirin alone or in combination on the infarct volumes are shown in Fig. 1A, B. Compared with the group treated with distilled water (group 2), the animals treated with TRCQT alone showed a significant decrease in their infarct volume ($P < 0.001$). In contrast, the group treated with aspirin alone (group 3) did not show any significant effects. A similar effect was also found in rats treated with aspirin combined with TRCQT (group 5) ($P < 0.001$) for 30 days after MCAO compared with the sham-operated (group 1).

Neurobehavioral assessment

Neurological deficit was examined at 24 h after reperfusion and scored on a 4-point scale according to the method described by Bederson's group [13]. The changes observed in the neurological deficit scores of the different groups are shown in Fig. 2. Rats treated with aspirin (group 3) for 30 days after MCAO exhibited a moderate reduction in their neurobehavioral scores compared with the sham-operated group at 24 h after ischemia ($P = 0.0525$). However, rats treated with TRCQT alone (group 4) for 30 days showed a significant reduction in their neurobehavioral deficit score compared with the sham-operated group at 24 h after thromboembolic occlusion ($P = 0.0537$). Notably, rats treated with a

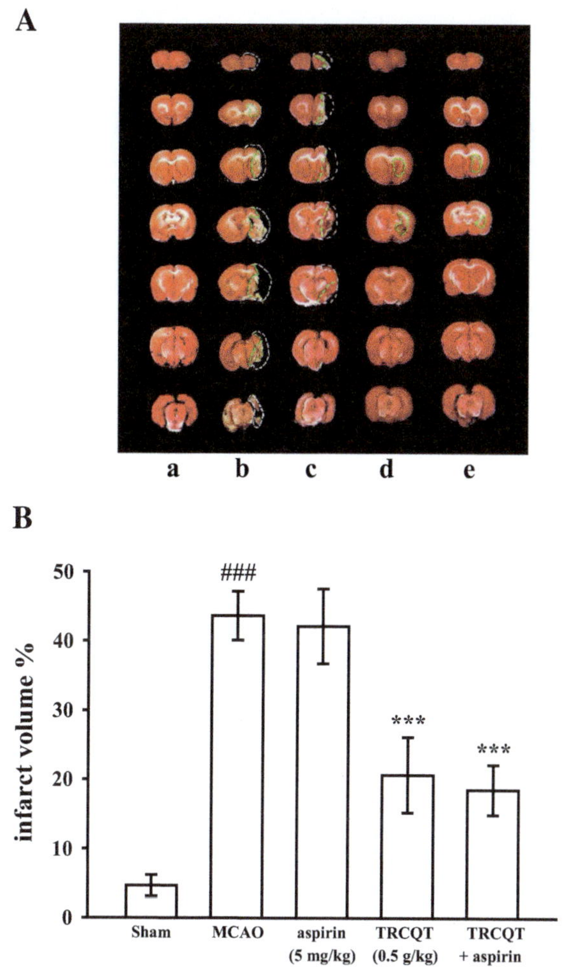

Fig. 1 Effects of TRCQT with aspirin against thromboembolic stroke in rats. The infarct volume was measured after 30 days of treatment with TRCQT, aspirin or a combination of TRCQT and aspirin after middle cerebral artery occlusion (MCAO). **A** TTC (2,3,5-triphenyltetrazolum chloride solution) staining of the brain slices showing the infarct areas in the sham (*a*), thromboembolic occlusion-induced untreated (*b*), aspirin (5 mg/kg) (*c*), TRCQT (0.5 g/kg) (*d*) and combination-treated groups (*e*). **B** Histogram showing the quantification of the infarct volumes in the sham, thromboembolic occlusion-induced untreated, aspirin, TRCQT and combination-treated groups. These data represent the mean ± SD of three independent experiments. $^{###}P < 0.001$ compared with sham group, $^{***}P < 0.001$ compared with the thromboembolic occlusion-induced untreated group ($n = 5$)

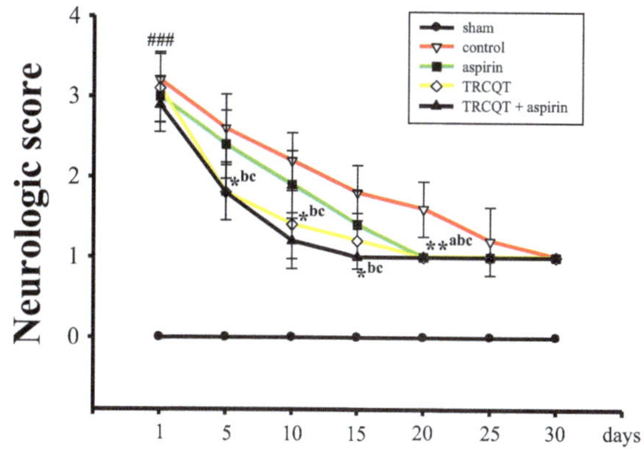

Fig. 2 Effects of TRCQT and aspirin on the neurological deficit. The panel shows the neurological deficit scores after stroke in the five experimental groups: sham, thromboembolic occlusion-induced untreated, aspirin, TRCQT and combination-treated. These data represent the mean ± SD of three independent experiments. $^{###}P < 0.001$ compared with the sham group, $^{*}P < 0.05$ compared with the thromboembolic occlusion-induced untreated group ($n = 5$)

combination of aspirin and TRCQT showed a better neurobehavioral outcome than those treated those treated with TRCQT or aspirin alone ($P = 0.0119$).

TRCQT enhanced aspirin's inhibitory effect on TNF-α and p-JNK in the ischemic brain

As shown in Fig. 3a, there was a significant increase in the expression levels of TNF-α in the MCAO-induced group, whereas the groups treated with aspirin ($P = 0.043$) or TRCQT ($P = 0.021$) alone showed significant decreases in the expression of this protein. Moreover, a significant inhibitory effect was observed in the expression of TNF-α in the rats treated with aspirin (0.5 g/kg) combined with TRCQT ($P = 0.02$).

The effects of the TRCQT, aspirin and TRCQT/aspirin combination on the levels of p-JNK are shown in Fig. 3b. Compared with the MCAO-induced group, the rats treated with TRCQT or aspirin alone showed a significant decrease in their p-JNK levels ($P < 0.001$). The rats treated with a combination of aspirin and TRCQT also showed a significant decrease in their expression of p-JNK compared with those from the individual treatment groups ($P < 0.001$).

TRCQT inhibited the apoptosis-related proteins Bax and activated caspase-3 in the ischemic brain tissues

As shown in Fig. 4a, there was a significant increase ($P = 0.015$) in the levels of Bax protein in the MCAO-induced group compared with the sham group. Although the rats treated with aspirin or TRCQT alone showed a significant decrease in the expression of Bax ($P = 0.018$ and 0.013, respectively), this effect was potentiated when these treatments were combined ($P = 0.011$).

The expression of activated caspase-3 did not change in the sham, MCAO-induced or aspirin treated rats (Fig. 4b), but there was significant decrease in the expression levels of this protein in the rats treated with a combination of aspirin and TRCQT ($P = 0.048$). The rats treated with TRCQT alone also showed a considerable decrease in their activated caspase-3 expression, although this effect was not significant.

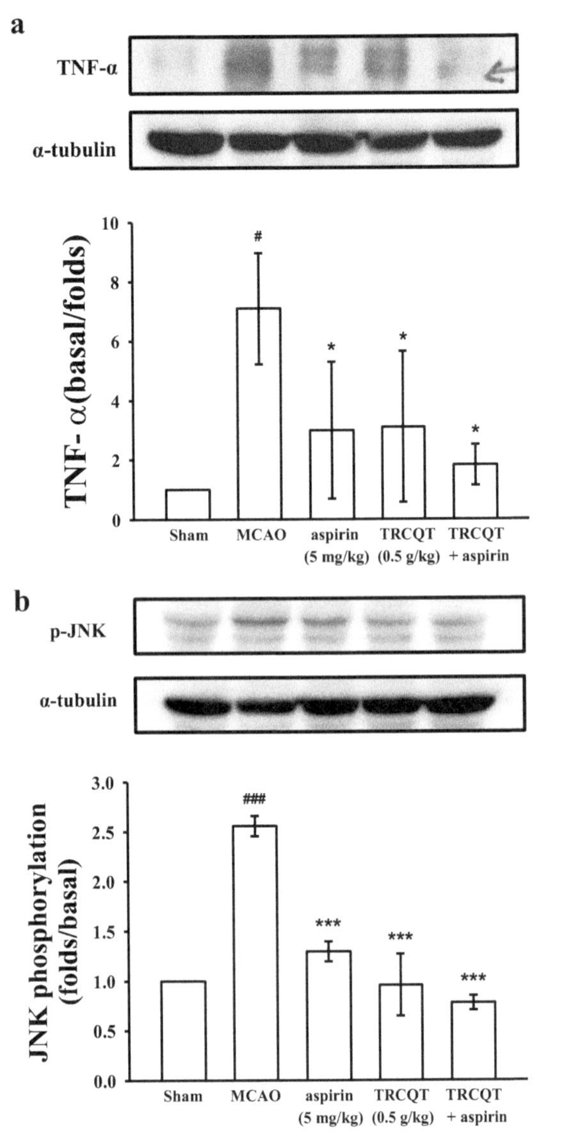

Fig. 3 Effects of TRCQT combined with aspirin on the expressions of TNF-α (**a**) and p-JNK (**b**) in cerebral homogenates 30 days after thromboembolic stroke in rats. The data represent the mean ± SD of three independent experiments. # and ###$P < 0.01$ compared with the sham-operated group, * and ***$P < 0.05$ compared with the thromboembolic occlusion-induced untreated group. Equal loading in each lane was demonstrated by similar intensities of α-tubulin ($n = 5$)

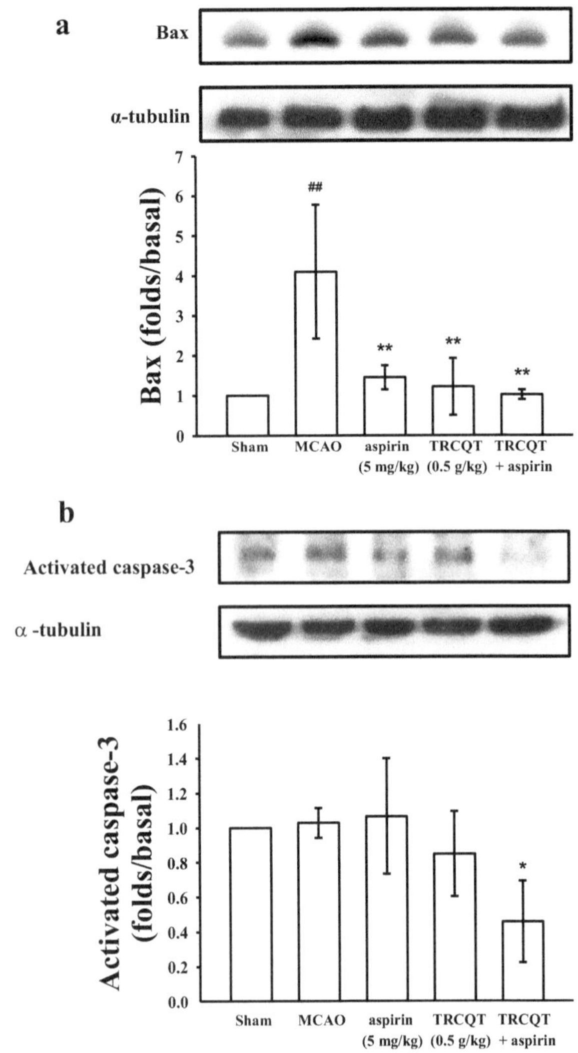

Fig. 4 Effects of TRCQT combined with aspirin on the expression levels of Bax (**a**) and activated caspase-3 (**b**) in cerebral homogenates 30 days after thromboembolic stroke in rats. The data represent the mean ± SD of three independent experiments. ##Compared with the sham-operated group, **compared with the thromboembolic occlusion-induced untreated group. Equal loading in each lane was demonstrated by similar intensities of α-tubulin ($n = 5$)

Effect of combination of TRCQT and aspirin on DNA fragmentation

Although no TUNEL-positive cells were identified in the sham-operated group (Fig. 5), we did observe a considerable increase in the number of TUNEL-positive cells in the MCAO-induced group. Rats treated with a combination of TRCQT and aspirin showed a noticeable reduction in the number of TUNEL-positive cells, although this effect was not statistically significant.

TRCQT attenuated the in vitro formation of HO· radicals

TRCQT significantly attenuated the Fenton reaction-induced formation of HO· radicals in a concentration-dependent manner (0.3, 0.7 and 1.3 mg/mL) (Fig. 6). Moreover, TRCQT inhibited the formation of HO· radicals to a much greater extent at a concentration of

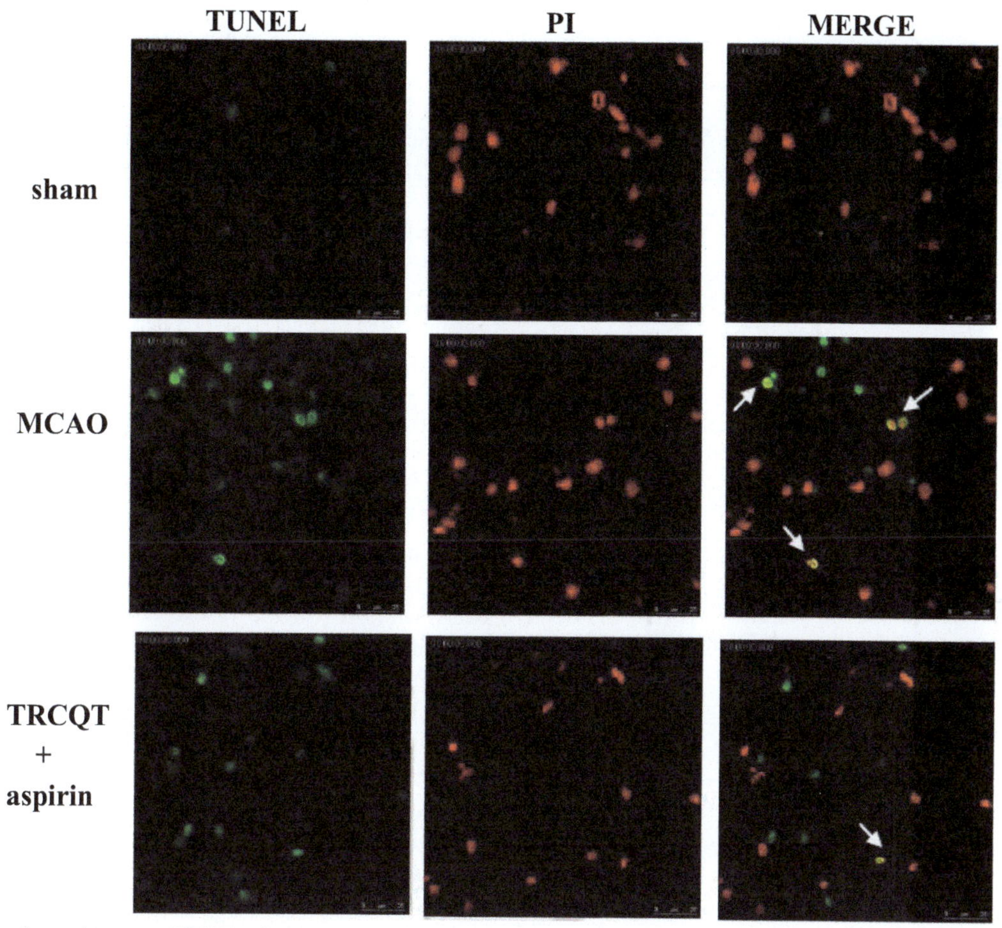

Fig. 5 Effects of a combination of TRCQT and aspirin on DNA fragmentation after MCAO injury in rats. TUNEL staining images of damaged cortex samples collected from each group after TRCQT combined with aspirin administration at high magnification (25 μm). The TUNEL-positive material was localized in the nuclei of the neurons. Numerous TUNEL-positive cells were identified in the thromboembolic occlusion-induced untreated group compared with the sham group and the group treated with a combination of TRCQT and aspirin

1.3 mg/mL compared with a concentration of 0.3 mg/mL ($P < 0.001$).

Discussion

This study demonstrated that the oral treatment with TRCQT or aspirin suppressed thromboembolic stroke in rats and led to an improved neurological outcome by reducing the infarct volume. The treatment of rats with TRCQT or aspirin alone inhibited the expression of TNF-α, p-JNK, activated caspase-3 and Bax, as well as reducing the number of TUNEL positive cells in the ischemic brain regions of these animals. Although the treatment of the rats with TRCQT or aspirin alone resulted in neuroprotective effects, the combination of these two drugs was much more effective. Treatment with TRCQT (0.3, 0.7 and 1.3 mg/mL) led to a significant reduction in the formation of HO· radicals.

Vascular inflammation is mediated by pro-inflammatory cytokines, such as TNF-α [16, 17]. The administration of TNF-α leads to an increase in tissue damage and neurological deficits, thereby aggravating ischemic brain injury [18]. Anti-TNF neutralizing antibodies [19] and the inhibition of soluble TNF-α receptor type 1 [20] have been reported to reduce ischemic damage and improve functional outcome after stroke [21]. The results of our previous study demonstrated that the oral administration of *Tao-Hong-Si-Wu Tang* (THSWT) attenuated the effects of embolic stroke by inhibiting the expression of TNF-α [22]. In this study, the treatment of MCAO-induced rats with TRCQT or aspirin alone led to a reduction in the TNF-α levels. Cerebral ischemia results in an increase in the levels of mitogen activated protein kinases (MAPKs) [23, 24]. Inhibition of the JNK MAPK pathways could therefore improved outcomes in ischemic

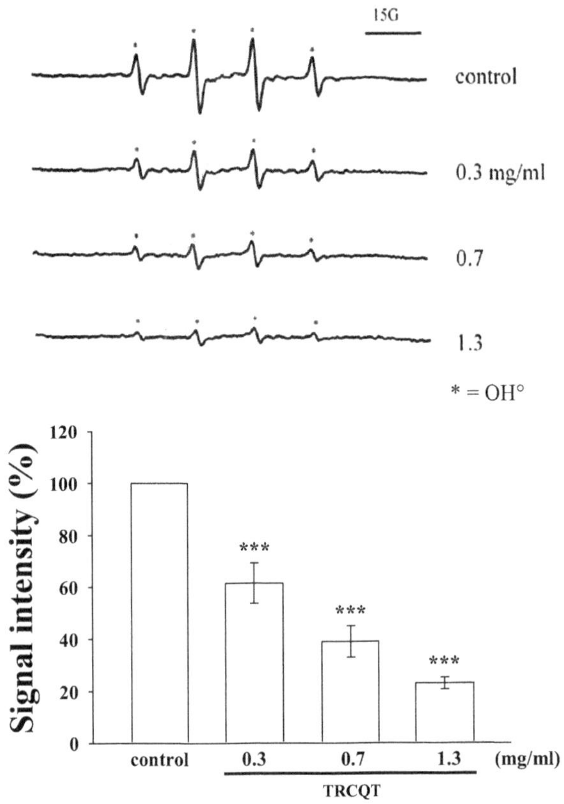

Fig. 6 Effects of TRCQT on the formation of hydroxyl radicals; the ESR spectra showed that TRCQT significantly inhibited the formation of hydroxyl radicals at concentrations of at 0.3, 0.7 and 1.3 mg/mL in the Fenton reaction. These data represent the mean ± SD of three independent experiments. ***$P < 0.001$ compared with the control group ($n = 3$)

brain injury by suppressing the production of inflammatory cytokines [25, 26]. The phosphorylation of JNK can promote stress-induced cell death and regulate the downstream signaling events associated with apoptosis during ischemic injury [27]. In this study, we observed increases in the activation of TNF-α and p-JNK in rats with MCAO-induced brain injury. Notably, the treatment of these rats with TRCQT or aspirin alone led a significant decrease in the activation of these proteins.

Activated caspase-3 occurs following apoptosis in the hippocampus after transient cerebral ischemia-mediated neuronal death [28, 29]. The levels of activated caspase-3 and Bax observed at 30 days after ischemia were higher than those found in the sham rats. Furthermore, the number of TUNEL-positive cells found in the ischemic region increased after MCAO ischemia. The oral administration of TRCQT in combination with aspirin led to significant decreases in the expression levels of Bax and activated caspase-3, as well as a reduction in the number of TUNEL-positive cells.

The production of reactive oxygen species (ROS) is a significant factor in the neuropathology of stroke [30]. During acute ischemic stroke, ROS can be generated through multiple injury mechanisms, including mitochondrial inhibition, Ca^{2+} overload and reperfusion injury [31]. H_2O_2 is the source of HO· radicals, which can contribute to neuronal injury after cerebral ischemic reperfusion, resulting in neuronal death [32, 33]. The hydroxyl radical-scavenging activity of TRCQT was directly evaluated using an ESR method, and the results revealed that TRCQT scavenged HO· radicals in a concentration-dependent manner.

The screening of traditional Chinese medicines to identify potential neuroprotective agents by evaluating their neuroprotective effects using in vivo and in vitro experimental models of stroke is highly desired. A large amount of clinical information has been gathered over the years pertaining to the use of Chinese medicines treat stroke using indigenous herbal materials [34]. The results of this study should provide researchers with a better understanding of the mechanisms underlying the therapeutic value of using a combination of TRCQT and aspirin to treat thromboembolic stroke.

Conclusions

TRCQT reduced brain infarct volume and improved neurological outcomes by reducing apoptosis, attenuating the expression of TNF-α and p-JNK, and reducing the formation of HO· radicals in MCAO-induced embolic stroke of rats.

Abbreviations

CCA: common carotid artery; ESR: electron spin resonance spectrometry; ICA: internal carotid artery; JNK: c-Jun N-terminal kinases; MCAO: middle cerebral artery occlusion; MTT: 2,5-diphenyl tetrazolium bromide; OH^-: hydroxyl radical; PA: pterygopalatine artery; ROS: reactive oxygen species; TdT: terminal deoxynucleotidyl transferase; TNF-α: tumor necrosis factor-α; TRCQT: *Tao-Ren-Cheng-Qi Tang*; TTC: 2,3,5-triphenyltetrazolium chloride; TUNEL: terminal deoxynucleotidyl transferase dUTP nick end labeling.

Authors' contributions

LWH and WCS perceived the study. MCY and TLY designed the study. LWH performed ESR study and WCS performed TUNEL assay. NCC performed the Western blot analysis. MCY, TLY, TJ and PAT performed the statistical analysis. TJ and JRS wrote the manuscript. All authors read and approved the final manuscript.

Author details

[1] Graduate Institute of Medical Sciences, College of Medicine, Taipei Medical University, Taipei, Taiwan. [2] Department of Internal Medicine, Yuan's General

Hospital, Kaohsiung, Taiwan. [3] Department of Internal Medicine, School of Medicine, Taipei Medical University, Taipei, Taiwan. [4] Department of Microbiology, Institute of Ophthalmology, Joseph Eye Hospital, Tiruchirappalli, Tamil Nadu 620 001, India. [5] Department of Pharmacology, School of Medicine, Taipei Medical University, Taipei, Taiwan.

Acknowledgements
This work was supported by Grants (MOST104-2622-B-038-003 and MOST 104-2320-B-038-045-MY2) from the Ministry of Science and Technology of Taiwan and Yuan's General Hospital-Taipei Medical University (103-YGH-TMU-04).

Competing interests
The authors declare that they have no competing interests.

References

1. Feigin VL, Lawes CMM, Bennett DA, Barker-Collo SL, Parag V. Worldwide stroke incidence and early case fatality reported in 56 population based studies: a systematic review. Lancet Neurol. 2009;8:355–69.
2. Lo EH, Moskowitz MA, Jacobs TP. How brain cells die after stroke. Stroke. 2005;36:189–92.
3. Jiang B, Wang WZ, Chen H, Hong Z, Yang QD, Wu SP, Du XL, Bao QJ. Incidence and trends of stroke and its subtypes in China. Stroke. 2006;37:63–8.
4. Fisher M. Characterizing the target of acute stroke therapy. Stroke. 1997;28:866–72.
5. Zhu XH, Li SJ, Hu HH, Sun LR, Das M, Gao TM. Neuroprotective effects of Xiao-Xu-Ming decoction against ischemic neuronal injury in vivo and in vitro. J Ethnopharmacol. 2010;127:38–46.
6. Li XM, Bai XC, Huang H, Xiao ZJ, Gao TM. Neuroprotective effects of Buyang Huanwu decoction on neuronal injury in hippocampus after transient forebrain ischemia in rats. Neurosci Lett. 2003;346:29–32.
7. Wang L, Zhou GB, Liu P, Song JH, Liang Y, Yan XJ, Xu F, Wang BS, Mao JH, Shen ZX, Chen SJ, Chen Z. Dissection of mechanisms of Chinese medicinal formula *Realgar-Indigo naturalis* as an effective treatment for promyelocytic leukemia. Proc Natl Acad Sci USA. 2008;105:4826–31.
8. Gong X, Sucher NJ. Stroke therapy in traditional Chinese medicine (TCM): prospects for drug discovery and development. Phytomed. 2002;9:478–84.
9. Shi H, Shi L. The clinical effect of modified Taohongsiwu decoction on diabetes peripheral neuropathy. J Henan Univ Chin Med. 2006;21:38–9.
10. Yang JM. Therapeutic effect observation of 154 cases of coronary artery disease angina using Taohongsiwutang (THSW). China J Mol Med. 2007;17:2268–75.
11. Hsiao G, Lin KH, Chang Y, Chen TL, Tzu NH, Chou DS, Sheu JR. Protective mechanisms of inosine in platelet activation and cerebral ischemic damage. Arterioscler Thromb Vasc Biol. 2005;25:1998–2004.
12. Lee YM, Chang CY, Yen TL, Geraldine P, Lan CC, Sheu JR, Lee JJ. Extract of *Antrodia camphorata* exerts neuroprotection against embolic stroke in rats without causing the risk of hemorrhagic incidence. Sci World J. 2014;2014:1–8.
13. Bederson JB, Pitts LH, Germano SM, Nishimura MC, Davis RL, Bartkowski HM. Evaluation of 2,3,5-triphenyltetrazolium chloride as a stain for detection and quantification of experimental cerebral infarction in rats. Stroke. 1986;17(6):1304–8.
14. Rodrigo J, Alonso D, Fernandez AP, Serrano J, Richart A, López JC, Santacana M, Martínez-Murillo R, Bentura ML, Ghiglione M, Uttenthal LO. Neuronal and inducible nitric oxide synthase expression and protein nitration in rat cerebellum after oxygen and glucose deprivation. Brain Res. 2001;909:20–45.
15. Chou DS, Hsiao G, Shen MY, Tsai YJ, Chen TF, Sheu JR. ESR spin trapping of a carbon-centered free radical from agonist-stimulated human platelets. Free Rad Biol Med. 2005;39:237–48.
16. Chamorro A, Hallenbeck J. The harms and benefits of inflammatory and immune responses in vascular disease. Stroke. 2006;37:291–3.
17. Barone FC, Feuerstein GZ. Inflammatory mediators and stroke: new opportunities for novel therapeutics. J Cereb Blood Flow Metab. 1999;19:819–34.
18. Barone FC, Arvin B, White RF, Miller A, Webb CL, Willette RN, Lysko PG, Feuerstein GZ. Tumor necrosis factor-alpha. A mediator of focal ischemic brain injury. Stroke. 1997;28:1233–44.
19. Hosomi N, Ban CR, Naya T, Takahashi T, Guo P, Song XY, Kohno M. Tumor necrosis factor-alpha neutralization reduced cerebral edema through inhibition of matrix metalloproteinase production after transient focal cerebral ischemia. J Cereb Blood Flow Metab. 2005;25:959–67.
20. Nawashiro H, Martin D, Hallenbeck JM. Inhibition of tumor necrosis factor and amelioration of brain infarction in mice. J Cereb Blood Flow Metab. 1997;17:229–32.
21. Wang X, Feuerstein GZ, Xu L, Wang H, Schumacher WA, Ogletree ML, Taube R, Duan JJ, Decicco CP, Liu RQ. Inhibition of tumor necrosis factor-alpha-converting enzyme by a selective antagonist protects brain from focal ischemic injury in rats. Mol Pharmacol. 2004;65:890–6.
22. Wu CJ, Chen JT, Yen TL, Jayakumar T, Chou DS, Hsiao G, Sheu JR. Neuroprotection by the traditional Chinese medicine, Tao-Hong-Si-Wu-Tang, against middle cerebral artery occlusion-induced cerebral ischemia in rats. Evid Based Complement Altern Med. 2011;2011:1–9.
23. Irving EA, Barone FC, Reith AD, Hadingham SJ, Parsons AA. Differential activation of MAPK/ERK and p38/SAPK in neurones and glia following focal cerebral ischaemia in the rat. Brain Res Mol Brain Res. 2000;77:65–75.
24. Hayashi T, Sakai K, Sasaki C, Zhang WR, Warita H, Abe K. c-Jun N-terminal kinase (JNK) and JNK interacting protein response in rat brain after transient middle cerebral artery occlusion. Neurosci Lett. 2000;284:195–9.
25. Okami N, Narasimhan P, Yoshioka H, Sakata H, Kim GS, Jung JE, Maier CM, Chan PH. Prevention of JNK phosphorylation as a mechanism for rosiglitazone in neuroprotection after transient cerebral ischemia: activation of dual specificity phosphatase. J Cereb Blood Flow Metab. 2012;33:106–14.
26. Wallace BK, Jelks KA, O'Donnell ME. Ischemia-induced stimulation of cerebral microvascular endothelial cell Na-K-Cl cotransport involves p38 and JNK MAP kinases. Am J Physiol Cell Physiol. 2012;302:505–17.
27. Tournier C, Hess P, Yang DD, Xu J, Turner TK, Nimnual A, Bar-Sagi D, Jones SN, Flavell RA, Davis RJ. Requirement of JNK for stress-induced activation of the cytochrome c-mediated death pathway. Science. 2000;288:870–4.
28. Chen J, Nagayama T, Jin K, Steler RA, Zhu RL, Graham SH, Simon RP. Induction of caspase-3-like protease may mediate delayed neuronal death in the hippocampus after transient cerebral ischemia. J Neurosci. 1998;18:4914–28.
29. Iijima T, Mishima T, Akagawa K, Iwao Y. Mitochondrial hyperpolarization after transient oxygen-glucose deprivation and subsequent apoptosis in cultured rat hippocampal neurons. Brain Res. 2003;993:140–5.
30. Coyle JT, Puttfarcken P. Oxidative stress, glutamate, and neurodegenerative disorders. Science. 1993;262:689–95.
31. Cuzzocrea S, Riley DP, Caputi AP, Salvemini D. Antioxidant therapy: a new pharmacological approach in shock, inflammation, and ischemia/reperfusion injury. Pharmacol Rev. 2001;53:135–59.
32. Zhu DY, Deng Q, Yao HH, Wang DC, Deng Y, Liu GQ. Inducible nitric oxide synthase expression in the ischemic core and penumbra after transient focal cerebra lischemia in mice. Life Sci. 2002;71:1985–96.
33. Ikonomidou C, Kaindl AM. Neuronal death and oxidative stress in the developing brain. Antioxid Redox Signal. 2011;14:1535–50.
34. Gong X, Sucher NJ. Stroke therapy in traditional Chinese medicine (TCM): prospects for drug discovery and development. Phytomedicine. 2002;9:478–84.

21

Electroacupuncture for the prevention of postoperative gastrointestinal dysfunction in participants undergoing vascular laparotomy under general anesthesia: a randomized controlled trial

Meng-yue Liu[1†], Cheng-wei Wang[1†], Zhou-peng Wu[2] and Ning Li[1*]

Abstract

Background: Postoperative gastrointestinal dysfunction (PGD) is a common complication following laparotomy under general anesthesia (GA). Abdominal distension occurs in 8–28% of surgeries within 24 h postoperatively. The present study aimed to analyze the efficacy of electroacupuncture (EA) for the prevention of PGD by applying pre-operative EA stimulation of PC6 (*Neiguan*), ST36 (*Zusanli*), and ST37 (*Shangjuxv*) bilaterally twice within 24 h prior to surgery, compared with no acupuncture treatment.

Methods: The study participants were assessed and selected from participants undergoing vascular laparotomy under GA at the Liver and Vascular Surgery Unit in West China Hospital of Sichuan University. The selected participants were randomly allocated to two groups: routine-treatment (RT) and EA group receiving EA at PC6, ST36, and ST37. A computer-generated list of random numbers was used to determine the allocation of the participants, with numbered opaque sealed envelopes containing the randomization schedule. Eligible participants were all adults aged 18 years or above who were scheduled to undergo vascular laparotomy under GA within 24 h and had no history of EA treatment. The exclusion criteria included participants with serious systemic disease and history of EA treatment. While the RT group received standard treatments, the EA group received additional EA treatments. During each treatment session, EA stimulation was performed for a duration of 20 min at a frequency of 15 Hz with a continuous wave. All such participants received two EA treatments within 24 h before surgery. The outcomes were measured in three metrics: incidence and degree of abdominal distension; first times of flatus and defecation; and duration of hospitalization.

Results: Forty-three participants were recruited, of whom 42 participants successfully completed the study. Each group contained 21 participants. The incidence of abdominal distension (42.8, 76.2%) and degree of abdominal distension were significantly reduced in the EA group ($P = 0.03$ and $P = 0.03$, respectively). In comparisons of the first times of flatus (3.05 ± 0.58, 3.29 ± 0.42 days) and defecation (2.81 ± 0.51, 3.20 ± 0.55 days) and duration of hospitalization (5.33 ± 0.68, 5.75 ± 0.66 days), the EA group was superior to the RT group to some extent ($P = 0.13$, $P = 0.02$, and $P = 0.04$, respectively).

*Correspondence: zhenjiuhuaxi@163.com
†Meng-yue Liu and Cheng-wei Wang contributed equally to this work
[1] Department of Integrated Traditional Chinese and Western Medicine, West China Hospital of Si-chuan University, Chengdu, Sichuan, China
Full list of author information is available at the end of the article

Conclusions: Preoperative EA at PC6, ST36, and ST37 might be useful for preventing PGD, thereby improving gastrointestinal function recovery.

Trial registration This study is registered with the Chinese Clinical Trial Registry: ChiCTR-TRC-13003649

Background

Postoperative gastrointestinal dysfunction (PGD) is a complication in participants undergoing major surgical procedures under general anesthesia (GA) [1]. Opioid-induced gastrointestinal dysfunction is as high as 81% in the United States [2]. Abdominal distension within 24 h of surgery occurs in 8–28% of all operations [3]. PGD causes longer hospital stays, greater medical cost [4], and higher risks for other complications, such as infections. In China, the rate of PGD remained the same between 1974 and 2011 [5]. In Japan, the rate increased by 10% over a 5-year period at the turn of the twenty-first century [6]. Internationally, an analysis was conducted on the records of more than 5000 participants undergoing major vascular surgery in 206 National Surgical Quality Improvement Program hospitals from 2008 to 2009 [7]. The results showed that >25% of participants with endovascular treatment, regardless of severity, suffered from postoperative complications, postoperative intestinal obstruction, and other gastrointestinal dysfunctions within 30 days of surgery. Although the 30-day survival rate of thoracoabdominal aortic operations was 92% [8], gastrointestinal dysfunction was ranked 4th among the causes for death [9].

Currently, there are four major methods of treatment for PGD: diet and nutritional support, drug treatment, operative procedure, and complementary medicine. Most of these treatments are open-label treatment trials with small samples [10]. Acupuncture is widely used in obstetrics and gynecology [11], gastrointestinal surgery [12], and orthopedics [13].

As a potential alternative therapy, acupuncture has gradually gained acceptance from physicians following the demonstration of its efficacy in clinical and basic research. For example, a 165-patient clinical study demonstrated that electroacupuncture (EA) reduced the duration of operative ileus [14]. Another small-sample-size trial found EA useful for postoperative recovery of abdominal distension [15], and a similar study showed that acupressure improved the recovery of stomach distension [16]. Animal experiments identified the factors contributing to PGD, including reduction in the number of interstitial cells of Cajal and atrophy of their structure [17], activation of the sympathetic nervous system and postoperative inflammatory cytokines [18], and leukocyte cell-induced nitrous oxide release, which restrained gastrointestinal peristalsis and causes intestinal inflammation [19]. Other animal studies showed that acupuncture ameliorated PGD by regulating these pathological changes [20].

The present study aimed to analyze the efficacy of EA for preventing PGD by applying preoperative EA stimulation of PC6 (*Neiguan*), ST36 (*Zusanli*), and ST37 (*Shangjuxv*) bilaterally twice within 24 h prior to surgery, compared with no acupuncture treatment.

Methods

Ethics approval

This study was approved by the Ethics and Research Committee of West China Hospital of Sichuan University (WCHSU), China [No. 2013 (105); Additional file 1]. The Ethics and Research Committee of WCHSU is an ethical approval committee organized by leading professors in their own fields. The study strictly followed the principles for medical ethics outlined in the Declaration of Helsinki [21]. The study was registered with the Chinese Clinical Trial Registry: ChiCTR-TRC-13003649. All participants were provided with information regarding the study and signed a written consent form in advance (Additional file 2). The Chinese Cochrane Center was responsible for the whole trial including the randomization, blinding, statistical analyses, and data management. The study was performed according to the CONSORT 2010 checklist (Additional file 3).

Trial design

This was a single-center, single-blind, pragmatic randomized controlled study. With balanced randomization (1: 1), the participants were assigned to two groups: EA group and RT group (routine-treatment group).

Participants

All participants were recruited from the WCHSU, China, after meeting the eligibility criteria and signing the informed consent forms. Chengdu is a major business city in the west of China, with a population of 14,047,600, and WCHSU is the primary health care provider in the west of China. Eligible participants were all adults aged 18 years or above who were scheduled to undergo vascular laparotomy under GA within 24 h and had no history of EA treatment.

The exclusion criteria were as follows: participants undergoing endovascular surgery; participants with a history of hypothyroidism, hyperthyroidism, cardiopulmonary disease, diabetes, or psychological disorder; participants with a history of EA treatment; participants with a cardiac pacemaker; participants in the menstruating phase of the menstrual cycle; participants who refused to accept acupuncture; participants who were unconscious before surgery; participants with inability to communicate; participants participating in another clinical trial that could interfere with the primary endpoint of the study; participants with a bleeding disorder (hemophilia or fibrinogenemia); participants with serious systemic disease (AIDS or sepsis); participants with initial body temperature of above 38.0 °C or below 36.0 °C; participants with a known history of alcohol or substance abuse; participants requiring systemic sedation for other reasons; participants needing emergency procedures; participants who were pregnant or lactating women.

The withdrawal criteria were as follows: at the patient's own request or at the request of their legal representative; if, in the opinion of the investigator or the specialized physician performing the acupuncture or examination, continuation of the trial would be detrimental to the patient's wellbeing (e.g. strong pain at insertion points, allergic reactions, other independent acute health problems).

Interventions

For prevention of PGD by EA, three acupuncture points, PC6 (*Neiguan*), ST36 (*Zusanli*), and ST37 (*Shangjuxv*), were selected.

The participants receiving EA therapy were treated bilaterally at the above three distal acupuncture points. PC6 is an acupuncture point of the pericardium meridian, which is located between the palmaris longus tendon and the flexor carpi radialis muscle tendon, 2 cun above the rasceta (Fig. 1). ST36 in a point between the tibialis anterior and extensor digitorum longus, which is located on the anterolateral side of the lower leg, 3 cun below *Dubi* and one finger width lateral of the anterior border of the tibia. ST37 is a point in the tibialis anterior, which is located 3 cun below ST36 (Fig. 2). The anterior tibial artery and anterior tibial vein are present around both ST36 and ST37, while there are the lateral sural cutaneous nerve and cutaneous branch of the saphenous nerve. The locations of these acupuncture points are described in *The National Standards for Acupoint Location* [22].

The participants in EA group were given the following EA treatment. After each insertion site was disinfected with 75% alcohol, sterile single-use 0.25 × 38-mm needles (Wuxi Jiajian Medical Instrument Co. Ltd., Jiangsu, China) were inserted vertically to a depth of 4–10 mm. At the appropriate depth, the acupuncturist manipulated the needles for *Deqi* sensation, defined as a feeling of heaviness around the acupoint [23], and then bilaterally connected a Nerve and Muscle Stimulator (Suzhou Medical Appliance Factory, Suzhou, China) to PC6 (positive electrode) and ST36 (negative electrode) on the ipsilateral limbs. In each treatment session, EA stimulation was performed for a duration of 20 min at a frequency of 15 Hz with a continuous wave. The participants received two EA treatments within 24 h before surgery, one at 10:00 a.m. and another at 16:00 p.m.

All participants in 2 groups received similar routine treatments after surgery, including gastrointestinal

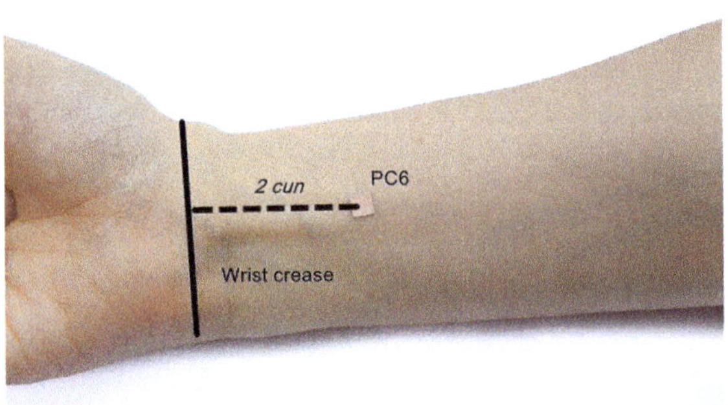

Fig. 1 Location of PC6

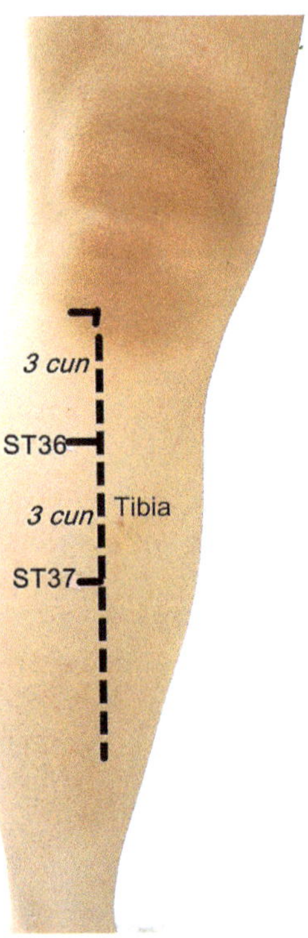

Fig. 2 Locations of ST36 and ST37

decompression, maintenance stabilization of homeostasis (especially maintenance of electrolyte balance), routine nursing care, and early walking, with no further EA treatments in EA group. The only combination therapy received by all participants was 1500 mL of physiological saline with 1.5 g Potassium Chloride Injection (China Otsuka Pharmaceutical Co. Ltd., Tianjin, China) for 2 days postoperatively.

All participants underwent preoperative and postoperative supervision and evaluation of curative effects by a blinded observer at 10:00 a.m. daily, until they were discharged. A third party performed all data treatments and analyses. The study was performed as shown in the flowchart (Fig. 3).

The participating acupuncturist had more than 2000 h of acupuncture training before participating in the trial and received their diploma 6 years ago. The physician had applied acupuncture in practice for more than 6 years and had treated about 1000 participants with acupuncture in the year before the trial.

Outcomes

A blinded observer obtained the postoperative data including the degree of abdominal distension, times of first flatus and defecation, and duration of hospitalization after surgery. As a subjective sensation, abdominal distension was measured by a Likert-type scale (Table 1) [24]. Postoperative abdominal distension was defined as a postoperative gastrointestinal motility change leading to invalid transfer of gastrointestinal contents [25], caused by intraoperative wound traction, abdominal adhesions, or lack of visceral perfusion [2]. In this study, the incidence and degree of abdominal distension after surgery were the main outcome indicators, while the times of first flatus and defecation and duration of hospitalization were secondary outcomes. The study focused on the prevention of PGD; therefore, the incidence of PGD was the primary endpoint.

Table 1 Presentation of the Likert-type scale

Score	Explanation
0	I feel no abdominal distension at all
1	I feel a little of abdominal distension
2	I feel abdominal distension but I can bear
3	I feel obvious abdominal distension that I cannot bear but it doesn't affect my life
4	I feel horrible abdominal distension and need it addressed

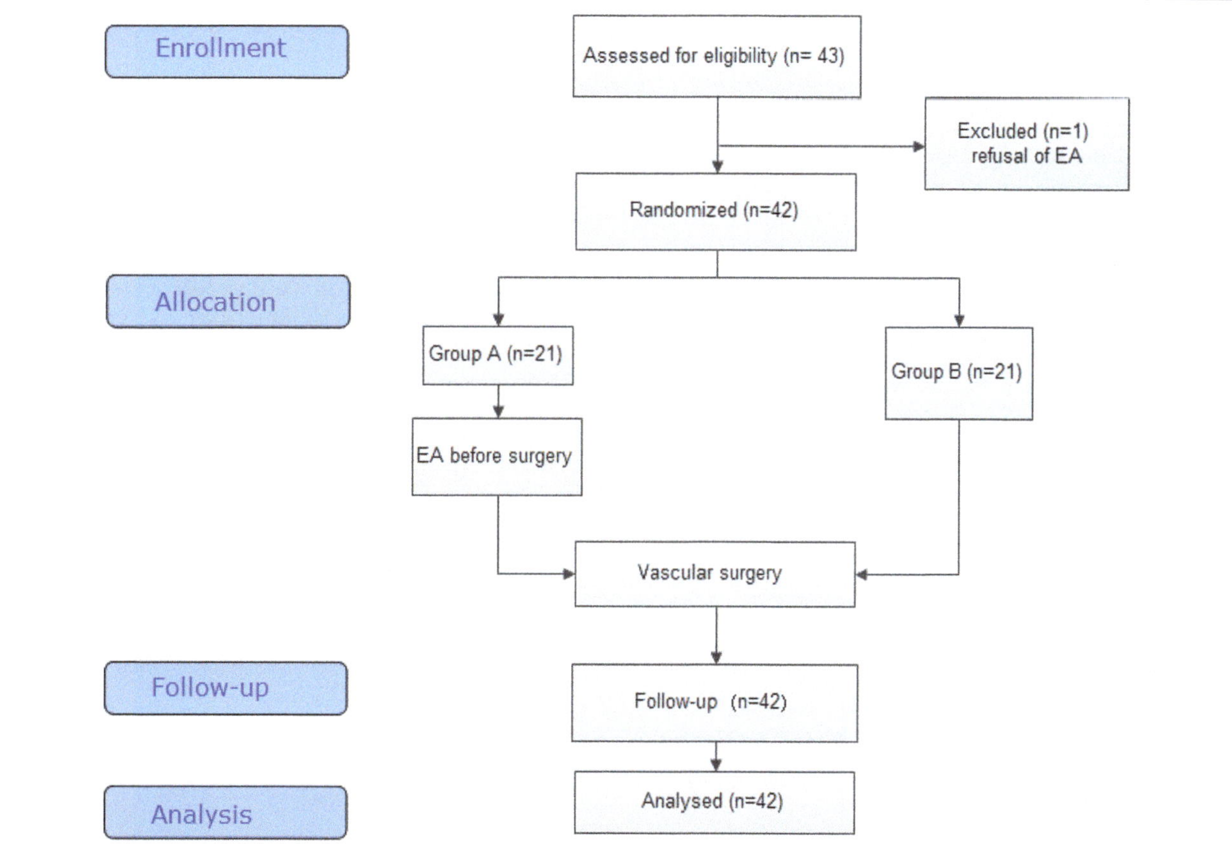

Fig. 3 Flowchart of the study

The study included a period from 24 h preoperatively to 7 days postoperatively. A graduate student, who did not participate in patient management, recorded the treatment details, including demographic data, anesthesia time, surgery duration, and dosage of opioids. The demographic data collected included: age; sex; race; marital status; job status; educational background; weight; and telephone number. Considering that the type of intravenous fluid given during and after surgery is a factor in postoperative recovery, we specified that all participants enrolled in the study were only under GA perioperatively and that all of their postoperative routine treatments, especially the combination therapy, were the same to avoid any bias conferred by administration of a different intravenous fluid.

Sample size calculation

Owing to a lack of previous reports on PGD-related acupuncture and vascular surgery, the study was designed to include a minimum of 20 cases [26] in each group following the minimum sample-size requirements. With consideration of selecting an appropriate sample size, controlling random errors, and achieving a certain effect, the lower limit of the sample size was set at 20 cases (20–30 cases per group stipulated by the China Food and Drug Administration, 20–50 cases in the European Union, 20–80 cases in the United States [26]).

Randomization and blinding

All participants were randomly assigned to the two groups on the basis of a concealed allocation approach using statistical analysis PROCPLAN statements (SAS 9.4; World Headquarters SAS Institute Inc., Cary, NC, USA). A computer-generated list of random numbers was used to determine the allocation of the participants, with numbered opaque sealed envelopes containing the randomization schedule. The envelopes were kept by an investigator who was not an assessor in the study, and who was informed of the outcomes at the end of the study. The researchers recording the outcomes and those making the conclusions were all blinded to patients' assessments.

Statistical analysis

All continuous data, including the incidence of abdominal distension, all secondary outcomes, and some of the baseline data, were expressed as mean ± standard deviation (SD). For these data, a *t* test used to compare normally distributed data between the two groups, while the Wilcoxon rank sum test applied for non-normally distributed data. Nominal variables, including the degree of abdominal distension and the remaining baseline data, were presented as frequency and percentage and analyzed using the Chi square (χ^2) test. Values of $P < 0.05$ were considered statistically significant. All the efficacy and safety analyses were performed using the intent-to-treat population. A third person performed blinded estimation and statistics of the curative effect.

Adverse events

All adverse events, such as hematoma, stuck needle, and fainting, were reported. In participants with serious adverse events, the experimental intervention was ceased immediately, and proper treatments were provided.

Results

Selection of participants

Recruitment for the study began on 10 February 2014 and finished on 14 July 2014, while follow-up was completed on 17 July 2014. During the 8-month-study, 43 participants were recruited, and 42 participants completed the study, with 21 participants in each group. One participant was excluded because of refusal to receive EA. The baseline demographic data and clinical characteristics of the two groups did not differ significantly and were comparable (Table 2). The mean morbidity age

Table 2 Demographic data for all participants

	EA group (N = 21)	RT group (N = 21)	*t*	χ^2	*P*
Age (years), mean ± SD	56.0 ± 11.31	56.8 ± 12.16	0.221		0.826
Gender (F), %	23.8%	23.8%	–	0.130	0.641
Race (Han), %	90.5%	85.7%	–	0.000	0.500
Married, %	95.2%	100%	–	0.000	0.235
Retirement, %	23.8%	23.8%	–	0.000	0.280
Illiteracy/yes, %	4.8%	19.0%	–	0.980	0.472
Weight (kg), mean ± SD	65.6 ± 2.56	64.7 ± 1.16	1.467	–	0.150
Anesthesia time (h), mean ± SD	4.03 ± 0.35	4.19 ± 0.38	1.419	–	0.164
Surgery duration (h), mean ± SD	3.52 ± 0.28	3.43 ± 0.31	0.987	–	0.329
Opioids' dosage (g), mean ± SD	0.86 ± 0.48	0.67 ± 0.66	1.067	–	0.292

EA electroacupuncture, *RT* routine treatment

was 56.40 ± 11.61 years, and the participants comprised 23.8% women and 76.2% men.

Outcomes and estimations

Primary endpoints

As shown in Table 3, there were significant differences in the incidence and degree of abdominal distension between the two groups ($P = 0.03$ and $P = 0.03$, respectively). The percentage of participants suffering from abdominal distension was 42.8% in EA group and 76.2% in RT group. The number of participants who could not stand the distension was 14.3% in EA group and 33.3% in RT group, as well as 28.6% in EA group and 37.9% in RT group were with sustainable abdominal distension which don't need any pharmacotherapy.

Secondary endpoints

As shown in Table 4, the time of first defecation (2.81 ± 0.51, 3.20 ± 0.55 days) and duration of hospitalization (5.33 ± 0.68, 5.75 ± 0.66 days) showed significant differences between the two groups ($P = 0.02$ and $P = 0.04$, respectively), while the time of first flatus (3.05 ± 0.58, 3.29 ± 0.42 days) showed no significant difference ($P = 0.13$). Among the three items, the reduction in first defecation time was most noticeable (12.18%), while the time of first flatus, showing the beginning of gastrointestinal function recovery, was reduced by 7.29% and the duration of hospitalization was shortened by 6.98%.

Table 3 Outcomes for incidence and degree of abdominal distension

	EA group (N = 21)	RT group (N = 21)	*t*	Z	*P*
AD's incidence	9 (42.8%)	16 (76.2%)	4.842		0.029
AD's degree				−2.109	0.035
0	12 (57.1%)	5 (23.8%)			
1	0 (0%)	2 (4.6%)			
2	6 (28.6%)	7 (33.3%)			
3	3 (14.3%)	4 (19.0%)			
4	0 (0%)	3 (14.3%)			

Data are shown as *n* (%)

EA electroacupuncture, *RT* routine treatment, *AD* abdominal distension

Table 4 Outcomes of the secondary endpoints

	EA group (N = 21)	RT group (N = 21)	*t*	*P*
First time flatus (d)	3.05 ± 0.58	3.29 ± 0.42	1.536	0.132
First time Defecation (d)	2.81 ± 0.51	3.20 ± 0.55	2.383	0.022
Hospitalization (d)	5.33 ± 0.68	5.75 ± 0.66	2.031	0.049

Data are shown as mean ± SD

EA electroacupuncture, *RT* routine treatment, *AD* abdominal distension

Table 5 Descriptions of the four common methods of sham-acupuncture

Advantages	Limitations	Indications
Sham-acupuncture		
Fine masking	Not suitable	Insistent estimation
Low stimulation	For all acupoints	Without EA history
		Acupoints on back
Non-acupoints		
Fine masking	Can't avoid	Different ganglion segment
Better feasibility	Physiological effect	Without EA history
		Study on acupoints' specificity
Shallow acupuncture		
Better masking	Narrow indication	Study on depths of needling
Low stimulation		
Non-disease-related acupuncture		
Better masking	Low feasibility	Without EA history
Lowest bias		Study on acupoints' specificity

Adverse events

There were no participants with needle breakages, unbearable pain, and other acupuncture-related adverse events during the study.

Discussion

This study was carried out to determine whether a preventive intervention program can reduce PGD after vascular surgery under GA. In WCHSU, gastrointestinal decompression or early walking is usually used for treatment of PGD, and these methods were applied to all study participants. For prevention of PGD, a previous study stated that EA should be applied from anesthesia induction to surgery completion [27]. However, application of EA was chosen during the 24-h period before surgery for four reasons: research purposes; safety; easy isolation of control and treatment groups; and efficacy. As a pre-validation study, the present study focused on whether this preventive intervention had an impact on PGD, while rehabilitation or acupuncture is often prescribed after surgery. In addition, this study used EA, which may interfere with other equipment used intraoperatively, such as an electric knife. In traditional Chinese medicine theory and human research [28], *Deqi* is a prerequisite for effective treatment. During or after surgery, GA and postoperative incision pain can cause a needling sensation, resulting in reduced levels of patient compliance.

The anesthetic items for both groups were compared, and only laparotomy was included to mitigate the experimental bias caused by different operative methods and anesthetic concentrations, especially opioids [29]. As the anesthetic concentration was proportional to weight, and there was no significant difference in weight between the two groups, the anesthetic dosages for both groups were comparable.

All secondary outcomes, used extensively for evaluating functional recovery, indicated that EA could accelerate the rehabilitation program for PGD. Among the three endpoints, the reduction of first defecation time showed the largest effect. Studies in the literature have used varying endpoints, such as bowel sounds, flatus, and bowel movements [30, 31]. Among these three endpoints, bowel movements are the most reliable endpoint [32].

To mitigate the potential bias among consenting participants induced by the Hawthorne effect, many studies have required inclusion of a sham acupuncture group. There are four methods in common use [33], as shown in Table 5. However, researchers rarely use placebo-controlled trials when comparing interventions with general routine therapy [34]. Acupuncture treatments are complex, multicomponent interventions. In sham-controlled trials that attempt to control only certain potentially therapeutic acupuncture-specific components, such as location, insertion depth, stimulation, needle size, and number [35], the moderately large nonspecific effects of sham acupuncture can decrease the reliability and the usefulness of the test results [36].

The incidence and degree of abdominal distension determined that EA was useful for preventing PGD and helped in the drawing of accurate conclusions. The Likert-type scale was used to measure the degree of abdominal distension, and the sustainable uncomfortable, which don't influent sleep, is 1′–2′ and the uncomfortable need pharmacotherapy is 3′–4′. In our study, EA could alleviate abdominal distension more. However, the Likert-type scale is only a rough estimation, although there is no specialized abdominal-distension personnel. Therefore, regarding validity of the findings, a comparison of objective parameters is necessary in a future study. The latest animal and human studies have demonstrated that not only a leukocytic pathway and subsequent injury-specific local inflammatory responses [37, 38], but also secondary lymphoid organs 0, are involved in the progression of postoperative ileus. It is indispensable to add an inflammatory cytokine test to a future study. There is also a necessity for a comparison of abdominal circumference as an objective factor 0.

There is a bias to the present study that cannot be ignored, namely that EA group had more doctor–patient contact hours and might experience placebo effects, even though the acupuncturist was not their surgeon. Considering that the acupuncturist performed EA only twice, the acupuncturist was recommended to get in contact with the participants in RT group in a future study.

Conclusions

Preoperative EA at PC6, ST36, and ST37 might be useful for preventing PGD, thereby improving gastrointestinal function recovery.

Abbreviations

EA: electroacupuncture; GA: general anesthesia; PGD: postoperative gastrointestinal dysfunction; WCHSU: West China Hospital of Sichuan University.

Authors' contributions

MYL, ZPW and NL designed the study. CWW performed the data analysis. MYL and CWW wrote the manuscript. All authors read and approved the final manuscript.

Author details

[1] Department of Integrated Traditional Chinese and Western Medicine, West China Hospital of Si-chuan University, Chengdu, Sichuan, China. [2] Department of Liver and Vascular Surgery, West China Hospital of Si-chuan University, Chengdu, Sichuan, China.

Acknowledgements

We must give our acknowledgement to Qian Wen, Physician-in-charge of WCHSU, for her performing the experiment and Jianghua Yan for data collection. We would like to thank Yu Zhao and Jian-Qin Lv from the Department of Integrated Traditional and Western Medicine, WCHSU, Chengdu, China for their support in designing the study. We also need to thank Si-jia Li, Maryland University, and Sha wang, National University of Singapore for their greatly help in language issues.

Competing interests

The authors declare that they have no competing interests.

References

1. Steinbrook RA. Epidural anesthesia and gastrointestinal motility. Anesth Analg. 1998;86:837–44.
2. Bell TJ, Panchal SJ, Miaskowski C. The prevalence, severity, and impact of opioid-induced bowel dysfunction: results of a US and European Patient Survey (PROBE 1). Pain Med. 2009;10:35–8.
3. Gu KM, Zeng M, Liu M. Comparison of several methods in treating postoperative abdominal distension. Harbin Yi Yao. 2007;27:22–3.
4. Eappen S, Lane BH, Rosenberg B. Relationship between occurrence of surgical complications and hospital finances. JAMA. 2013;309:1599–608.
5. Sheng DJ, Jun DY, Fang L. The development situation and tendency of vascular surgery in China. Hebei Med J. 2002;24:397–402.
6. Nowygrod R, Egorova N, Greco G. Trends, complications, and mortality in peripheral vascular surgery. J Vasc Surg. 2006;43:205–12.
7. Ma X, Yuan QH, Yu ZX. Efficacy comparison between endovascular aneurysm repair versus open surgery for patients with abdominal

aortic aneurysms: a meta-analysis. Zhonghua Xin Xue Guan Bing Za Zhi. 2012;40:878–86.
8. Yamamoto H, Yamamoto F, Ishibashi K. Long-term outcomes of open surgical repair for ruptured iliac artery aneurysms. Ann Vasc Surg. 2011;25:740–8.
9. Girotti ME, Ko CY, Dimick JB. Hospital morbidity rankings and complication severity in vascular surgery. J Vasc Surg. 2013;57:158–67.
10. Svensson LG, Crawford ES, Hess KR, Coselli JS, Safi HJ. Experience with 1509 patients undergoing thoracoabdonimal aortic operations. J Vasc Surg. 1993;17:357–68.
11. Zerbino DD. Kuzyk Iul. Aortic dissecting aneurysms: clinical masks, differential diagnosis. Klin Med. 2002;80:58–62.
12. Van Noord BA, Roffey P, Thangathurai D. Abdominal compartment syndrome following opioid-induced postoperative ileus. J Clin Anesth. 2013;25:146–54.
13. Camilleri M, Parkman HP, Shafi MA. Clinical guideline: management of gastroparesis. Am J Gastroenterol. 2013;108:18–20.
14. Wan Q. Auricular-plaster therapy plus acupuncture at zusanli for postoperative recovery of intestinal function. J Tradit Chin Med. 2000;20:134–42.
15. Kexin L. One hundred and forty-six cases of postoperative abdominal distention treated by electroacupucnture. World J Acu Mox. 2009;19:60–1.
16. Wanting H, Yichuan C, Meiling Y, et al. Acupressure improves the postoperative comfort of gastric cancer patients: a randomized controlled trial. Complement Ther Med. 2015;23:339–46.
17. Forster J, Damjanov I, Lin Z. Absence of the interstitial cells of Cajal in patients with gastroparesis and correlation with clinical findings. J Gastrointest Surg. 2005;9:102–7.
18. Kalff JC, Carlos TM, Schraut WH. Surgically induced leukocytic infiltrates within the rat intestinal muscularis mediate postoperative ileus. Gastroenterology. 1999;117:378–87.
19. Kalff JC, Schraut WH, Billiar TR. Role of inducible nitric oxide synthase in postoperative intestinal smooth muscle dysfunction in rodents. Gastroenterology. 2000;118:316–27.
20. Senna-Fernandes V, França DL, Souza D. Acupuncture at "Zusanli" (St.36) and "Sanyinjiao" (SP.6) points on the gastrointestinal tract: a study of the bioavailability of (99 m)Tc-sodium pertechnetate in rats. Evid Based Compl Alt. 2011;2011:823941.
21. Allen TK, Habib AS. P6 stimulation for the prevention of nausea and vomiting associated with cesarean delivery under neuraxial anesthesia: a systematic review of randomized controlled trials. Anesth Analg. 2008;107:1308–14.
22. Ouyang MW, Qin ZS, Lin CS. Prophylactic effect of acupuncture on nausea and vomiting after laparoscopic operation. Zhongguo Zhen Jiu. 2009;29:915–24.
23. Molsberger A. Acupuncture in orthopedics. ORTHOPADE. 2012;41:100–1.
24. General administration of quality supervision, inspection and quarantine of the People's Republic of China, standardization administration of the People's Republic of China. Nomenclature and location of acupuncture points. (GB/T 12346-2006).
25. Langevin HM, Churchill DL, Fox JR. Biomechanical response to acupuncture needling in humans. J Appl Physiol. 2001;91:2471–8.
26. Xuezhong Z, Xuerui T, Hongxing P. The sample size of clinic trials. Shi Jie Hua Ren Xiao Hua Za Zhi. 2006;14:1339–40.
27. Klaus L, Karin N, Antonius S, et al. How large are the nonspecific effects of acupuncture? A meta-analysis of randomized controlled trials. BMC Med. 2010;8:75–6.
28. Andrew L, Edward L, Yvette T. Mechanisms and treatment of postoperative ileus. Arch Surg. 2003;138:206–14.
29. Lee A, Chan S. Acupuncture and anesthesia. Best Pract Res Clin Anaesthesiol. 2006;20:303–12.
30. Chen TY, Zhou J, Wang K, Xu JJ, Ma W, Wu YY. Electroacupuncture intervention combined with anesthetics for analgesia and post-surgical gastrointestinal recovery in pneumectomy patients. Zhen Ci Yan Jiu. 2015;40:461–4.
31. Huanqin L, Huilin L, Cunzhi L. Effect of "Deqi" during the study of needling "Wang's Jiaji" acupoints treating spasticity after stroke. Evid Based Compl Alt. 2014;2014:715351.
32. Helene M, Langevin L, Peter M. Paradoxes in acupuncture research: strategies for moving forward. Evid Based Compl Alt. 2011;2011:180805.
33. Oh DS, Jung SY, Kim AR. A crossover clinical trial to determine the effect of Siguan (four gates) points on gastrointestinal motility suppressed by loperamide administration. J Korean Oriental Med. 2008;29:1–6.
34. Schmidt J, Stoffels B, Chanthaphavong RS. Differential molecular and cellular immune mechanisms of postoperative and LPS-induced ileus in mice and rats. Cytokine. 2012;59:49–58.
35. Yin J, Chen JD. Gastrointestinal motility disorders and acupuncture. Auton Neurosci. 2010;157:31–7.
36. Koscielny A, Engel D, Maurer J. The role of lymphoid tissue in the attenuation of the postoperative ileus. Am J Phys. 2012;304:401–12.
37. Van Bree SHW, Cailotto C. Systemic in flammation with enhanced brain activation contributes to more severe delay in postoperative ileus. Neuro-Gastroent Motil. 2013;25:540–50.
38. Magalhães FJ, Mendonça LB, Rebouças CB. Risk factors for cardiovascular diseases among nursing professionals: strategies for health promotion. Rev Bras Enferm. 2014;67:394–7.

PERMISSIONS

All chapters in this book were first published in CM, by BioMed Central; hereby published with permission under the Creative Commons Attribution License or equivalent. Every chapter published in this book has been scrutinized by our experts. Their significance has been extensively debated. The topics covered herein carry significant findings which will fuel the growth of the discipline. They may even be implemented as practical applications or may be referred to as a beginning point for another development.

The contributors of this book come from diverse backgrounds, making this book a truly international effort. This book will bring forth new frontiers with its revolutionizing research information and detailed analysis of the nascent developments around the world.

We would like to thank all the contributing authors for lending their expertise to make the book truly unique. They have played a crucial role in the development of this book. Without their invaluable contributions this book wouldn't have been possible. They have made vital efforts to compile up to date information on the varied aspects of this subject to make this book a valuable addition to the collection of many professionals and students.

This book was conceptualized with the vision of imparting up-to-date information and advanced data in this field. To ensure the same, a matchless editorial board was set up. Every individual on the board went through rigorous rounds of assessment to prove their worth. After which they invested a large part of their time researching and compiling the most relevant data for our readers.

The editorial board has been involved in producing this book since its inception. They have spent rigorous hours researching and exploring the diverse topics which have resulted in the successful publishing of this book. They have passed on their knowledge of decades through this book. To expedite this challenging task, the publisher supported the team at every step. A small team of assistant editors was also appointed to further simplify the editing procedure and attain best results for the readers.

Apart from the editorial board, the designing team has also invested a significant amount of their time in understanding the subject and creating the most relevant covers. They scrutinized every image to scout for the most suitable representation of the subject and create an appropriate cover for the book.

The publishing team has been an ardent support to the editorial, designing and production team. Their endless efforts to recruit the best for this project, has resulted in the accomplishment of this book. They are a veteran in the field of academics and their pool of knowledge is as vast as their experience in printing. Their expertise and guidance has proved useful at every step. Their uncompromising quality standards have made this book an exceptional effort. Their encouragement from time to time has been an inspiration for everyone.

The publisher and the editorial board hope that this book will prove to be a valuable piece of knowledge for researchers, students, practitioners and scholars across the globe.

LIST OF CONTRIBUTORS

Xin Zhang, Zhi-Chao Xu, Ai-Jia Ji, Hong-Mei Luo and Chao Sun
Institute of Medicinal Plant Development, Chinese Academy of Medical Sciences and Peking Union Medical College, Beijing 100193, China

Shi-Lin Chen
Institute of Medicinal Plant Development, Chinese Academy of Medical Sciences and Peking Union Medical College, Beijing 100193, China
Institute of Chinese Materia Medica, China Academy of Chinese Medical Sciences, Beijing 100700, China

Jiang Xu
Institute of Chinese Materia Medica, China Academy of Chinese Medical Sciences, Beijing 100700, China

Jing-Yuan Song
Institute of Medicinal Plant Development, Chinese Academy of Medical Sciences and Peking Union Medical College, Beijing 100193, China
Chongqing Institute of Medicinal Plant Cultivation, Chongqing 408435, China

Yuan-Lei Hu
State Key Laboratory of Protein and Plant Gene Research, College of Life Sciences, Peking University, Beijing 100871, China

Sin Bond Leung, Hongwei Zhang and Zhi-Xiu Lin
School of Chinese Medicine, Faculty of Medicine, The Chinese University of Hong Kong, Shatin, N.T., Hong Kong, People's Republic of China

Chi Wai Lau
School of Biomedical Sciences, Faculty of Medicine, The Chinese University of Hong Kong, Shatin, N.T., Hong Kong, People's Republic of China

Fang Liu, Xiao-Jing Zhang, Yuanjia Hu, Peng Li and Jian-Bo Wan
State Key Laboratory of Quality Research in Chinese Medicine, Institute of Chinese Medical Sciences, University of Macau, Macao, People's Republic of China

Xu Bai
Waters Technologies (Shanghai) Ltd., Shanghai, People's Republic of China

Feng-Qing Yang
School of Chemistry and Chemical Engineering, Chongqing University, Chongqing 400030, People's Republic of China

Xiao-Qing Ma, Su-Mei Li, Chi Leung Chan, Tao Su, Wei-Dong Li, Wang-Fun Fong and Zhi-Ling Yu
School of Chinese Medicine, Hong Kong Baptist University, Kowloon Tong, Hong Kong, China

Hui Cao
National Engineering Research Center for Modernization of Traditional Chinese Medicine, Zhuhai, Guangdong, China

Hui-Hui Xiao and Man-Sau Wong
State Key Laboratory of Chinese Medicine and Molecular Pharmacology (Incubation), Shenzhen Research Institute of The Hong Kong Polytechnic University, Shenzhen 518057, China

Raymond Cooper
Department of Applied Biology and Chemical Technology, The Hong Kong Polytechnic University, Hung Hom, Kowloon, Hong Kong, China

Yan Zhang
Spine Research Institute, Longhua Hospital, Shanghai University of Traditional Chinese Medicine, Shanghai 200032, China

Xin-Sheng Yao
Institute of Traditional Chinese Medicine & Natural Products, College of Pharmacy, Jinan University, Guangzhou 510632, China

Rong Ji, Anqi Wang, Haixia Shang and Liu Chen
College of Acumox and Tuina, Shanghai University of Traditional Chinese Medicine, Shanghai 201203, China

Chunhui Bao, Luyi Wu, Huangan Wu and Yin Shi
Shanghai Research Institute of Acupuncture-Moxibustion and Meridian, Shanghai 200030, China.

Yao Fong
Department of Thoracic Surgery, Chi-Mei Medical Center, Tainan 710, Taiwan

Chia-Chun Tang
Division of Chest, Ten Chan General Hospital, Chung-Li 320, Taiwan, ROC

Huei-Ting Hu and Yen-Chun Chen
Department of Biotechnology, Kaohsiung Medical University, Kaohsiung 807, Taiwan

Bing-Hung Chen
Department of Biotechnology, Kaohsiung Medical University, Kaohsiung 807, Taiwan
The Institute of Biomedical Sciences, National Sun Yat-Sen University, Kaohsiung 804, Taiwan

Chang-Yi Wu
Department of Biotechnology, Kaohsiung Medical University, Kaohsiung 807, Taiwan
Department of Biological Sciences, National Sun Yat-sen University, Kaohsiung 804, Taiwan

Hsin-Yu Fang
Department of Food Nutrition, Chung-Hwa University of Medical Technology, Tainan 701, Taiwan

Shyng-Shiou Yuan
Translational Research Center, Kaohsiung Medical University Hospital, Kaohsiung 807, Taiwan

Hui-Min David Wang
Graduate Institute of Biomedical Engineering, National Chung Hsing University, Taichung 402, Taiwan

Yen-Ni Teng
Department of Biological Sciences and Technology, National University of Tainan, Tainan 700, Taiwan

Chien-Chih Chiu
Department of Biotechnology, Kaohsiung Medical University, Kaohsiung 807, Taiwan
Department of Biological Sciences, National Sun Yat-sen University, Kaohsiung 804, Taiwan
Translational Research Center, Kaohsiung Medical University Hospital, Kaohsiung 807, Taiwan
Research Center for Environment Medicine, Kaohsiung Medical University, Kaohsiung 807, Taiwan

Natthida Weerapreeyakul
Faculty of Pharmaceutical Sciences, Khon Kaen University, Khon Kaen 40002, Thailand

Sasipawan Machana
Graduate School, Khon Kaen University, Khon Kaen 40002, Thailand

Sahapat Barusrux
Faculty of Associated Medical Sciences, Khon Kaen University, Khon Kaen 40002, Thailand.

Ahmad Zaim Mat Pauzi, Adam Leow Thean Chow, Nadiah Abu Tamilselvan Subramani, Soon Guan Tan and Noorjahan Banu Alitheen
Department of Cell and Molecular Biology, Faculty of Biotechnology and Biomolecular Sciences, Universiti Putra Malaysia, 43400 Serdang, Selangor, Malaysia

Swee Keong Yeap and Abdul Rahman Omar
Institute of Bioscience, Universiti Putra Malaysia, Serdang, Malaysia

Kian Lam Lim
Faculty of Medicine and Health Sciences, Universiti Tunku Abdul Rahman, Sungai Long Campus, Jalan Sungai Long, Bandar Sungai Long, Cheras, 43000 Kajang, Selangor, Malaysia

Suraini Abdul Aziz
Department of Bioprocess Technology, Faculty of Biotechnology and Biomolecular Sciences, Universiti Putra Malaysia, Serdang, Selangor, Malaysia

Jia Wen Xian, Angus Yiu-Ting Choi, Wing Nang Leung and Chun Wai Chan
School of Chinese Medicine, The Chinese University of Hong Kong, Shatin, New Territories, Hong Kong, People's Republic of China

Chun Fai Ng
Institute of Chinese Medicine, The Chinese University of Hong Kong, Shatin, New Territories, Hong Kong, People's Republic of China

Clara Bik-San Lau
Institute of Chinese Medicine, The Chinese University of Hong Kong, Shatin, New Territories, Hong Kong, People's Republic of China
State Key Laboratory of Phytochemistry and Plant Resources in West China, The Chinese University of Hong Kong, Shatin, New Territories, Hong Kong, People's Republic of China

Won Kyung Kim, Yuna Pyee, Tae Jun Choi, Hyen Joo Park, Ji-Young Hong and Sang Kook Lee
College of Pharmacy, Seoul National University, Seoul 151-742, Republic of Korea

Hwa-Jin Chung
College of Pharmacy, Seoul National University, Seoul 151-742, Republic of Korea
Jaseng Spine and Joint Research Institute, Jaseng Medical Foundation, Seoul 135-896, Republic of Korea

Joon-Shik Shin, Jin Ho Lee and In-Hyuk Ha
Jaseng Spine and Joint Research Institute, Jaseng Medical Foundation, Seoul 135-896, Republic of Korea

Charlotte Southern, Charlie Lloyd, Tingting Zhang, Martin Bland and Hugh MacPherson
Department of Health Sciences, University of York, York, UK

Jianping Liu and Congcong Wang
Centre for Evidence-Based Chinese Medicine, Beijing University of Chinese Medicine, Beijing, China

Linda L. D. Zhong, Cheng Yuan Lin, Tao Huang, Ling Zhao and Zhao Xiang Bian
School of Chinese Medicine, Hong Kong Baptist University, 7 Baptist University Road, Kowloon Tong, Hong Kong, China
Hong Kong Chinese Medicine Study Centre, Hong Kong Baptist University, Hong Kong SAR, China

Guang Zheng
School of Chinese Medicine, Hong Kong Baptist University, 7 Baptist University Road, Kowloon Tong, Hong Kong, China
School of Information Science and Engineering, Lanzhou University, Lanzhou, China

Li Da Ge
Department of Surgery, The First People's Hospital of Xiaoshan District, Hangzhou, China

Cheng Lu
School of Chinese Medicine, Hong Kong Baptist University, 7 Baptist University Road, Kowloon Tong, Hong Kong, China
Institute of Basic Research in Clinical Medicine, China Academy of Traditional Chinese Medicine, Beijing, China

Ai Ping Lu
School of Chinese Medicine, Hong Kong Baptist University, 7 Baptist University Road, Kowloon Tong, Hong Kong, China
Hong Kong Chinese Medicine Study Centre, Hong Kong Baptist University, Hong Kong SAR, China
Institute of Basic Research in Clinical Medicine, China Academy of Traditional Chinese Medicine, Beijing, China

Natthida Weerapreeyakul and Thaweesak Thitimetharoch
Faculty of Pharmaceutical Sciences, Khon Kaen University, Khon Kaen 40002, Thailand

Cholpajsorn Junhom
Graduate School, Faculty of Pharmaceutical Sciences, Khon Kaen University, Khon Kaen 40002, Thailand

Sahapat Barusrux
Faculty of Associate Medical Sciences, Khon Kaen University, Khon Kaen 40002, Thailand

Shi-Lin Chen
Institute of Chinese Materia Medica, China Academy of Chinese Medical Sciences, Beijing 100700, China

Hong-Mei Luo and Chun-Fang Li
Institute of Medicinal Plant Development, Chinese Academy of Medical Sciences, Beijing 100193, China

Hua Yu
Institute of Medicinal Plant Development, Chinese Academy of Medical Sciences, Beijing 100193, China
Shandong Center of Crop Germplasm Resources, Jinan 250100, China

Qiong Wu
Institute of Medicinal Plant Development, Chinese Academy of Medical Sciences, Beijing 100193, China
School of Pharmacy, Guilin Medical University, Guilin 541004, China

André Steinmetz
Plant Molecular Biology Laboratory, Centre de Recherche Public-Sante´, 1526 Luxembourg, Luxembourg.

Zhe Cai, Jie Dong, Delong Jiao and Man Chu
Department of Chemical Pathology, The Chinese University of Hong Kong, Prince of Wales Hospital, Shatin, N.T., Hong Kong, China
Shenzhen Research Institute, The Chinese University of Hong Kong, Shenzhen, China

Chun Kwok Wong
Department of Chemical Pathology, The Chinese University of Hong Kong, Prince of Wales Hospital, Shatin, N.T., Hong Kong, China
Shenzhen Research Institute, The Chinese University of Hong Kong, Shenzhen, China
Institute of Chinese Medicine and State Key Laboratory of Phytochemistry and Plant Resources in West China, The Chinese University of Hong Kong, Hong Kong, China

Ping Chung Leung, Clara Bik San Lau and Ching Po Lau
Institute of Chinese Medicine and State Key Laboratory of Phytochemistry and Plant Resources in West China, The Chinese University of Hong Kong, Hong Kong, China

Lai Shan Tam
Shenzhen Research Institute, The Chinese University of Hong Kong, Shenzhen, China
Department of Medicine and Therapeutics, Prince of Wales Hospital, The Chinese University of Hong Kong, Shatin, Hong Kong, China

Christopher Wai Kei Lam
State Key Laboratory of Quality Research in Chinese Medicine, Macau Institute for Applied Research in Medicine and Health, Macau University of Science and Technology, Taipa, Macau, China

Lai Lai Wong
School of Chinese Medicine, Hong Kong Baptist University, Kowloon, Hong Kong Special Administrative Region, People's Republic of China

Zhitao Liang, Hubiao Chen and Zhongzhen Zhao
School of Chinese Medicine, Hong Kong Baptist University, Kowloon, Hong Kong Special Administrative Region, People's Republic of China
Research Center for Pharmacognosy, Institute of Chinese Materia Medica, Academy of Chinese Medical Sciences, Beijing, People's Republic of China

Run-sheng Zheng, Wen-li Wang, Jing Tan, Hui Xu, Ruo-ting Zhan and Wei-wen Chen
Research Centre of Chinese Herbal Resource Science and Engineering, Guangzhou University of Chinese Medicine, Guangzhou, China
Key Laboratory of Chinese Medicinal Resource from Lingnan, Ministry of Education, Guangzhou University of Chinese Medicine, Guangzhou, China

Rui Di, Wing-Leung Hsu and Ye-Qing Huang
Research Group for Bioactive Products, Department of Biomedical Sciences, City University of Hong Kong, Hong Kong SAR, China

Hon-Yeung Cheung
Research Group for Bioactive Products, Department of Biomedical Sciences, City University of Hong Kong, Hong Kong SAR, China
Key Laboratory of Biochip Technology, Shenzhen Biotech and Health Centre, City University of Hong Kong, Shenzhen 518057, China

Yuan-Yuan Li
Research Group for Bioactive Products, Department of Biomedical Sciences, City University of Hong Kong, Hong Kong SAR, China
Present Address: System and Translational Science Center, RTI International, Research Triangle Park, NC 27709, USA

Ling-Wei Hsu, Meng-Che Yu, Ting-Lin Yen and Thanasekaran Jayakumar
Graduate Institute of Medical Sciences, College of Medicine, Taipei Medical University, Taipei, Taiwan

Wei-Cheng Shiao
Graduate Institute of Medical Sciences, College of Medicine, Taipei Medical University, Taipei, Taiwan
Department of Internal Medicine, Yuan's General Hospital, Kaohsiung, Taiwan

Nen-Chung Chang
Department of Internal Medicine, School of Medicine, Taipei Medical University, Taipei, Taiwan

Philip Aloysius Thomas
Department of Microbiology, Institute of Ophthalmology, Joseph Eye Hospital, Tiruchirappalli, Tamil Nadu 620 001, India

Joen-Rong Sheu
Graduate Institute of Medical Sciences, College of Medicine, Taipei Medical University, Taipei, Taiwan
Department of Pharmacology, School of Medicine, Taipei Medical University, Taipei, Taiwan

Meng-yue Liu, Cheng-wei Wang and Ning Li
Department of Integrated Traditional Chinese and Western Medicine, West China Hospital of Si-chuan University, Chengdu, Sichuan, China

Zhou-peng Wu
Department of Liver and Vascular Surgery, West China Hospital of Si-chuan University Chengdu, Sichuan, China

Index

A
Acetylcholine, 18, 20, 22, 33
Acupuncture, 18-19, 21-35, 76, 84-85, 133, 142-153, 164, 238-241, 243-245
Acute Stroke, 121, 130, 237
Anti-inflammatory, 2, 29, 42, 56, 60-62, 67, 110, 133, 139-140, 166, 172-173, 185-186, 196, 204
Anti-tumor, 2, 42, 110, 174
Antifungal Effects, 60, 62, 66, 72
Antioxidant Enzymes, 121, 126, 129, 131
Antioxidative Activity, 34
Antitumor, 16, 48, 60, 67, 74, 173
Aortic Rings, 18-21
Aortic Tissue, 18, 20, 29
Apoptosis, 16, 67, 69, 72, 75-77, 84-89, 92-93, 95-99, 101, 103, 105, 107-109, 111, 113-119, 121, 129-130, 165-167, 169, 171-174, 196, 230, 233, 236-237
Apoptotic Cells, 96, 101, 103, 105, 113, 168-169, 230, 232
Articular Cartilage, 132-133, 135-136, 139, 141

B
Blood Flow, 123, 131, 133, 230, 237
Blood Pressure, 18-19, 21-23, 25-27, 29, 31, 33-35, 196
Bone Fractures, 60-62, 72
Bone Loss, 132, 134-135, 139
Breast Cancer, 66, 74, 91, 94, 97-98, 109-111, 113, 115, 117-119, 172

C
Capillary Electrophoresis, 37, 45
Cardiovascular Diseases, 35, 67
Carotid Arteries, 18-19, 21-22, 24, 26, 28-29
Cell Proliferation, 62, 73, 91, 96, 98, 172
Cellular Metabolism, 1
Cerebral Artery Occlusion, 120-121, 123, 130-131, 230, 233, 236-237
Cerebral Ischemia, 19, 120-121, 129-131, 235-237
Chemotherapeutic Drug, 99-100
Chromatography, 16, 36-37, 45-48, 58-59, 63, 69, 99-100, 131, 133, 165-166, 168, 172-173, 186, 199, 212-214, 217, 220-221, 228
Colonic Tissues, 76-78, 81-82
Connective Tissues, 19, 24
Constipation, 154-164
Cortical Bone, 63
Crohn's Disease, 76-77, 84-85
Cyclooxygenase, 98, 133, 140-141
Cysteine Endopeptidase, 109-110, 117

D
Dehydrogenase, 1, 3, 16-17, 79, 120, 122, 130, 133, 140
Diabetes, 34, 67, 75, 87, 97, 166, 193, 197, 222, 231, 237, 240
Dihydroethidium, 18, 20, 33, 86, 88, 96
Dimethylsulfoxide, 107, 122, 167

E
Endothelial Dysfunction, 18-19, 27, 34-35
Endothelial Function, 18-19, 33-35
Ethanol Extract, 16, 62-63, 196

F
Ferulic Acid, 67, 74, 86-87, 89, 91, 93, 95-98
Fungal Contamination, 214-215, 217-219, 221

G
Gastrointestinal Tract, 119, 133, 163, 245
Gelatin Zymography, 86, 89, 95
Glycosides, 47-48, 54, 56, 58, 67, 73, 198, 204
Gradient Elution, 37, 49, 201, 222

H
Hepatocellular Carcinoma, 96, 98, 100, 103, 107, 165, 167, 169, 171, 173-174
Herbal Medicines, 36-37, 46, 157-158, 160, 164, 173, 214, 229
Hypertension, 18-19, 26-27, 32-35, 130, 222

I
Immune Responses, 48, 56, 59, 76, 192, 237
Intestinal Epithelial, 76-78, 83-85
Ischemic Injury, 120-121, 129, 236-237

L
Lipopolysaccharide, 59, 133, 140, 186, 197
Lung Cancer, 17, 86-87, 89-98, 107

M
Medicinal Plants, 46, 130, 164, 166, 173, 175-184, 221, 228
Mesenchymal Stem Cells, 66, 95, 98
Mitochondrial Membrane, 109, 111, 114, 116, 118, 171
Monosodium Iodoacetate, 132-133, 135, 137, 139-141

Mucosal Hyperemia, 79, 81
Muscular Tissues, 80, 82

N
Neuronal Cell, 121
Nitric Oxide, 18-19, 31, 33-35, 133, 140-141, 237, 245
Nitrotyrosine, 18, 20, 22, 24, 27, 29-30

O
Osteoarthritis, 74, 132-133, 135, 137, 139-141
Oxidative Stress, 18-19, 27, 29, 31, 34, 69, 85, 87, 97, 121, 127, 129-131, 137, 237

P
Phenolic Acids, 60, 62-63, 66-67, 72, 74, 222
Phytochemicals, 41, 60-61, 63, 65, 67, 69, 71, 73-75, 169, 199, 222
Plant Hormones, 1
Plant Materials, 37, 199, 212, 223
Plant Species, 36, 167, 175-177, 179-180, 182-183
Platycodin, 47-56, 59
Platycodonis Radix, 47, 49, 51, 53, 55, 57, 59
Potential Health, 60-63, 65, 67, 69, 71, 73, 75

R
Reactive Oxygen Species, 18-20, 24, 66, 75, 86, 97-98, 121, 126-127, 130-131, 236
Reperfusion Injury, 59, 129, 131, 236
Rheumatoid Arthritis, 140-141, 164, 196
Ribosomal Protein, 2-3, 16

S
Sulfur Fumigation, 47-49, 51, 53-59

T
Terpenoids, 60, 62, 67-68
Therapeutic Effects, 37, 63, 67, 186, 196
Thin Layer Chromatography, 37, 45-46, 186
Trabecular Bone, 61, 63, 132, 134-135, 139
Triterpenoids, 16, 59, 62-63, 67, 73
Tumor Necrosis, 67, 77, 84-85, 119, 135, 140, 166, 174, 186, 195-196, 230, 236-237
Tumor Necrosis Factor, 67, 77, 84-85, 119, 140, 166, 174, 186, 195-196, 230, 236-237

V
Vascular Function, 19
Vascular Structure, 24, 29-30